Medical Response to Terrorism
Preparedness and Clinical Practice

Editor-in-Chief

Daniel C. Keyes, MD, MPH

Associate Professor and Chief
Section of Toxicology, Emergency Medicine
The University of Texas Southwestern Medical Center at Dallas
Director, Southwestern Toxicology Training Program
The University of Texas Southwestern Medical Center at Dallas
Medical Director, North Texas Poison Center
Dallas, Texas

Editors

Jonathan L. Burstein, MD, FACEP

Assistant Professor of Emergency Medicine, Harvard Medical School
Assistant Professor of Population and International Health, Harvard School of Public Health
Medical Director, Center for Emergency Preparedness, Massachusetts Dept.
of Public Health
Boston, Massachusetts

Richard B. Schwartz, MD, FACEP

Chairman, Department of Emergency Medicine
Director, Center of Operational Medicine
Medical College of Georgia
Augusta, Georgia

Raymond E. Swienton, MD, FACEP

Assistant Professor, Emergency Medicine
Co-Director, Section of EMS, Homeland Security and Disaster Medicine
The University of Texas Southwestern Medical Center at Dallas
Dallas, Texas

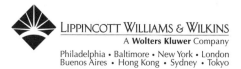
LIPPINCOTT WILLIAMS & WILKINS
A **Wolters Kluwer** Company
Philadelphia • Baltimore • New York • London
Buenos Aires • Hong Kong • Sydney • Tokyo

Acquisitions Editor: Anne Sydor
Developmental Editor: Scott Scheidt
Project Manager: Alicia Jackson
Senior Manufacturing Manager: Benjamin Rivera
Marketing Manager: Adam Glazer
Production Service: Nesbitt Graphics, Inc.
Printer: Maple Press

© 2005 by LIPPINCOTT WILLIAMS & WILKINS
530 Walnut Street
Philadelphia, PA 19106 USA
LWW.com

Printed in the USA

Library of Congress Cataloging-in-Publication Data

Medical response to terrorism / editor-in-chief, Daniel C. Keyes; editors, Jonathan L. Burstein, Richard B. Schwartz, Raymond E. Swienton.
    p. ; cm.
  Includes bibliographical references and index.
  ISBN 0-7817-4986-7
 1. Terrorism. 2. Medical emergencies. I. Keyes, Daniel C.
  [DNLM: 1. Terrorism. 2. Communicable Disease Control. 3. Disaster Planning.
4. Emergency Medical Services. 5. Poisoning. 6. Radiation Injuries. WA 295 M489 2005]
RC88.9.T47M43 2005
362.18--dc22

                                      2004020228

We collectively dedicate this work to the victims of terrorism and their families, their friends, and their communities—they are not forgotten. You are our motivation and inspiration.

The editors and contributors

To my father, Professor W. Noel Keyes, a wise and learned role model for writing, teaching, and life itself; to my prayerful mother; to my wife, truly a woman of valor, who summons great patience and support; to my wonderful children: Asher, Avi, and Yaeli, who give special purpose to my life.

DCK

To my wife and family, whose love sustains me.
JLB

This book is dedicated to the Special Operations Medic. Whether serving in the military or civilian law enforcement communities, your selfless service keeps us safe and strong.

RBS

To the citizens of every local community, I pray that you, by trust and hope, will have the courage, strength, and insight to sustain during the war on terrorism and to maintain peace.

To everyone who serves to protect our citizens, provide care for the victims, and manage the consequences of terrorism; I pray that you will have the deliverable skills, that you will be willing and able to participate, that you will respond when alerted, and that you will share yourself with your community when needed.

To my wife, Anne, my son, Kyle, and my daughter, Heather; I thank you for your love, unwavering support, and encouragement during the preparation of this book. I pray that God is our refuge and fortress, in Him we trust.

RES

CONTENTS

CONTRIBUTORS

Richard V. Aghababian, MD, FACEP
Professor and Chair
Department of Emergency Medicine
University of Massachusetts Medical School
Worcester, Massachusetts

Yedidia Bentur, MD
Senior Lecturer, Faculty of Medicine
Technion-Israel Institute of Technology
and
Director, Israel Poison Information Center
Rambam Medical Center
Haifa, Israel

Richard N. Bradley, MD, FACEP
Clinical Associate Professor
Department of Emergency Medicine
University of Texas Medical School
and
Medical Director, Emergency Center
Memorial Hermann Hospital
Houston, Texas

Jonathan L. Burstein, MD, FACEP
Assistant Professor of Emergency Medicine,
    Harvard Medical School
Assistant Professor of Population and International Health,
    Harvard School of Public Health
Medical Director, Center for Emergency Preparedness
Boston, Massachusetts

F. Marion Cain III, PE, LTC, U.S. Army (Ret)
Deputy Director
US Department of Homeland Security
The Center for Domestic Preparedness
Anniston, Alabama

Anthony J. Carbone MD, MS, MPH
Research Fellow in Biosecurity
Harvard Center for Public Health Preparedness
Harvard School of Public Health
Boston, Massachusetts

Teriggi J. Ciccone, MD
Resident
Harvard Affiliated Emergency Medicine Residency
Harvard Medical School
and
Chief Resident
Department of Emergency Medicine
Beth Israel Deaconess Medical Center
Boston, Massachusetts

Darren F. Collins
Director, Center for Public Health Preparedness
Dekalb County Board of Health
Decatur, Georgia

Joanne Cono, MD, ScM
Senior Medical Officer
Bioterrorism Preparedness and Response Program
Centers for Disease Control and Prevention
Atlanta, Georgia

Phillip L. Coule, MD, FACEP
Assistant Professor, Department
    of Emergency Medicine
Medical College of Georgia
Augusta, Georgia
and
Director, Emergency Communications Center
MCG Medical Center
Augusta, Georgia

Seric S. Cusick, MD
Clinical Fellow, Harvard Medical School
and
Resident, Emergency Medicine
Beth Israel Deaconess Medical Center
Boston, Massachusetts

Cham E. Dallas, MD
Director, Interdisciplinary Toxicology Program
Department of Pharmaceutics and
    Biomedical Sciences
College of Pharmacy
University of Georgia

Inger Damon, MD, PhD
Chief, Poxvirus Program
Division of Viral and Rickettsial Diseases
Centers for Disease Control and Prevention
Atlanta, Georgia

K. Sophia Dyer, MD
Assistant Professor of Emergency Medicine
Department of Emergency Medicine
Boston University School of Medicine
and
Assistant Medical Director, Boston EMS
Toxicologist, Boston Medical Center
Boston, Massachusetts

Marc Eckstein, MD
Assistant Professor, Department
    of Emergency Medicine
Keck School of Medicine
University of Southern California
and
Medical Director of EMS
Los Angeles Fire Department
Los Angeles, California

Keith Edsall, MB, BS, MRCS, LRCP, MSc
Consultant in Radiation Medicine (Retired)
Former Head of Tri-Service Radiation Medicine,
    Research and Training
Consultant Advisor to the Royal Air Force
Staff Physician to the Radiation Emergency Assistance
    Centre/Training Site
Oak Ridge, Tennessee

William P. Fabbri, MD, FACEP
Medical Director
Emergency Medical Support Program
Federal Bureau of Investigation, U.S. Department of Justice
Washington, District of Columbia

Raymond L. Fowler, MD, FACEP
Assistant Professor of Emergency Medicine
Department of Surgery
University of Texas Southwestern Medical Center
and
Faculty Member
Department of Emergency Medicine
Parkland Memorial Hospital
Dallas, Texas

Jennifer Gil Almanza, MD
Assistant Professor
School of Medicine
Universidad Nacional de Columbia, Bogotá
Bogotá, Columbia

Melissa L. Givens, MD
Clinical Toxicology Fellow and Clinical Instructor
Department of Emergency Medicine
University of Texas Southwestern, Dallas
Dallas, Texas

John Gomez, MD
Clinical Toxicology Fellow
University of Texas Southwestern Medical Center
Dallas, Texas

Rebeca Gracia, PharmD
Clinical Instructor
Department of Surgery, Emergency Medicine
University of Texas Southwestern, Dallas
and
Clinical Toxicologist, North Texas Poison Center
Parkland Health and Hospital Systems
Dallas, Texas

David W. Gruber, MMAS
Assistant Commissioner
New Jersey Department of Health and Senior Services
Trenton, New Jersey

Stacey L. Hail, MD
Clinical Instructor, Emergency Medicine
University of Texas Southwestern Medical Center
and
Toxicology Fellow, Department of Toxicology
Parkland Hospital
Dallas, Texas

Robert S. Hoffman, MD
Associate Professor, Emergency Medicine
New York University School of Medicine
and
Director, New York City Poison Center
New York, New York

Karelene Hosford, MD
Attending Physician
Lincoln Medical and Mental Health Center
South Bronx, NY
and
Instructor in Emergency Medicine
Cornell University Medical School

Gila Hyams, RN, MA
Director, Teaching Center for Trauma, Emergency
    and Mass Casualty Situations
Director of Nursing, Surgical Division
Trauma Coordinator
Rambam Medical Center
Haifa, Israel

Daniel C. Keyes, MD, MPH
Associate Professor and Chief
Section of Toxicology, Emergency Medicine
The University of Texas Southwestern
    Medical Center at Dallas
and
Director, Southwestern Toxicology Training Program
The University of Texas Southwestern Medical Center at Dallas
Medical Director, North Texas Poison Center
Dallas, Texas

Brian Alan Krakover, MD
Resident, Division of Emergency Medicine
University of Texas Southwestern Medical Center
Parkland Memorial Hospital
Dallas, Texas

Gregory Luke Larkin, MD, MS, MSPH, FACEP
Professor, Surgery and Public Health
Division of Emergency Medicine
University of Texas Southwestern Medical Center
Dallas, Texas

K. Edwin Leap II, MD, FACEP
Staff Physician, Emergency Department
Oconee Memorial Hospital
Seneca, South Carolina

Richard Linsky, MD
Former Fellow, Government Emergency Medical Security Services
Division of Emergency Medicine
University of Texas Southwestern Medical Center at Dallas
Dallas, Texas
and
Emergency Physician, Department of Emergency Medicine
Baylor Medical Center at Irving
Irving, Texas

Mariann Manno, MD, FAAP
Associate Professor of Clinical Pediatrics and Emergency Medicine
University of Massachusetts Medical School
Division Director, Pediatric Emergency Medicine
Children's Medical Center
UMASS Memorial Health Care
Worcester, Massachusetts

C. Crawford Mechem, MD
Associate Professor, Department of
    Emergency Medicine
University of Pennsylvania School of Medicine
and
Attending Physician, Department of Emergency Medicine
Hospital of the University of Pennsylvania
Philadelphia, Pennsylvania

Carl Menckhoff, MD
Assistant Professor and Residency Director
Department of Emergency Medicine
Medical College of Georgia
Augusta, Georgia

Moshe Michaelson, MD
Director, Department of Emergency Medicine
Director, Trauma Unit
Chair, Israel National Committee
for Trauma Disaster Preparedness
Rambam Medical Center
Haifa, Israel

Adam H. Miller, MD, MSc, FACEP
Assistant Professor, Department of Surgery
Division of Emergency Medicine
University of Texas Southwestern Medical Center
and
Associate Medical Director, Emergency Department
Parkland Hospital
Dallas, Texas

Paul E. Moore, MS, EMT
Business Manager, Administrator
Department of Surgery
Division of Emergency Medicine
University of Texas Southwestern Medical Center
Dallas, Texas

Peter Moyer, MD, MPH
Professor of Emergency Medicine
Department of Emergency Medicine
Boston University School of Medicine
and
Medical Director, Boston EMS, Fire Police
Boston, Massachusetts

John Munyak, MD
Attending Physician
Lincoln Medical and Mental Health Center
South Bronx, NY
and
Instructor in Emergency Medicine
Cornell University Medical School

Madison W. Patrick, MD
Contract Medical Director
Washington Group International
Chemical Demilitarization Facility Clinic
Pine Bluff Arsenal
Pine Bluff, Arkansas

Paul E. Pepe, MD, MPH
Professor of Medicine, Surgery, Public Health
Chair, Emergency Medicine
University of Texas Southwestern Medical Center
and
Medical Director
Dallas Metropolitan Medical Response System
Dallas Metropolitan Biotel (EMS) System
Dallas, Texas

Timothy D. Peterson, MD, MPH
Adjunct Faculty, Department of Preventative Medicine
University of Iowa
Iowa City, Iowa
and
Staff Physician, Emergency Department
Polk County Hospital
Des Moines, Iowa

Kathy J. Rinnert, MD, MPH
Assistant Professor, Department of Surgery
Division of Emergency Medicine
University of Texas Southwestern at Dallas
and
Senior Emergency Medicine Faculty
Emergency Services Department
Parkland Health and Hospital System
Dallas, Texas

Wilfredo Rivera, MD
Instructor
Department of Surgery, Emergency Medicine
University of Texas Southwestern Medical Center
and
Assistant Medical Director
Parkland Health and Hospital Systems
Dallas, Texas

Lynn Roppolo, MD
Assistant Professor and Assistant Residency Director
Department of Surgery
Division of Emergency Medicine
University of Texas Southwestern
Dallas, Texas

Lisa D. Rotz, MD
Acting Director
Bioterrorism Preparedness and Response Program
National Center for Infectious Diseases
Centers for Disease Control and Prevention
Atlanta, Georgia

Timothy Rupp, MD, FACEP
Asst. Professor, Emergency Medicine
Asst. Residency Director, Emergency Medicine
Division of Emergency Medicine
University of Texas Southwestern Medical Center
Dallas, Texas

Josh Schier, MD
Assistant Professor
Department of Emergency Medicine
Emory University School of Medicine
and
Medical Toxicology Attending and Consultant
Georgia Poison Control Center
Atlanta, Georgia

Seth Schonwald, MD
Attending Physician and Director of Toxicology
Urgent Care
East Boston Neighborhood Health Center
East Boston, Massachusetts

Richard B. Schwartz, MD, FACEP
Chairman, Department of Emergency Medicine
Director, Center of Operational Medicine
Medical College of Georgia
Augusta, Georgia

Michael D. Shaw, DO
Chief Resident, Emergency Medicine
Medical College of Georgia
Augusta, Georgia

John Greene Shepherd, PharmD
Clinical Associate Professor, Clinical and Administrative
Pharmacy
University of Georgia, College of Pharmacy

and
Clinical Associate Professor
Department of Emergency Medicine
Medical College of Georgia
Augusta, Georgia

William S. Smock, MD
Associate Professor, Emergency Medicine
University of Louisville
Louisville, Kentucky

Myra M. Socher, BS, EMT/P
Assistant Professor, Department of Emergency Medicine
The George Washington University School of Medicine and
    Health Sciences
Washington, District of Columbia

Raymond E. Swienton, MD, FACEP
Assistant Professor, Emergency Medicine
Co-Director, Section of EMS, Homeland Security and Disaster
    Medicine
The University of Texas Southwestern Medical Center at Dallas
and
Department of Emergency Medicine
Parkland Memorial Hospital
Dallas, Texas

Nelson Tang, MD, FACEP
Assistant Professor, Department of Emergency Medicine
Johns Hopkins University
Baltimore, Maryland
and
Medical Director, United States Secret Service
Department of Homeland Security
Washington, District of Columbia

Nelson Téllez, MD
Assistant Professor, Department of Pathology
Universidad Nacional de Columbia, Bogotá
and
Forensic Pathologist, Dirección Regional Oriente
Instituto Nacional de Medicina Lagal y Ciencias
Bogotá, Columbia

Robert Abe Timmons, DO, MPH
Chief Resident
Occupational & Environmental Medicine Program
Harvard School of Public Health
Boston, Massachusetts

Stephen Traub, MD
Lecturer in Medicine, Department of Emergency Medicine
Harvard Medical School
and
Associate Director of Toxicology
Beth Israel Deaconess Medical Center
Boston, Massachusetts

Scott F. Wetterhall, MD, MPH
Adjunct Associate Professor, Department of Epidemiology
    Emory Rollins School of Public Health
Atlanta, Georgia
and
Assistant Director for Epidemiology & Public Health
    Preparedness
DeKalb County Board of Health
Decatur, Georgia

Warren L. Whitlock, MD, COL, MC
Assistant Professor, Department of Medicine
Medical College of Georgia
Augusta, Georgia
and
Director, Center for Total Access
Applied Research, Medical Informatics and Telemedicine
Southeastern Region Medical Command
Fort Gordon, Georgia

Eric J. Won, DO, MPH
Chief Resident
Department of Occupational and Environmental Medicine
Harvard School of Public Health
Boston, Massachusetts
and
Physician, Department of Occupational and Environmental
    Medicine
St. Jude Heritage Medical Group
Fullerton, CA

Jay Robert Woody, MD, FACEM
Clinical Instructor, Emergency Medicine
Department of Surgery, Division of Emergency Medicine
University of Texas Southwestern Medical Center
Dallas, Texas
and
Instructor Emergency Medicine
Department of Emergency Medicine
Parkland Memorial Hospital
Dallas, Texas

Shane Zatkalik, MD
Resident Physician, Department of Emergency Medicine
University of Texas Southwestern Medical Center
Dallas, Texas
and
Resident Physician, Department of Emergency Medicine
Parkland Hospital
Dallas, Texas

PREFACE

Even two decades ago, few would have imagined that terrorism would be planned and carried out on such an enormous scale as it is today. Terrorist attacks rely on horror and surprise, invoking different times, places, victims, and methods. Their purpose is to cause widespread confusion, fear, injury, and death. They disrupt security, and even more importantly the *perception* of security, which is essential to the success of civilization. A framework of certainty and trust allows individuals to carry out the activities of normal life; loss of that belief can lead to distrust, fear, and even civil disruption.

Success against terrorism ultimately will result from exercising the fundamental strengths of society. Political and religious leaders must provide true leadership to their communities by openly condemning these activities. Children will be taught that no cause justifies inflicting pain and death upon the innocent. Of course there is the need to capture the perpetrators and plan to respond to the consequences of their attacks. This fight belongs to all civilized societies. However, today we do not have the necessary complete cooperation for such efforts across all geopolitical regions.

Terrorism pushes the limits of engagement to the extreme, justifying the killing of young children, for example. This loss of ethical boundaries also threatens the health care system. Precisely because it is unacceptable behavior to attack hospitals, ambulances, and health care personnel, they are at especially high risk. In addition, whether or not they are the targets, health care workers are the key agents of response to terrorism. It is critical that clinicians be able to diagnose, triage, decontaminate, and treat victims of terror attacks of all types.

The entire medical system must work together for successful consequence management. Statistics show that in mass chemical attacks, (such as occurred in the mid-1990s in Japan), a majority of victims present directly to hospitals, without triage or decontamination. It is no longer possible to assume that our colleagues who are hazardous materials (HAZMAT) experts, paramedical professionals, or military teams will conduct all triage, decontamination, and initial treatment prior to arrival at the hospital. Biological terrorism is similar in that victims are likely to present directly to hospitals and clinics. Therefore, both EMS professionals *and* hospital personnel must be prepared to conduct all aspects of care for the victims of terrorism.

We have learned that terrorists plan extensively to find vulnerable targets, and will likely avoid sites where there is a strong preparation. Hence, *a prepared community is less likely to ever need to implement the principles contained in this text.* By training in terrorism response, you are directly protecting your community and yourself from the pain, suffering, and death caused by those who no longer value the sanctity of human life.

One experienced author on hospital preparedness in this book teaches that responding to terrorism is "like a military ambush." This means that the most important decisions must be made and practiced prior to the event. One half of this text is devoted to providing practical tools for the administrator, disaster planner and key health provider-leaders to *prepare and plan* for terrorism response at their clinical site.

Terrorism is an unfortunate reality of our time. This text is written by leading authorities on this topic from around the world, and we trust that the reader will find it to provide the most relevant and updated information to respond to this threat.

Daniel C. Keyes, MD, MPH
Jonathan L. Burstein, MD, FACEP
Richard B. Schwartz, MD, FACEP
Raymond E. Swienton, MD, FACEP

ACKNOWLEDGMENTS

The authors and editors very much appreciate the efforts of Anne Sydor, Acquisitions Editor at Lippincott Williams & Wilkins, who took a personal interest in the success of this book, as well as the efforts of Scott Scheidt, Developmental Editor, who provided diligent coordination of the editorial team.

Dr. Keyes would like to acknowledge a grant from the Council of International Exchange of Scholars (CIES) and the United States-Israel Educational Foundation for support he received as a Fulbright Scholar and visiting professor to the Rambam Hospital, Technion-Israel Institute of Technology, which contributed to his completion of this text.

Part 1

Agents of Terrorism and Medical Management

Chemical Terrorism

1

Chemical Nerve Agents

Daniel C. Keyes

INTRODUCTION

Terrorism has become a reality of life in many parts of the world. News reports frequently remind us of those individuals and groups who are intent on injuring and killing noncombatants in the name of a cause, for personal satisfaction, or for power. The March 1995 sarin nerve agent attack on the Tokyo subway system resulted in a heightened level of concern in the United States for such an attack on domestic soil. Since the attacks on the World Trade Center in 1993 and September 2001, the United States has entered into a new era of awareness of the terrorism threat.

Although there are a variety of potential weapons for terrorism, only a few are currently thought to be likely for use in a nonmilitary setting. Dr. Alexei Yablokov, an expert on nuclear security and former science advisor to President Boris Yeltsin, testified before the National Security House Subcommittee in 1997 about the existence of "nuclear suitcase bombs" in the former Soviet Union and the lack of knowledge of their current location (1). Each suitcase is attributed a 1-kiloton nuclear weapon. It is assumed that nuclear weapons might be difficult for a terrorist group to bring into the United States and detonate. Radioactive materials could, however, be incorporated into an explosive device and thus constitute a greater threat.

Chemical and biological agents are considered much more likely to be used and thus are considered to be highly

significant threats by the U.S. Federal Bureau of Investigation. Both of these have now been used in a nonmilitary setting with significant consequences. It is now considered a question of *when,* not *if* a terrorist using chemical weapons will strike in many countries.

HISTORY OF BIOLOGICAL AND CHEMICAL WARFARE

Nonconventional weapons have been used throughout history. The Greeks used animal corpses to pollute the water wells used by the enemy. In the Middle Ages, invading armies catapulted bodies laden with plague and other diseases against besieged populations (2). The United States, Britain, and France have all used blankets laden with smallpox to infect Native Americans. In World War I, biological and chemical weapons became important tools of the continental armies. At Ypres, Belgium, the Germans instituted the first use of chemical agents in warfare. In April 1915, they released 168 tons of chlorine gas along enemy lines. Five miles of Allied lines were opened, but the Germans did not expect such a result, and they did not take advantage of the success. They later implemented mustard gas also. There were approximately 1 million chemical casualties in World War I, with approximately 5% of those being fatalities.

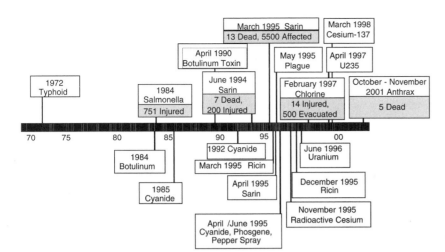

Figure 1–1. Chemical, biological, and nuclear terrorist incidents in the United States and abroad since 1970. [Adapted from Soldier Biological and Chemical Command (SBCCOM), 2003. Domestic Preparedness Training Program Materials.]

The number of terrorist acts and attempts have been increasing since the 1970s. Many of these have involved the use of explosive devices; however, there have been several notable attempts to use chemical and biological agents (Fig. 1-1). In 1972, a group called the Order of the Rising Sun was found to have 30 to 40 kg of typhoid bacteria cultures with which they intended to attack the water supplies of Chicago, St. Louis, and other cities in the Midwest. In 1984 the Bhagwan cult located in a small town in Oregon, sprayed salmonella onto restaurant salad bars in an attempt to influence local elections. In that event, 45 victims were admitted to area hospitals, and 751 people became ill. No fatalities were reported. These two events were more isolated in nature.

In the early 1980s, a man named Chizuo Matsumoto changed his name to Asahara and established the Aum Association of Mountain Wizards. After a trip to meet the Dalai Lama, he decided to establish a world religion and changed the name of his organization to Aum "Supreme Truth" or *Aum Shinrikyo*. This organization grew to a membership of 20,000 members and an estimated wealth of $1 billion. The group became increasingly authoritative, requiring absolute submission to its leader, Asahara. The group carried out assassinations of opponents and developed facilities to manufacture nerve agents and biological terrorist weapons.

In June 1994, the group attempted to assassinate three judges in Matsumoto, Japan. The assassination team released sarin nerve agent in the residential community where the judges lived. The attack involved a truck with a special device to release sarin. Although the judges were not killed, seven people died, and 280 were injured.

On March 20, 1995, Aum Shinrikyo launched a chemical attack on the Tokyo subway (3). They put dilute sarin nerve agent into lunch boxes and other containers disguised as lunch bags. The terrorists used umbrellas with sharpened points to puncture the containers during the morning rush hour on three subway lines. This tragic event caused 11 deaths and approximately 5,500 injuries among the commuters and emergency responders (4). The nearest acute care facility, St. Luke's International Hospital, saw 641 of the victims. Approximately 85% of the victims bypassed the emergency medical system and presented directly to hospitals without decontamination. Fortunately, the weekly grand rounds were taking place at St. Luke's hospital and a large part of the medical staff was present when patients began arriving (5).

During this event, the identity of the poison involved was not initially known, and there was a delay in reporting this information to the hospitals. Medical personnel contacted the poison center, but this agency had not been informed of the nature of the toxin. Initially, it was assumed that the victims had been exposed to carbon monoxide or possibly cyanide vapor. A physician from Matsumoto correctly noted from news coverage that this was similar to the incident that had occurred in his city several months previously. He contacted colleagues in Tokyo with the identity of the agent within 2 hours of the subway attack (6).

The Tokyo sarin incident demonstrated a concept commonly discussed by disaster response planners. A great majority of victims presented directly to hospitals without the intervention of hazmat or other Emergency Medical Services (EMS) personnel. A typical time for response and set-up for a hazmat incident is 1 hour. This is the time realistically required because of the sequence of activities that must occur: notification, response, hot-zone and perimeter setup, assembly of decontamination stations, and initiation of victim triage. In most cases, ambulatory victims are not willing to wait so long for treatment or transportation to a medical facility. The most realistic option for an individual on the scene would be to obtain private transportation to the nearest emergency room. As a result of this public self-referral to area hospitals, health facilities must be prepared with decontamination facilities, personal protective equipment (PPE), antidotes, and disaster plans to respond to such an incident; they cannot rely on EMS for these actions.

Physicians are key participants in the response to a chemical agent attack. After a terrorist incident, the great majority of patients present to hospitals without the benefit of decontamination or treatment at the scene by emergency medical system personnel. This means that medical personnel and hospitals must plan to be able to respond to such an incident. The agents that are discussed here include tabun, sarin, soman, and VX.

| TABLE 1-1 | Physical and Chemical Properties of the Nerve Agents |

AGENT	MOLECULAR FORMULA, MOLECULAR WEIGHT (G/MOL), CAS REGISTRY NO.	LCt$_{50}$ (MG/MIN/M^3)	VOLATILITY (MG/M^3 AT 25°C)	VAPOR DENSITY (AIR = 1)	TOPICAL LD$_{50}$ (MG)
Tabun (GA)	$C_5H_{11}N_2O_2P$; 162.12; 77-81-6	400	610	5.63	1,000
Sarin (GB)	$(CH_3)_2CHOP(CH_3)OF$; 140.11; 107-44-8	100	22,000	4.86	1,700
Soman (GD)	$C_7H_{16}FO_2P$; 182.17; 96-64-0	50	3,900	6.33	100
VX	$C_{11}H_{26}NO_2PS$; 267.37; 50782-69-9	10	10.5	9.20	10

LCt$_{50}$, the does that kills 50% of unprotected humans expressed as a concentration per cubic meter and with a 1-minute exposure. Modified from Holstege CP, Kirk M, Sidell FR. Chemical warfare. Nerve agent poisoning. *Crit Care Clin.* 1997;13:923–42.

Abbreviation	Common Name	Proper Name
GA	Tabun	Ethyl N-dimethylphosphoramidocyanidate 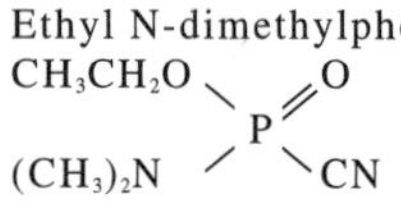
GB	Sarin	Isopropyl methylphosphonofluoridate 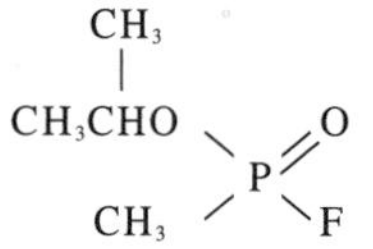
GD	Soman	1,2,2-trimethylpropyl methylphosphonofluoridate (Pinacolyl methylphosphonofluoridate) 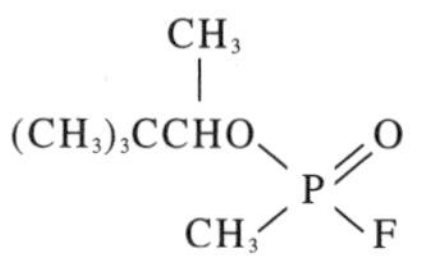
GE	Ñ	Isopropyl ethylphosphonofluoridate 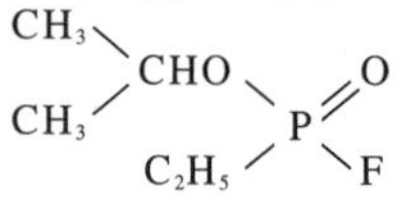
GF	Ñ	Cyclohexyl methylphosphonofluoridate 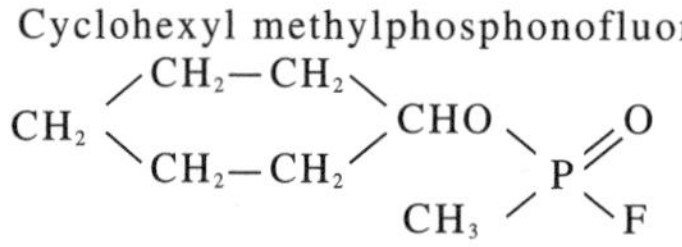
VX	Ñ	O-Ethyl S-[2-(diisopropylamino)ethyl] methylphosphonothioate 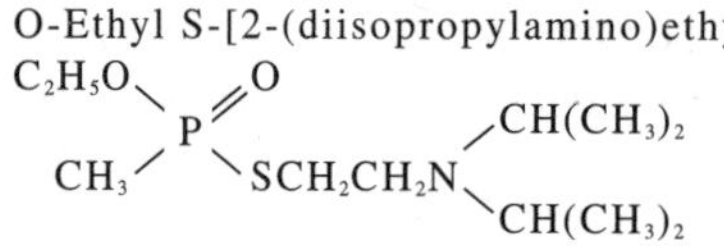
VE	Ñ	O-Ethyl S-[2-(diethylamino)ethyl] ethylphosphonothioate 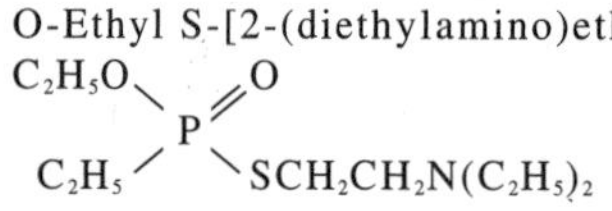
VG	Ñ	O O-Diethyl S-[2-(diethylamino)ethyl] phosphorothioate 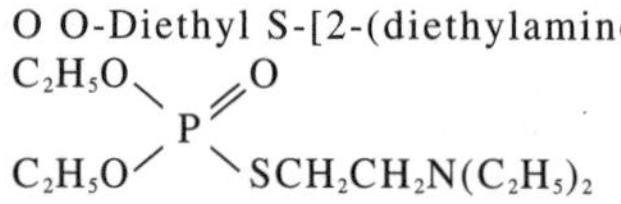
VM	Ñ	O-Ethyl S-[2-(diethylamino)ethyl] methylphosphonothioate 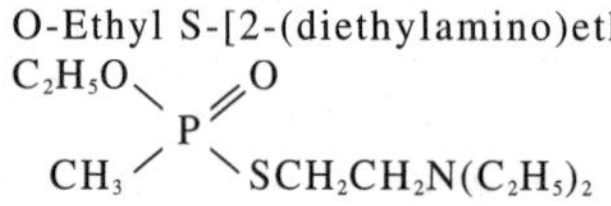

Figure 1–2. Structures and nomenclature of nerve agents. Ñ = No common name assigned. (Adapted from Ballantyne B, Marust C, eds. Clinical and experimental toxicology of organophosphates and carbamates. Oxford: Butterworth-Heinemann, 1992.).

HISTORY OF THE NERVE AGENTS

The nerve agents include the German products tabun (GA), sarin (GB), and soman (GD), known as the "volatile agents," and VX, a "persistent agent." The biologic and physical properties of these agents and several others are provided in Table 1-1 and Fig. 1-2.

The modern use of nerve agents began in World War II (7). A chemist named Gerhard Schrader was working on the development of organophosphate (OP) insecticides in 1936 when he developed the first nerve agent, tabun. This was followed by SARIN, named for the initials of the scientists involved in its creation (8). The German Ministry of Defense established a large production facility at Dyhernfurth. This facility produced tabun and sarin beginning in 1942 (8). Toward the end of the war, the Soviets captured the Dyhernfurth facility, dismantled it, and moved it to the former Soviet Union where production continued.

THEORETICAL AND SCIENTIFIC BACKGROUND

The nerve agents differ in their potential toxicities (Table 1-1). The LCt_{50} refers to the dose that kills 50% of unprotected humans expressed as a concentration per cubic meter and with a 1-minute exposure. The first three agents (tabun, sarin, and soman) are considered volatile agents, with characteristics that allow their suspension in air from a properly designed dissemination device. The highly viscous VX has a consistency similar to motor oil.

Nerves communicate with each other by secreting chemical neurotransmitters in the synapse (nerve terminal). The neurotransmitter in the cholinergic subset of the autonomic nervous system, and also in autonomic ganglia is *acetylcholine* (Fig. 1-3). Nerve agents and other organophosphate chemicals inhibit this neurotransmitter and cause an excess of cholinergic symptoms.

The neurotransmitter acetylcholine becomes attached to acetylcholinesterase (AChE) by weak ionic bonds. At the esteratic site, acetylcholine is cleaved into two simple molecules: acetate and choline. This enzyme has a high turnover number (number of substrate molecules that it catalyzes per unit time). Acetate goes into intermediate metabolism, and choline is taken up presynaptically and recycled by combination with acetyl CoA to make more acetylcholine.

Organophosphorus and *carbamate* compounds are attracted to this esteratic site of AChE, and, as a result of this attraction, acetylcholine cannot enter. This blocks the cleaving of the neurotransmitter and causes acetylcholine accumulation in the synapse. Carbamates attach to both the anionic and esteratic sites. A portion of the carbamate is immediately cleaved off. The enzyme remains inactive during the time in which the carbamate remains carbamoylated to this esteratic site. This hydrolysis step may take 1 hour in the case of the pharmaceutical agent physostigmine, or several hours in the case of pyridostigmine. Carbamate inactivation of AChE is always reversible.

In contrast to the carbamates, most OPs attach only to the esteratic site of AChE. Nerve agents and organophosphorus insecticides combine with the hydroxyl group of a serine residue, leaving an inactive phosphorylated form of the enzyme. Depending on the size of the alkyl group on the OP molecule, hydrolytic cleavage may take a long time to occur, or it may not occur at all. If this bond becomes permanent, the enzyme remains inactivated definitively. When the AChE enzyme has become permanently inactivated, this is referred to as *aging* of the enzyme. New enzyme must be synthesized for the synapse to function normally once again. In the case of red blood cells, this period of regeneration corresponds to the life of the cell, or 120 days. A series of antidotes, known as *oximes,* can reverse the inhibition of the AChE enzyme if given before the permanent bond has formed (known as *aging*). Examples of these oxime antidotes include *pralidoxime* and *obidoxime.* They will be discussed in more detail later.

Wherever AChE excess is found, there are symptoms of cholinergic excess. Acetylcholine is the neurotransmitter at the neuromuscular endplate and for the parasympathetic nervous system. It is also the neurotransmitter at the ganglionic level for the sympathetic and parasympathetic nervous systems. As a result, neurotransmitter excess is manifested in the sympathetic and parasympathetic nervous system. Ganglionic, nicotinic cholinergic excess can result in tachycardia, hypertension, and mydriasis, which may be misleading for the clinician who expects to see the classic cholinergic (muscarinic) findings.

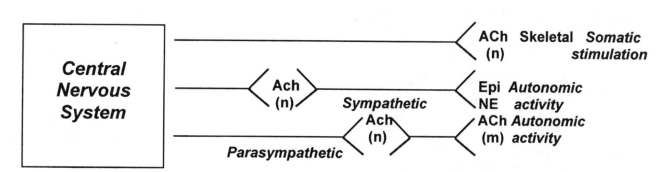

Figure 1–3. Acetylcholine neurotransmission. [From Texas Terrorism Response and Emergency Care (Texas TREC) Course syllabus 2003. With permission.]

CHARACTERISTICS OF SPECIFIC AGENTS

SARIN

A 52-year-old man was exposed to sarin nerve agent and developed the following signs: cyanosis, seizures, labored respirations, miosis, muscle fasciculations, marked salivation, and rhinorrhea. He was treated with atropine (14 mg in 1 day), pralidoxime chloride (2 g in 150 ml normal saline IV) given three times over the first 2 hours, oxygen, assisted ventilation, and nasogastric suction. The patient recovered within several days after a period of emotional lability but died of an acute myocardial infarction 18 months later (9).

Three adults experienced a sudden onset of rhinorrhea and slight respiratory discomfort, miosis, eye pain, increase in salivation, scattered wheezes, and rhonchi. Symptoms were mild and no treatment was given. The AChE levels were depressed, with full recovery occurring in 20 to 90 days (9,10).

Two adults accidentally exposed to sarin vapor (0.09 mg/m^3) exhibited RBC-ChE levels of 19% and 84%, respectively, and developed fixed extremely miotic pupils (11). No other signs or symptoms developed, and neither man required treatment. Recovery to normal cholinesterase activity was gradual over a 90-day period. Pupillary reflexes were not detectable 11 days after exposure. The miotic pupils dilated slowly over a 30- to 45-day period (12). Inhibition of red cell cholinesterase activity appears to be directly related to the dose of sarin. After exposure to sarin at a concentration of 2.73 mg/m^3 for 2 minutes, one of two subjects manifested a 23% RBC-ChE inhibition. Contraction of the pupils persisted for 24 hours (13). Workers exposed to sarin three or more times within the previous 6 years developed long-term brain abnormalities reflected in the electroencephalogram (14–16).

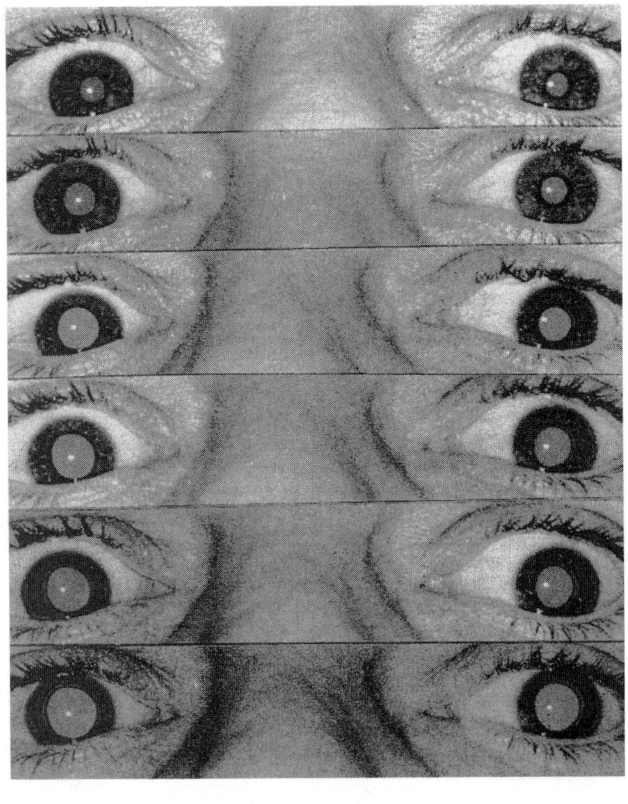

SOMAN

There are few reported cases of soman poisoning. One such case is reported from over 30 years ago. A 33-year-old male laboratory technician was working with 1 ml of 25% (V/V) soman solution and broke the pipette, splashing a small amount into and around his mouth. "He immediately washed his face and rinsed his mouth with water and was brought to the emergency room . . . about 5 to 10 minutes after the accident. He complained of impending doom and immediately collapsed. His physical examination revealed him to be comatose with labored respirations and he was slightly cyanotic. He had miosis, which persisted for over 2 months (Fig. 1-4), markedly injected conjunctiva, marked oral and nasal secretions, moderate trismus and nuchal rigidity, prominent muscular fasciculations, and hyperactive deep-tendon reflexes. Except for tachycardia, his heart, lungs, and abdomen were normal" (9).

After a total of 12 mg of atropine as well as pralidoxime, his bronchoconstriction became less severe; however, he could not be intubated because of trismus. He received a tracheostomy and awoke after approximately 30 minutes. His hospital course was described as difficult with persistent fasciculations, nausea, weakness, and restlessness. Although previous publications suggested the possibility of worsening cholinergic symptomatology with the use of phenothiazines, he was given a dose of Phenergan®. He later developed torticollis that responded to diphenhydramine (17,18). A remarkable feature of this case was the requirement of anticholinergic therapy for 5 more weeks (Fig. 1-3). Scopolamine was administered with varying effects during the hospital course. The drug seemed beneficial at the beginning of his medical care but detrimental toward the end (19).

TOXIC DOSE

In experiments conducted some 45 years ago, a sarin dose of 2 mg/kg IV produced no symptoms in human subjects. The red cell cholinesterase (RBC-ChE) was depressed to 28% of control values. No spontaneous recovery was seen. The antidote 2-PAM Cl was administered (2.5 to 25 mg/kg) 1 to 5 hours after sarin exposure, resulting in reactivation of approximately 40% of the RBC-ChE (20,21).

Figure 1–4. Prolonged miosis after accidental exposure to soman. As with other volatile agents, miosis tends to be predominant and is prolonged. This fascinating series of photographs was taken by Dr. Frederick Sidell to demonstrate the long duration of miosis after soman exposure. These photographs were taken over a 62-day period in which the patient was maximally dark-adapted, then a flash photograph was taken of the pupil faster than its ability to constrict. (From Sidell FR, 1974. With permission.).

Oral VX administration of 0.004 mg/kg resulted in a few symptoms (diarrhea, transient nausea) within 3 to 4 hours (10). The RBC-ChE was depressed to 70% below normal values in this experiment. Spontaneous recovery occurred in some subjects within 24 to 48 hours. Pralidoxime chloride (5 to 30 mg/kg IV) was administered at 5 to 48 hours after VX. All subjects exhibited reactivation of 70% of the inhibited enzyme. With a VX infusion of 1.5 mg/kg IV, most subjects experienced some lightheadedness and dizziness; some had nausea and vomiting within 1 hour. An increase in heart rate and blood pressure was observed at 3 hours. Erythrocyte cholinesterase was depressed to approximately 20% of normal in subjects with symptoms and to 28% of normal in asymptomatic subjects. Spontaneous recovery of RBC-ChE was observed at 1% per hour over 70 hours. Pralidoxime chloride (2.5 to 25 mg/kg IV) at 0.5 to 24 hours after VX resulted in reactivation of 70% of the inhibited enzyme.

SIGNS, SYMPTOMS, AND LABORATORY: DIAGNOSIS OF AGENT EXPOSURE

The primary diagnosis of exposure to nerve agents is based on the signs and symptoms of victims. The majority of exposed patients present with miosis (small pupils) in the case of the volatile agents. It is interesting that victims of VX exposure usually do not manifest miosis. With any of these agents, the more severely intoxicated patients present with vomiting and seizures. Observation of these effects should provoke the inclusion of nerve agent exposure in the mind of the treating physician. The combination of miosis and muscle fasciculation is considered pathognomonic of organophosphate exposure. If several patients present with the same symptoms, this should cause the physician and hospital staff to consider the possibility of a terrorist attack with these agents. If a chemical attack occurs, one would expect that the majority of victims would arrive within a short period of time (hours) during the same day as the exposure.

The cholinergic symptoms are listed in Table 1-2. It is of special importance to include the important findings of bronchorrhea and bronchoconstriction in one's effort to remember this toxic syndrome. These are the principal causes of death in organophosphate poisoning. The resolution of pulmonary and bronchial complications constitutes the primary endpoint of treatment. The common mnemonic SLUDGE (salivation, lacrimation, urination, diaphoresis, defecation, GI motility, emesis) leaves out this important endpoint and should not be used for teaching health care providers the characteristics of the cholinergic (muscarinic) toxic syndrome. A better mnemonic for this purpose is DUMBELS (diarrhea, urination, miosis, bronchoconstriction and bronchorrhea, emesis, lacrimation, salivation).

Vapor exposures tend to primarily affect the areas they have contact with, eyes (miosis) or lungs (bronchoconstriction) (Table 1-3). In contrast, dermal application of the same agent often produces local effects of fasciculation and sweating. Systemic effects may follow and may be delayed (Table 1-4).

DIFFERENCE BETWEEN ORGANOPHOSPHORUS NERVE AGENTS AND INSECTICIDES

Many people are familiar with insecticide poisoning, which occurs with much greater frequency than nerve agent exposure. Although many similarities exist between the OP insecticides and the nerve agents in terms of their pathophysiology and treatment, there are some differences. In cases of *volatile* nerve agent exposure, patients who do not present to the hospital with symptoms are not likely to become ill later. Several of the OP insecticides differ in this respect. Some OP insecticides such as fenthion and chlorfenthion may cause late onset of symptoms 12 or more hours after exposure due to their strong lipophilicity. The nerve agent VX can also cause severe symptomatology late after the exposure; however, the *G agents (tabun, sarin, soman) typically have an onset of symptoms within minutes.*

Another difference associated with the OP insecticides is the type of complications that the patients develop. A syndrome called *organophosphate-induced delayed neuropathy* (OPIDN) occurs with some insecticides. It occurs following acute exposure to some OP insecticides, and includes weakness or paralysis, usually in the lower extremities. Sometimes there is also pain or numbness. This is possibly due to the action of these insecticides on *neuropathy target esterase* (NTE), an enzyme located in the distal nerve. Such chronic neuropathy does not appear to occur with the nerve agents. Another difference between OP insecticides and the nerve agents is with respect to the dosing of atropine, which is needed to treat exposed victims. The OP insecticides may require extremely large doses of atropine, sometimes over 1,000 mg, in small doses. The nerve agents rarely require more than 20 to 30 mg of atropine.

CHARACTERISTICS AND CASE REPORTS OF SOME SPECIFIC NERVE AGENTS

DIAGNOSTIC TESTING: CHOLINESTERASE MEASUREMENT

There are two types of cholinesterases in the blood. These blood cholinesterase levels do not exactly reflect the effect of nerve agents inside target cells throughout the body. But they do provide an indirect way of measuring the activity of this enzyme, and the seriousness of exposure to the nerve agents. The two types are (a) serum or butyrylcholinesterase (BChE) and (b) RBC-ChE. The first, BChE, is the easiest one to measure and is also described as serum or *pseudocholinesterase*. The second cholinesterase, RBC-ChE or "true" cholinesterase, is thought to be a more representative marker for tissue AChE activity, but it is more difficult to determine because it is inside of the red cell. Cholinesterase levels may vary depending on ethnicity and other genetic factors, nutritional status, and underlying disease states. Considerable variation occurs between individuals.

TABLE 1-2 Signs and Symptoms of Nerve Agent Poisoning

SITE OF ACTION	SIGNS AND SYMPTOMS
After local exposure	
Muscarinic	
Pupils	Miosis, marked, usually maximal (pinpoint), sometimes unequal
Ciliary body	Frontal headache, eye pain on focusing, blurring of vision
Nasal mucous membranes	Rhinorrhea, hyperemia
Bronchial tree	Tightness in chest, bronchoconstriction, increased secretion, cough
Gastrointestinal	Occasional nausea and vomiting
After systemic absorption (depending on dose)	
Bronchial tree	Tightness in chest, with prolonged wheezing expiration suggestive of bronchoconstriction or increased secretion, dyspnea, pain in chest, increaseed bronchial secretion, cough, cyanosis, pulmonary edema
Gastrointestinal	Anorexia, nausea, vomiting, abdominal cramps, epigastric and substernal tightness (cardiospasm) with "heartburn" and eructation, diarrhea, tenesmus, involuntary defecation
Sweat glands	Increased sweating
Salivary glands	Increased salivation
Lacrimal glands	Increased lacrimation
Heart	Bradycardia
Pupils	Miosis, occasionally unequal, later maximal miosis (pinpoint)
Ciliary body	Blurring of vision, headache
Bladder	Frequency, involuntary micturition
Nicotinic	
Striated muscle	Easy fatigue, mild weakness, muscular twitching, fasciculations, cramps, generalized weakness/flaccid paralysis (including muscles of respiration) with dyspnea and cyanosis
Sympathetic ganglia	Pallor, transitory elevation of blood pressure followed by hypotension
Central nervous system	Immediate (acute) effects: generalized weakness, depression of respiratory and circulatory centers with dyspnea, cyanosis, and hypotension; convulsions, loss of consciousness, and coma
	Delayed (chronic) effects: giddiness, tension, anxiety, jitteriness, restlessness, emotional lability, excessive dreaming, insomnia, nightmares, headaches, tremor, withdrawal and depression, bursts of slow waves of elevated voltage in electroencephalogram (especially on hyperventilation), drowsiness, difficulty concentrating, slowness of recall, confusion, slurred speech, ataxia

Adapted from Army FM8-285, Navy NAVMED P-5041, Air Force AFM 160-11 Field Manual. The treatment of chemical agent casualties and conventional military chemical injuries. Washington DC: Departments of the Army, the Navy, and the Air Force; February 28, 1990.

TABLE 1-3 Effects of Vapor Exposure to Nerve Agents[a]

Exposure to small amount (local effects)
    Miosis
    Rhinorrhea
    Slight bronchoconstriction/secretions (slight dyspnea)
Exposure to moderate amount (local effects)
    As above plus the following:
Loss of consciousness
Convulsions (seizures)
Generalized fasciculations
Flaccid paralysis
Apnea
Involuntary micturition/defecation

[a]Onset within seconds to several minutes after onset of exposure.
Adapted from Sidell FR. In: Somani SM ed. Chemical warfare agents. San Diego: Academic Press, 1992: 155–94.

TABLE 1-4	Effects of Dermal Exposure to Nerve Agents

Minimal exposure
   Increased sweating at site of exposure
   Muscular fasciculations at site of exposure
Moderate exposure
   Increased sweating at site
   Muscular faciculations at site
   Nausea, vomiting, and diarrhea
   Feeling of generalized weakness
   May be precipitant in onset after lone (4–18 h) asymptomatic interval
Severe exposure
   The previous may be present
   Loss of consciousness (may be precipitous in onset after asymptomatic interval)
   Convulsions (seizures)
   Generalized fasciculations
   Flaccid paralysis
   Apnea
   Involuntary micturition/defecation
Adapted from Sidell FR. In: Somani SM ed. Chemical warfare agents. San Diego: Academic Press, 1992: 155–94.

Studies that have attempted to relate symptoms of toxicity to AChE levels have found a greater correlation to RBC-ChE than to BChE (19,22). Many OP insecticides preferentially inhibit BChE, whereas nerve agents such as VX tend to inhibit RBC-ChE to a greater degree (10,23). Once inhibited, BChE is resynthesized more rapidly than RBC cholinesterase, which takes approximately 120 days to return to normal, or 1% per day (24). BChE requires approximately 50 days to return to normal levels. BChE less than 20% of predicted was a useful prognostic indicator for poor outcome in the Tokyo sarin terrorist attack (25).

Symptoms vary in the degree that they relate to serum cholinesterase levels. Eye and airway signs are caused principally by direct exposure and have little correlation to RBC-ChE levels (26–28).

DIAGNOSTIC TESTS TO IDENTIFY NERVE AGENTS

A capillary column gas chromatography-mass spectrometry method is available for tabun determinations. Gas chromatography retention indices have been determined for 22 chemical warfare agents (29).

MEDICAL MANAGEMENT: DECONTAMINATION AND TREATMENT

Treatment of nerve agents generally follows proper decontamination of the victims (discussed in the following section). If contaminated patients are brought into the hospital, many of the staff members may become secondarily contaminated and develop injury from exposure to the nerve agent involved (30). Where autoinjectors are available (discussed later), treatment simultaneous with decontamination may be considered.

DECONTAMINATION

Personal protective equipment refers to special garments designed to protect the members of the decontamination team against exposure to the toxic materials. The components of PPE include suits, eye protection, boots, gloves, and respiratory devices. Various types of PPE are available depending on the agent involved and the risk of exposure. Not all hospital staff members require sophisticated PPE, provided that victims are adequately decontaminated before entering the hospital. However, all personnel who work with decontaminated patients should work in a well-ventilated environment and use basic universal precautions including the use of a face mask. "Universal" precautions (also known as *Body Substance Isolation* or BSI), do not prevent the inhalation of a nerve agent; however, they do minimize the risk of secondary contamination from splash and small amounts of contaminants that might not be removed from the victim.

The use of more sophisticated PPE is required by any personnel who is involved in decontamination and also for those involved with the initial triage of victims. Those who use this type of equipment are required to receive appropriate training as mandated by the U.S. Occupational Safety and Health Administration (29 CFR 1910.120 and 19410.134), and also in some cases by the National Institute for Occupational Safety and Health (NIOSH), the U.S. Environmental Protection Agency (EPA), and the Joint Commission on Accreditation of Healthcare Organizations (JCAHO).

Decontamination is the process of physically removing toxic substances from a victim, equipment, or supplies. In the hospital setting, it is imperative to avoid the introduction of contaminated elements into the clinical setting. In most cases, victims arrive at the hospital nearest to the incident with no prior decontamination. Institutions should have a plan for decontaminating victims of hazardous material incidents, including those involving terrorist nerve agents. In the 1995 terrorist sarin incident of Tokyo, many hospital personnel were secondarily contaminated due to their involvement in removing clothing or working in poorly ventilated environments. At one research institution, the Keio University School of Medicine, 13 people developed symptoms of secondary contamination from off-gassing of the nerve agent (30).

For the volatile nerve agents such as sarin, decontamination is nearly complete with the simple removal of clothing and jewelry by the decontamination team. Use of large amounts of low-pressure water adequately completes the decontamination, along with the use of soap and a gentle brush to assist in the removal of fat-soluble substances. Decontamination is most ideally undertaken outdoors near the hospital emergency department. This outdoor setting is especially suitable for areas with milder weather. Indoor facilities are necessary in conditions of severe winter weather. Security personnel should have a plan to direct traffic to the decontamination area, and to prevent entry of persons into other parts of the hospital. Signs, the presence of security personnel, and locking incorrect access points help to ensure the proper flow of traffic.

Bleach solutions have sometimes been advocated for use in decontamination, particularly after mustard exposures. However, bleach may be irritating when used on human skin, and is more challenging to store and use properly. It is no longer routinely recommended for use on living victims of a chemical agent attack. Cadavers exposed to nerve agents may require special hypochlorite treatment, however. Simple soap and water are adequate for large-scale exposure such as the sarin attack in Tokyo—in which more than 600 patients arrived within the first hours after the incident. With an event such as this, it is not appropriate to be concerned over use of hypochlorite solution. The simple removal of clothing and jewelry outside of the facility by properly protected decontamination personnel would have essentially eliminated the secondary contamination problems experienced in the Tokyo incident.

SUPPORTIVE CARE

The acute management of the patient with nerve agent exposure involves rapid establishment of a patent airway. The major cause of death in nerve agent poisoning is hypoxia resulting from pulmonary and bronchial involvement with the toxin. In cases of severe bronchoconstriction and bronchorrhea, it may be necessary to provide atropine before other interventions are attempted. Endotracheal intubation may be difficult without first administering atropine, due to the very high airway resistance associated with bronchoconstriction. This can be on the order of 50 to 70 cm, higher than the pressure allowed by the "pop-off" valve of most bag-valve mask devices.

Patients who respond to treatment initially begin to show small skeletal muscle movements. They progress to spontaneous, random movements of the limbs and then a struggle against the mechanical ventilation. There may be alternating periods of spontaneous breathing and apnea. Weakness and obtundation may persist for 1 or more days. Miosis and subtle mental change may persist for weeks (31–33).

ANTIDOTES

Three classes of pharmaceuticals are considered essential in the management of nerve agent exposure and OP insecticide intoxication: atropine, pralidoxime (or other oximes), and diazepam (or other benzodiazepines).

Atropine. *Atropine* is an agent with both systemic and central effects to combat the consequences of acetylcholine excess at muscarinic sites. Atropine dosing should begin with typical advanced cardiac life support doses of 1 to 3 mg, but may require much more than the usual amounts after this initial test-dose (Table 1-5). Lack of response to normal doses of atropine supports the diagnosis of nerve agent or other OP toxicity. Patients with severe muscarinic effects require larger amounts of atropine. *The endpoint of atropine administration is the clearing of bronchial secretions and a decrease in ventilatory resistance.* This is an essential point to remember because heart rate and pupil diameter are not useful parameters for monitoring the response to treatment with this antidote. Nebulized bronchodilators such as albuterol are not as effective as atropine at treating nerve agent exposure due to the need for an anticholinergic effect (7).

Typical doses for atropine in severely intoxicated nerve agent casualties are in the range of 5 to 15 mg (9,34). This is in sharp contrast to the much larger doses required in organophosphate insecticide intoxication, in which several grams of atropine may be required in the first days of treatment (35,36). In cases of severe OP poisoning, an IV drip is implemented to meet the continuing requirement for atropinization (37). This is not usually needed for the nerve agents.

The U.S. military supplies kits containing the two most important antidotes for nerve agent exposure, atropine and pralidoxime. The military kit, known as the *Mark I*, consists of two autoinjector pens. The smaller autoinjector contains 2 mg of atropine for intramuscular administration. The autoinjector mechanism provides remarkable rapid absorption (Fig. 1-4). After the atropine is administered, the pralidoxime is administered in the same fashion either to the same thigh or to the opposite side. The atropine autoinjectors each contain 2 mg of atropine citrate. Such kits are also available commercially for civilian use (Meridian Medical Technologies, St. Louis, MO). These autoinjectors permit rapid intramuscular injection of antidote through protective clothing and underlying garments. Experience shows these autoinjectors to be effective at administering certain medications, such as atropine (Fig. 1-5 and reference). Military medical personnel carry additional atropine autoinjectors and are trained to add more atropine as required based on the endpoints of good control of respiratory secretions and adequate respiratory effort (38). In the hospital setting, most planners have concluded that intravenous pharmaceutical preparations should be used instead of autoinjectors. This is also the case with the *oximes,* which are discussed next.

TABLE 1-5	Recommended Nerve Agent Treatment		
TYPE OF EXPOSURE	**PRESENTATION**	**ANTIDOTAL THERAPY**	**OBSERVATION**
Mild vapor (GA, GB, BD) exposure	Nasal congestion with mild shortness of breath, miosis	One Mark I kit or 2 mg atropine, 1 g 2PAMCl	Miosis may not reverse with treatment
Mild liquid (VX) exposure	Localized sweating and fasciculations	One Mark I kit or 2 mg atropine, 1 g 2PAMCl	—
Moderate vapor or liquid exposure	More severe respiratory distress, muscular weakness	One or two Mark I kits or 2–4 mg atropine, 1 g 2PAMCl intravenous drip over 30 min	—
Severe vapor or liquid exposure	Unconscious, possibly seizing or flaccid, possibly apneic or severe symptoms	Three Mark I kits or 6 mg atropine and 1 g 2PAMCl initially	May repeat atropine as needed and 2PAMC1 in 1 h

Soldier Biological and Chemical Command, 2003.

Oximes. The oximes (pralidoxime, obidoxime) are nucleophilic substances that reactivate the acetylcholinesterase inhibited by OP toxins. An oxime should be administered before *aging*, permanent disabling of the cholinesterase enzyme, occurs. Aging occurs at different time intervals from exposure for different nerve agents. For example, sarin requires several hours to age, whereas soman ages in only 2 to 6 minutes, and VX takes more than 2 days (Table 1-6). The time for complete aging is approximately 10 times the half-life, and treatment with an oxime may be useful up to this point.

After the oxime has regenerated acetylcholinesterase, the enzyme resumes its critical role in the breakdown of acetylcholine, normalizing neurotransmission. This brings about the improvement of nicotinic symptoms, such as fasciculations, muscle twitching, and the return to normal muscle strength. *Pralidoxime* is the oxime used currently in the United States. Other countries use obidoxime or other oximes to treat nerve agent victims. Pralidoxime as the chloride (2PAMC1) or mesylate (P2S) probably is best administered in a dose of 30 mg/kg body weight over a 30-minute period every 4 to 6 hours, preferably by IV injection, but it can also be given by intramuscular injection (Table 1-5). Oxime concentrations more than 4 mg/ml can be maintained for 3 to 6 hours after intramuscular injections of 30 mg/kg body weight of either oxime (chloride or mesylate). Alternatively, 2-PAM (chloride or mesylate) can be given as a continuous infusion at a rate of 550 mg/hour (8 mg/kg/hour) after the injection of 30 mg/kg/body weight on two occasions 4 hours apart (35), but this is usually done for OP insecticide exposure, and not necessarily for the nerve agents. In principle, PAM should be continued as long as the OP compound or its active metabolite is present in the body.

Benzodiazepines. Benzodiazepines (diazepam, lorazepam, and others) should be used to treat the seizures induced by the nerve agents. This can be administered IV or through the use of an autoinjector. Military sources suggest that for patients manifesting symptoms of severe toxicity, benzodiazepines should be administered even before seizures are evident. If three of the Mark I kits are administered due to severe symptoms in the victim, diazepam should be administered immediately after completing the administration with the autoinjector kits. With the exception of benzodiazepines, phenytoin and other conventional treatment modalities for seizures are considered ineffective in this setting (39).

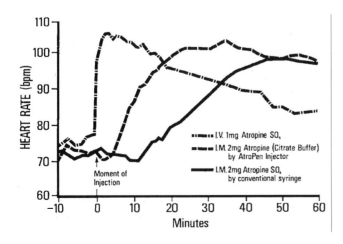

Figure 1–5. Absorption of atropine administered by autoinjector device. Heart rate was used to demonstrate the effect of atropine administration given either intravenously, intramuscularly, or by autoinjector. The graph illustrates the effectiveness of the device. Intravenous administration causes an effect more rapidly but has a shorter duration of action. (Modified from Martin TR, Kastor JA, Kershbaum KL, Engelman K. The effects of atropine administered with standard syringe and self-inductor device. American Heart Journal, 1980, 99(3): 282-88, and the Domestic Preparedness Program, Soldier Biological and Chemical Command (SBCCOM), Hospital Provider Course, DPT 8.0, 2002 with data provided by Frederick R. Sidell, MD.

TABLE 1-6	Aging

AGENTS	AGING HALF-LIFE
Tabun	46 h
Sarin	5.2–12 h
VX	50–60 h
Soman	40 sec to 10 min
Paraxon	2.1–5.4 d

Adapted from Dunn MA, Sidell RF. *JAMA.* 1989;262:649–52

Treatment of nerve agent casualties should be based on the initial signs and symptoms and modified appropriately when the actual agent is defined. If the exposure was a volatile agent, such as sarin or soman, the patients will be symptomatic within the first several minutes of exposure to the toxin. This means that patients who are not symptomatic when they are evaluated at the hospital are not likely to become serious exposure victims. For the case of the liquid exposure of VX, patients may not become symptomatic for up to 18 hours and therefore should be observed for a much longer period of time. If one does not know to which agent the patient was exposed, it is prudent to carry out a longer observation period in the ER or ICU. The severity of symptoms determines the dose of the antidotal therapy (Table 1-5).

THE SPECIAL CASE OF PYRIDOSTIGMINE PRETREATMENT

The use of atropine and the oximes may be insufficient for protection against the toxic effects of GD (soman), even if they are administered immediately after the agent. Soman **ages** extremely rapidly within minutes. As Dunn and Sidell have emphasized (40), even with training and the ability to don a mask rapidly, soldiers on a chemical battlefield may be at risk for absorbing up to five times the lethal dose of GD during a chemical attack. The *protective ratio* (40,41) is the factor by which a treatment raises the lethal dose of a toxic agent. Currently available antidotes do not raise the protective ratio sufficiently high in humans to couteract the lethal effects of soman (GD), although a new oxime antidote, HI-6, shows much promise. A preexposure treatment with the reversible agent *pyridostigmine* has been used to solve this problem with soman. Pretreatment is not effective against sarin and VX challenge. When used for soman challenge, it should be followed by atropine and an oxime.

Pyridostigmine is a *carbamate* compound that binds to acetylcholinesterase. Like the nerve agents, it causes acetylcholine to build up and cholinergic symptoms (DUMBELS) to occur. The difference is that with carbamate compounds like pyridostigmine, the binding to the AChE is reversible. Organophosphates, like the nerve agents, cause irreversible, permanent binding to the enzyme. For this reason, pyridostigmine was given to soldiers in the Gulf War of 1991 to temporarily bind to AChE, and to prevent the attachment of the much more dangerous nerve agent. Some controversy exists with its use, however. Some authors have partially attributed the symptoms of the "Gulf War Syndrome" to use of this agent (42).

Pyridostigmine by itself does not provide protection without the use of the antidotes (atropine/oximes). It is an antidote *enhancer* rather than a *true* treatment. It appears to enhance the efficacy of the antidotes within 1 to 3 hours after taking the first tablet. Maximal benefit appears to develop with time and may be reached when a tablet is taken every 8 hours (38).

The U.S. Army provides a pyridostigmine bromide (30 mg) pretreatment set of tablets (21 total) packaged in a blister pack, to be taken one every 8 hours, enough for 7 days. One tablet is taken orally with water (38).

TRIAGE OF NERVE AGENT VICTIMS

Methods of triage of nerve agent victims are usually based on military experience. An understanding of the principles involved in nerve agent action can aid considerably in guiding the triage officer at the time of an exposure incident. A general approach to the triage of victims of nerve agent exposure follows (39). Each patient is divided into one of four groups based on a system agreed upon in advance: immediate, delayed, minimal, or expectant.

IMMEDIATE

All patients who are symptomatic with more than just miosis are triaged to an "immediate" category and require immediate decontamination and application of antidotes, airway control, and other supportive measures. If the patient has two or more systems involved (for example miosis and wheezing), the patient should be considered an "immediate" and should receive treatment. Rapid treatment should result in a successful resuscitation for these victims.

DELAYED

Patients who have received an initial treatment in the field or in the triage area of the hospital, and are improving, will need to be reassessed at a later time. Such patients may be deferred from the initial group of patients requiring treatment. These patients may still have miotic pupils. Pupil size alone is not sufficient clinical information to triage patients who have been exposed to nerve agents properly.

MINIMAL

Patients who are ambulatory and conversant and have no symptoms or only miosis will usually require no immediate medical treatment. They may require counseling and social support, however. For more efficient care of the sicker patients, these individuals may be moved to a low acuity environment.

EXPECTANT

Patients who present with apnea greater than 5 minutes in duration, or whose vital signs are not detectable, may be considered in the "expectant" category and do not receive treatment in the high-volume multicasualty incident (MCI). This is particularly true when there are more than just a very small number of victims.

PLANNING FOR TERRORIST EVENTS AND FUTURE ANTIDOTAL CONSIDERATIONS

Treatment of nerve agent exposure should follow proper decontamination of victims. It is essential for institutions to prepare for large numbers of casualties because experience dictates that most victims will bypass EMS and come directly to nearby acute care facilities.

Planning for nerve agent attack will require stocking of antidotes, including atropine, diazepam, and the oximes. Atropine may be obtained as a powdered form, which may be compounded in the hospital pharmacy. The powdered drug has a much longer shelf life than does the atropine-containing solution. One alternative is to have enough atropine solution on hand for 30 to 40 casualties and to use the powdered form after the initial stock is completed. Compounding of atropine solution from the powdered form can be initiated in the pharmacy after the first cases arrive at the hospital.

In the United States, the only oxime widely available is pralidoxime. The data for pralidoxime with soman are rather unique. In an experiment using rat, monkey, and human muscle tissue, Clement demonstrated that pralidoxime is ineffective in the treatment of soman poisoning, and that survival after oxime administration was not due to reactivation of acetylcholinesterase (43). Hence, the agent most commonly used in the United States would not be useful for treatment of this particular poison. The lethal dose for soman is approximately 50 mg. One problem with soman is the extremely rapid aging time. Aging occurs in approximately 2 minutes, making the application of an agent such as pralidoxime essentially useless.

The bispyridinium oximes offer promise as a treatment for soman. The structure includes an additional oxime ring: a nitrogen-substituted benzene ring with a side group. By combining oximes into larger molecules, antidotes that are effective against nerve agents have been developed. One such agent is HI-6 (Fig. 1-6). Hamilton investigated the efficacy of the bispyridinium agent HI-6 after giving monkeys five times an LD_{50} of soman. Three out of four monkeys survived using the newer oxime (44). One of the interesting aspects of this case was the fact that acetylcholinesterase inhibition was the same for the monkeys that survived and those that died. Thus, some factor is involved in the efficacy

of the bispyridinium agent other than acetylcholinesterase reactivation. Some have suggested that the brain cholinesterase makes the difference in survival. However, in a study involving rat brain homogenate cholinesterase activity, essentially no improvement enzyme reactivation could be found from pralidoxime (45). The mechanisms involved in oxime antidotal efficacy are still to be fully elucidated (46). There is not a perfect oxime reactivator that is effective for all agents. However, a combination of oxime agents would offer a more complete spectrum of protection (47).

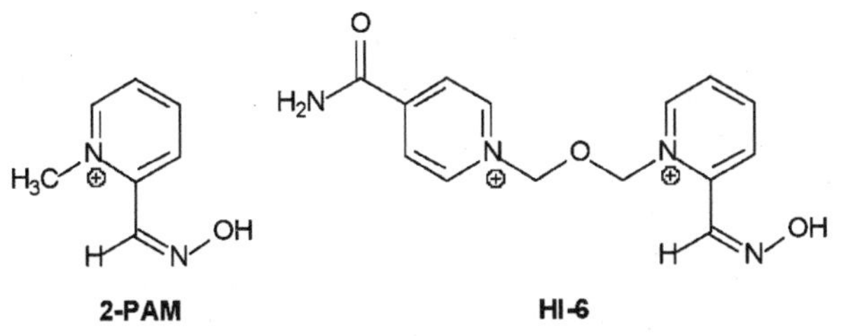

SUMMARY

- The volatile agents—tabin (GA), sarin (GB), and soman (GD)—cause rapid onset of toxicity after aerosol exposure.

- For the volatile agents, removal of clothes and jewelry constitutes essentially complete decontamination, but copious irrigation is suggested if uncertain of the identity of the agent.

- VX is a persistent agent, which may cause either immediate or delayed symptoms.

- Full decontamination with soap and water is necessary for VX. Some authorities suggest irrigation for volatile agents also, if time and circumstances permit.

- Antidotes for the nerve agents include atropine, oximes (pralidoxime, obidoxime), and diazepam.

- Health care facilities must be prepared to receive the majority of patients without the benefit of EMS intervention.

QUESTIONS AND ANSWERS

1. **Which of the following nerve agents is a persistent agent (i.e., presents a danger in the environment for a long time)?**
   A. Sarin
   B. Soman
   C. Tabun
   D. VX
   E. Pyrethroid insecticides

2. **Which is not a feature of the cholinergic toxic syndrome?**
   A. Diarrhea
   B. Urination
   C. Bronchorrhea
   D. Dry skin
   E. Lacrimation

3. **What is the most appropriate and sufficient decontamination measure for a victim of a confirmed vapor nerve agent exposure?**

Figure 1–6. Oxime acetylcholinesterase reactivators. 2-PAM, pralidoxime.

2-PAM   HI-6

A. Wash with copious amounts of soap and water
B. Remove all clothing and jewelry
C. Wash with a hypochlorite solution
D. Wash with soap and water and then with a hypochlorite solution
E. No decontamination is needed

4. What is the endpoint of atropine administration in the setting of a nerve agent exposure?
A. Pupil size
B. Drying of respiratory secretions and ease of ventilation
C. Drying of skin
D. Control of seizures
E. Control of vomiting

ANSWERS

1: **D.** *VX*
2: **D.** *Dry skin*
3: **B.** *Remove all clothing and jewelry*
4: **B.** *Drying of respiratory secretions and ease of ventilation*

REFERENCES

1. Public Broadcasting System (PBS). An interview with Alexei 1999. PBS online and WGBH/FRONTLINE. Complete interview available at http://www.PBS.org.
2. Newardk T. Medieval warfare. London: Bloomsbury Books; 1988.
3. Kaplan DE, Marshall A. The cult at the end of the world: the terrifying story of the Aum Doomsday Cult, from the subways of Tokyo to the nuclear arsenals of Russia. New York, NY; Crown Publishing, 1996.
4. Morita H, Yanagisawa N, Nakajima T, et al. Sarin poisoning in Matsumoto, Japan. Lancet. 1995;346:290-93.
5. Okumura T, Suzuki K, Fukuda A, et al. The Tokyo subway sarin attack: disaster management, part 2: hospital response. Acad Emerg Med. 1998;5(6):618-24.
6. Okumura T, Suzuki K, Fukuda A, et al. The Tokyo subway sarin attack: disaster management, part 1: community emergency response. Acad Emerg Med. 1998;5(6):613-17.
7. Sidell FR. Nerve agents. In: Zajtchukk R, Bellamy RF eds. Textbook of military medicine. Washington DC: Office of the Surgeon General; 1997.
8. Paxman HR. A higher-form of killing. New York: Hill and Wang; 1982:53.
9. Sidell FR. Soman and sarin: clinical manifestations and treatment of accidental poisoning by organophosphates. Clin Toxicol. 1974;7:1-17.
10. Sidell FR, Groff WA. The reactivatibility of cholinesterase inhibited by VX and sarin in man. Toxicol Appl Pharmacol. 1974;27:241-52.
11. Rengstorff RH. Accidental exposure to sarin : vision effects. Arch Toxicol. 1985;56:201-3.
12. Oberst FW, Koon WS, Christensen MK, et al. Retention of inhaled sarin vapor and its effect on red blood cell cholinesterase activity in man. Clin Pharmacol Ther. 1968;9:421-27.
13. Rubin LS, Goldberg MN. Effect of sarin on dark adaptation in man. Threshold change. J Appl Physiol. 1957;11:439-44.
14. Duffy FH, Burchfiel JL, Bartels PH, et al. Long-term effects of an organophosphate upon the human electroencephalogram. Toxicol Appl Pharmacol. 1979;47:161-76.
15. Burchfield JL, Duffy FH. Organophosphate neurotoxicity: chronic effects of sarin on the electroencephalogram of monkey and man. Neurobehav Toxicol Teratol. 1982;4:767-78.
16. Burchfield JL, Duffy FH, Sim VM. Persistent effects of sarin

and dieldrin upon the primate electroencephalogram. Toxicol Appl Pharmacol. 1976;35:365-79.
17. Arterberry JD, Bonifaci RW, Nash EW, et al. Potentiation of phosphorus insecticides by phenothiazine derivative. JAMA. 1962;182:848.
18. Weiss LIZ, Orzel RA. Enhancement of toxicity of anticholinesterases by central depressant drugs in rats. Toxicol Appl Pharm. 1967;10:334.
19. Kechum JS, Sidell FR, Crowell EB, et al. Atropine, scopolamine and Ditran: comparative pharmacology and antagonists in man. Psychopharmacology (Berlin). 1973;28:121.
20. Grob D. The manifestations and treatment of poisoning due to nerve gas and other organic phosphate anticholinesterase compounds. Arch Intern Med. 1956;98:221-38.
21. Grob D, Harvey JC. Effects in man of the anticholinesterase compound sarin (isopropyl methyl phosphorofluoridate). J Clin Invest. 1958;37:350-68.
22. Grob D, Lilienthal JL Jr, Harvey AM, et al. The administration of di-isopropyl fluorophosphate (DFP) to man, I: effect on plasma and erythrocyte cholinesterase; general systemic effects; use in study of hepatic function and erythropoieses; and some properties of plasma cholinesterase. Bull Johns Hopkins Hosp. 1947;81:217-44.
23. Sim VM. Variability of different intact human skin sites to the penetration of VX. Edgewood Arsenal, MD: Medical Research Laboratory; 1962. Chemical Research and Development Laboratory Report 3122.
24. Grob D, Harvey AM. The effects and treatment of nerve gas poisoning. Am J Med. 1953;14:52-63.
25. Okumura T, Takasu N, Ishimatsu S, et al. Report on 640 victims of the Tokyo subway sarin attack. Ann Emerg Med. 1996;28:129-35.
26. Harvey JC. Clinical observations on volunteers exposed to concentrations of GB. Edgewood Arsenal MD: Medical Research Laboratory; 1952. Medical Laboratory Research Report 144.
27. Craig AB, Woodson GS. Observations on the effects of exposure to nerve gas, I: clinical observations and cholinesterase depression. Am J Med Sci. 1959;238:13-7.
28. Sidell RF. Clinical considerations in nerve agent intoxication. In: Somani SM, ed. Chemical warfare agents. New York: Academic Press; 1992:163.
29. D'Agostino PA, Provost LR. Gas chromatographic retention indices of chemical warfare agents and stimulants. J Chromatogr. 1985;331:47-54.
30. Nozaki H, Hod S, Shinozawa Y, et al. Secondary exposure of medical staff to sarin vapor in the emergency room. Intens Care Med. 1995;21:1032-35.
31. Fischetti M. Gas vaccine. Bioengineering immunization could shield against nerve gas. Sci Am. 1991;153-54.
32. Orma PS, Middleton RK. Aerosolized atropine as an antidote to nerve gas. Ann Pharmacother. 1992;26:937-38.
33. Doctor BP, Blick DW, Recht KM, et al. Protection of rhesus monkey against soma toxicity by pretreatment with cholinesterase. Proceedings of the 4th International Symposium: Protection against Chemical Warfare Agents. Stockholm, Sweden: June 8-12,1992; 335-40.
34. Ward JR. Case report: exposure to a nerve gas. In: Whittenberger JL, ed. Artificial respiration: theory and applications. New York: Harper & Row; 1962:258-65.
35. Vale JA, Meredith TJ, Health A. High dose atropine in organophosphorus poisoning. Postgrad Med J. 1990;66:881.
36. Chew LS, Chee KT, Leo JM, et al. Continuous atropine infusion in the management of organophosphorus insecticide poisoning. Singapore Med J. 1971;12:80-85.
37. LeBlanc FN, Benson BE, Gilg AD. A severe organophosphate poisoning requiring the use of an atropine drip. Clin Toxicol. 1986;24:69-76.
38. Departments of the Navy, Army, and Air Force. Potential mili-

tary chemical biological agents and compounds. December 12, 1990; FM 3-9, NAV/ FAC:467.

39. Soldier Biological and Chemical Command (SBCCOM). Domestic Preparedness Training Program materials; 2003.

40. Dunn MA, Sidell FR. Progress in medical defense against nerve agents. JAMA. 1989;262:649-52.

41. Munro NB, Watson AP, Ambrose KR, Griffin GD. Treating exposure to chemical warfare agents: implications for health care providers and community emergency planning. Environ Health Perspect. 1990;89:205-15.

42. Haley RW, Billecke S, La Du BN. Association of low PON1 type Q (type A) arylesterase activity with neurologic symptom complexes in Gulf War veterans. Toxicol Appl Pharmacol. 1999;157(3):227–33.

43. Clement JG. Survivors of soman poisoning: recovery of the soman LD50 to control value in the presence of extensive acetylcholinesterase inhibition. Arch Toxicol. 1989;63(2):150-54.

44. Hamilton MG, Lundy PM. HI-6 therapy of soman and tabun poisoning in primates and rodents. Arch Toxicol. 1989;63(2): 144-49.

45. Kassa J, Cabal J. A comparison of the efficacy of a new asymmetric bispyridinium oxime BI-6 with currently available oximes and H oximes against soman by in vitro and in vivo methods. Toxicol. 1999;132(2-3):111-18.

46. Van Helden HP, Busker RW, Meichers BP, et al. Pharmacological effects of oximes: how relevant are they? Arch Toxicol. 1996;70(12):779-86.

47. Kassa J. Review of oximes in the antidotal treatment of poisoning by organophosphorus nerve agents. J Toxicol Clin Toxicol. 2002;40(6):803-16.

2

Vesicating Agents Including Mustard and Lewisite

Stacey L. Hail and Daniel C. Keyes

MUSTARDS

Vesicating agents are chemicals named for causing blistering; they have a long military history. The mustards include mainly sulfur mustard and nitrogen mustard. Nitrogen mustard will not be discussed as it has not been stockpiled for military use and is largely used for chemotherapeutic purposes. Sulfur mustard (2,2-dichloroethyl sulfide) has been the most commonly used mustard compound.

Known also as mustard, mustard gas, "the king of war gases," Yperite, H, and HD, sulfur mustard is one of the most powerful vesicants used as a chemical weapon (1,2). The chemical warfare agent H is an agent containing 70% sulfur mustard and 30% sulfur impurities. HD, however, is sulfur mustard purified by distillation and washing (3).

The term "mustard gas" is a misnomer because the agent is a liquid at typical environmental temperatures. Mustards are oily, yellow-brown, fat-soluble substances that are heavier than water. Mustard vapor has been described to smell like mustard, onion, garlic, or horseradish. Due to its low volatility, mustard concentrates in low-lying trenches and may persist in the environment for up to five days (3,4). At temperate climates with little wind, mustard may remain in the environment for more than a week. However, in areas with temperatures above 37.7°C, the agent may persist for only one day (2) (Table 2-1).

Sulfur mustard was discovered in 1822 by Belgian scientist Cesar-Mansuete Despretz (5) , but was not used in battle until 1917 near Ypres, Belgium. That is how mustard earned the name Yperite. During World War I, mustard was responsible for as many as 400,000 battlefield injuries and 8,000 deaths (4). Interestingly, mustard accounted for 77% of World War I casualties (4). Thus, casualties from mustard gas were more numerous than those from any other agent used in World War I (6). Although several warring nations during World War II stockpiled sulfur mustard, there is little evidence that it was used in combat. In December 1943, an Allied ship carrying 100 tons of mustard was attacked by German planes and exploded near Bari, Italy. This attack caused mustard to disseminate over a large area producing mysterious ocular and dermal

TABLE 2-1 Mustard Characteristics

- Liquid at normal environmental temperatures
- Boiling point 215° to 217.2°C
- Melting point 14.4°C
- Oily, yellow-brown, fat-soluble
- Heavier than water
- Odor of mustard, onion, garlic, or horseradish
- Low volatility
- Vapor pressure 0.9 mm Hg at 30°C
- Odor threshold <1.3 mg/m^3

vesicant effects. This attack resulted in over 600 mustard casualties and numerous respiratory deaths (2,7). More recently, Iraqi forces during the Iran-Iraq conflict (1980 to1988) used mustard causing as many as 3,000 Kurdish deaths (7). Iranian soldiers were evacuated to Europe where they were treated for classic mustard poisoning in the Iran-Iraq war (1,8). As recently as 1998, three American workers sustained mustard burns while collecting routine chemical samples from a storage site. All three individuals presented with blisters (9).

THEORETICAL AND SCIENTIFIC BACKGROUND

Approximately 20% of sulfur mustard is rapidly absorbed through the skin (7,10). Due to the mustard's fat solubility and its penetration down hair follicles and sweat glands, absorption occurs within 2 minutes. Twelve to 50% will react or remain "fixed" with skin components. The remainder will enter the systemic circulation and be absorbed by other tissues or solid organs. Once the sulfur mustard diffuses across a cell membrane, cell injury and cell death occurs. Although the exact mechanisms of sulfur mustard-induced cell death have yet to be elucidated, there are four proposed theories: (a) alkylation of deoxyribonucleic acid (DNA), (b) oxidative stress upon cell components, (c) depletion of glutathione, and (d) inflammatory responses (10).

16

Alkylation of DNA

An alkylating agent is an agent that replaces a proton on another molecule with an alkyl group (i.e., a simple chain of carbon atoms). DNA is cross-linked as a result of alkylation. The mustard alkylates the DNA, creating DNA strand breaks. This precipitates an increase in activity of various proteinases that may cause cellular damage and blister formation. DNA cross-linking also greatly inhibits further DNA synthesis. As DNA synthesis is inhibited, unbalanced growth of the cell occurs. Unbalanced cell growth triggers apoptosis, or programmed cell death (7,10).

Mustard changes the structure of DNA, cellular membranes and proteins through alkylation. After the mustard alkylates complementary strands of DNA, the molecules cannot separate. Separation of DNA molecules is needed for normal replication of DNA; therefore cell division is disturbed. Mustards exert their greatest effect on rapidly dividing cells (7).

Oxidative Stress

It is known that numerous biochemical reactions in the body and environmental sources generate highly reactive oxygen species (ROS) and free radicals that may cause cellular damage (11). Sulfur mustard is also believed to lead to oxidative stress upon intracellular molecules. As mustard diffuses across the cell membrane, it enters the aqueous environment of the cytosol. Within this aqueous media, sulfur mustard undergoes intramolecular cyclization creating a highly reactive *episulfonium* intermediate. This episulfonium ion reacts with functional groups on molecules, especially sulfhydryl-containing compounds. The episulfonium ion also reacts with the sulfhydryl groups on enzymes maintaining calcium homeostasis, thus leading to increased intracellular calcium. Increased cytosolic calcium leads to death in two ways. First, the calcium disrupts microfilaments that maintain cell integrity. The loss of cell integrity leads to cell death. Additionally, calcium induces apoptosis or programmed cell death (PCD) by activating endonucleases, proteases, and phospholipases (10).

Formation of this highly reactive episulfonium intermediate is greatly enhanced in an aqueous environment. Thus, moist regions such as mucosal tissues of the eye and respiratory tract are very susceptible to mustard injury (1).

Depletion of Glutathione

Another theory of how mustard exposure causes injury is through depletion of glutathione. Reactive oxygen species (ROS) are normally detoxified by glutathione. However, in the setting of mustard, these ROS are left unchecked to react with membrane phospholipids forming lipid peroxidases. Lipid peroxidases cause loss of membrane function, membrane fluidity, and membrane integrity (10).

Inflammatory Response

After exposure to sulfur mustard, cells are stimulated to produce cytokines in response to the chemical stress. These cytokines are small peptides secreted by white blood cells and endothelial cells that cause immunologic reactions and further tissue damage (10).

SIGNS AND SYMPTOMS

Potentially, all organs can be affected by mustard exposure. However, the skin, eye, airway, bone marrow, gastrointestinal, and nervous system are particularly susceptible. One of the hallmarks of mustard intoxication is that it produces not only skin and eye effects but also systemic toxicity to internal organs such as the bone marrow. Clinical manifestations occur 2 to 48 hours after exposure, but typically are observed within 4 to 8 hours. The earlier signs and symptoms manifest, the more severe the exposure (4).

Skin

Skin is an important target for mustard since it contains frequently dividing cells. Eighty percent of mustard applied to human skin evaporates, with the remaining one-fifth of the agent penetrating and causing toxicity (7,10). Since sweat glands seem to facilitate mustard's penetration through the skin, moist areas including the groin and axillae are particularly affected (12). In fact, scrotal and perianal burns were noted in nearly half of American survivors of World War I mustard gas attacks (2). Acute exposure is not associated with immediate discomfort or pain since the mustard has a long latency period (13).

Sulfur mustard produces cutaneous blisters and erythema in humans on areas directly exposed to the agent, often in areas covered by clothing. Burns may develop from exposure to the vapor or the liquid. The skin effects from vapor are dependent upon the ambient temperature and concentration. The concentration time (C_t) needed to produce erythema is 100 to 400 mg-min/m^3, while onset of burns is about 200 to 1,000 mg-min/m^3, and severe incapacitating burns result from 750 to 10,000 mg-min/m^3. Erythema appears in affected areas within 2 to 4 hours and causes extreme pruritus. As the blisters appear, this itching diminishes. The blisters do not generally appear for 18 to 24 hours and contain large volumes of fluid. The fluid in the blister does not contain active mustard since the mustard completely reacts with the skin in the first several minutes (12).

Skin response to sulfur mustards has been described to have two phases: an *immediate phase* and a *delayed phase*. In the immediate phase, there is injury to the endothelium of superficial capillaries and venules due to direct damage to the cell membrane. Vascular leakage and infiltration with basophils may occur. The delayed phase is characterized by death of basal epidermal cells secondary to DNA damage, vascular leakage, neutrophilic immigration, and ulceration (7).

Human skin consists of two layers: a superficial layer, the epidermis, rests upon the dermis. The deepest layer of the epidermis is the stratum basale, which contains mitotically active keratinocytes. Between the epidermis and dermis is the basement membrane. This basement membrane is anchored to the keratinocytes in the epidermis by *hemidesmosomes* (Fig. 2-1). Sulfur mustard spares the basement membrane but disrupts the hemidesmosomes. Thus, a blister forms between the epidermis and the dermis leaving the basement membrane on the dermal side (12) (Fig. 2-2). Interestingly, there is racial variation in the severity of vesicant burns. Increased melanin appears to offer some protection (14).

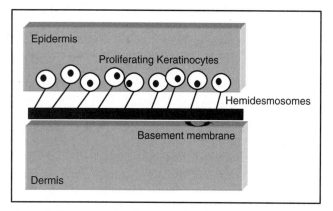

Figure 2–1. Schematic of normal skin. The basement membrane is located between the epidermis and the dermis. The proliferating keratinocytes are located at the base of the epidermis. They are anchored to the basement membrane by hemidesmosomes.

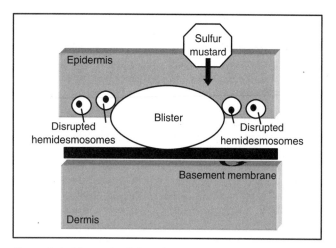

Figure 2–2. Schematic of skin after exposure to sulfur mustard. The sulfur mustard is rapidly absorbed. Injury occurs to the keratinocytes, and the hemidesmosomes are disrupted. Thus, a blister forms between the epidermis and the dermis. The basement membrane remains attached to the dermis.

The burn caused by sulfur mustard behaves similarly to thermal burns in terms of depth, but it does not penetrate the skin as deeply as an acid burn. The skin effects can be classified as mild, moderate, or severe. Mild injuries involve erythema, edema, and first-degree burns and occur after exposure to doses of 50 mg-min/m^3 or direct skin application 0.1 to 1.0 μg/cm^2 liquid mustard. Moderate injury involves exposure to 1.0 to 2.5 mg/cm^2 and leads to severe edema and vesication. Severe injury occurs after doses of 200 to 1,000 mg-min/m^3 or direct skin application of more than 2.5 μg/cm^2. At these doses, areas of necrosis are seen with surrounding vesication (2).

Mustard burns take twice the time to heal as thermal burns since the proliferating cells have been damaged (12). Experience with mustard gas casualties from the Iran-Iraq war demonstrated the slow resolution of these burns. Five soldiers with skin burns were managed with saline baths twice daily and dressings with silver sulfadiazine cream with paraffin gauze. Pain was severe and required opioids. None required skin grafting, but the healing process took 4 to 6 weeks (15). A characteristic brown pigmentation may

be observed during the healing process and may even persist afterward (13).

Eye

In World War I and the Iran-Iraq war, 80% to 90% of casualties suffered ocular injuries. Injuries ranged from mild conjunctivitis to moderate and severe keratoconjunctivitis, which often lead to corneal damage. A World War I military physician documented: "12 hours after exposure, the patient's eyes were inflamed and lacrimation, blepharospasm, and photophobia were present, … by the end of 24 hours the most distressing symptom was pain in the eyes, which was very severe. The patient was virtually blinded, with tears oozing from between the bulging, edematous eyelids, over his reddened blistered face" (16).

Mustard reacts rapidly after contact with eye tissues. In fact, mustard penetrates the cornea more rapidly than it does the skin (13). Symptoms, however, may be delayed for several hours (2,16). The aqueous-mucous surface of the cornea and conjunctiva facilitates absorption. Additionally, mustard solution is lipophilic so it concentrates in the oily moiety of the tears where it interacts with corneal epithelial cells. *Because these corneal epithelial cells have a high turnover rate, they are some of the most vulnerable cells in the body.* Initial symptoms include eye pain, photophobia, lacrimation, and blurred vision. Physical examination reveals blepharospasm (spasmodic winking), periorbital edema, conjunctival injection, and inflammation of the anterior chamber (9,16). For several days, the intraocular pressure may be elevated. Several hours later, the corneal epithelium begins to vesicate and slough. Visual acuity is decreased with worsening corneal injury. Ocular damage is classified as mild, moderate, or severe (2,16).

Mild injury occurs at doses of 12 to 70 mg/min/m^3. At these doses, there is ocular irritation but little lacrimation, blepharospasm, or photophobia. On physical examination, there is mild erythema of the eyelids and conjunctiva. There is no corneal involvement. Complete recovery is often seen in several days (16).

Moderate ocular injuries are seen with doses of 100 to 200 mg/min/m^3. Injury involves the eyelids, conjunctiva, and corneal epithelium with occasional iritis. Six hours after exposure, the patient complains of eye pain, eye dryness, photophobia, and possibly blindness. On examination, there is marked edema of the eyelids with blepharospasm. The conjunctiva is also edematous and congested. The cornea is edematous and fluorescein staining reveals punctate lesions at the palpebral fissure. There is gradual recovery after 48 hours. The corneal epithelium regenerates within 4 to 5 days. Complete symptomatic recovery takes at least 6 weeks (16).

Severe ocular injuries occur at doses higher than 200 mg/min/m^3 and involve full-thickness corneal lesions. Symptoms include severe ocular pain, blepharospasm, and blurred vision. On physical examination, the eyelids are swollen, and there is conjunctival chemosis and loss of blood vessels at the nasal and temporal limbal areas. The cornea has been described to have an "orange peel appearance" and corneal sensation is weak or absent. Other findings in severe ocular injuries are pupillary constriction, iris vasodilatation, hemorrhages, and necrosis with development of chemical anterior uveitis leading to the formation of posterior iridolenticular synechiae, increased intraocular pressure, and opacification of the lens. Resolution does not occur for 1 to 2 weeks. In 0.5% of casualties, delayed ulcerative keratitis leading to blindness may develop. These effects may be seen in patients up to 40 years after the mustard exposure (16).

Battlefield mustard exposure results in the rapid visual incapacitation of large numbers of persons. During the Iran-Iraq conflict, 90% of individuals with mustard ocular injury were visually disabled for 10 days with conjunctivitis, photophobia, and minimal corneal swelling. The conjunctivitis and photosensitivity persisted in many patients for several months. Ninety percent of patients recovered completely from their ocular injuries (17).

Lungs and Airways

After eye lesions, the greatest acute discomfort produced by exposure to mustard is from injury to the respiratory system (13). Respiratory symptoms are also the most common cause of mortality (9). Pulmonary complications such as edema and airway obstruction are most responsible for deaths that occur soon after mustard exposure (4).

Low-dose inhalation of mustard gas causes chest tightness. Larger exposures result in sneezing, rhinorrhea, nasal bleeding, sore burning throat, hoarseness, and hacking cough. Cough may persist for 10 to 48 hours. Early signs of pulmonary edema, aphonia, and tachypnea may then occur. After 48 hours, bronchopneumonia appears (7). Fibrinous pseudomembranes can form, peel off, and lead to further airway obstruction (9,10).

In 1985 and 1986, European doctors treated 39 Iranian soldiers who had been exposed to mustard gas. The most commonly reported respiratory effect was a severe cough, which did not respond to cough suppressants, steam, bronchodilators, or corticosteroids. Some patients had a dry cough while others produced plentiful sputum. Even in the presence of a normal chest radiograph, low PaO_2 was quite common as was airflow obstruction. Three of these patients required ventilation and two patients died 7 and 14 days after exposure. Fiberoptic bronchoscopy revealed marked sloughing of the tracheal and bronchial mucosa that produced adherent plugs, which could not be removed by suction. In some cases, removal of such tissue plugs with forceps resulted in improved ventilation (18).

Chronically, mustard gas exposure can lead to the development of airway hyperreactivity, chronic bronchitis, bronchiectasis, pulmonary fibrosis, and upper airway obstruction (19,20). Long-term effects of mustard on the respiratory tract were studied in 220 Iran-Iraq war victims. These patients were evaluated 7 to 13 years after their exposure. At the time of examination, nearly all the victims complained of cough and dyspnea. Six victims experienced hemoptysis. Four patients were observed to have respiratory distress. About two-thirds of the patients had wheezing or coarse rales. Radiographic findings were essentially normal, and spirometry was found to be the most useful, revealing an obstructive pattern (21). High-resolution computed tomography (HRCT) of the chest has been shown to be useful in evaluating long-term sequelae from mustard exposure. Bronchial wall thickening, interstitial lung disease, and emphysema were common findings on HRCT (19). Bronchoalveolar lavage fluid in patients with sulfur mustard-induced asthma or chronic bronchitis had the same cellular constituents as patients with asthma or chronic bronchitis from other causes (20). Finally, evidence suggests that World War I battlefield exposure of mustard gas resulted in a slightly increased incidence of lung cancer at least 20 years later (22).

Gastrointestinal Tract

The mucosal membrane of the gastrointestinal tract can be damaged after mustard exposure. This may result in nausea, vomiting, abdominal pain, bloody diarrhea, or dehydration (23). Nausea, vomiting, and abdominal pain may be seen 4 to 16 hours after mustard exposure. In fact, violent, frequent, and prolonged vomiting has been reported in four cases of experimental mustard burns in which only the skin was exposed. These men were wearing respirators and exposed to a C_t of 660 mg/min/m^3 under tropical conditions (13).

Blood

Bone marrow suppression results from mustard exposures exceeding 1,000 mg/min/m^3. Development of mustard-induced hematological effects is a poor prognostic sign (2). Half of the severely injured casualties from the Iran-Iraq conflict experienced leukopenia as a result of bone marrow suppression. Serious infections may occur, further complicating the management of these patients (9).

Leukocyte precursors die 3 to 5 days after exposure. Depending upon the severity of exposure, a leukopenic nadir occurs from 3 to 14 days. Anemia and thrombocytopenia are late findings (24).

Gonads

Various experiments with mice in the 1940s involved intravenous and intraperitoneal injections of mustards into male mice resulting in the inhibition of spermatogenesis (13,25). Damage, however, was usually transient as testicular recovery was observed at 2 weeks and mature sperm were seen at 4 weeks after exposure (13,26,27).

Eighty-one patients exposed to sulfur mustard after the Iran-Iraq conflict were evaluated in terms of their infertility. Azoospermia (absence of living spermatozoa in semen) and severe oligospermia were found in 42.5% and 57.5% of patients, respectively. Testicular biopsy showed atrophy of the germinal epithelium, intact Sertoli cells, and normal-appearing Leydig cells. There was an elevated plasma follicle-stimulating hormone level. Luteinizing hormone and testosterone concentrations were normal (28).

Administration of mustards did not seem to have the same effects on female mice. There were no injurious effects observed in the ovaries, and their reproductive potential was not altered (13,25).

Carcinogenicity and Other Long-Term Effects

The Veteran's Administration and the Institute of Medicine released a report January 6, 1993 entitled *Veterans at Risk: The Health Effects of Mustard Gas and Lewisite.* The report cites respiratory cancers (especially nasopharyngeal, laryngeal, and lung), skin cancer, pigmentation abnormalities of the skin, chronic skin ulceration and scar formation, recurrent ulcerative disease of the eye (including opacities), bone marrow depression (after exposure but infections left secondary permanent damage to organs), psychological disorders, and sexual dysfunction (caused by scarring of the scrotum or penis) (29). A 50-year mortality follow-up study was performed on World War II Navy veterans who experienced low-level mustard exposure, and the results were compared to those who had not been exposed. These veterans had voluntarily participated in mustard gas chamber tests in Bainbridge, Maryland, between 1944 and 1945. They had worn protective clothing and masks. The levels to which they had been exposed were sufficient to have caused erythema, vesicles, and ulceration. However, 50 years later, these levels of exposure were not associated with any increased risk of cause-specific mortality (30).

Sulfur mustard was the first chemical with proven genotoxic effects. After prolonged or repeated exposures, humans have shown increased risk of cancer (2). There is evidence of a link between *nitrogen* mustard and nonlymphocytic leukemia. Currently, evidence suggests a link between nonlymphocytic leukemia and *sulfur* mustard exposure (29).

MEDICAL MANAGEMENT

Currently, there are no antidotes to treat mustard toxicity. Several agents are under investigation. These include antioxidants (vitamin E), antiinflammatory drugs (corticosteroids), mustard scavengers (glutathione, *N*-acetylcysteine), and nitric oxide synthase inhibitors (L-nitroarginine methyl ester) (24). In animal studies, increased survival and fewer pathological organ effects were noted after administration of sodium thiosulfate, vitamin E, or dexamethasone within 15 minutes of exposure (31). Therefore, some experts recommend postexposure treatment with some of these agents. One regimen recommends intravenous sodium thiosulfate 500 mg/kg per day for 48 hours, followed by 10 days of oral *N*-acetylcysteine and vitamin C (4,32). Investigation with an agent known as amifostine has also shown promise. Also known as WR-271, amifostine is a drug used to prevent the effects of cancer chemotherapy, and it seems to provide protection against alkylating agents. It has been suggested that this agent may be useful if administered prophylactically to avoid mustard toxicity (33).

Preventing exposure to mustard agents, however, is most important. Protective equipment and barrier creams are discussed in the section entitled "Personal Protection." Early decontamination after exposure is priority. Additionally, unique management strategies exist for dermal, ocular, and respiratory problems after exposure to mustards.

Decontamination

Decontamination within 2 minutes of exposure is the most pressing and necessary intervention after dermal exposure. Mustard rapidly fixes to tissues, and its effects are then irreversible. Early after mustard exposure, patients typically lack any signs or symptoms. It is important to remember that this delay in symptomatology should not delay decontamination (24).

Sulfur mustard may persist as a liquid on contaminated skin, clothing, and equipment for hours to days. Thus medical personnel are at risk for skin blistering and other effects if they come into contact with contaminated victims. First, all contaminated clothing should be removed as quickly as possible. Thickened mustard agent can be removed with a wooden spatula. The exposed skin should be powdered with antigas powder containing calcium chloride and magnesium oxide. Then washing with household bleach (hypochlorite) diluted to 0.5% is a traditionally recommended military medical strategy. However, one should not delay early decontamination to locate or reconstitute hypochlorite. Soap and water are likely to be sufficient. Vigorous scrubbing should be avoided as this may allow deeper penetration of the mustard. Mustard is relatively insoluble in water, thus water alone probably has limited value as a decontaminant. Household products such as flour, talcum powder, salad oil, Dutch powder, dry tissue paper, and wet tissue paper may be used, as they are commonly available and can be effective (13). Eyes should be irrigated with water for at least 5 minutes and must occur within several minutes of exposure to prevent subsequent damage. Decontamination after several minutes may not prevent injury to the victim; however, it does protect emergency care personnel from further contact exposure (9,17,24).

Skin

Mustard-induced skin lesions often require aggressive burn management. Because these burns heal slowly and are prone to infection, careful wound care is essential. In the early stages of mustard toxicity, pain is not a major problem. However, intense itching is associated with the erythematous stage. This itching is best treated with a benzodiazepine or chlorpromazine. Once the blister appears, there are two options for treatment. Experience from World War I suggests that in the early phase, the blister fluid may be aspirated and the epidermal layer allowed to act as a dressing until it separates naturally. If the victim is encountered at a later stage, the blister can be deroofed and dressed with silver sulfadiazine (12).

Surgical debridement of blisters and necrotic tissue may be warranted after a severe exposure (2). If burns cover 20% to 25% of the body, the patient has potentially been exposed to a lethal dose of mustard and should be admitted to a critical care unit (9). Burns should be irrigated several times daily and washed with soap and water. Topical antibiotics are also recommended. Pain may be severe and require opiates. Experience with mustard gas casualties in the Iran-Iraq war emphasized the efficacy of carbamazepine during skin healing in controlling severe pain not relieved by analgesics or antihistamines (15). Recently, novel techniques have been studied to facilitate healing of deep partial thickness mustard-induced burns. Such techniques include the use of enzymatically active dressings to induce debridement, CO_2 laser debridement, and dermabrasion; they have been very effective in animal models (14,34). Finally, overhydration should be avoided, as fluid losses are generally less than with thermal burns (24).

Eye

After the eyes are irrigated with water for 5 minutes, visual acuity testing, inspection of the eye, fluorescein staining, and slit-lamp examination should be performed. If fluorescein uptake is noted in the cornea, the eyes should be treated with an antibiotic, a corticosteroid ointment, and a mydriatic. Petroleum jelly may be used to keep the eyelids from sticking. Dark glasses can be used for the photophobia, but eye padding should be avoided. In victims with severely inflamed nonnulcerated keratitis and hemorrhagic conjunctivitis, it has been recommended to use dexamethasone and ascorbate drops every 3 hours. However, ocular burns should be managed in conjunction with an ophthalmologist (2,9,12,17,24).

Respiratory Support

Airway control should always be considered first while managing a patient exposed to mustard. Endotracheal intubation may be necessary if dysphonia, stridor, or respiratory distress are noted. Sloughing epithelium may obstruct smaller endotracheal tubes; therefore, the largest tube that can pass through the vocal cords should be utilized. A rapidly developing upper airway pseudomembrane may require emergent tracheotomy to prevent complete obstruction. Bronchoscopy may be required to assess damage and to remove any necrotic debris. Humidified air, cough suppressants, or the use of mucolytics can help soothe inhalational injury. Inhaled sympathomimetics and corticosteroids may help relieve bronchospasm (2,9,24). In an animal model, N-acetylcysteine (NAC) administered intraperitoneally to rats had lower indices of lung injury after exposure to mustard. This suggests that NAC may be useful as a treatment compound for mustard-induced lung injury (35).

TRIAGE CONSIDERATIONS

Depending on the severity of exposure, signs and symptoms after exposure to mustards are typically delayed because the serious manifestations of toxicity from these agents do not occur immediately. However, these patients must be observed carefully for the delayed effects of the mustard. Very few patients will be classified as *expectant* since mustard use is generally chosen to incapacitate. Victims of a severe exposure may manifest early respiratory signs and symptoms. These victims should be classified as *immediate* due to potential impending airway obstruction. Most importantly, decontamination is most effective if instituted within the first several minutes to avoid toxicity. Even after that time, decontamination should still occur, primarily to protect all personnel who come in contact with the patient.

PERSONAL PROTECTION

Chapter 30 of this book provides a thorough overview of personal protection against the chemical agents. Prevention of secondary mustard contamination is extremely important, particularly in light of the lack of specific antidotes for this class of agents. Prevention involves wearing protective garments and equipment and the use of topical barrier compounds.

Street clothing and battle fatigues provide little skin protection against the mustard agents, as seen in the World War I casualties with scrotal, perianal, and auxiliary burns. Special military garments such as CPOG (chemical protective overgarment), BDO (battle dress overgarment), and MOPP (mission-oriented protective posture), possess a charcoal layer to absorb any penetrating mustard. Such garments provide 6 hours of protection after exposure. However, these garments are not generally available outside the military (2). Civilian first responders and hospital-based emergency care personnel involved in direct exposure or decontamination of victims should wear level A personal protective equipment (PPE) (24).

Protective clothing and masks provide protection; however, they limit physical agility. Thus, various topical barrier creams are under investigation. Such a cream is difficult to develop since sulfur mustard is absorbed and fixes to skin so rapidly. The U.S. Army has developed a cream that contains perfluoroalkylpolyether (PFAPE) oil and polytetrafluoroethylene. The new preparation should be applied in a thin layer to the skin (0.15 mm). This product and other topical agents still need to undergo clinical trials prior to validating their widespread clinical use. Another product, S-330 (a chloroamide) has also been shown to provide protection from sulfur mustard in preliminary studies (10). Other work has focused on the development of highly reactive nanoparticles of metals and metal oxides that are incorporated into skin creams. Experiments have shown that prepared MgO nanoparticles destroyed 50% of the sulfur mustard (36). A recent study was conducted to evaluate various commercially available barrier creams against sulfur mustard. In some cases barrier creams appear to interfere with decontamination. It has been generally concluded that currently available barrier creams may reduce exposure to chemical agents, but they should not replace protective clothing or decontamination (37).

LEWISITE

Lewisite (Agent L) is an arsenical vesicant (dichloro[2-chlorovinyl]arsine). In its pure form, Lewisite is a colorless and odorless liquid. However, impurities may give it an amber or brownish color. It has been described as having an odor of geraniums. Lewisite is heavier than mustard and poorly soluble in water (Table 2-2). Although it is a vesicating agent, Lewisite also has systemic effects, causing pulmonary edema, diarrhea, restlessness, weakness, low temperature, and low blood pressure. If inhaled in high concentrations, Lewisite may be fatal in as little as 10 minutes (38,39).

TABLE 2-2 Lewisite Characteristics
• Liquid at normal environmental temperatures
• Boiling point 190°C
• Freezing point -18°C
• Oily, colorless liquid
• Poorly soluble in water
• Heavier than mustard
• Odor of geraniums
• Low volatility
• Vapor pressure 0.394 mm Hg at 20°C
• Odor threshold 20 mg-min/m^3

European chemists discovered that organic chloroarsines caused destructive effects on insects and human tissue in the mid-19th century. German chemists began to explore and develop these compounds as chemical weapons. American chemists developed the most notorious agent among these warfare agents—2-chlorovinyldichloroarsine—which they named Lewisite after Captain Lewis, the leader of the scientists' team. Lewisite has never been used on a large scale; however, it has been stockpiled in the United States, Russia, and China. Additionally, Lewisite is easy to produce and has a rapid onset of action. Thus, Lewisite is considered a potential threat for use as a chemical warfare agent (40).

THEORETICAL AND SCIENTIFIC BACKGROUND

Lewisite is not only a lethal vesicant but also a systemic poison when absorbed into the bloodstream. In contrast to sulfur mustard, exposure to Lewisite is quite painful, and the onset of symptoms occur much more rapidly (40). Lethal exposures can occur via inhalation, skin or eye contact, or ingestion.

Inhalation of Lewisite vapor causes immediate burning pain of the respiratory tract at concentrations of 8 mg-min/m^3. At 20 mg-min/m^3, the odor can be detected. It is described as the odor of geraniums. The LCt_{50} is approximately 1,500 mg-min/m^3. Absorption of Lewisite across the skin occurs within minutes. Lewisite is faster acting and more toxic via direct skin contact than mustard. The LD_{50} of liquid on the skin is about 30 to 50 mg/kg. Thus, 2 ml of liquid Lewisite on the skin can be fatal to an adult. Additionally, liquid and vapor Lewisite causes severe eye damage within minutes of contact. Ingestion of Lewisite is a very uncommon route of exposure. However, it can lead to local effects and systemic absorption (38).

When absorbed into the bloodstream, Lewisite becomes a systemic poison. The liver, gallbladder, and bile duct are particularly susceptible. At very high doses, the kidneys and urinary tract can be affected. Lewisite acts in a different manner than mustard by directly affecting enzyme systems (3). However, the exact mechanism by which Lewisite damages cells is unclear. It inhibits a variety of enzymes, including pyruvic oxidase, alcohol dehydrogenase, succinic oxidase, hexokinase, and succinic dehydrogenase. Lewisite appears to have a high affinity for these enzymes, which contain thiol groups (38,40). Immediate death from systemic absorption of Lewisite has been termed Lewisite shock. It is hypothesized that loss of blood plasma results from the increased permeability of capillaries damaged by the circulating Lewisite (3).

SIGNS AND SYMPTOMS

In order of appearance and severity of symptoms, Lewisite acts as a blister agent and a toxic lung irritant, and then it is absorbed by tissues and becomes a systemic poison.

Skin

Liquid Lewisite produces more rapid, severe lesions of the skin than liquid mustard. Within 10 to 20 seconds after contact, stinging pain is usually felt. As penetration of the agent occurs, the pain increases in severity and then becomes a deep, aching pain. After contact with the skin, erythema occurs within 15 to 30 minutes. Vesication fully develops within 12 to 18 hours and usually expands over the entire area of erythema. Unlike mustard burns, there is deeper injury to connective tissue and muscle, greater vascular damage, and more severe inflammation. There may even be necrosis of tissue and gangrene (38,39).

Eye

Lewisite vapor and liquid cause pain and blepharospasm on contact followed by edema of the conjunctiva and the eyelids. The eyes may be swollen shut within an hour. Higher doses may cause corneal damage and iritis. After a few hours, edema of lids subsides and haziness of the cornea develops (38,39).

Lungs and Airways

Conscious casualties will usually rapidly put on a mask since the vapors of arsenical vesicants are so irritating to the respiratory tract. Therefore, severe respiratory injuries are less likely to occur except among those who do not have masks or those who are too wounded to put one on. Lewisite produces a burning sensation in the nasal passages and sinuses followed by profuse nasal secretion, epistaxis, and sneezing. Longer exposure causes coughing productive of frothy mucus, laryngitis, and dyspnea. Pseudomembrane formation may also occur leading to airway obstruction. Respiratory injury from vapor exposure to Lewisite is similar to that with mustard; however, pulmonary edema is often more severe and accompanied by pleural fluid (38,39).

Gastrointestinal Tract

Nausea and vomiting may follow ingestion or inhalation of Lewisite.

Cardiovascular

Lewisite shock is a condition resulting from high-dose exposure to Lewisite. This is likely from increased capillary permeability leading to intravascular fluid loss, hypovolemia, and organ congestion. Hepatic necrosis may occur due to the shock and hypoperfusion. Renal failure may be caused by decreased renal function secondary to hypotension (38).

Carcinogenicity and Long-Term Effects

The literature is limited regarding potential delayed or latent effects of Lewisite exposure and there is only anecdotal evidence regarding potential carcinogenicity (3,38).

MEDICAL MANAGEMENT

Decontamination

Unlike mustard agents, Lewisite exposure is characterized by immediate onset of pain. Therefore, most patients will immediately seek decontamination and treatment (3). To significantly reduce tissue damage, the eyes and skin must be decontaminated within 1 or 2 minutes of exposure. The eyes should be flushed with water for 5 to 10 minutes. If exposure to the liquid agent is suspected, all clothing and jewelry should be removed. The skin should be washed immediately with soap and water. Alternative forms of decontamination include 0.5% sodium hypochlorite solution, flour, talcum powder, or Fuller's earth (38).

Antidotes

There is an antidote for Lewisite known as British Anti-Lewisite (BAL) or dimercaprol. BAL is a chelating agent that has been shown to reduce the systemic effects seen after Lewisite exposure. *However, due to potentially toxic side effects, BAL should only be administered to patients who have shock or significant pulmonary injury.* Chelation therapy should be initiated in consultation with the regional poison center. The standard dosage regimen is 3 to 5 mg/kg intramuscularly every 4 hours for four doses. Contraindications include renal disease, pregnancy (except in life-threatening circumstances), and concurrent use of medicinal iron. It has been suggested that alkalinization of the urine stabilizes the BAL-arsenic complex and protects the kidneys during chelation therapy. Hemodialysis to remove the BAL-arsenic complex may be necessary if acute renal insufficiency develops.

At 3 mg/kg, the most common side effect of BAL is pain at the injection site. At 5 mg/kg, the effects may include nausea and vomiting; headache; burning sensation of the lips, mouth, throat, and eyes; lacrimation; salivation; rhinorrhea; muscle aches; burning and tingling extremities; tooth pain; diaphoresis; chest pain; anxiety; and agitation (38).

Skin

A patient presenting with a small area of erythema that began 12 hours after exposure is unlikely to progress farther. Such patients may be treated with a soothing lotion and an analgesic and allowed to go home with warnings. Patients with significant erythema with or without blistering should be admitted for further evaluation.

Burns may be second or third degree. In general, it has been recommended that blisters smaller than 1 cm should remain roofed while larger than 1 cm should be unroofed. The wound should be irrigated two to three times a day followed by application of a topical antibiotic. As with mustards, these skin lesions may take weeks to months to heal. Larger burns should be managed in a burn unit (38). Current investigation has shown promise for treating Lewisite burns with laser debridement. This "lasablation" has been shown to possibly accelerate the rate of healing of burns caused by Lewisite (41).

Eye

Mild conjunctivitis that starts more than 12 hours after exposure is unlikely to become more severe. The patient should undergo a thorough eye examination, be treated with a soothing eye solution, and be advised to return home with warnings to return if symptoms progress. Conjunctivitis beginning less than 12 hours after exposure or associated with lid edema or inflammation will need inpa-

tient care and observation.

More severe eye injuries should be treated in conjunction with an ophthalmologist. These patients may require a topical mydriatic, a topical antibiotic, and Vaseline applied to the lid edges. Topical steroids within the first 24 hours may reduce inflammation, but this is controversial. Pain may require systemic antibiotics. Dark glasses may help with photophobia (38).

Respiratory Support

Patients with mild, nonproductive cough, nasal irritation, or sore throat that began more than 12 hours after exposure may use vaporizers, lozenges, or cough drops to ease their symptoms. Any patient with more severe effects such as laryngitis, dyspnea, productive cough, pulmonary edema, or pseudomembrane formation should undergo prompt endotracheal intubation (38). Further care is supportive.

Cardiovascular

Since Lewisite causes systemic capillary leakage, hypovolemic shock may occur. These patients require closely monitored blood pressure, volume, and hepatic and renal function (38).

TRIAGE CONSIDERATIONS

In the setting of Lewisite exposure, the patient should be triaged as *immediate* if they demonstrate lower respiratory signs such as dyspnea or productive cough. *Delayed* patients are those with impaired vision, moderate-sized skin lesions, or cough with sputum production. *Minimal* patients include those with minor eye lesions with no vision impairment, small skin lesions, cough, or sore throat. Any patient with dyspnea or signs of airway necrosis, or skins lesions covering more than half of the body surface area are typically categorized as *expectant* (38), since survival is very unlikely in these patients.

PERSONAL PROTECTION

Lewisite is readily absorbed by inhalation and by ocular and dermal contact. Therefore, pressure-demand, self-contained breathing apparatus (SCBA) is recommended in situations that involve Lewisite exposure. Level A PPE and butyl rubber chemical protective gloves are recommended at all times (38).

SUMMARY

MUSTARDS

- Produce dermal, ocular, and respiratory effects

- Effects are typically delayed several hours

- Decontamination is only effective if done within 1-2 minutes

- Decontamination performed later is useful to protect personnel who contact the patient

- Systemic toxicity includes bone marrow suppression and low white cell counts.

- Burns are slow to heal

- Eye injuries should be treated aggressively to avoid permanent sequelae

- Respiratory effects may be severe and require prompt airway management

- No specific antidote exists

LEWISITE

- Limited combat experience

- Produce dermal, ocular, and respiratory effects

- Effects are immediate

- Decontamination is ideally performed within 1-2 minutes

- Burns are slow to heal

- Eye injuries should be treated aggressively to avoid permanent sequelae

- Respiratory effects may be severe and require prompt airway management

- BAL may be an effective antidote for systemic effects

RESOURCES

1. U.S. Soldier Biological and Chemical Command (SBC-COM), Edgewood Research Development and Engineering Center
Provides assistance if proper PPE is not available, if rescuers have not been trained in its use, or if information related to local emergency operations is not available. From 0700–1630 EST, call 410-671-4411 and ask for staff duty officer. From 1630–0700 EST, call 410-278-5201 and ask for staff duty officer.

2. Centers for Disease Control and Prevention
Analyzes and identifies agents suspected in biological and chemical terrorism and warfare.
Phone: 301-619-2833. Web address: http://www.cdc.gov or http://www.hopkins-biodefense.org

3. Virtual Naval Hospital
Offers textbook information on the chemical agents.
Web address: *http://www.vnh.org*

4. National Response Center
Sole point of federal government contact for reporting chemical releases.
Phone: 800-424-8802.
Web address: http://www.nrc.uscg.mil/index.htm

5. Mayo Clinic
Provides patient-related information on biological and chemical weapons.
Web address: http://www.mayoclinic.com

6. Poison Center
Provides information regarding chemical exposures and provides toxicological consultation for management of poison-related injuries. Phone: 1-800-222-1222.

QUESTIONS AND ANSWERS

1. **Which is NOT a characteristic of dermal sulfur mustard toxicity?**
   A. Erythema and blistering of the skin hours after exposure
   B. Predilection for warm moist areas such as the axillae or groin
   C. Blistering forms at the epidermal-dermal junction
   D. The skin lesions from sulfur mustard heal quickly with silver sulfadiazine application
   E. Mustard reacts with skin constituents within 2 minutes and is irreversible

2 **Sulfur mustard produces toxicity by which of the following mechanisms?**
   A. Alkylation of DNA
   B. Oxidative stress upon cell component
   C. Depletion of glutathione
   D. Increased inflammatory response
   E. All of the above

3. **What is most important in the treatment of casualties exposed to sulfur mustard?**
   A. Rapid administration of Vitamin C and thiosulfate
   B. Clothing removal and decontamination within 2 minutes
   C. Endotracheal intubation even if they have a minor cough
   D. Prompt ophthalmologic consultation to prevent permanent blindness
   E. Administration of intravenous antibiotics to prevent skin infection

4. **Concerning Lewisite, which of the following is FALSE?**
   A. BAL should be administered to patients with skin lesions, conjunctivitis, and minor cough
   B. Lewisite has been described as having the odor of geraniums
   C. Lewisite produces toxicity more rapidly than sulfur mustard
   D. Lewisite contains arsenic
   E. Lewisite may be absorbed systemically and cause shock

ANSWERS

1: D. *The skin lesions from sulfur mustard heal quickly with silver sulfadiazine application*
2: E. *All of the above*
3: B. *Clothing removal and decontamination within 2 minutes*
4: A. *BAL should be administered to patients with skin lesions, conjunctivitis, and minor cough*

REFERENCES

1. Wormser U. Toxicology of mustard gas. Trends Pharmacol Sci. 1991;12(4):164-67.
2. Borak J, Sidell FR. Agents of chemical warfare: sulfur mustard. Ann Emerg Med. 1992;21(3):303-08.
3. Watson AP, Griffin GD. Toxicity of vesicant agents scheduled for destruction by the Chemical Stockpile Disposal Program. Environ Health Perspect. 1992;98:259-80.
4. Devereaux A, Amundson DE, Parrish JS, Lazarus AA. Vesicants and nerve agents in chemical warfare: decontamination and treatment strategies for a changed world. Postgrad Med. 2002;112(4):90-96; quiz 4.
5. Chemical weapons: history and controls. Web site: www.stimson.org
6. Blanc PD. The legacy of war gas. Am J Med. 1999;106(6):689-90.
7. Somani SM, Babu SR. Toxicodynamics of sulfur mustard. Int J Clin Pharmacol Ther Toxicol. 1989;27(9):419-35.
8. Requena L, Requena C, Sanchez M, et al. Chemical warfare: cutaneous lesions from mustard gas. J Am Acad Dermatol. 1988;19(3):529-36.
9. Davis KG, Aspera G. Exposure to liquid sulfur mustard. Ann Emerg Med. 2001;37(6):653-56.
10. Smith KJ, Hurst CG, Moeller RB, et al. Sulfur mustard: its continuing threat as a chemical warfare agent, the cutaneous lesions induced, progress in understanding its mechanism of action, its long-term health effects, and new developments for protection and therapy. J Am Acad Dermatol. 1995;32(5 Pt 1):765-76.
11. Naghii MR. Sulfur mustard intoxication, oxidative stress, and antioxidants. Mil Med. 2002;167(7):573-75.
12. Mellor SG, Rice P, Cooper GJ. Vesicant burns. British Journal of Plastic Surgery. 1991;44:434-37.
13. Dacre JC, Goldman M. Toxicology and pharmacology of the chemical warfare agent sulfur mustard. Pharmacol Rev. 1996;48(2):289-326.
14. Rice P, Brown RF, Lam DG, et al. Dermabrasion—a novel concept in the surgical management of sulphur mustard injuries. Burns. 2000;26(1):34-40.
15. Newman-Taylor AJ, Morris AJ. Experience with mustard gas casualties. Lancet. 1991;337(8735):242.
16. Solberg Y, Alcalay M, Belkin M. Ocular injury by mustard gas. Surv Ophthalmol. 1997;41(6):461-66.
17. Safarinejad MR, Moosavi SA, Montazeri B. Ocular injuries caused by mustard gas: diagnosis, treatment, and medical defense. Mil Med. 2001;166(1):67-70.
18. Rees J, Harper P, Ellis F, Mitchell D. Mustard gas casualties. Lancet. 1991;337(8738):430.
19. Bagheri MH, Hosseini SK, Mostafavi SH, Alavi SA. High-resolution CT in chronic pulmonary changes after mustard gas exposure. Acta Radiol. 2003;44(3):241-45.
20. Emad A, Rezaian GR. Characteristics of bronchoalveolar lavage fluid in patients with sulfur mustard gas-induced asthma or chronic bronchitis. Am J Med. 1999;106(6):625-28.
21. Bijani K, Moghadamnia AA. Long-term effects of chemical weapons on respiratory tract in Iraq-Iran war victims living in Babol (North of Iran). Ecotoxicol Environ Saf. 2002;53(3):422-24.
22. Norman JE, Jr. Lung cancer mortality in World War I veterans with mustard-gas injury: 1919–1965. J Natl Cancer Inst. 1975;54(2):311-17.
23. Aasted A, Darre E, Wulf HC. Mustard gas: clinical, toxicological, and mutagenic aspects based on modern experience. Ann Plast Surg. 1987;19(4):330-33.
24. Arnold JL. Chemical warfare agents. In: Hooker, Edmond; 2001. Web site: www.emedicine.com/emerg/topic852.htm
25. Graef I, Karnofsky DA, Jager VB, et al. The clinical and pathological effects of nitrogen and sulfur mustards in laboratory animals. Am J Pathol. 1948;24:1-47.
26. Landing B, Eisenberg F. Statistical analysis of effects on sarcoma 180 and viscera of normal mice in relation to toxicity and structure. Cancer. 1949;2:1083-86.
27. Landing B, Goldin A, Noe H. Testicular lesions in mice following parenteral administration of nitrogen mustards. Cancer. 1949;2:1075-82.
28. Safarinejad MR. Testicular effect of mustard gas. Urology 2001;58(1):90-4.
29. Pechura CM. From the Institute of Medicine. JAMA. 1993;269(4):453.
30. Bullman T, Kang H. A fifty year mortality follow-up study of veterans exposed to low level chemical warfare agent, mustard gas. Ann Epidemiol. 2000;10(5):333-38.
31. Vojvodic V, Milosavljevic Z, Boskovic B, Bojanic N. The protective effect of different drugs in rats poisoned by sulfur and nitrogen mustards. Fundam Appl Toxicol. 1985;5(6 Pt 2):S160-68.
32. Medical management of chemical casualties handbook. 3rd ed. USAMRICO. Aberdeen Proving Ground, MD; 2000.
33. Vijayaraghavan R, Kumar P, Joshi U, et al. Prophylactic efficacy of amifostine and its analogues against sulfur mustard toxicity. Toxicol. 2001;163:83-91.
34. Eldad A, Weinberg A, Breiterman S, et al. Early nonsurgical removal of chemically injured tissue enhances wound healing in partial thickness burns. Burns. 1998;24:166-72.
35. Anderson DR, Byers SL, Vesely KR. Treatment of sulfur mustard (HD)-induced lung injury. J Appl Toxicol. 2000;20 Suppl 1:S129-32.
36. Koper O, Lucas E, Klabunde KJ. Development of reactive topical skin protectants against sulfur mustard and nerve agents. J Appl Toxicol. 1999;19 Suppl 1:S59-70.
37. Chilcott RP, Jenner J, Hotchkiss SA, Rice P. Evaluation of barrier creams against sulphur mustard. I. In vitro studies using human skin. Skin Pharmacol Appl Skin Physiol. 2002;15(4):225-35.
38. DeRosa CT, Holler JS, Allred M, et al. Managing hazardous materials incidents. In: Agency for Toxic Substances and Disease Registry; 2002. Web site: www.atsdr.cdc.gov
39. Chemical warfare agents. In: Federation of American Scientists; 1998. Web site: www.fas.org/nuke/intro/cw/agent.htm
40. Noort D, Benschop HP, Black RM. Biomonitoring of exposure to chemical warfare agents: a review. Toxicol Appl Pharmacol. 2002;184(2):116-26.
41. Lam DG, Rice P, Brown RF. The treatment of Lewisite burns with laser debridement—"lasablation". Burns. 2002;28:19-25.

3

Cyanide

Rebeca Gracia
Pharm. D.

THEORETICAL AND SCIENTIFIC BACKGROUND

HISTORY

Cyanide was used as a poison for centuries before the chemical was isolated and identified. Ancient records from Egypt make reference to poisoning from a natural food source of cyanide in reports detailing "the penalty of the peach" (1). The use of cyanide also dates back to the first century where, in Rome, the Emperor Nero supposedly used the cyanogenic plant cherry laurel to poison opponents. The Swedish scientist Scheele first chemically isolated cyanide in 1782, and it has been reported that he was the first person to become a victim of the purified chemical four years later in a laboratory accident (2). Historically, cyanide has been a relatively uncommon agent of warfare, although it is highly lethal. Napoleon III suggested its use as a weapon by coating bayonets in the 1870 Franco-Prussian war. The French military made an unsuccessful attempt at utilizing hydrocyanic acid early during World War I but, through continued experimentation, finally did create the more effective cyanogen chloride. The rate of development of chemical weapons increased greatly during the following years with subsequent design and use of additional cyanogens. Most notoriously, Zyklon B was the form of cyanide reportedly used in Nazi death camps during World War II. Zyklon B was hydrocyanic acid adsorbed onto a pharmaceutical base that was initially developed as a pesticide and rodenticide (3a). Although cyanide has not frequently been used for military purposes, several attempts have been made to utilize it as a poison and contaminant (Fig. 3-1). As a chemical weapon, it is not easy to disseminate upon a large number of people. However, cyanide is both widely available and easily accessible throughout the world, making it very attractive as a potential terrorist agent (4). It also possesses the ability to cause significant social disruption and public panic and demands special attention to public health preparedness (i.e., antidote stocking). Although cases of

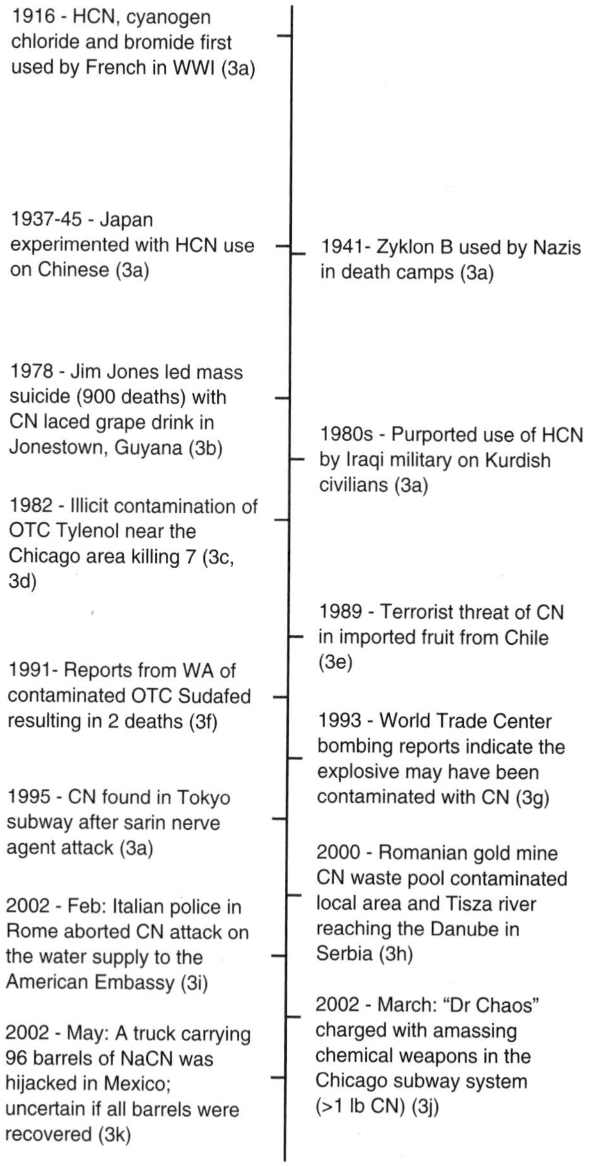

1916 - HCN, cyanogen chloride and bromide first used by French in WWI (3a)

1937-45 - Japan experimented with HCN use on Chinese (3a)

1941- Zyklon B used by Nazis in death camps (3a)

1978 - Jim Jones led mass suicide (900 deaths) with CN laced grape drink in Jonestown, Guyana (3b)

1980s - Purported use of HCN by Iraqi military on Kurdish civilians (3a)

1982 - Illicit contamination of OTC Tylenol near the Chicago area killing 7 (3c, 3d)

1989 - Terrorist threat of CN in imported fruit from Chile (3e)

1991- Reports from WA of contaminated OTC Sudafed resulting in 2 deaths (3f)

1993 - World Trade Center bombing reports indicate the explosive may have been contaminated with CN (3g)

1995 - CN found in Tokyo subway after sarin nerve agent attack (3a)

2000 - Romanian gold mine CN waste pool contaminated local area and Tisza river reaching the Danube in Serbia (3h)

2002 - Feb: Italian police in Rome aborted CN attack on the water supply to the American Embassy (3i)

2002 - March: "Dr Chaos" charged with amassing chemical weapons in the Chicago subway system (>1 lb CN) (3j)

2002 - May: A truck carrying 96 barrels of NaCN was hijacked in Mexico; uncertain if all barrels were recovered (3k)

Figure 3–1. Timeline illustrating the use of cyanide over the past 100 years (3a-3k).

cyanide toxicity from industrial sources and poisonings are currently the most commonly encountered exposures, the potential impact of an attack with cyanide warrants preparation. Health care providers should be equipped with the knowledge and resources necessary to manage a mass casualty incident involving this agent.

SOURCES

Cyanide is most likely to be used in the volatile, water-soluble, and liquid forms of hydrogen cyanide and cyanogen chloride (NATO designation AC and CK, respectively). Hydrogen cyanide (HCN) may also be referred to as hydrocyanic acid, blauseare (German for Berlin blue acid), and prussic acid (due to its origination from Prussian blue). The highly reactive salt forms are exploited for numerous industrial applications including chemical synthesis, electroplating, tanning, metallurgy (especially silver and gold), printing, agriculture, photography, and manufacture of paper and plastics, as well as fumigants and insecticides. Water-soluble salt forms such as calcium cyanide (CaCN), sodium cyanide (NaCN), and potassium cyanide (KCN) are most often utilized. These salts produce HCN gas when mixed with strong acid and thus pose a significant risk in industrial accidents as well as intentional exposures (5,6). The insoluble salt forms, mercury cyanide (HgCN), copper cyanide (CuCN), gold cyanide (AuCN), and silver cyanide (AgCN), also can be found in the industrial setting (7). Waste products from mining processes produce vast amounts of cyanide complexes including ferrocyanide. These chemicals are significantly less toxic than their salt counterparts; however, they do pose a considerable risk to the environment due to accumulation (8). The use of these cyanide waste products as terrorist agents may be appealing due to their abundance and relative ease of acquisition. In fact, ferrocyanide was implicated in the aborted attempt to poison a water supply in Rome in 2002.

A noteworthy form of cyanide is the chemical group referred to as nitriles (R-CN); acetonitrile and propionitrile are the most frequently encountered forms (9–15). Nitriles are easily accessible over the counter as acrylic nail and glue removers. These chemicals are also commonly encountered in industry as solvents. As parent compounds, nitriles are not significantly toxic, but slowly release cyanide into the body as they are metabolized. This occurs via cytochrome p450 (cyp 450) enzyme 2E1 where the resulting cyanohydrin metabolite then is converted into the actively toxic cyanide molecule (16–18). Exposure to these organic cyanides results in a delay in the onset of signs and symptoms as a latent period of several hours passes during transformation and liberation of the toxin. This delay has been implicated in several case reports of missed diagnosis and fatal outcomes and poses a significant risk to responding personnel who may not accurately perceive the risk in the situation.

Structural fires, as a source of cyanide, pose a looming threat in any disaster situation. HCN gas may be released in the combustion of many synthetic polymers, such as nylon and plastics, as well as natural materials including wool and silk. Any material that contains carbon and nitrogen may release cyanide during pyrolysis (19). Victims of fire inhalation especially from domestic fires are at an additional risk

for cyanide toxicity as well as carbon monoxide effects (20). Because cyanide has a considerably limited residential time in the blood, levels may be decreased significantly by the time the victim arrives to a health care facility. Both carbon monoxide and cyanide will cause hypoxic damage and the effects will be additive and possibly synergistic (21). Cyanide toxicity may be more contributory to death in some fire victims than the carbon monoxide itself (22). Early initiation of empiric treatment and management of probable cyanide exposure may be warranted in many cases of fire exposures (23–27).

Medically important sources of iatrogenic cyanide toxicity include nitroprusside (Nipride) and Laetrile. Each molecule of nitroprusside can release up to four or five CN groups, and patients may develop toxicity as cyanide accumulates. It is recommended to avoid prolonged administrations of high dose nitroprusside (28,29). Laetrile was used as a chemotherapeutic medication and is the purified form of the natural cyanide compound, amygdalin. When these products are ingested, the enzyme beta-glucosidase in the gastrointestinal tract metabolizes the amygdalin into hydrogen cyanide, resulting in toxicity. Many case reports have been published on the devastating use of Laetrile (30–33).

Additional sources of cyanide include tobacco smoke and food sources, although these rarely pose risk as acute toxicity (34). Smokers can average about 0.17 μg/ml of cyanide in their blood as compared to 0.06 μg/ml of cyanide in nonsmokers. Food sources of the cyanogenic glycoside, amygdalin, include apple seeds and fruit pits from the Prunus sp. Of these, the bitter almonds and apricot pits contain the highest concentrations. Food sources rarely cause toxicity as they must be consumed in large amounts or in purified forms to accumulate enough cyanide. Dietary staples such as cassava and lima beans have been implicated in chronic cyanide poisonings (37). Not only can long-term exposure to large amounts of these cyanide-containing food sources result in toxicity, but acute cyanide toxicity can occur from exposure to the wastewater from these food-processing factories (38,39).

CHEMICAL CHARACTERISTICS

Key features determining the effectiveness of a chemical as a warfare agent include not only the toxicity of the specific agent but also chemical characteristics such as volatility, persistence, and latency (40–42). Volatility is the tendency of a liquid to evaporate and form a vapor or gaseous form. Cyanide is one of the most volatile chemical warfare agents and as a liquid can readily transform into a more potent gas form. HCN is extremely volatile to such an extent as to limit its use as an effective weapon because it is, in fact, lighter than air. The HCN gas too readily dissipates and is difficult to deliver in high concentrations unless in an enclosed space. Cyanogen chloride was specifically formulated to be slightly heavier than air and provide a more persistent weapon. Persistence is inversely related to volatility; a balance is needed between these chemical characteristics in order to result in the most effective distribution. Agents with increased persistence are also more likely to remain on site available for contamination, penetrate the skin, and pose the greatest risk for rescue and medical personnel. Latency is the time delay between absorption of the agent and onset of symptoms. Cyanide can cause symptoms within seconds to minutes, or the presentation may be delayed up to hours depending on the form. Agents with prolonged latency times not only pose a risk to exposed victims who may go undiagnosed and untreated but also pose an increased risk to responding teams who may not be aware of the need for decontamination.

TOXIC DOSE

Cyanide is notorious for its high degree of lethality. This potency is a product of its rapid diffusion into tissues and irreversible binding to target sites. It is the rapidity of action rather than the minuteness of a lethal dose that makes cyanide effective as a chemical weapon. The toxic dose of cyanide is relatively high when compared to other agents used in chemical warfare. Because the most likely exposure to cyanide is via inhalation rather than the intravenous route, the lethal dose is expressed in a product of the concentration (C) of the agent in the air and exposure time (t). The amount determined to be lethal to 50% of a population is signified as the LCt_{50}. The LCt_{50} for HCN is 2,500 to 500 mg x min/m^3 and the LCt_{50} for CK is 1.1g x min/m^3 (43). Cyanide does not produce a constant effect of lethality; exposure to a high dose of cyanide gas even for a very short period of time will be fatal in comparison to smaller doses over a longer time. Inhalation of a concentration of cyanide at 300 mg/m^3 (270 ppm) will result in immediate death. In contrast, it would take several hours of exposure to a concentration of 20 mg/m^3 (18 ppm) before even mild symptoms would be seen (44). The form of cyanide significantly influences the toxic dose. The LD_{50} for IV CK is 1 mg/kg, and the estimated LD_{50} for dermal CK is 100 mg/kg. The lethal dose of an ingested cyanide salt is between 50 and 200 mg, depending on the specific salt form (43).

The severity and time to onset of clinical symptoms depend on the amount and mode of exposure as well as the type of cyanide. Intravenous and inhalational exposures to cyanide produce the most rapid onset of symptoms. Death can occur within seconds to minutes. Ingestion of cyanide salts may result in a delayed presentation of toxicity as the cyanide must first be absorbed. Presentation may be further delayed after dermal exposures to intact skin. Exposure to the gaseous form of cyanide results in immediate toxicity. Signs of poisoning from exposure to the salt forms of cyanide will be delayed to varying degrees depending on the specific salt. Exposure from the cyanide salts elicits a less dramatic progression of signs and symptoms. The soluble salts display a reduced onset to action time as compared to insoluble salts. One important exception to this would be the case of mercurial salts of cyanide. The mercury content in these chemicals is highly caustic and immediately elicits noxious injury to tissue. Significant cyanide poisoning may follow, but the clinical presentation is confounded by the concurrent mercury poisoning. The delay in clinical presentation of toxicity from cyanogens and cyanide compounds such as the nitriles will be even more pronounced. Cyanide can be transferred into breast milk and therefore can pose a significant risk to children through secondary transmission (45).

MECHANISM OF TOXICITY

Sulfane and cyanocobalamin reactions primarily within the liver metabolize the low levels of cyanide encountered normally. In the acute poisoning situation, endogenous pathways of cyanide metabolism are rapidly overwhelmed, and conjugate substrates are depleted allowing for accumulation and progression of toxic effects. Although cyanide inhibits many additional metabolic processes, the commonly cited mechanism of toxicity involves binding of cytochrome oxide within the mitochondria (46) (Fig. 3-2). The cyanide avidly binds to the ferric ion (Fe^{3+}) on the a3 complex. Subsequently, oxygen no longer is able to re-oxidize the reduced cytochrome a3, effectively bringing electron transport to a halt. This uncoupling of oxidative phosphorylation in essence terminates the synthesis pathway of adenosine triphosphate (ATP). The mitochondria exhibit impaired oxygen extraction and utilization despite adequate exposure to the oxygen supply (47). In response to this disruption of the primary metabolic aerobic pathway, the rate of glycolysis via anaerobic pathways increases.

The binding to the mitochondrial oxidase system can be delayed by a few minutes, but early signs of cyanide poisoning are seen within seconds. This observation leads to the theory of additional mechanisms of toxicity. Because cyanide exists predominantly in the un-ionized form within the body, it readily diffuses across membranes. Rapid effects seen after inhalation may be due to the near instantaneous diffusion across the blood brain barrier. Cyanide appears to alter neuronal transmission following absorption into the central nervous system (CNS) possibly through a glutamate pathway. It also appears to increase vascular resistance early in poisoning and to increase cerebral blood flow further potentiating penetration. These additional mechanisms represent just a few of the potential toxicities and open the door to experimentation with new therapies (8).

SIGNS AND SYMPTOMS

ACUTE CLINICAL MANIFESTATIONS

Exposure to high concentrations of cyanide can result in death within seconds to minutes leaving inadequate opportunity to recognize toxic symptoms and initiate management (34,48). Cyanide is often classified as a blood agent although it manifests primarily as CNS and cardiac toxicity. In cases of more prolonged onset of toxicity, signs and symptoms reflect a progressive intracellular hypoxia. Clinical hypoxia with cyanosis in the case of a worsening acidosis is a hallmark of cyanide poisoning. Initial symptoms are nonspecific and transient. The early symptoms of dizziness, headache, weakness, diaphoresis, dyspnea, and hypernea may be misinterpreted as anxiety. Without a reasonable index of suspicion, the diagnosis may be missed (49). The effects on respiration are thought to be mediated via direct stimulation of the carotid body and peripheral chemoreceptor bodies (8). This immediate stimulation of chemoreceptor

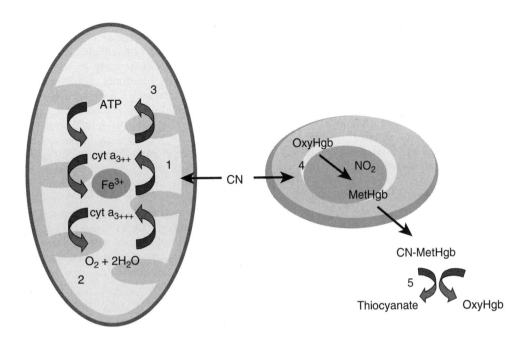

Figure 3–2. The binding of the cytochrome oxidase within the mitochondria resulting in abrupt cessation of cellular respiration (1). Cyanide binds to the iron in the cytochrome a3 complex (2). Oxidative phosphorylation is blocked and oxygen no longer is utilized (3). Electron transport chain is uncoupled resulting in loss of aerobic metabolism/generation of ATP (4). Nitrites form methemoglobin, which draws cyanide out of mitochrondria (5). Thiosulfate combines with cyanomethemoglobin and cyanide and is converted to the less toxic thiocyanate, which is excreted in the kidney.

bodies also mediates a transient rise in blood pressure. HCN and cyanogen chloride gas may cause mucous membrane irritation as well. Cyanide is purported to have an odor of bitter almonds, but only around 40% to 60% of the population have the gene necessary to detect this odor. The presence of a bitter almond odor is not a reliable sign of cyanide exposure (50,51). Although cyanide historically is associated with a cherry red flush, the dramatic color alteration is not always present. Visualization of equally red retinal arteries and veins can be used as an easy and rapid indicator of cyanide toxicity. The venous blood supply will have a similar oxygen concentration as the cells are no longer able to extract oxygen efficiently (52). As cellular hypoxia worsens, victims will experience loss of consciousness progressing to coma with fixed dilated pupils, hemodynamic compromise, arrhythmias, seizures, apnea, secondary cardiac arrest, and finally death. Those organs such as the heart and brain with high oxygen demands are the most sensitive to cyanide poisoning.

LABORATORY ABNORMALITIES

The most prominent laboratory finding in cyanide toxicity is a metabolic acidosis with dramatically elevated lactate levels. The shift from aerobic to anaerobic metabolism ultimately results in marked production of lactate as a profound high anion gap acidosis ensues. Several reports indicate that lactate levels may be utilized as markers of severity of cyanide toxicity (24,53). This correlation may be confounded by numerous processes in a critically ill patient, therefore its utility is limited. Later in the course, the meta-

bolic acidosis may be compounded by the addition of a respiratory acidosis from worsening apnea.

In the case of an unknown exposure, check venous blood gases as well as arterial blood gases to determine if there is a supranormal venous oxygen content or "arteriolization of venous blood," which would strongly indicate cyanide toxicity (54–56). The pulse oximetry will remain high as the blood has good oxygen content; consequently, the problem will lie in oxygen utilization and extraction. Note that once therapy has been initiated to induce methhemoglobinemia, the pulse oximetry will in fact depict a higher than actual oxygen concentration as both entities deflect light at similar wavelengths (57,58).

Although cyanide does target cardiac tissue, no prominent electrocardiogram (EKG) changes are noted. The patient may demonstrate a variety of conduction abnormalities including junctional rhythms, heart block, atrial fibrilliation, and premature beats. Case reports have described nonspecific ST-T segment elevation and depression, but this is not characteristic of cyanide poisoning. As the clinical picture worsens, the poisoned patient may eventually develop shock with profound hypotension, bradyarrhythmias, and possibly noncardiogenic pulmonary edema (49).

Cyanide tests are not readily available and often require a few days as turnaround time. Cyanide levels should be used only to verify toxicity; management of the victim should be based upon index of suspicion and clinical presentation. Levels may not necessarily correlate with clinical manifestations due to frequent, but unavoidable interferences. Red blood cells have the highest concentration of cyanide, and whole blood specimens should be collected for analysis.

Cyanide levels tend to decrease over time, and even the most carefully handled specimens may underestimate true peak concentrations (59). Note that moderately elevated cyanide levels probably indicate a severe toxicity due to the extreme extent the cyanide molecules adhere to the cytochrome oxidase (47). Reported toxic concentrations of cyanide range from levels as small as 0.5 µg/ml. A conversion factor of 0.026 should be used when interpreting traditional units and International System units (µg/mL = µmol/L x 0.026). Cyanide levels may be misleading and patient care should be based on clinical presentation.

CHRONIC EXPOSURE

Long-term effects from an acute cyanide exposure can contribute a significant morbidity. The effects seem to be related to and are synonymous with those effects seen from hypoxia as with carbon monoxide poisoning. Cyanide induces cellular hypoxia leading to oxidative stress and lipid membrane peroxidation (60,61). Long-term manifestation reports include anoxic encephalopathy, dystonia, and a parkinson-like syndrome (62–67). Some authors recommend to follow up with magnetic resonance imaging (MRI) to evaluate the extent of damage in those highly oxygen-dependent areas of the brain most sensitive to cyanide intoxication (68).

Several neurological diseases thought to be due to chronic cyanide toxicity include tobacco amblyopia, retrobulbar neuritis, Leber optic atrophy (a disorder of defective cyanide metabolism), and Nigerian nutritional ataxic neuropathy otherwise known as tropical ataxic neuropathy (TAN) and Konzo (34,47,69,70). Consumption of cyanogens from natural food sources rarely produces acute signs and symptoms, but long-term repeated exposure is associated with a clinically independent cluster of ailments. Cassava (Manihot sp.) contains a number of antinutritional agents that are cyanogenic glucosides, the most common ones being linamaris and lotaustralin. Populations with limited intake of food sources other than cassava often demonstrate TAN/Konzo (71). Controversy exists over the exact etiology of these chronic syndromes; additional purported causes include malnourishment and vitamin B_{12} deficiency (72,73). Clinical manifestations of this disorder involve mucous membrane lesions as well as neuropathy of not only peripheral nerves but also optic, auditory, and spinal nerve involvement. Reported associated symptoms from chronic industrial/occupational cyanide exposures also include thyroid enlargement, intellectual deterioration, confusion, and even parkinsonism (74). Chronic exposure from, for example, undetected contamination of an environmental source such as a well water supply could occur, and treatment recommendations for these situations have not been established.

DETECTION AND IDENTIFICATION

The only widely available method of identification of cyanide is measuring a level from the poisoned victim or surrounding environment. Industrial technologies, such as wastewater tests, vary in specificity and have a limited range of detected agents. There are significant time limitations to this process of collecting, handling, transporting, and analyzing as it is intended to be a background environment quality control type of check rather than an emergency measurement. In the early 1970s, a rapid chemical test was developed by Lee-Jones, but it was not widely used (75). Continued research has been done in an effort to develop a reliable rapid method of detection. There was a microdiffusion spectrophotometric method developed in Japan for analysis of suspected contaminated beverages. These new tests are not currently approved for use and are not easily accessible (76,77). The military does have several handheld devices for investigation of contaminated areas including the Chemical Agent Monitor (vapor), M8 Detection Paper (liquid), and the M256 Detection Kit (vapor and liquid). Hazmat investigations in the case of an area wide contamination will, of course, include sampling of air, soil, water, biological sources, other exposed materials, munitions, and other potential contaminated sources. Results will invariably be delayed.

MEDICAL MANAGEMENT

TRIAGE CONSIDERATIONS AND PERSONAL PROTECTION

Cyanide is extremely quick to act, and there is an alarmingly narrow time window of opportunity to initiate treatment before the victim is deemed nonsalvageable. The initial step in the management of an acute cyanide poisoning is to ensure termination of exposure and containment of contaminated environment. Prevention of secondary contamination is paramount throughout all processes. Use of full chemical protective clothing and a self-contained positive pressure breathing apparatus is recommended for activities within the contaminated area (43). Otherwise, standard personal protection equipment is warranted.

DECONTAMINATION

Patients should undergo decontamination appropriate to the type of exposure. Remove clothing and accessories for inhalational exposures. Proceed to dermal decontamination with water for liquid and solid exposures. A mild detergent or hypochlorite solution can be used if available. In the case where there may not have been adequate decontamination of the victim, it is recommended to utilize double gloves, replacing them often, and a mask (42,43,78). Several case reports describe secondary contamination due to off-gassing from victims. The cyanide may be exhaled from the effected individual's lungs or emanate from heavily soaked clothing, skin, or toxic vomitus (42). Any ocular exposure should be treated with a thorough flush with fluids. Tap water or saline are most commonly used, although the patient may find a flush with Lactated Ringers solution more tolerable. Decontamination of the victim must be performed rapidly. Cyanide is rapidly absorbed from the gastrointestinal (GI) tract, and GI decontamination measures may prove futile.

However, some forms of cyanide such as the organic nitriles may demonstrate prolonged absorption kinetics. If the patient presented within one hour of an ingestion, it would be reasonable to consider performing an orogastric lavage in an attempt to recover any amount of the cyanide. One gram of activated charcoal only binds to 35 mg of cyanide, but because only 50 to 200 mg of cyanide is considered lethal, administration of charcoal may be adequate as a decontamination measure (79). Due to the risk of rapid demise, inducing emesis is contraindicated. Any toxic vomitus or gastric washings should be isolated as well.

SUPPORTIVE CARE

Initial stabilization of the victim involves the standard airway, breathing, and circulation assessment triad. Intubate the patient to protect airway when needed and immediately obtain intravenous access and institute cardiac monitoring. These steps are common to any emergency situation, but many cases report successful treatment of cyanide poisoning with supportive therapy alone (47,80,81).

Supplemental oxygen is a crucial part of supportive care in cyanide poisoning. Ventilation with 100% oxygen would of course increase tissue oxygen delivery. It may seem superfluous to employ enhanced oxygen as a therapy seeing as the mechanism of toxicity of oxygen utilization rather than availability (82). Even in a case of normal measured pO_2, oxygen should be utilized because it may enhance antidote efficacy (83,84). Theoretically, increased oxygen could afford synergistic effect with antidotes. Oxygen may serve to increase respiratory excretion of cyanide, restore the cytochrome oxidase activity by displacing cyanide, stimulate activation of other oxidative systems (such as those enzymes not yet poisoned by cyanide), and perhaps facilitate the rhodenase enzyme indirectly (85).

The use of hyperbaric oxygen for cyanide toxicity remains controversial. The published literature on the topic offers little corroboration as some investigations find positive effects and other studies fail to demonstrate correlations with improved clinical status (86–89). The use of hyperbaric oxygen may be especially warranted in the case of exposure to nitriles due to the delayed and prolonged production of cyanide (88). Most literature reports a 3 to 4 hour latent period before the onset of symptoms, although times as much as 12 hours have been reported. These patients should be monitored for at least 24 to 48 hours after exposure to ensure that ample time has expired to allow for all cyanide to be released. The Undersea and Hyperbaric Medicine Society recommends treating carbon monoxide-induced hypoxia complicated with cyanide poisoning with hyperbaric oxygen (90).

Additional supportive therapies addressing acidosis, hemodynamic compromise, and seizures should be employed as needed throughout the clinical course. Seizures resulting from cyanide poisoning may be refractory and require aggressive management. Any chemical burn requires aggressive wound treatment and additional guard against opportunistic infection. Cyanide casualties should not be excluded as organ donors because not all organs are affected, and cyanide levels may fall to undetectable. Hemodialysis has been advocated in some cases of cyanide toxicity and would be beneficial especially in the face of worsening acidosis and failing renal function where the concentrations of therapeutic agents could accumulate to induce their own additional toxicity (91).

ANTIDOTE

Although supportive care is considered foremost in the management of cyanide toxicity, the antidote should be considered as part of the "A" in the "ABCs." Delay in administration should be avoided. The cyanide antidote kit should be used in the advent of a suspected or unknown exposure resulting in rapid onset of respiratory and neurological symptoms (47). The differential diagnosis for acute cyanide poisoning is relatively small, and administration of the antidote should be administered empirically (Table 3-1). This antidote was among the emergency antidotes recommended for stocking (92). The current cyanide antidote kit is now supplied from Acorn Inc. It contains three constituents: amyl nitrite, sodium nitrite, and sodium thiosulfate. Although other countries have access to alternative antidotes, this combination is the only antidote available in the United States, and it has proven to be adequately beneficial (93, 94).

Nitrites are utilized to induce methemoglobinemia. The cyanide will preferentially bind to the iron of the methemoglobin rather than in the mitochondria. It is thought that an increased amount of cyanide will then transfer to the extracellular space and be displaced from the cytochrome. The mitochondria can then reactivate electron transport (93). It has been proposed that the formation of methemoglobin may not be the sole mechanism of action of nitrites (95). Several studies have demonstrated that many agents with vasoactive properties, presumably via nitrous oxide, also afford protection against cyanide toxicity (96). They may, in fact, alleviate toxicity through a vasodilatory mechanism. Cyanide may be bound and inactivated by nitrous oxide. Several other vasodilatory agents, including promethazine and chlorpromazine, have been proven to have beneficial effects a well (97). The nitrites are by no means the ideal antidote; they do cause significant adverse side effects, namely vasodilatation and hypotension. These side effects are quite problematic and can be compounded by other cardioactive agents such as calcium channel blockers and ethanol or preexisting cardiovascular disease. Although methemoglobinemia is the desired endpoint to therapy, it may exacerbate the condition of certain patients including those with poor cardiopulmonary reserve and those with concomitant carbon monoxide poisoning. It is recommended to avoid nitrites in smoke inhalation victims due to the risk of worsening the oxygen-carrying-capacity deficit (98). The antidote for methemoglobinemia is methylene blue and will counteract excess methemoglobinemia formation, but it may subsequently release the cyanide.

The amyl nitrite is supplied in ampules for rapid access to a liquid that can be wafted and inhaled. They may be referred to as "pearls" or "poppers." These are intended to be a temporizing measure before IV access is gained. Administer by crushing 1 ampule (pearl) in gauze and placing it under the nose for inhalation for 30 seconds every minute. Replace with a new pearl every 3 minutes as the effect lasts for about 2 to 3 minutes. This initial step is designed to achieve a methemoglobin

TABLE 3-1	Differential Diagnoses for Treating Acute Cyanide Poisoning and Other Poisonous Gases
AGENT	**DIFFERENTIAL DIAGNOSIS**
Hydrogen sulfide	Mechanism of toxicity very similar to that of cyanide
	Presents with often indistinguishable signs and symptoms
	Treat with supportive care, oxygen, and nitrites (no thiosulfate)
Carbon monoxide	Frequent concurrent toxicity especially in fire victims
Azide compounds	Metabolized to cyanide and produce toxicity in a delayed fashion
Methanol	Produces similar degree of profound acidosis
Methemoglobinemia	Affects oxygen utilization in a similar fashion
Isoniazid, theophylline, hemlock, and htrychnine	Induce refractory seizures (strychnine does not cause true seizures but antagonizes glycine in the spinal cord)
Additional nontoxin etiologies and/or complications	Ischemic stroke and encephalitis
	Pediatric patients may not present with an apparent toxidrome
	Consider meningitis, encephalitis, and gastroenteritis

level of about 5%, but it is rather unpredictable. Amyl nitrite is a pregnancy category X medication and should be omitted in the case of pregnancy.

Sodium nitrite is dosed as 10 ml of a 3% solution (300 mg) IV over at least 5 minutes. Some reports indicate that this dose can be given over a shorter period of time as long as is tolerated. However, the administration rate may need to be slowed to avoid severe hypotension. The goal of therapy with sodium nitrite is to maintain the methemoglobin around 20% to 30%. An additional half dose may be given if needed. The pediatric dose is 0.12 to 0.33 ml/kg (max 10 cc) of the 10% solution given over at least 3 minutes. This dose may also be repeated if needed. It is also difficult to predict methemoglobin level with this agent and significant risk of compromised oxygen-carrying capacity develops when methemoglobin levels reach 40%. Adverse drug reactions may be as minor as headache and dizziness but can progress to significant vasodilation and orthostatic hypotention, especially with higher does and rapid infusions. There is specific dosing adjustment in severe anemia as the risk of methemoglobinemia increases with decreasing baseline oxyhemoglobin concentrations. Sodium nitrite is in Pregnancy Class C and should only be used when the benefit of treatment outweighs the risk of complications due to adverse drug events.

The third component of the cyanide antidote kit is sodium thiosulfate. This agent enhances clearance of cyanide by acting as a sulfur donor. Thiosulfate reversibly combines with cyanide in the extracellular space to form the minimally toxic and renally excreted thiocyanate. It may also augment mitochronrial sulfurtransferase reactions. The enzyme rhodanase is the catalyst for the direct conversion of cyanide to thiocyanate. The reactions between 3-meraptopyruvate sulfurtransferase, thiosulfate reductase (in the liver), and cystathionase indirectly convert cyanide to thiocyanate. The body can detoxify about 0.017 mg of cyanide/kg/min (3). These enzymatic routes are highly effective, but they are insufficient for

large amounts of cyanide encountered in poisonings due to depletion of sulfur donors. The effectiveness of sodium thiosulfate as an antidote is limited by its delay to onset of action, short half life, and small volume of distribution. In contrast to its counterparts, the nitrites, sodium thiosulfate has very few side effects. The only significant adverse reaction is the rare hypersensitivity reaction and infusion rate dependent hypotension. It is to be administered intravenously as 50 ml of a 25% solution (12.5 g) over 10 minutes. If there is no response in 30 minutes, a half dose may be repeated. The pediatric dose is 1.65 ml/kg of the 25% solution given over 10 minutes. Individuals with glucose-6-phosphate dehydrogenase (G6PD) deficiency should not receive sodium thiosulfate treatment due to the risk of hemolysis. Sodium thiofulate is listed as a Pregnancy Class C, but the benefit of treatment usually outweighs the risk of drug utilization. Chronic exposure to thiocyanates does cause toxicity because thiocyanates and cyanide exist in equilibrium. The effects seen from acute treatment of cyanide exposure are virtually nonexistent, but they should be kept in mind. Note that thiosulfate toxicity may be pronounced in renal insufficiency, but it is dialyzable (99).

ADDITIONAL CYANIDE ANTAGONISTS

The ideal antidote is one that is quick to act and highly effective with no side effects. Hydroxycobalamin is probably the best antidote used so far (100). Although it is not yet available as a cyanide antidote in the United States, it has been used as an antidote in other countries, predominantly France, for over 40 years with reportedly great success. Hydroxycobalamin is vitamin B_{12a} and acts as a chelating agent to bind cyanide in equimolar amounts directly forming cyanocobalamin, vitamin B_{12} (101,102). This antidote has proven to be highly effective due to its increased affinity for cyanide as compared to the cytochrome oxidase moiety. Adverse reactions to this therapy are rare and not severe and include allergic reactions (102). The treatment dose is relatively high due to the large molar amounts needed to be effective. It is dosed as 4 to 5 g IV in acute exposures but is virtually nontoxic even at high doses (103). Its utility is only limited by the large dose required and a relatively short half life due to light instability (104). Tachyphylaxis has been reported. This agent is Pregnancy Class A, and the only precaution is a transient (4 to 5 days) reddish discoloration of mucous membranes and urine (105,106). It is currently only available in the United States with an investigational license. There may be a synergistic protection if the hydroxycobalamin therapy is augmented by sodium thiosulfate. Cyanocobalamin (vitamin B_{12}) is readily available but does not afford the same degree of protection in cyanide toxicity. It lacks a key hydroxyl group and is relatively ineffective at trapping cyanide molecules. Treatment with hydroxycobalamin should not be substituted with cyanocobalamin (107).

A different methemoglobin inducer, 4-dimethylaminophenol (DMAP), is used as an intramuscular (IM) injection for rapid treatment of cyanide toxicity by German military and civilians. It is reported to be highly effective but limited by problematic adverse drug reactions such as necrosis at the injection site and the increased potential of causing excessive methemoglobinemia (108). Other investigated methemoglobin inducers include compounds similar to DMAP, p-aminopropiophenone (PAPP), p-aminoheptanoylphenone (PAHP), p-aminooctanoylphenone (PAOP), and hydroxylamine (109). A novel methemoglobin-inducing agent, stromafree methemoglobin, has been investigated in a few animal studies and would, in essence, bind cyanide without compromising oxygen-carrying capacity (110).

Various cobalt salts have been considered as cyanide antagonists, but their therapeutic benefit is limited by their pronounced toxicity profile. Dicobalt edentate, a cobalt salt of ethylrnrdiaminetetraacetic acid (EDTA) is available commercially in Europe as Kelocyanor. The chelation of cyanide is thought to form cobalticyanide ($CoCN_6$), a relatively stable chemical with a low toxic profile. Comparison studies thus far have provided conflicting reports on efficacy. The innate toxicity of the cobalt salts even after resolution of cyanide toxicity limits their use and further experimentation as potential cyanide antidotes. Cobalt salts cause a myriad of adverse reactions including hypotension, gastrointestional distress, and chest pain. Severe effects of ventricular arrhythmias and respiratory failure leading to death have been reported following their use (111).

Many agents are being explored as prophylactic cyanide antagonists. Amyl nitrite and sodium nitrite possess much too potent of side effects to be utilized safely as prophylactic agents (99). Sodium thiosulfate, although quite safe, acts too slowly to be of prophylactic benefit. The aminophenol derivatives that induce methemoglobinemia, PAPP, its metabolite, PAHP, and PAOP have been shown to reduce cyanide within the red blood cells and their antagonism may be enhanced by the addition of sodium thiosulfate (112). Other agents that induce methemoglobinemia including the 8-aminoquinoline analog of primaquine have been studied. Further studies of these agents as antidotes have been complicated by the fact that cyanide toxicity changes the pharmacokinetics of the agent. Cyanohydrin-forming drugs including alpha-ketoglutarate, pyruvate, glyoxal, and other carbonyl related agents

may improve the protection provided by the nitrites. The glyoxal trimer seems to elicit the greatest activity when comparing the group, but these agents are plagued by similar limitations such as short half lives and large required doses. Alpha-ketoglutarate may have a promising future as a prophylactic and/or adjunctive therapy in cyanide toxicity. It is an endogenous scavenger of amino groups throughout the body. Several animal studies have demonstrated a significant protective effect especially when used in conjunction with the current antidote regimen (113, 114). It has also been investigated with other potential antidotes, including the sulfur donor N-acetylcysteine (NAC) (115). The most significant effect was seen when it was administered prior to cyanide insult, and it may even provide significant protection up to 60 minutes before an exposure. Alpha-ketoglutarate boasts of a limited side-effect profile, specifically a lack of vasoactive properties. Development of a form approved for human use would render benefit in cases of cyanide toxicity where nitrites are contraindicated, such as fire victims, and for emergency personnel anticipating exposure. This may also serve as an antidote in the chronic occupational/environmental exposures. Dihydroxyacetone (DHA) administered both IV and orally (PO) has demonstrated benefit in animal studies. DHA readily, but reversibly, binds cyanide and may enhance ATP formation through glycosis because DHA-p is a component of the glycolysis pathway. Preliminary reports indicate that the onset of benefit after oral dose is about 10 to 15 minutes and it lasts only 30 minutes. This estimates DHA quicker to onset of action than sodium thiosulfate but shorter in duration (116). Anticipated synergistic effects are being investigated.

Because cyanide inhibits numerous enzyme systems, there are many other potential mechanisms of detoxification yet to be exploited. Exogenous administration of enzymes or subtrates normally involved in cyanide metabolism and detoxification may prove beneficial (117). A few investigations report novel treatments like utilizing carrier erythrocytes containing rhodanase and thiosulfate to reverse cyanide toxicity (118,119). Future research aims to find a faster acting, more effective, and better tolerated treatment for cyanide toxicity.

CONCLUSION

Cyanide poses a threat to society due to its propensity to be used as a chemical weapon and widespread usage in industry. Concerns about acute exposures from a mass casualty incident may seem foremost in the minds of health care providers. However, very real risks exist from chronic exposures in the occupational setting and also from environmental contamination. Health care facilities are urged to acquire supplies of antidote kits in preparation for a large-scale exposure. As detailed in the April 21, 2000, issue of the *Morbidity and Mortality Weekly Report*: "The public health infrastructure must be prepared to prevent illness and injury that would result from biological and chemical terrorism. Recent threats and use of biological and chemical agents against civilians have exposed U.S. vulnerability and highlighted the need to enhance our capacity to detect and control terrorist acts. The U.S. must be protected from an extensive range of critical biological and chemical agents, including some that have been developed and stockpiled for military use. Even without threat of war, investment in national defense ensures preparedness and acts as a deterrent against hostile acts." (40)

SUMMARY

- Cyanide, widely available, is notorious for its lethality and use as a chemical weapon, and can potentially cause significant social and public health disruption.

- Cyanide can be found in a multitude of forms, but it is most effective as a chemical weapon in a gaseous state that can be inhaled.

- The hallmark sign of cyanide toxicity is evidence of cellular hypoxia and acidosis. Cyanosis may develop later in the course, but it is not typically an initial finding.

- Treatment is based on index of suspicion and presenting signs and symptoms and consists of supportive care and the antidote kit (nitrites, thiosulfate).

QUESTIONS AND ANSWERS

1. **Cyanide toxicity causes which of the following presenting signs and symptoms?**
   - A. Anxiety
   - B. Seizures
   - C. Arteriolization of venous blood supply
   - D. Bitter almond-like odor
   - E. All of the above

2. **What laboratory abnormality is a hallmark sign of cyanide poisoning?**
   - A. Lactic acidosis
   - B. Cyanosis
   - C. Prominent EKG changes
   - D. Elevated cyanide level
   - E. All of the above

3. **How does cyanide cause toxicity?**
   - A. Binding to cytochrome oxidase
   - B. Uncoupling oxidative phosphorylation
   - C. Altering neuronal transmission possibly through a glutamate pathway
   - D. Increasing vascular resistance cerebral blood flow potentiating absorption
   - E. All of the above

4. **Which medications are not currently included in the cyanide antidote kit?**
   - A. Amyl nitrite
   - B. Sodium thiosulfate
   - C. Sodium nitrate
   - D. Sodium nitrite
   - E. All of the medications are included

ANSWERS

1: *E. All of the above*
2: *A. Lactic acidosis*
3: *E. All of the above*
4: *C. Sodium nitrate*

REFERENCES

1. Gettler AO, St. George AV. Cyanide poisoning. Am J Clin Pathol. 1934;4(5):429-37.
2. Kunkel D. The toxic emergency—cyanide: looking for the source. Emerg Med. 1987;115-25.
3a. Baskin SI. Cyanide poisoning: medical aspects of chemical and biological warfare. In: Textbook of military medicine. Washington DC: Office of the Surgeon General; 1997.
3b. Thompson RL, Manders WW, Cowan RW. Postmortem findings of the victims of the Jonestown tragedy. J Forensic Sci. 1987;32(2):433-43.
3c. Wolnick KA, Fricke FL, et al. The Tylenol tampering incident—tracing the source. Anal Chem. 1984;56(3):466A–70A, 474A.
3d. Dunea, G. Death over the counter. Br Med J (Clin Res Ed). 1983;286(6360):211-12.
3e. Grigg B, Modeland V. The cyanide scare: a tale of two grapes. FDA Consumer. Jul-Aug 1989:7-11.
3f. Howard J, Pouw TH, et al. Cyanide poisonings associated with over-the-counter medication—Washington State, 1991. MMWR Morb Mortal Wkly Rep. 1991;40(10):161, 167-68.
3g. Parachini JV. The World Trade Center bombers (1993). In: Tucker JB ed. Toxic terror: assessing terrorist use of chemical and biological weapons. Cambridge: MIT Press; 2000.
3h. Kovac C. Cyanide spill threatens health in Hungary. BMJ. 2000;320(7234):536.
3i. BBC News - BBC web page (http://news.bbc.co.uk/1/hi/world/europe/1831511.stm).
3j. CNN web page (http://www.cnn.com/2002/US/03/12/chicago.cyanide/).
3k. CNN web page (http://www.cnn.com/2002/WORLD/americas/05/16/mexico.cyanide/).
4. Burklow TR, Yu CE, Madsen JM. Industrial chemicals: terrorist weapons of opportunity. Pediatr Ann. 2003;32(4):230-34.
5. Kovac C. Cyanide spill threatens health in Hungary. BMJ. 2000;320(7234):536.
6. Kovac C. Cyanide spill could have long term impact. BMJ. 2000;320(7245):1294.
7. Blanc, P., et al. Cyanide intoxication among silver-reclaiming workers. JAMA. 1985;253(3):367-71.
8. Way JL. Cyanide intoxication and its mechanism of antagonism. Annu Rev Pharmacol *Toxicol*. 1984;24:451-81.
9. Willhite CC. Inhalation toxicology of acute exposure to aliphatic nitriles. Clin Toxicol. 1981;18(8):991-1003.
10. Vogel RA, Kirkendall WM. Acrylonitrile (vinyl cyanide) poisoning: a case report. Tex Med. 1984;80(5):48-51.
11. Caravati EM, Litovitz TL. Pediatric cyanide intoxication and death from an acetonitrile-containing cosmetic. JAMA. 1988;260(23):3470-73.
12. Kurt TL, et al. Cyanide poisoning from glue-on nail remover. Am J Emerg Med. 1991;9(3):271-72.

13. Geller RJ, Ekins BR, Iknoian RC. Cyanide toxicity from acetonitrile-containing false nail remover. Am J Emerg Med. 1991;9(3):268-70.

14. Losek JD, Rock AL, Boldt RR. Cyanide poisoning from a cosmetic nail remover. Pediatrics. 1991;88(2):337-40.

15. Bismuth C, et al. Cyanide poisoning from propionitrile exposure. J Emerg Med. 1987;5(3):191-95.

16. Wang H, Chanas B, Ghanayem BI. Cytochrome P450 2E1 (CYP2E1) is essential for acrylonitrile metabolism to cyanide: comparative studies using CYP2E1-null and wild-type mice. Drug Metab Dispos. 2002;30(8):911-17.

17. Freeman JJ, Hayes EP. Microsomal metabolism of acetonitrile to cyanide: effects of acetone and other compounds. Biochem Pharmacol. 1988;37(6):1153-59.

18. Feierman DE, Cederbaum AI. Role of cytochrome P-450 IIE1 and catalase in the oxidation of acetonitrile to cyanide. Chem Res Toxicol. 1989;2(6):359-66.

19. Symington IS, et al. Cyanide exposure in fires. Lancet. 1978;2(8080):91-92.

20. Silverman SH, et al. Cyanide toxicity in burned patients. J Trauma. 1988;28(2):171-76.

21. Pitt BR, et al. Interaction of carbon monoxide and cyanide on cerebral circulation and metabolism. Arch Environ Health. 1979;34(5):345-49.

22. Lundquist P, Rammer L, Sorbo B. The role of hydrogen cyanide and carbon monoxide in fire casualties: a prospective study. Forensic Sci Int. 1989;43(1):9-14.

23. Hall AH, Rumack BH, Karkal SS. Increasing survival in acute cyanide poisoning. Emerg Med Rep. 1988;9(17):129-36.

24. Baud FJ, et al. Elevated blood cyanide concentrations in victims of smoke inhalation. N Engl J Med. 1991;325(25):1761-66.

25. Koschel MJ. Where there's smoke, there may be cyanide. Am J Nurs. 2002;102(8):39-42.

26. Clark CJ, Campbell D, Reid WH. Blood carboxyhaemoglobin and cyanide levels in fire survivors. Lancet. 1981;1(8234):1332-35.

27. Becker CE. The role of cyanide in fires. Vet Hum Toxicol. 1985;27(6):487-90.

28. Curry SC, Arnold-Capell P. Toxic effects of drugs used in the ICU: nitroprusside, nitroglycerin, and angiotensin-converting enzyme inhibitors. Crit Care Clin. 1991;7(3):555-81.

29. Rindone JP, Sloane EP. Cyanide toxicity from sodium nitroprusside: risks and management. Ann Pharmacother. 1992;26(4):515-19.

30. Rauws AG, Olling M, Timmerman A. The pharmacokinetics of amygdalin. Arch Toxicol. 1982;49(3-4):311-19.

31. Beamer WC, Shealy RM, Prough DS. Acute cyanide poisoning from laetrile ingestion. Ann Emerg Med. 1983;12(7):449-51.

32. Braico, KT, et al. Laetrile intoxication. Report of a fatal case. N Engl J Med. 1979;300(5):238-40.

33. Shragg TA, Albertson TE, Fisher CJ Jr. Cyanide poisoning after bitter almond ingestion. West J Med. 1982;136(1):65-69.

34. Baumeister RG, Schievelbein H, Zickgraf-Rudel G. Toxicological and clinical aspects of cyanide metabolism. Arzneimittelforschung. 1975;25(7):1056-64.

35. Rubino MJ, Davidoff F. Cyanide poisoning from apricot seeds. JAMA. 1979;241(4):359.

36. Morse DL, Harrington JM, Heath CW Jr. Laetrile, apricot pits, and cyanide poisoning. N Engl J Med. 1976;295(22):1264.

37. Akintonwa A, Tunwashe OL. Fatal cyanide poisoning from cassava-based meal. Hum Exp Toxicol. 1992;11(1):47-49.

38. Okafor PN, Okorowkwo CO, Maduagwu EN. Occupational and dietary exposures of humans to cyanide poisoning from large-scale cassava processing and ingestion of cassava foods. Food Chem Toxicol. 2002;40(7):1001-05.

39. Oliveira MA, Reis EM, Nozaki J. Biological treatment of wastewater from the cassava meal industry. Environ Res. 2001;85(2):177-83.

40. Biological and chemical terrorism: strategic plan for preparedness and response. Recommendations of the CDC Strategic Planning Workgroup. MMWR Recomm Rep. 2000;49(RR-4):1-14.

41. Brennan RJ, et al. Chemical warfare agents: emergency medical and emergency public health issues. Ann Emerg Med. 1999;34(2):191-204.

42. Shenoi R. Disaster medicine: chemical warfare agents. Clin Ped Emerg Med. 2002;3(4):239-47.

43. Bogucki S, Weir S. Pulmonary manifestations of intentionally released chemical and biological agents. Clin Chest Med. 2002;23(4):777-94.

44. Hall AH, Rumack BH. Clinical toxicology of cyanide. Ann Emerg Med. 1986;15(9):1067-74.

45. Soto-Blanco B, Gorniak SL. Milk transfer of cyanide and thiocyanate: cyanide exposure by lactation in goats. Vet Res. 2003;34:213-20.

46. Way JL, et al. The mechanism of cyanide intoxication and its antagonism. Ciba Found Symp. 1988;140:232-43.

47. Vogel SN, Sultan TR, Ten Eyck RP. Cyanide poisoning. Clin Toxicol. 1981;18(3):367-83.

48. Stewart R. Cyanide poisoning. Clin Toxicol. 1974;7(5):561-64.

49. Mokhlesi B, et al. Adult toxicology in critical care: Part II: specific poisonings. Chest. 2003;123(3):897-922.

50. Dhamee MS. Letter: acute cyanide poisoning. Anaesthesia. 1983;38(2):168.

51. Gonzalez ER. Cyanide evades some noses, overpowers others. JAMA. 1982;248(18):2211.

52. Peters CG, Mundy JV, Rayner PR. Acute cyanide poisoning. The treatment of a suicide attempt. Anaesthesia. 1982;37(5):582-86.

53. Baud, FJ, et al. Value of lactic acidosis in the assessment of the severity of acute cyanide poisoning. Crit Care Med. 2002;30(9):2044-50.

54. Johnson RP, Mellors HW. Arteriolization of venous blood gases: a clue to the diagnosis of cyanide poisoning. J Emerg Med. 1988;6(5):401-04.

55. Yeh MM, Becker CE, Arieff AI. Is measurement of venous oxygen saturation useful in the diagnosis of cyanide poisoning? Am J Med. 1992;93(5):582-83.

56. Vegfors M, Lennmarken C. Carboxyhaemoglobinaemia and pulse oximetry. Br J Anaesth. 1991;66(5):625-26.

57. Barker SJ, Tremper KK. The effect of carbon monoxide inhalation on pulse oximetry and transcutaneous PO2. Anesthesiology. 1987;66(5):677-79.

58. Gonzalez A, Gomez-Arnau J, Pensado A. Carboxyhemoglobin and pulse oximetry. Anesthesiology. 1990;73(3):573.

59. Ballantyne B, Bright J, Williams P. An experimental assessment of decreases in measurable cyanide levels in biological fluids. J Forensic Sci Soc. 1973;13(2):111-17.

60. Johnson JD, et al. Peroxidation of brain lipids following cyanide intoxication in mice. Toxicology. 1987;46(1):21-28.

61. Ardelt BK, et al. Cyanide-induced lipid peroxidation in different organs: subcellular distribution and hydroperoxide generation in neuronal cells. Toxicology. 1994;89(2):127-37.

62. Uitti RJ, et al. Cyanide-induced parkinsonism: a clinicopathologic report. Neurology. 1985;35(6):921-25.

63. Rachinger J, et al. MR changes after acute cyanide intoxication. AJNR Am J Neuroradiol. 2002;23(8):1398-1401.

64. Carella F, et al. Dystonic-Parkinsonian syndrome after cyanide poisoning: clinical and MRI findings. J Neurol Neurosurg Psychiatr. 1988;51(10):1345-48.

65. Grandas F, Artieda J, Obeso JA. Clinical and CT scan findings in a case of cyanide intoxication. Mov Disord. 1989;4(2):188-93.

66. Rosenow F, et al. Neurological sequelae of cyanide intoxication—the patterns of clinical, magnetic resonance imaging, and positron emission tomography findings. Ann Neurol. 1995;38(5):825-28.

67. Messing B, Storch B. Computer tomography and magnetic resonance imaging in cyanide poisoning. Eur Arch Psychiatr Neurol Sci. 1988;237(3):139-43.

68. Rosenberg NL, Myers JA, Martin WR. Cyanide-induced parkinsonism: clinical, MRI, and 6-fluorodopa PET studies. Neurology. 1989;39(1):142-44.

69. Freeman AG. Optic neuropathy and chronic cyanide intoxication: a review. J R Soc Med. 1988;81(2):103-06.

70. Bismuth C, Baud FJ, Pontal PG. Hydroxocobalamin in chronic cyanide poisoning. J Toxicol Clin Exp. 1988;8(1):35-38.

71. Tylleskar T, et al. Konzo in the Central African Republic. Neurology. 1994;44(5):959-61.

72. Oluwole OS, et al. Low prevalence of ataxic polyneuropathy in a community with high exposure to cyanide from cassava foods. J Neurol. 2002;249(8):1034-40.

73. Soto-Blanco B, Marioka PC, Gorniak SL. Effects of long-term low-dose cyanide administration to rats. Ecotoxicol Environ Saf. 2002;53(1):37-41.

74. El Ghawabi SH, et al. Chronic cyanide exposure: a clinical, radioisotope, and laboratory study. Br J Ind Med. 1975;32(3):215-19.

75. Lee-Jones M, Bennett MA, Sherwell JM. Cyanide self-poisoning. Br Med J. 1970;4(738):780-81.

76. Tsuge K, Kataoka M, Seto Y. Rapid determination of cyanide and azide in beverages by microdiffusion spectrophotometric method. J Anal Toxicol. 2001;25(4):228-36.

77. Fligner CL et al. Paper strip screening method for detection of cyanide in blood using CYANTESMO test paper. Am J Forensic Med Pathol. 1992;13(1):81-84.

78. Brueske PJ. ED management of cyanide poisoning. J Emerg Nurs., 1997;23(6):569-73.

79. Lambert RJ, Kindler BL, Schaeffer DJ. The efficacy of superactivated charcoal in treating rats exposed to a lethal oral dose of potassium cyanide. Ann Emerg Med. 1988; 17(6):595-98.

80. Brivet F, et al. Acute cyanide poisoning: recovery with non-specific supportive therapy. Intensive Care Med. 1983;9(1):33-35.

81. Graham DL, et al. Acute cyanide poisoning complicated by lactic acidosis and pulmonary edema. Arch Intern Med. 1977;137(8):1051-55.

82. Way JL. Cyanide antagonism. Fundam Appl Toxicol. 1983;3(5):383-86.

83. Way JL, Gibbon SL, Sheehy M. Cyanide intoxication: protection with oxygen. Science. 1966;152(3719):210-11.

84. Sheehy M, Way JL. Effect of oxygen on cyanide intoxication. 3. Mithridate. J Pharmacol Exp Ther. 1968;161(1):163-68.

85. Isom GE, Way JL. Effect of oxygen on cyanide intoxication. VI. reactivation of cyanide-inhibited glucose metabolism. J Pharmacol Exp Ther. 1974;189(1):235-43.

86. Litovitz TL, Larkin RF, Myers RA. Cyanide poisoning treated with hyperbaric oxygen. Am J Emerg Med. 1983; 1(1):94-101.

87. Goodhart GL. Patient treated with antidote kit and hyperbaric oxygen survives cyanide poisoning. South Med J. 1994; 87(8):814-16.

88. Scolnick B, Hamel D, Woolf AD. Successful treatment of life-threatening propionitrile exposure with sodium nitrite/sodium thiosulfate followed by hyperbaric oxygen. J Occup Med. 1993;35(6):577-80.

89. Trapp WG. Massive cyanide poisoning with recovery: a boxing-day story. Can Med Assoc J. 1970;102(5):517.

90. Weiss LD, Van Meter KW. The applications of hyperbaric oxygen therapy in emergency medicine. Am J Emerg Med. 1992;10(6):558-68.

91. Wesson DE, et al. Treatment of acute cyanide intoxication with hemodialysis. Am J Nephrol. 1985;5(2):121-6.

92. Dart RC, et al. Combined evidence-based literature analysis and consensus guidelines for stocking of emergency antidotes in the United States. Ann Emerg Med. 2000:36(2):126-32.

93. Chen KK, Rose C L. Nitrite and thiosulfate therapy in cyanide poisoning. JAMA. 1952;149(2):113-15.

94. Hall AH, et al. Nitrite/thiosulfate treated acute cyanide poisoning: estimated kinetics after antidote. J Toxicol Clin Toxicol. 1987;25(1-2):121-33.

95. Way JL, et al. Recent perspectives on the toxicodynamic basis of cyanide antagonism. Fundam Appl Toxicol. 1984;4(2 Pt 2):S231-S239.

96. Baskin SI, Nealley EW, Lempka JC, Cyanide toxicity in mice pretreated with diethylamine nitric oxide complex. Hum Exp Toxicol. 1996;15(1):13-18.

97. Way JL, Burrows G. Cyanide intoxication: protection with chlorpromazine. Toxicol Appl Pharmacol. 1976;36(1):93-97.

98. Moore SJ, et al. Antidotal use of methemoglobin forming cyanide antagonists in concurrent carbon monoxide/cyanide intoxication. J Pharmacol Exp Ther. 1987;242(1):70-73.

99. Baskin SI, Horowitz AM, Nealley EW. The antidotal action of sodium nitrite and sodium thiosulfate against cyanide poisoning. J Clin Pharmacol. 1992;32(4):368-75.

100. Sauer SW, Keim ME. Hydroxocobalamin: improved public health readiness for cyanide disasters. Ann Emerg Med. 2001;37(6):635-41.

101. Brouard A, Blaisot B, Bismuth C. Hydroxocobalamine in cyanide poisoning. J Toxicol Clin Exp. 1987;7(3):155-68.

102. Hall AH, Rumack BH. Hydroxycobalamin/sodium thiosulfate as a cyanide antidote. J Emerg Med. 1987;5(2):115-21.

103. Houeto P, et al. Relation of blood cyanide to plasma cyanocobalamin concentration after a fixed dose of hydroxocobalamin in cyanide poisoning. Lancet. 1995;346(8975):605-08.

104. Zerbe NF, Wagner BK. Use of vitamin B_{12} in the treatment and prevention of nitroprusside-induced cyanide toxicity. Crit Care Med. 1993;21(3):465-67.

105. Forsyth JC, et al. Hydroxocobalamin as a cyanide antidote: safety, efficacy and pharmacokinetics in heavily smoking normal volunteers. J Toxicol Clin Toxicol. 1993;31(2):277-94.

106. Cottrell JE, et al. Prevention of nitroprusside-induced cyanide toxicity with hydroxocobalamin. N Engl J Med. 1978;298(15):809-11.

107. Mushett C, Kelley KL, Boxer GE, et al. Antidotal efficacy of vitamin B_{12} (hydroxocobalamin) in experimental cyanide poisoning. Proc Soc Exp Biol. 1952;81:234-37.

108. Weger NP. Treatment of cyanide poisoning with 4-dimethylaminophenol (DMAP)—experimental and clinical overview. Middle East J Anesthesiol. 1990;10(4):389-412.

109. Bhattacharya R, et al. Protection against cyanide poisoning by the coadministration of sodium nitrite and hydroxylamine in rats. Hum Exp Toxicol. 1993;12(1):33-36.

110. Breen PH, et al. Protective effect of stroma-free methemoglobin during cyanide poisoning in dogs. Anesthesiology. 1996;85(3):558-64.

111. Nagler J, Provoost RA, Parizel G. Hydrogen cyanide poisoning: treatment with cobalt EDTA. J Occup Med. 1978;20(6):414-16.

112. Bhattacharya R. Antidotes to cyanide poisoning: present status. Indian J Pharmacol. 2000;32:94-101.

113. Bhattacharya R, Vijayaraghavan R. Promising role of alpha-ketoglutarate in protecting against the lethal effects of cyanide. Hum Exp Toxicol. 2002;21(6):297-303.

114. Hume AS, et al. Antidotal efficacy of alpha-ketoglutaric acid and sodium thiosulfate in cyanide poisoning. J Toxicol Clin Toxicol. 1995;33(6):721-24.

115. Dulaney MD Jr, et al. Protection against cyanide toxicity by oral alpha-ketoglutaric acid. Vet Hum Toxicol. 1991;33(6):571-75.

116. Niknahad H, Ghelichkhani E. Antagonism of cyanide poisoning by dihydroxyacetone. Toxicol Lett. 2002;132(2):95-100.

117. Schwartz C, et al. Antagonism of cyanide intoxication with sodium pyruvate. Toxicol Appl Pharmacol. 1979;50(3):437-41.

118. Cannon EP, et al. Antagonism of cyanide intoxication with murine carrier erythrocytes containing bovine rhodanese and sodium thiosulfate. J Toxicol Environ Health. 1994;41(3):267-74.

119. Petrikovics I, et al. Encapsulation of rhodanese and organic thiosulfonates by mouse erythrocytes. Fundam Appl Toxicol. 1994;23(1):70–75.

4

Phosgene and Toxic Gases

Melissa L. Givens

NAME AND DESCRIPTION OF AGENT

Toxic gases, also known as choking agents, are the forerunners of modern chemical warfare. Chlorine gas was first deployed during World War I. On April 22, 1915, the Germans released 150 tons of chlorine gas along the battlefront in Ypres, Belgium, creating multiple casualties who taxed medical resources. The novel use of toxic gas created widespread fear of this new chemical weaponry. Subsequently, battle stress precipitated by this horrific threat compounded the treatment challenges faced by medical professionals. Phosgene was also used during World War I, both alone and mixed with chlorine gas. Phosgene was the likely culprit in nearly 80% of poison gas deaths that occurred during the war (1,2). Use of phosgene on the battlefield was estimated to have resulted in 311,000 man-days lost to hospitalization during the war, the equivalent of 852 man-years (3). This degree of hospitalization only underscores the potential for toxic gas exposure to strain hospital resources in the event of a terrorist attack.

Toxic gas use is not isolated to World War I. The use of phosgene by Egyptian bombers has been reported in attacks against the Yemeni royalist forces in the Yemeni civil war during the 1980s (4). More recently, on April 20, 1995, the Aum Shrinrikyo ("Supreme Truth") cult, the same organization linked to the sarin release in the Tokyo subway, was implicated in the release of a phosgene-type gas in a train station in Yokohama, resulting in the hospitalization of over 300 people.

Chlorine and phosgene are produced in large quantities worldwide and used extensively in multiple industries. Chlorine is commonly used in cleaning products, in water purification, and as an intermediate in the manufacturing of plastics and synthetics. Chlorine is the most common cause of accidental industrial and household inhalational injury in the United States, and the release of toxic amounts of chlorine has occurred worldwide more than 200 times since the early 20th century (5–7).

Phosgene is also used extensively in industry as a chemical precursor in the production of dyes, pesticides, plastics, polyurethane, isocyanates, and pharmaceuticals. Phosgene is also formed by combustion of chlorinated fluorocarbons, which are found in refrigeration units, and toxicity has been reported in refrigeration workers who were welding refrigeration conduits and welders using chlorinated solvents (8,9). Over 1 million tons of phosgene are used yearly in the United States (10). An estimated 5 billion pounds are produced worldwide (11). Identification of phosgene can be confusing because there are many other nomenclatures including: carbonyl chloride, carbon oxychloride, carbonic acid chloride, D-Stoff, and green cross (2,12). The military designation for phosgene is CG. The widespread availability of phosgene and chlorine makes them attractive agents of terror. Both agents are mass-produced and are stored and transported in large-volume containers that could have devastating effects if vaporized. The ease of attainment and distribution, coupled with the significant strain on medical resources that accompanies injury with these agents makes toxic gases potential terrorist agents of warfare. The psychological harm that can be inflicted with a chemical attack is only a bonus feature in terms of terrorist potential.

There are other agents that also may produce toxic injury to the airways such as smoke and obscurants, including zinc oxide, phosphorous smokes, sulfur trioxide-chlorosulfonic acid, and perfluoroisobutylene (a combustion product of Teflon). These agents are less likely to be used in a direct chemical attack. They are very irritating to victims, causing them to evacuate the smoke cloud quickly, thus limiting exposure. Consequently, these agents are considered less desirable as offensive weapons. The discussion of such agents is beyond the scope of this chapter. This chapter will focus mainly on the acute and the delayed injury pattern associated with phosgene exposure. Chlorine will be discussed briefly to highlight the clinical differences that can occur when dealing with a patient exposed to a toxic gas.

THEORETICAL AND SCIENTIFIC BACKGROUND

Toxic gas injury is determined by the chemical properties of the toxic gas and the conditions in which the exposure occurs. Phosgene is a gas at temperatures above 47°F (8°C) (13). At temperatures below the boiling point, phosgene is a liquid and has limited toxicity. Chlorine enters the gaseous state at F (−34°C) (13). It is often stored in a compressed state because of its low boiling point. The ambient heat, humidity, and air currents can all affect the properties of these gases and the clinical response generated by the exposure. A drop in ambient pressure may result in an increase of the toxin in the gaseous state. Strong wind currents can dissipate the gas to nontoxic levels and changes in wind patterns can result in the gas distributing in an unpredictable direction.

Once an individual is exposed to a toxic gas, the extent of injury is defined by the exposure characteristics. Exposure is defined by duration (t) and intensity or concentration (C) where Ct = concentration in mg/m^3 multiplied by time in minutes. Confounding variables that alter the concentration over time include respiratory rate, depth of respirations (minute ventilation), and even body position. Of note, all can be affected by the sympathetic discharge likely to occur in the event of a terrorist attack. Patients are likely to be breathing rapidly and deeply and may not think to protect their airway as a first line of defense. Also, one cannot forget to consider underlying conditions such as history of hyperreactive airways and tobacco use when trying to predict the clinical outcome of a toxic gas exposure. The presence of underlying disease can magnify the clinical response and can result in severe symptoms at even negligible concentration exposures.

The effects of toxic gases on the human airway depend on the chemical properties of the gas. The anatomic site of injury is related to the solubility of the gas in water. Gases that are more water-soluble, such as chlorine, primarily affect upper airways and central airways. Less soluble gases, like phosgene, penetrate deeper into lungs and affect peripheral airways and alveoli. The end result of this deep injury is damage to the capillary-alveolar wall and leakage of plasma into the alveoli.

Chlorine (Cl_2), discovered in 1774, is a greenish-yellow gas, with an offensive, pungent odor that fortunately acts as a warning signal at concentrations below lethal exposures (14). Coughing occurs at 30 parts per million (ppm) and exposures of 40 to 60 ppm for more than 30 minutes may cause severe damage. Lethality has been reported at exposures of 500 ppm for 5 minutes (13). Once chlorine reaches the respiratory tract, it reacts with water to form hydrochloric and hypochlorous acids. Hypochlorous acid reacts with sulfhydryl groups of cysteine, and also causes enzyme inhibition (15). Additionally, chlorine hydrolysis generates free radicals capable of penetrating cell membranes that can result in cell injury and death. The formation of hydrochloric acid is most likely to occur in the moist areas of the eyes, mouth, and upper airways, thus chlorine is much more irritating when compared to phosgene, which undergoes little hydrolysis. However, the exact mechanisms of chlorine toxicity in the respiratory tract cannot entirely be attributed to this formation of hydrochloric acid, and pathogenesis is still controversial (14).

Phosgene ($COCl_2$), which was first manufactured in 1812 by Sir Humphrey Davey in Great Britain, is a colorless, volatile gas that is heavier than air; it has an odor of freshly mown hay. Toxic exposure occurs below the odor

threshold which is 0.4 ppm (16). This is important because *victims may be exposed to dangerous levels without even realizing that they are in danger.* Estimated LCt_{50} for phosgene is 500 to 800 ppm for a 2-minute exposure (2,17). Once phosgene is inspired, hydrolysis occurs upon contact with water resulting in the formation of carbon dioxide and hydrogen chloride.

$$COCl_2 + H_2O \rightarrow CO_2 + 2HCl$$

This liberation of hydrogen chloride was once thought to be the mechanism of injury; however, the amount of hydrogen chloride released is miniscule and cannot account for the pulmonary damage incurred by phosgene exposure (18). The formation of hydrogen chloride may account for the small degree of mucous membrane irritation similar to that seen in chlorine exposure.

Phosgene also reacts with sulfhydryl, amine, and hydroxyl groups, which are cellular constituents of biological molecules, in a process known as acylation(19).

$$COCl_2 + 2R-NH_2 \rightarrow C=O(NH-R)_2 + 2HCl$$
$$R-OH \rightarrow C=O(O-R)_2 + 2HCl$$
$$R-SH \rightarrow C=O(S-R)_2 + 2HCl$$

Acylation results in protein and lipoid denaturation, changes in membrane structure, and disruption of enzymes (2). Phosgene also disrupts the surfactant layer, thus impairing mechanical performance that depends on adequate surface tension for alveolar gas exchange (20). Phosgene can undergo heterolytic and/or homeolytic cleavage into a reactive carbamoyl monochloride radical. This may be responsible for its reactivity with lung tissue components (21).

Animal studies of phosgene show changes in energy metabolism. Cyclic adenosine triphosphate (cATP) and cyclic adenosine monophophate (cAMP) are decreased, which may result in inadequate energy to maintain fluid homeostasis within the lung (22,23). Decreases in oxygen uptake and depressed cellular glycolysis are also observed. Phosgene additionally causes disruption of the glutathione redox cycle (glutathione acts as a natural antioxidant), with subsequent increase in opportunities for oxidant injury by free radicals (24–26). The oxidant stress of phosgene is demonstrated by elevated antioxidant enzyme levels for days after acute exposure (24–27). Phosgene exposure has also been shown to cause lipid peroxidation and release of arachidonic acid metabolites to include sulfidopeptide leukotrienes TC4/LTD4/LTE4. These leukotrienes are of interest because they are the primary components of SRS-A. SRS-A is the slow reacting substance of anaphylaxis. Leukotrienes can be tied to vasoconstriction of bronchial smooth muscle, coronary vasoconstriction, and increased vascular permeability. LTB4 is a neutrophil chemotactic agent and is elevated in rats exposed to phosgene, and subsequent neutrophil migration is noted in conjunction with elevated levels of this leukotriene. The exact role of these mediators in phosgene-induced injury is still unclear, and there are conflicting animal studies in regards to how leukotrienes may modulate or incite injury. The inflammatory process may be the cause of toxin-mediated injury or a response to the direct toxic effects (28–31).

In extremely high concentrations (greater than 200 ppm), phosgene's effects may no longer be isolated to the lungs. Phosgene may cross the blood air barrier in the lung and cause hemolysis and red blood cell hyperaggregation (32). This causes pulmonary sludging, which in turn may cause cor pulmonale and subsequent death (18).

SIGNS AND SYMPTOMS

Toxic gases can produce clinical signs and symptoms in several ways. If the gas is released in an enclosed space, the gas can displace oxygen and result in asphyxia from lack of oxygen. Toxic gases may also cause direct damage to the respiratory tract resulting in airway obstruction, interstitial damage, and alveolar-capillary damage, all with impaired oxygen exchange. Additionally, an allergic response that results in cellular damage or tissue swelling and possible systemic inflammatory damage may be initiated. Each of these sequelae of toxic gas exposure can affect how the patient presents clinically, and the clinician must be prepared to deal with a combination of clinical responses to toxic gas exposure. A comparison of chlorine and phosgene gas exposures is seen in Table 4-1 in the summary section of the chapter.

Chlorine is a highly irritating gas with an unpleasant odor. Exposure often causes rapid eye pain, blephorospasm, and lacrimation. The offensive nature of chlorine results in immediate symptoms after exposure and is often protective because it signals the patient to depart the area of exposure. Other early symptoms that can occur include headache, salivation, oropharyngeal pruritus, dyspnea, cough, hemoptysis, retrosternal burning, and vomiting (33). Symptoms are usually temporally related to the exposure, and delayed symptoms are uncommon.

Physical exam may reveal tachypnea, cyanosis, and tachycardia. Providers should exclude corneal burns or abrasions with a fluoroscein exam. Oropharyngeal secretions may be profound. Oropharyngeal erythema may signify more distal injury, and physicians can consider laryngoscopy or bronchoscopy to further evaluate the airway. Symptoms of upper airway irritation or pruritus should also prompt a more thorough oropharyngeal exam. Endoscopy should be done in conjunction with preparations for endotracheal intubation in the event of airway compromise. Laryngospasm may occur with a high dose exposure, and one should look for stridor, hoarseness, and aphonia as harbingers of impending upper airway obstruction. Often laryngospasm occurs at the time of exposure so emergency responders need to be prepared to provide emergent airway control. Highly toxic exposures may result in bronchospasm or pulmonary edema with wheezes and rhonchi heard on exam.

Phosgene is a far more subversive agent than chlorine. Initially, irritation to the eyes or respiratory system may occur, but often the patient has no early signs or symptoms related to the exposure. Toxicity occurs below the odor and irritant threshold, so the patient may have no warning triggers to exit the exposure area.

The following is an excerpt from Sir Wilmot Herringham's description of soldiers exposed to phosgene in the spring of 1915.

> *We gradually recognized three classes. a) The severest of all, which were either collapsed from the first or became collapsed after a day or two. When collapse was present the color was an ashy gray, the breathing was rapid and shallow, and the pulse was very small. These cases died rapidly. b) Those which were severely affected, but were purple in color and had a full though rapid pulse. Some of these cases became progressively worse and eventually became collapsed and gray, and then died. Others, if carefully treated, recovered. c) Slighter cases which showed little cyanosis or none, and only had a slight cough. Postmortem examination showed laryngitis, enormous edema of lungs, emphysema on edge of lung, and air under pleura.*
>
> *Lancet Feb 21, 1920*

Phosgene affects peripheral airways with corresponding symptoms of dyspnea and chest tightness. Chest pain and cough may also occur. Patients characteristically develop dyspnea 2 to 6 hours after exposure. However, the latency phase may last for up to 15 hours (2). Shorter latent periods suggest a more toxic exposure. Objective clinical findings such as decreased arterial oxygen saturation (PaO_2) and pulmonary edema may lag behind subjective symptoms. It is common for the patient to complain of dyspnea after the exposure, and the provider may be frustrated by lack of objective findings to explain the patient's complaints. Once clinical findings do develop, the patient may suffer significant clinical deterioration in rapid progression. Pulmonary edema may be profound. Significant pulmonary edema may result in hypotension secondary to volume depletion. Amazingly, fluid losses from alveolar capillaries may be as much as 1 L/h, underscoring the need for aggressive volume resuscitation (34). Pulmonary edema that occurs early (less than 4 hours after exposure) signifies a grave prognosis.

Although inhalational injury is the most commonly encountered form of toxic gas exposure, both phosgene and chlorine can result in injury when splash injury of the liquid occurs. Compressed gases may cause frostbite when skin contact occurs. Ocular exposure to liquid phosgene has caused corneal opacification and perforation in one exposure. Skin exposure to phosgene is usually manifested only as local irritation and erythema (35).

MEDICAL MANAGEMENT

PREHOSPITAL

Toxic gas exposures pose significant risk to rescue workers who must enter the scene to extricate patients. Rescue workers entering an area with unknown concentrations of a toxic gas should wear a self-contained breathing apparatus (SCBA) with a full face-piece that operates on pressure demand or other positive pressure mode to prevent toxic injury while engaging in rescue activities (13).

Prehospital providers should remove the patients from the exposure area before engaging in medical interventions. Simple decontamination can be done with soap and water. Patients with eye exposure should undergo copious irrigation with water or normal saline. The first priority after removing the toxin is to evaluate airway patency and establish airway control. As noted earlier, laryngospasm may occur at high gas concentrations, and significant edema may result in airway compromise necessitating early endotracheal intubation or even surgical cricothyroidotomy. Meticulous control of airway secretions may be necessary in the case of upper airway irritants such as chlorine. Fortunately, patients often do very well once they are removed from the reaches of the toxic gas. Supplemental oxygen can be given to all patients exposed to toxic gases. Beta-agonist therapy may be required in the event of bronchospasm.

Once airway control has been established, rescue personnel can provide supportive therapy with intravenous (IV) fluids. Fluids should be administered in the setting of volume depletion, but empiric fluid boluses by field personnel are not indicated. Patients with toxic gas exposure should also be kept at rest. One of the most striking historical features of phosgene poisoning is the clinical decline described in patients who undertake physical activity. Herringham wrote about his World War I experience: "We rapidly learnt also that exertion, sometimes even slight exertion, made the patients worse. Men who had been comfortable while lying became rapidly worse and sometimes died suddenly if they walked or sat about" (36). We already know that physical exertion can stress the body and uncover subclincial compromise that is not obvious at rest. In the case of phosgene poisoning, there is ongoing pulmonary damage even when the patient is asymptomatic that may be revealed with even the slightest increase in oxygen requirement. Furthermore, there is concern that physical activity may further exacerbate the lung injury causing a deterioration that might not have occurred if the patient had stayed at rest. Phosgene has not been thoroughly studied, but the literature suggests that moderate exercise shortly after exposure does not affect survival; however, strenuous exercise postexposure or even slight exercise after the onset of pulmonary edema can be deleterious (37). Cautious management would be to *keep patients with expected phosgene exposure at rest during observation even when they are asymptomatic* and show no clinical signs of pulmonary damage. The damage may be brewing in their lungs, and exertion may only serve to accelerate or worsen the consequences of the exposure. In the setting of a bioterrorist attack, it may be difficult to contain these asymptomatic patients. Once they have entered into the medical system, they need to be observed and discouraged against premature elopement. This may prove difficult if they are worried about their homes and loved ones who may have suffered in an attack.

HOSPITAL

Upon arrival at the hospital or treatment area, the patient's airway should be reassessed to ensure patency. The patient should be intubated immediately if there is stridor or other findings that suggest upper airway obstruction or respiratory distress. Place the patient on a monitor and provide supplemental oxygen to maintain adequate oxygen saturation (PaO$_2$ greater than 60 mmHg). The patient should be kept at bed rest. Vital signs and lung exam should be repeated every 30 minutes to detect early changes.

Laboratory values are of little diagnostic utility in the patient exposed to toxic gas. Lactate dehydrogenase (LDH) has been shown to elevate in animal studies, but case reports in humans have been inconsistent, and it cannot be considered a reliable indicator of exposure or injury (38). Arterial blood gases (ABGs) are important when following oxygenation, but a normal PaO$_2$ early in the course of phosgene exposure is not reassuring. It may take several hours for hypoxemia to develop. A normal ABG upon patient presentation may falsely reassure the clinician, and care should be taken not to dismiss patients with possible exposure prematurely. It is important to recognize that the PCO$_2$ may be elevated in patients with reactive airways and bronchospasm. Patients with findings of hypercarbia or wheezing are good candidates for bronchodilators and steroids.

The same precaution in interpreting early ABGs also applies when interpreting a chest x-ray (CXR) done on arrival of a patient with suspected toxic gas exposure. The initial CXR may be normal, and the patient may go on to develop profound pulmonary edema only a few hours later. Fortunately, the CXR can often detect pulmonary edema sooner than the clinical exam. There are findings other than pulmonary edema on CXR that the physician can use when evaluating a patient with a toxic gas exposure. Atelectasis is a more common finding in exposures that affect the upper airways (chlorine). Hyperinflation signifies air trapping due to injury to smaller peripheral airways, which can occur with phosgene exposure. Damage to the alveolar-capillary membranes may result in the characteristic "batwing" appearance of pulmonary edema, but one should watch for more subtle findings such as blurred enlargement of the hila and patchiness in the central lungs (2). A baseline CXR can be useful for comparison, and subtle changes may be indicators of impending pulmonary edema (Fig. 4-3). The time of onset of radiographic findings is inversely proportional to the inhaled phosgene dose—patients with higher doses become sicker earlier. Radiographic findings may appear as early as to 1 to 2 hours in moderate to high exposures but may be delayed in lower dose exposures. If the CXR is normal at 8 hours, it is unlikely the patient will develop pulmonary edema (38).

Management of pulmonary edema parallels that of adult respiratory distress syndrome (ARDS). ARDS is also a vascular permeability-based pathologic process that involves cellular damage and inflammatory mediators and is dissimilar to volume overload pulmonary edema such as congestive heart failure. There is little use for diuretics when dealing with pulmonary edema that is not a result of volume overload. Patients with toxic gas injury are often intravascularly volume depleted as the fluid shifts from the vascular to lung compartments. *Diuresis will only serve to worsen volume depletion* early on in the setting of fluid shifts secondary to a damaged capillary-alveolar membrane. It is more likely that the patient will require mechanical ventilatory support for adequate oxygenation. Positive end-expiratory pressure (PEEP) may be necessary to maintain PaO$_2$ over 60 mmHg. It is essential to ensure intravascular volume replacement in the setting of PEEP as PEEP may decrease preload and result in subsequent hypotension.

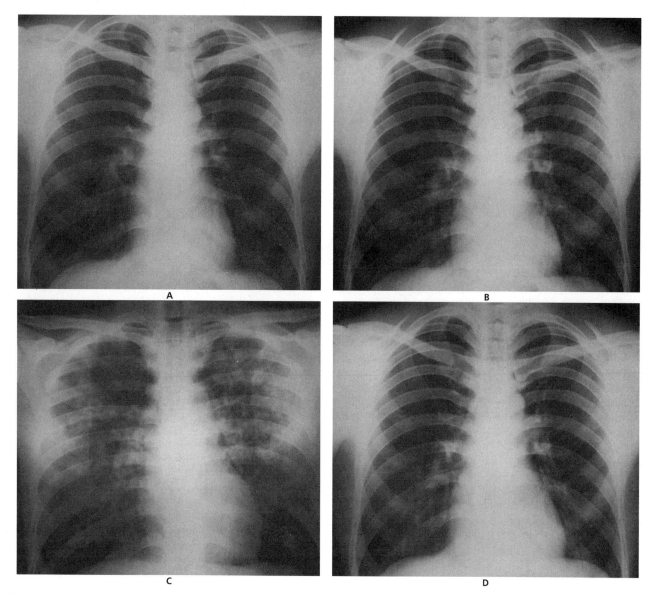

Figure 4–3. Series of chest radiographs after an acute phosgene exposure. **A:** Normal chest x-ray 1 year prior to exposure. **B:** 6 h after phosgene exposure (blurring of hila and slight enlargement of pulmonary vessels, ill-defined patchiness in central lung regions). **C:** 10 h after exposure (overt pulmonary edema). **D:** 5 days after exposure with complete resolution and a normal x-ray. Radiographs are courtesy of Jonathon Borak and Werner Diller (deceased).

Toxic gases may cause transient cardiac arrhythmias that are usually self-limited once the patient is removed from the toxic environment and receives supplemental oxygen (12). Cardiac dysrhythmias that occur after toxic gas exposure can be treated with standard Advanced Cardiac Life Support (ACLS) protocols with extra attention given to ensure the patient is adequately oxygenating.

Symptoms of bronchospasm and obstructive airway disease manifested by wheezing and increased PCO_2 should be aggressively treated with beta-agonists. There is little data to support the use of steroids for all toxic gas exposures. However, patients with airway hyperreactivity may benefit from steroids in conjunction with beta-agonist therapy. Empiric steroid therapy for chlorine- and phosgene-exposed patients is controversial. Animal studies in swine show decreased severity of symptoms when inhaled steroids were given shortly after chlorine exposure. This suggests some benefit can be obtained even in patients without reactive airways (39). Animal

studies examining the utility of steroids in phosgene exposure show decreased lung edema and decreased mortality (28,40,41). There is no human data supporting these animal studies, but some sources do recommend either IV or inhaled steroids (42,43). Further studies need to be done to clarify the role of steroids in toxic gas exposure. Nebulized bicarbonate has also been used to theoretically neutralize the hydrochloric acid in the respiratory tract after chlorine exposure, but the studies are limited, and further exploration needs to be done before it can be considered first-line therapy (44,45).

Exposures to both chlorine and phosgene may cause fever, elevated white blood cell counts, and infiltrates on CXR in the first 3 to 4 days postexposure. These findings do not reliably indicate bacterial infection; therefore, antibiotics should not be given routinely in this period. Prophylactic antibiotics may only serve to select for more virulent organisms. Sputum cultures may aid in determining the need for antimicrobial therapy. Pathogen identification along with sensitivity analysis can help appropriately guide antibiotic choice (12). The CXR should show improvement 3 to 5 days postexposure, so a worsening CXR suggests a superinfection, and antibiotic use is warranted along with surveillance for viral organisms.

Many other treatment modalities for phosgene exposure are currently under investigation. They are described as prophylactic treatment because they are most effective when given after exposure but before clinical signs or symptoms develop. Animal studies showed reduced pulmonary edema formation after phosgene exposure in those animals treated with medications that cause increased cAMP such as aminophylline, B-adreneric agents, or cAMP analogs (dibutyryl adenosine 3'5'cyclic monophosphate, DbcAMP) (29). DbcAMP may also act as an antioxidant and retain reduced glutathione. Aminophylline may act as a phosphodiesterase inhibitor. The animals in the combined study of aminophylline, beta-adrenergic agents, and Db-cAMP received medications within 10 minutes after exposure so further studies need to be done to determine efficacy of this type of intervention in a more realistic clinical timeframe. A separate study of aminophylline was conducted at 80 to 90 minutes postexposure. Decreased lung weight, increased reduced glutathione, and phosphodiesterase inhibition was observed in the treatment group (24). Isoproterenol, which elevates intracellular cAMP was studied 50 to 60 minutes postexposure and showed some benefit in terms of reduced vascular pressure, decreased leukotriene-mediated vascular permeability, and a favorable redox state in lung tissue when given both IV and via the intratracheal route (46).

Ibuprofen has been studied as both pre- and postexposure treatment for phosgene exposure and showed some benefit in reducing pulmonary edema in rats. Ibuprofen may act as a free radical scavenger and inhibit arachidonic acid metabolites (47). Ibuprofen is relatively safe and readily available making it a promising medication; its role in toxic gas exposure deserves further investigation.

N-acetylcysteine (NAC) has also been studied as a glutathione source to protect against the proposed free radical toxicity of phosgene. Rabbits given NAC via intratracheal bolus at 45- and 60-minutes post-phosgene-exposure showed less pulmonary edema, reduced lipid peroxidation, and decreased leukotriene production than controls (26). We can look toward the future for further delineation of the role of these mediators in toxic lung injury.

Once patients recover from toxic gas injury, they should be counseled regarding the anticipated symptoms that occur after recovery from toxic gas-induced acute pulmonary edema. Symptoms related to chlorine exposure typically resolve in 1 week to 1 month. However, prolonged symptoms and abnormal pulmonary function testing have been described (48,49). Patients with airway obstruction after exposure are more likely to have more chronic effects than similarly exposed patients with only complaints of dyspnea (50). Long-term effects of phosgene exposure have been described to include persistent exertional dyspnea and decreased physical fitness. It may take many years for complete recovery after exposure. A few patients may develop chronic bronchitis, emphysema, or generalized airway hyperreactivity (51). Chronic effects appear to be more common in patients who are smokers or have underlying pulmonary disease, and deterioration postexposure may occur. This underscores the need for close follow-up and pulmonary function testing in patients who continue to experience symptoms after recovery from the acute pulmonary edema.

TRIAGE CONSIDERATIONS

Patients exposed to toxic gases who display any respiratory symptoms should be triaged into an immediate category to obtain rapid airway control. Once airway control has been established and the patient is stable, the patient can be retriaged to a less urgent category. If patients present early, with few or no symptoms, they can be triaged into delayed category but should be watched carefully for signs of respiratory compromise. Patients should not be released from observation until at least 8 hours have passed since exposure and the patient has a clear CXR. Do not dismiss dyspnea in the face of few clinical findings as late sequelae may develop. Patients who present within a few hours after phosgene exposure may require more urgent triage as respiratory demise may occur rapidly.

PERSONAL PROTECTION

Rescue workers entering an area withunknown concentrations of phosgene or chlorine should wear an SCBA with a full face-piece that operates on pressure demand or other positive pressure mode to prevent toxic injury while engaging in rescue activities (13).

There is little chance of secondary exposure unless skin is contaminated with liquid phosgene. Because of phosgene's chemical properties, this can only occur below temperatures of 47°F (8°C). If liquid phosgene is present it can cause damage by direct contact or off-gassing.

SUMMARY

TABLE 4-1 Key Features of Chlorine and Phosgene

CHLORINE	PHOSGENE
Pungent odor	Odor of freshly mown hay
Highly irritating to mucous membranes	Little irritation to mucous membranes
Immediate symptoms	Delayed symptoms
Pulmonary edema	Pulmonary edema
Supportive treatment	Supportive treatment
Consider bronchodilators	Consider bronchodilators
Consider steroids	Consider steroids
No need for prophylactic antibiotics	No need for prophylactic antibiotics
Unlikely chronic sequelae	Potential for prolonged symptoms after recovery

RESOURCES

1. Centers for Disease Control and Prevention
   http://www.bt.cdc.gov/agent/phosgene/index.asp

2. National Library of Medicine and National Institute of Health Medlineplus
   http://www.nlm.nih.gov/medlineplus/biodefenseandbioterrorism.html

3. World Health Organization
   http://www.who.int

4. National Institute for Occupational Safety and Health
   http://www.cdc.gov/niosh/homepage.html

5. Agency for Toxic Substances and Disease Registry
   http://www.atsdr.cdc.gov/atsdrhome.html

QUESTIONS AND ANSWERS

Scenario #1

A 24-year-old male presents to the emergency department complaining of dyspnea for the past hour. He reports he was at an outdoor rally that was dispersed after an explosion. He recalls a musty odor that was present. He left the rally 3 hours prior to arrival in the ED.

1. **Which of the following studies would be most useful in the early management of this patient?**
   A. Complete blood count
   B. Serum LDH
   C. Chest x-ray
   D. EKG
   E. Serum electrolytes

2. **The patient in scenario #1 develops clinical signs of pulmonary edema and airway hyperreactivity. Which of the following treatment modalities is least appropriate?**
   A. Supplemental oxygen
   B. Positive pressure ventilation
   C. Bronchodilators
   D. Corticosteroids
   E. Diuretics

3. **The patient in scenario #1 should be kept at bed rest with minimal exertion. True or false?**
   A. True
   B. False

Scenario #2

A 43-year-old female is brought by EMS from her home. The patient lives near a railroad track and witnessed an explosion of a tanker on the tracks. At the time of EMS arrival, she had increased oral secretions and was mildly hypoxic with a SpO_2 of 86% on room air. She has improved during transport and is able to recall a pungent odor after the accident. She now has slight wheezes on exam and oropharyngeal erythema.

4. **Which of the following agents is the most likely cause of this patient's symptoms?**

   A. Carbon monoxide
   B. Chlorine
   C. Phosgene
   D. Organophosphate
   E. Cyanide

5. **Four hours after arrival in the ED, the patient in scenario #2 develops a fever of 101°F. Her white blood count is 16,000 and her chest x-ray shows infiltrates. She still has slight wheezes on exam. Which of the following treatment is least likely to improve her symptoms?**
   A. Broad spectrum antibiotics
   B. Systemic corticosteroids
   C. Supplemental oxygen
   D. Inhaled corticosteroids
   E. Inhaled beta-agonist

6. **Both chlorine and phosgene have a detectable odor or irritation at nontoxic concentrations. True or false?**
   A. True
   B. False

ANSWERS

1: C. *A chest x-ray would be most helpful in a case such as this with possible phosgene exposure.*

2: E. *Diuretics may worsen volume depletion and are not indicated. The use of corticosteroids is controversial.*

3: A. *A. True, exertion may worsen pulmonary symptoms from phosgene exposure.*

4: B. *Chlorine is the likely culprit given early symptoms with mixed upper and lower airway symptoms.*

5: A. *The early fever and elevated white blood count are likely directly due to the toxic gas exposure and not infection. Antibiotics are unlikely to provide any benefit.*

6: B. *False, phosgene may not be detectable at toxic levels.*

REFERENCES

1. Marrs TC MR, Sidell FR. Phosgene in chemical warfare agents. Chichester: John Wiley; 1996.
2. Borak J, Diller WF. Phosgene exposure: mechanisms of injury and treatment strategies. J Occupat Environ Med. 2001;43(2):110-9.
3. Jackson K. Phosgene. J Chem Educ. 1933;October:622-26.
4. Evison D, Hinsley D, Rice P. Chemical weapons. BMJ. 2002;324(7333):332-35.
5. Schonhofer B VT, Kohler D. Long term lung sequelae following accidental chlorine gas exposure. Respiration. 1996;63(3):155-59.
6. Baxter PJ DP, Murray V. Medical planning for toxic releases into the community: the example of chlorine gas. Br J Ind Med. 1989;46:277-85.
7. Davis DS DG, Ferland KA. Accidental release of air toxics. Park Ridge, NJ: NDC; 1989.
8. Wyatt JP, Allister CA. Occupational phosgene poisoning: a case report and review. J Acc Emerg Med. 1995;12(3):212-13.
9. Selden A SL. Chlorinated solvents, welding and pulmonary edema. Chest. 1991;99:263.
10. NIOSH. Criteria for a recommended standard: occupational exposure to phosgene. Washington, DC: National Institute of Occupational Safety and Health. Publication 76137.
11. WHO. Environmental health criteria 193: Phosgene. Geneva: World Health Organization; 1997.

12. Urbanetti J. Toxic inhalation injury. In: Zajtchukk R, Bellamy RF eds. Textbook of military medicine part I: medical aspects of chemical and biological warfare. Washington DC: Office of the Surgeon General; 1997.

13. NIOSH. NIOSH pocket guide to chemical hazards. Accessed 2003. http://www.cdc.gov/niosh/npg/npgd0504.html.

14. Das R BP. Chlorine gas exposure and the lung: a review. Toxicol Indus Health. 1993;9(3):439-55.

15. Knox WE SP, Green DE, Auerbach VH. The inhibition of sulfhydryl enzymes as the basis for bactericidal action of chlorine. J. Bacteriol. 1948;55:451-58.

16. AIHA. Odor thresholds for chemicals with established occupational health standard. Akron: American Industrial Hygiene Association; 1989.

17. Cucinell SA. Review of the toxicity of long-term phosgene exposure. Arch Environ Health. 1974;28:272-75.

18. Diller WF. Pathogenesis of phosgene poisoning. Toxicol Indus Health. 1985;1(2):7-15.

19. Babad H ZA. The chemistry of phosgene. Chem Rev. 1973;73:75-91.

20. Frosolono MF, Currie WD. Response of the pulmonary surfactant system to phosgene. Toxicol Indus Health. 1985;1(2):29-35.

21. Arroyo CM FF, Kolb DL, Keeler JR, Millette SR. Autoionization reaction of phosgene studied by electron paramagnetic resonance/spin trapping techniques. J Biochem Toxicol. 1993;8:107-10.

22. Currie WD HG, Frosolono MF. Changes in lung ATP concentration in the rat after low-level phosgene exposure. J Biochem Toxicol. 1987;2:105-14.

23. Currie WD PP, Frosolono MF. Response of pulmonary energy metabolism to phosgene. Toxicol Indus Health. 1985;1:17-27.

24. Sciuto AM, Strickland PT, Kennedy TP, Gurtner GH. Postexposure treatment with aminophylline protects against phosgene-induced acute lung injury. Exp Lung Res. 1997;23(4):317-32.

25. Sciuto AM. Assessment of early acute lung injury in rodents exposed to phosgene. Arch Toxicol. 1998;72(5):283-8.

26. Sciuto AM, Strickland PT, Kennedy TP, Gurtner GH. Protective effects of N-acetylcysteine treatment after phosgene exposure in rabbits. Am J Resp Crit Care Med. 1995;151(3 Pt 1):768-72.

27. Jaskot RH GE, Richards JH. Effects of inhaled phosgene on rat lung antioxidant system. Fundam Appl Toxicol. 1991;17:666-74.

28. Guo YL, et al. Mechanism of phosgene induced lung injury: role of arachidonate mediators. J Appl Physiol. 1990;69:1615-22.

29. Kennedy TP, Michael JR, Hoidal JR, et al. Dibutyryl cAMP, aminophylline, and beta-adrenergic agonists protect against pulmonary edema caused by phosgene. J Appl Physiol. 1989;67(6):2542-52.

30. Sciuto AM, Stotts RR. Posttreatment with eicosatetraynoic acid decreases lung edema in guinea pigs exposed to phosgene: the role of leukotrienes. Exp Lung Res. 1998;24(3):273-92.

31. Duniho SM, et al. Acute changes in lung histopathology and bronchoalveolar lavage parameters in mice exposed to the choking agent gas phosgene. Toxicol Pathol 2002;30(3):339-49.

32. Sciuto AM, Moran TS, Narula A, Forster JS. Disruption of gas exchange in mice after exposure to the chemical threat agent phosgene. Mil Med. 2001;166(9):809-14.

33. Sexton JD PD. Chlorine inhalation: the big picture. Clin Toxicol. 1998;36(1&2):87-93.

34. White SM. Chemical and biological weapons. Implications for anaesthesia and intensive care. Brit J Anaesth. 2002;89(2):306-24.

35. Lazarus AA, Devereaux A. Potential agents of chemical warfare: worst-case scenario protection and decontamination methods. Postgrad Med. 2002;112(5):133-40.

36. Herringham W. Gas poisoning. Lancet. 1920;1:423-24.

37. Diller WF. Medical phosgene problems and their possible solution. J Occupat Med. 1978;20(3):189-93.

38. Diller WF. Early diagnosis of phosgene overexposure. Toxicol Indus Health. 1985;1(2):73-80.

39. Gunnarsson M WS, Seidal T, Lennquist S. Effects of inhalation of corticosteroids immediately after experimental chlorine gas lung injury. J Trauma Injury, Infection Crit Care. 2000;48(1):101.

40. Frosolono MF SE, Holzman BH, Morecki R, Hurston E. Effect of aminophylline, hydrocortisone, and prostaglandin E1 on survival time and % lung water in rabbits after exposure to phosgene. Am Rev Respir Dis. 1978;117 (suppl):233-34.

41. Diller WF, Zante R. A literature review: therapy for phosgene poisoning. Toxicol Indus Health. 1985;1(2):117-28.

42. Registry AfTSaD. Medical management guidelines for acute chemical exposures. Washington DC: US Department of Health and Human Services; 1994.

43. Diller WF. Therapeutic strategy in phosgene poisoning. Toxicol Indus Health. 1985;1(2):93-99.

44. Vinsel PJ. Treatment of acute chlorine gas inhalation with nebulized sodium bicarbonate. J Emerg Med. 1990;8:327-29.

45. Bosse GM. Nebulized sodium bicarbonate in the treatment of chlorine gas inhalation. J Clin Toxicol. 1994;32:233-41.

46. Sciuto AM, Strickland PT, Gurtner GH. Post-exposure treatment with isoproterenol attenuates pulmonary edema in phosgene-exposed rabbits. J Appl Toxicol. 1998;18(5):321-29.

47. Sciuto AM, Stotts RR, Hurt HH. Efficacy of ibuprofen and pentoxifylline in the treatment of phosgene-induced acute lung injury. J Appl Toxicol. 1996;16(5):381-84.

48. RS B. The more common gases; their effects on the respiratory tract. Arch Int Med. 1919;24:678-84.

49. Gilchrist HL MP. The residual effects of warfare gases: the use of chlorine gas, with report of cases. Med Bull Vet Admins. 1933;9:229-70.

50. Hasan FM GA, Fuleihan FJD. Resolution of pulmonary dysfunction following acute chlorine exposure. Archiv Environ Health. 1983;38:76-80.

51. Diller WF. Late sequelae after phosgene poisoning: a literature review. Toxicol Indust Health. 1985;1(2):129-36.

5

Incapacitating Agents: BZ, Calmative Agents, and Riot Control Agents

Yedidia Bentur and John Gomez

3-QUINUCLIDINYL BENZILATE OR BZ

NAME AND DESCRIPTION OF AGENT

3-Quinuclidinyl benzilate, code named by the Army and widely known as BZ (or QNB), is a potent centrally acting glycolic acid ester anti-cholinergic. It has effects very similar to atropine, but it is much more potent in the central nervous system (CNS) and has a very long duration of action. It is primarily dispersed by aerosol or smoke-producing munitions, and the route of exposure is primarily respiratory. The British reportedly have a similar agent, known only as Agent 15. BZ was first tested commercially as a gastrointestinal antispasmodic, but when the extreme CNS effects were noted, civilian therapeutic research was abandoned. The U.S. Army conducted experiments from the 1960s to the 1980s with various anticholinergics and found BZ to be the most effective (1–3) The ICt50 (airborne concentration of BZ necessary to incapacitate 50% of exposed and unprotected individuals through inhalation during a set time period) is approximately 100 mg·min/m^3 (Figs. 5-1 and 5-2).

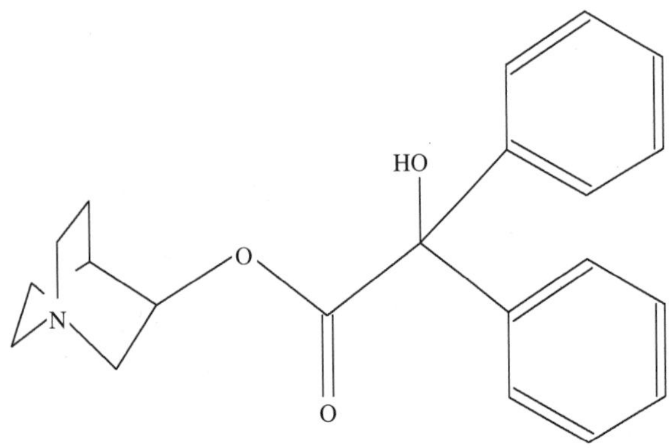

Figure 5–1. 3-Quinuclidinyl benzilate

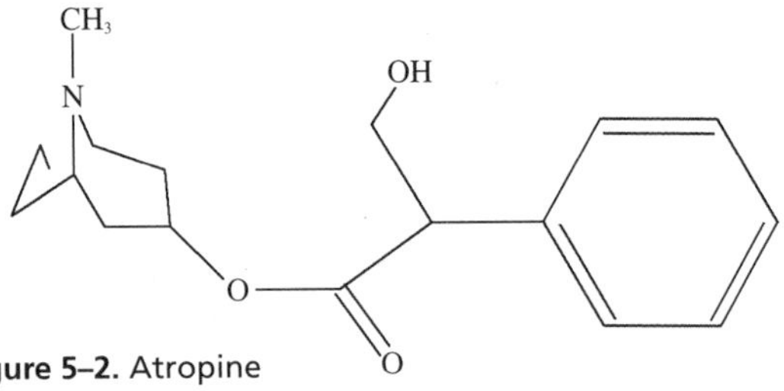

Figure 5–2. Atropine

THEORETICAL AND SCIENTIFIC BACKGROUND

The use of incapacitating agents is not limited to the 20th century. Instances of biologic and chemical warfare have been recorded in ancient times. Various alkaloid anticholinergics were used as early as 200 B.C. The infamous Roman enemy and Carthaginian General Hannibal used mandrake root to intoxicate or "incapacitate" rebel African tribes (3–5). A well-reported use of a belladonna (atropine-like) alkaloid was by the Bishop of Muenster who in 1672 used projectiles and grenades containing belladonna during his attack on the city of Groningen. Shortly after this occurrence in 1675, the French and Germans signed the first known treaty outlawing the use of chemical weapons (1,3,6).

The first recorded use of an incapacitating anti-cholinergic substance in the 20th century occurred in 1908 when a French unit in present-day Vietnam were poisoned with Datura placed in their evening meal. Several of the soldiers exhibited classic signs of anti-cholinergic delirium but recovered uneventfully (3,6). The former national Yugoslavian army was known to have weaponized and stockpiled BZ. There has been speculation that BZ was used during the conflict in Bosnia. In July of 1995, a contingent of a group of 15,000 people attempting to walk to Srebrenica reportedly suffered from hallucinations after an attack from Serbian forces using an unknown gas (7). There are also allegations that Serbian forces used BZ against Kosovo Liberation Army forces near the Albanian border. Iraq is suspected to have developed an agent similar or identical to BZ.

An incapacitating agent may be defined as a chemical that is temporary in its duration, is nonlethal, and has no permanent sequelae. From a military standpoint, an ideal incapacitating agent would be odorless, colorless, easily dispersed, and last a few hours to days, but longer than a few minutes as seen with the riot control agents. This substance should inhibit the cognitive functions of an enemy, keeping them from performing their task, and be easily dispersible, but still have a large margin of safety. It should be potent, and have an effective antidote known only to the user. Numerous agents were studied by the U.S. Army for this purpose, including atropine, scopolamine, lysergic acid diethylamide (LSD), phenothiazines, and delta-9 tetrahydrocannibinol (THC) (2). BZ offers several advantages over atropine and scopolamine as an incapacitating agent. BZ is said to have a very high safety profile and has 25 times more CNS anticholinergic potency than atropine (8). The incapacitating dose is defined to be roughly 0.5 mg in a typical adult compared to doses 20 to 25 times that for atropine. In addition, BZ also has less peripheral antimuscarinic effect than atropine, which makes it safer, and it is easier to weaponize/disperse. The onset of action is approximately one hour, and it peaks at about 8 hours, often persisting for 3 to 4 days (1,3,8).

Acetylcholine plays a vital role in cognitive function. This is why new centrally acting acetylcholinesterase inhibitors have been developed to improve memory and general cognitive function in patients with Alzheimer's dementia. Blockade of muscarinic receptors by BZ results in profound CNS dysfunction.

SIGNS AND SYMPTOMS

BZ crosses the blood brain barrier effectively and produces symptoms within 2 hours. Because of its ready penetration across the blood brain barrier, the predominant effects are CNS symptoms. Patients will have anticholinergic delirium and frequently will not be able to report many symptoms. If they are coherent enough to give a history, they may report hallucinations, peripheral effects including dry mouth, visual symptoms such as blurriness and inability to focus, as well as a feeling of warmth (1,3).

The symptoms of anticholinergic delirium range from a mild delirium to full-blown coma. At the mild end of the spectrum when a victim has received only a minimally effective dose, symptoms might include poor judgment, somnolence, impaired speech, and difficulty with complex task assignment. The more severely poisoned victim may manifest severe hallucinations from sensory stimuli, and agitation and even seizures. Consistent with the definition of delirium, there may be waxing and waning of the symptoms with occasional lucid intervals (1,3).

Anticholinergic delirium includes a few unique characteristics that may help identify poisoning with BZ. Patients may exhibit bizarre grasping movements where they may pick at the air, their skin, or clothing. The term "woolgathering" was once used to describe this peculiar feature. Shared hallucinations are described between two patients with anticholinergic delirium who are placed in the same room. Vivid hallucinations may occur that can be visual, auditory, or sometimes tactile. These undergo slow extinction as the CNS symptoms abate (1,3).

Like other anticholinergics, BZ can cause peripheral signs and symptoms; however, they may not be as pronounced as one would expect with the typical belladonna alkaloids such as atropine or Jimson weed (*Datura strammonium*), for example. Patients may manifest features of the classic anticholinergic toxic syndrome: "dry as a bone, red as a beet, hotter than Hades, and blind as a bat." Sinus tachycardia, mydriasis, flushed, dry warm skin, and diminished bowel sounds, hyperthermia, and urinary retention may be present. Seizures may occur in severe poisoning. It is important to note that pupillary dilatation may be mild or even absent at doses capable of causing delirium. BZ also causes fewer peripheral symptoms than other anticholinergic drugs. Absence of these symptoms, especially early in the course of the exposure, is not uncommon (3).

MEDICAL MANAGEMENT

Much like any other biologic or chemical warfare attack agent, treatment is contingent upon proper diagnosis and maintaining a high index of suspicion. An isolated exposure to BZ would not be expected, making the diagnosis more difficult. The combination of peripheral antimuscarinic effects described previously with the characteristic delirium suggests the diagnosis. Laboratory examinations are not clinically useful. They assist in ruling out other potential causes (such as metabolic derangements) and in diagnosing possible complications such as rhabdomyolysis and renal failure. Serum levels can be obtained from specific reference laboratories, although they are not helpful in the acute settings.

Patients with exposure to BZ should be decontaminated as soon as possible. All clothing should be removed and placed in sealed plastic bags. Skin should be thoroughly rinsed with copious amounts of water to prevent possible ongoing absorption. Staff members should be trained to prevent contamination of this potent agent.

Supportive care is paramount and intuitive. Delirious patients can certainly be a danger to themselves and others if not properly monitored. Victims should be temporarily restrained if necessary, and parenteral benzodiazepines should be used to control agitation. Although such sedatives are not specific antidotes, they can be useful measures to implement in an agitated patient and to decrease heat production.

Hyperthermia is an important concern due to the inability to sweat and increased psychomotor agitation. The patient's rectal temperature should be monitored closely to prevent the potential dangerous complications. Hyperthermic patients should be cooled rapidly by misting the patient with water and then applying fans for evaporation, or by implementing other effective techniques. Cold ice packs are not thought to be effective for this form of hyperthermia.

Anticholinergic agents cause drying of the secretions, and along with tachycardia mistakenly lead the treating physician to believe there is significant volume depletion when the patient is actually euvolemic. Hydration status and urine output should be closely monitored, particularly in warm weather (1,8). As with many stimulants and drugs of abuse, patients are at risk for rhabdomyolysis.

Acetylcholinesterase inhibitors are a classic but much maligned antidote for antimuscarinic poisonings. Neostigmine, pyridiostigmine, and physostigmine are all known as medicinal carbamates. They act by inhibiting the breakdown of acetylcholine at the synapse, increasing its level, and overcoming the blockade by competitive displacement. Unlike the other two agents listed, physostigmine has a tertiary amine group enabling it to cross the blood brain barrier. Due to its CNS penetration, it is the cholinesterase inhibitor of choice for delirium caused by BZ. There is controversy concerning the use of physostigmine due to reported adverse effects such as seizures and asystole (9–12). Wide use of physostigmine in the 1970s and 1980s for undifferentiated toxic delirium or coma was felt to be the cause of these reports of complications. Ketchum reports on military studies that show the safety and efficacy of physostigmine in the treatment of BZ-induced delirium (3). Other studies have showed the safety of physostigmine when used in patients with anticholinergic toxidrome who have not ingested drugs with fast sodium channel blocking activity such as tricyclic antidepressants (9–12). Some clinicians are still reluctant to recommend physostigmine use in this setting. However with BZ, it appears that physostigmine is safe and appropriate.

A typical adult dose of physostigmine would be 1 to 2 mg, IM or IV. The recommended pediatric dose of physostigmine is 20 µg/kg, up to 0.5 mg over 5 minutes. The dose may be repeated. Slow IV push over 5 to 10 minutes reportedly lowers the incidence of seizures and cardiac effects. All patients should have an electrocardiogram (ECG) prior to administration to check the QRS and PR width, and ECG monitoring is recommended. A QRS duration >100 milliseconds and a PR interval >200 milliseconds are contraindications to administration. Possible co-ingestions of tricyclic antidepressants or phenothiazines are relative contraindications, although this is highly unlikely in a suspected BZ exposure (8,9,13).

Physostigmine reversal of symptoms in BZ poisoning may not be immediate for reasons that are not completely understood (3). Once symptom reversal has been obtained, a similar dose should be repeated every 6 hours to prevent relapse. Much higher doses may be required for reversal of severe delirium. In one subject exposed to BZ, a total of 200 mg of physostigmine was given without the occurrence of adverse events (3). Oral dosing is also effective and is an option once the patient has been stabilized. Patients should be admitted for observation for 24 to 36 hours.

TRIAGE CONSIDERATIONS

When evaluating patients with suspected or known BZ poisoning, rapid triage of those with severe agitated delirium for safety issues is important. Those with hyperthermia, severe delirium, or seizures should intuitively take first priority in a mass exposure situation.

PERSONAL PROTECTION

Routine universal precautions should be used, including mask and eye goggles, a long sleeve gown and gloves to prevent contamination.

BZ Summary

- BZ is a potent centrally acting anticholinergic
- Anticholinergic delirium is the hallmark of BZ exposure; peripheral antimuscarinic effects may be delayed or less prominent.
- Diagnosis is historical, epidemiological, and clinical.
- Decontaminate all suspected patients, wear appropriate protective clothing.
- Restrain patients to protect them from harm when necessary, using loose netting. Use benzodiazepines liberally.
- Treat hyperthermia aggressively; monitor for rhabdomyolysis.
- The treatment of choice for patients with significant intoxication is physostigmine 30 to 45 µg/kg IV/IM.

SEDATIVE OR CALMATIVE AGENTS

NAME AND DESCRIPTION OF AGENTS

Opioids and volatile anesthetics are potential sedative or calmative agents. Opioids have been used for analgesia for over 100 years. Intuitively, opiates can serve as calmative and/or incapacitating agents. Morphine's tendency to cause severe respiratory depression, as well as other side effects and logistical concerns limit its use in this capacity. In this section, we will discuss fentanyl and n-4-substituted fentanyl derivatives used as incapacitating agents.

Carfentanil is an n-4 substituted fentanyl derivative that has high potency and a high therapeutic index (Figs. 5-3 and 5-4). Its safety has been well studied in large animal models, when used to immobilize wildlife. Other similar drugs in its class include sufentanil, alfentanil, and remifentanil. A detailed discussion follows later in the chapter.

Halothane is an example of an anesthetic gas that can also be considered as a potential calmative agent. However, its odor and safety profile may be of concern in this capacity.

THEORETICAL AND SCIENTIFIC BACKGROUND

The first and only reported modern use of a sedating incapacitating agent occurred in Russia. In late October of 2002, Chechen rebels took 800 civilian hostages attending a stage show. The rebels were armed with explosives and threatened to blow up themselves and their captives. A few days later, Russian special forces used a calmative gas to subdue the rebels and take control of the crisis. Victims were taken to local Moscow hospitals. In the tragic aftermath of the situation, 646 people were treated in local hospitals, and 118 of the victims died (16).

The victims were found to have signs and symptoms of opiate toxicity (15,16). After significant pressure from the families of the victims, the Russian government released a statement claiming that the gas used was a derivative of fen-

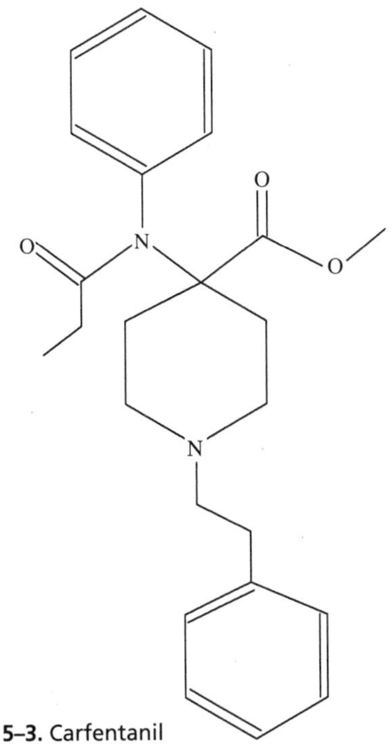

Figure 5-3. Carfentanil

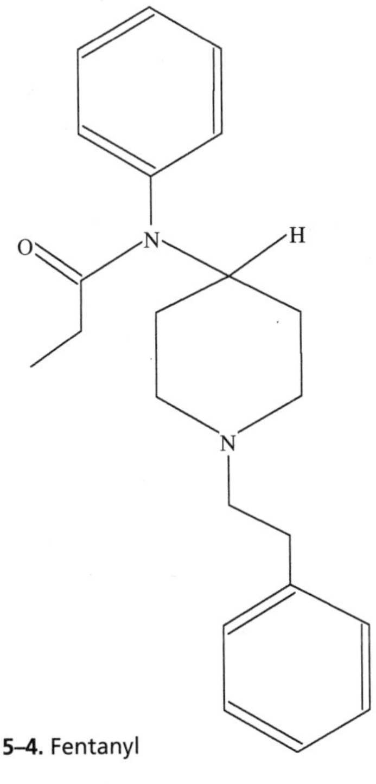

Figure 5-4. Fentanyl

tanyl. Wide speculation is that carfentanil, a substituted *n*-4 fentanyl derivative, was the most likely agent used. Etorphine has also been suggested as a possibility (16). Many experts believe that there was a concomitant use of an inhalational anesthetic. Evidence to support this comes from two German victims who were found to have traces of halothane when urine and blood samples were obtained (17).

The ideal *calmative agent* should have the potential to induce quick but easily reversible deep sedation or coma in an armed, dangerous, hostile situation, especially where innocent victims are involved. Its physical properties should en-

able quick removal from the environment and have a high therapeutic index. The episode described here has increased awareness of the potential use of calmative agents for use as incapacitating agents. In hostage situations such as the Chechnyan crisis, the potential advantages of calmative agents over a deliriant (BZ) or LSD become obvious.

Fentanyl is a synthetic opioid with a potency 100 times that of morphine, while having a much safer side-effect profile (18). It is a selective mu-agonist with an elimination half-life of 2 to 4 hours. Over the past two decades, more potent substituted *n*-4 fentanyl derivatives have been developed. These agents differ in the substitution of the *n*-4 position, classed as *n*-4 substituted 1-(2-arlethyl)-4 piperidinyl-*n*-phenylpropanamides. A few examples include sufentanil, alfentanil, remifentanil, and carfentanil. These agents have been used for intravenous analgesia used in conjunction with inhalational anesthetics. These agents are purported to have very high safety margins (19).

Trials of aerosolized fentanyl for analgesia have been performed in humans (20,21). These studies found a relatively low bioavailability and a wide variation in serum blood levels to achieve effective analgesia. This was believed to be due mainly to fentanyl's variable pharmacokinetics, lipid solubility, and high volume of distribution. Higgins noted that individual doses vary widely in part due to variability in each patient's respiratory pattern (20). These features, together with inconsistent aerosolized particle distribution, make fentanyl an improbable candidate for use as a calmative agent.

Carfentanil has been extensively used as a pareteral incapacitating agent for large animals (22–25). Carfentanil has a potency 10,000 times that of fentanyl (15). As mentioned previously, a high therapeutic ratio has been noted in all *n*-4 substituted fentanyl derivatives in rats (19). In theory this makes carfentanil a good candidate as an incapacitating or calming agent. One may doubt that carfentanil alone would be adequate as a calmative agent, perhaps explaining the possible use of halothane in the Russian hostage situation described previously.

There are several problems with the use of a fentanyl derivative as an incapacitating agent. Although carfentanil and its similar analogs have high potency and a high therapeutic index for other uses, the dose required to produce incapacitation of 99% of the target victims is significantly higher than what is likely safe, resulting in a high potential incidence of unintended mortality. Distribution of an aerosolized agent to a large group of people in equipotent doses is also logistically problematic. Some people may receive a substantially larger dose than desired while others may be underdosed. This is because of varying degrees of ventilation by various individuals and because of uneven dispersal patterns.

Halothane is a bromine-containing inhalational anesthetic (2-bromo-2-chloro-1,1,1-trifluoroethane). It is a highly volatile, colorless and lipid-soluble liquid that can be detected by its sweet odor. Halothane is a rapid and short-acting agent with a peak action at 1.3 to 3.5 minutes. It has an elimination half-life of 26 minutes with duration of action of 4 to 16 minutes. About two-thirds of the absorbed dose is excreted unchanged by the lung, the rest being metabolized. The main metabolites include bromine, trifluoroacetic acid, chloride salts, ethanolamine, and cysteine conjugates. The latter two metabolites may be involved in halothane-induced hepatotoxicity It is more potent than nitrous oxide and enflurane with minimum alveolar concentration of 0.6% to 1.0% (26,27).

SIGNS AND SYMPTOMS

The history may not be available from the patient, and Emergency Medical Services, bystanders, or the agency that used this agent should be recruited to assist in obtaining critical information. The clinical manifestations are those widely associated with opioid intoxication. At low doses, drowsiness and euphoria may be reported. Rapid induction of coma and respiratory depression may be the only history available.

Miosis, CNS depression or coma, and respiratory depression or arrest are all hallmarks of this toxidrome. Other findings may include bradycardia, hypotension, and hypothermia.

Urine drug screens are not likely to pick up the presence of synthetic opiates such as fentanyl. Serum levels of suspected exposure victims can be sent to a reference laboratory, but this will not be useful in the acute clinical setting (8).

The main toxic effects of halothane include a dose-dependent CNS and respiratory depression, including apnea, bradycardia, other arrhythmias, and hypotension. Halothane is known to sensitize the myocardium to catecholamines. Hepatotoxicity of Type I (transient enzyme abnormalities) and Type II (idiosyncratic reaction) have been reported (26,27).

MEDICAL MANAGEMENT

The critical component in the treatment of an opiate poisoning is support of the respiratory system. Even if the standard antidote is not available, oxygenation with early and aggressive support of ventilation is important to prevent hypoxic brain injury.

Naloxone is the antidote of choice for opiate poisoning or overdose. Unique to synthetic opiates is that high doses of this antidote are often required to reverse respiratory depression and coma (8). Experience with carfentanil in wildlife has shown higher than standard doses of naloxone are required to reverse clinical effects (28). Higher doses in the range of 0.3 mg/kg or higher may be required. It is important to remember that naloxone typically has a shorter duration of action than many opiates. The patient should be monitored for the potential of recurrent respiratory depression after administering this antidote. Fentanyl and 4 n-substitutes also undergo redistribution due to their highly lipophilic properties. At high doses the clinician should be vigilant to observe for recurrence of respiratory and CNS depression.

If an additional inhalational agent has been used, naloxone may not be completely effective. Aggressive support of oxygenation and ventilation with cardiovascular support should suffice until the effects have dissipated.

The treatment of halothane toxicity includes removal from exposure and support of the respiratory and cardiovascular systems. Vasopressors may induce cardiac arrhythmias and should be used cautiously. There is no antidotal treatment, although N-acetylcysteine has been suggested as a treatment modality based on animal studies (26,27).

TRIAGE CONSIDERATIONS

When triaging patients, those with any signs of hypoventilation or depressed mental status should take immediate priority. In a multicasualty incident, naloxone stores may not be sufficient to treat all victims. In all circumstances, however, it should be remembered that support of ventilation and oxygenation are the mainstays of treatment.

PERSONAL PROTECTION

Once the patient has been removed from the area to a well-ventilated space, significant contamination of staff is unlikely. Until the nature of the exposure is known, appropriate personal protection should be maintained.

Calmative Agents Summary

- Calmative agents such as potent short-acting opiates may become increasingly used in hostage situations.
- The most critical action is support of oxygenation and ventilation.
- Miosis, coma, and respiratory depression are the hallmarks of the intoxication.
- Large doses of naloxone may be required, and a continuous intravenous drip should be considered.
- In the event of a calmative agent use, adequate disaster response resources should be made available.

RIOT CONTROL AGENTS

NAME AND DESCRIPTION OF AGENT

In this section we will discuss the three most common riot control agents together and elucidate their individual characteristics. These agents include chloroacetophenone (CN), chlorobenzylidene malonitrile (CS), and oleoresin capsicum (OC). We will also include a fourth agent, diphenylaminochloroarsine (DM), out of historical interest only (Figs. 5-5 to 5-8). Other general descriptions used interchangeably are harassing agents or lacrimators. Details and actions of the individual agents are discussed in more detail later.

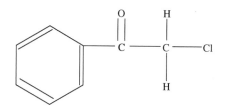

Figure 5–5. Chloracetophenone (CN)

Figure 5–6. Chlorobenzylidine malonitrile (CS)

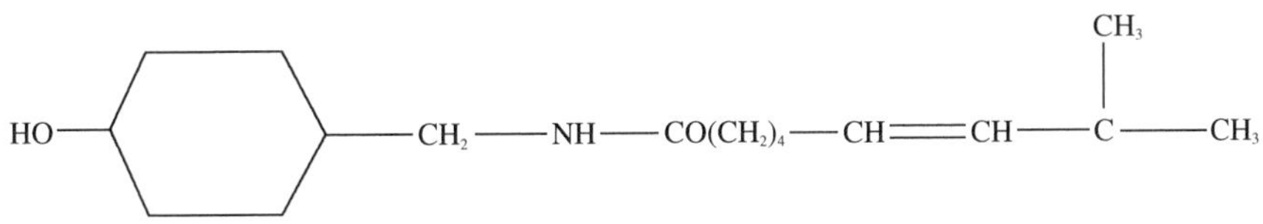

Figure 5–7. Capsaicin

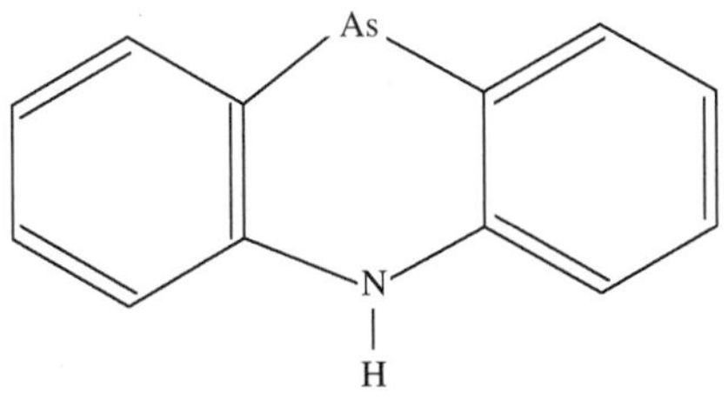

Figure 5–8. Adamsite (DM)

THEORETICAL AND SCIENTIFIC BACKGROUND

The use of irritant gases as nonlethal riot control agents is a fairly modern concept. There are several historical instances of irritant gas use worth mentioning. Several accounts of sulfur oxides, also known as Greek Fire, were used from ancient times through the Middle Ages. Hunyada Janos, a Hungarian national hero, used an arsenical smoke against the Ottoman Turks in the successful battle of Belgrade (29,30). The first modern use of irritant gas for the purpose of riot control came in 1914. In this year, the Paris police used ethylbromoacetate grenades to subdue prisoners (31). Both sides during World War I used harassing agents. The use and development of irritant gases for riot control expanded greatly in the 1950s and 1960s.

Riot control agents are by definition short-acting and nonlethal, and they temporarily incapacitate the target population very rapidly. Also known as sensory incapacitants, they cause severe irritation and discomfort and, therefore, reduce the ability and motivation of the target victim to cause harm. Their duration of action is short, usually less than 30 minutes. Ideally, they should have low and reversible toxicity. Although they all have common clinical manifestations, they are theoretically subdivided into lacrimators, sternutators, and vomiting agents. Lacrimators include agents that cause irritation and lacrimation, sternutators are products that induce violent coughing and sneezing, and vomiting agents cause vomiting.

The potencies of these agents are defined by the product of the concentration and exposure time sufficient to disable 50% of a group of unprotected individuals. This is otherwise known as the ICt_{50}. The LCt_{50} is a description of the time that is required to be lethal to 50% of the population. A higher LCt_{50} coupled with a lower ICt_{50} indicates a higher safety margin. Exact values for the agents are not important for our discussion and may be obtained from the reference section.

Chloroacetophenone or CN, more commonly known by its trade name Mace, was developed in 1871 and used in World War I. It became the most commonly used riot control agent by the U.S. military and police agencies through the 1950s and is still available today. CN was found to be relatively more harmful than some of the other agents and has largely been replaced.

Corson and Stoughton first synthesized o-chlorobenzylidene malonitrile (CS) in 1928, and their initials were used for its trade name. It has been used extensively in the past by the U.S. military, and currently it is being used worldwide as a sensory incapacitant (32). Relative to CN, the LCt_{50} for CS is higher and considered a safer riot control agent. It is up to ten times more potent than CN. There has been extensive experience with the use of this agent.

Oleoresin capsicum (OC) is also known as capsaicin and pepper spray. OC is derived from extracts of the peppers *Capsicum annum* and *Capsicum frutescence*. Numerous compounds are found in this extract; however, capsaicin is the primary and most irritating component. It is now the most commonly used sensory incapacitant in the United States, and its use is increasingly globally. Concentrations are available in 1% to 10% solutions, with lower concentrations for sale to the public. Capsaicin causes the release of the neuropeptide substance P, which causes vasodilatation, inflammation, and increased and prolonged pain through slow-acting c-fibers (31,33,34).

Diphenylarenamine (DM) also known as Adamsite is an irritant and vomiting agent. DM is more toxic than CN, CS, and OC. At lower concentrations, DM acts in similar fashion as the other harassing compounds with typical sensory irritant properties. At higher concentrations DM was known to cause vomiting in a delayed fashion (31,35). This delayed irritation caused by DM is considered an advantage in warfare in that by the time the target develops irritant symptoms and then puts on his/her mask, he/she may have already received a large dose. The victim will begin to vomit, remove his/her gas mask and be exposed, perhaps to nerve agents or other highly toxic substances. At lower concentrations irritant symptoms predominate, while higher doses are required for nausea and vomiting. Due to the propensity for victims to vomit, the use of DM has been widely discontinued in the civilian setting.

SIGNS AND SYMPTOMS

Riot control agents all affect the ophthalmologic, upper respiratory, lower respiratory, and integumentary systems to varying degrees. Table 5-1 summarizes the general clinical effects by organ system. The most pronounced effect of all these agents at low concentrations are the ophthalmologic symptoms of intense pain and involuntary blinking that temporarily will incapacitate the victim. Vomiting is very commonly associated with DM, as discussed previously. It has also been seen to a lesser extent with the use of CN.

TABLE 5-1 Effects of Riot Control Agents

- Ophthalmologic—stinging, pain, tearing, blepharospasm (involuntary blinking)
- Upper respiratory tract—pain/burning of the oropharynx and nasal passages, copious rhinorrhea
- Lower respiratory tract—cough, chest tightness, shortness of breath
- Dermal—stinging, burning, erythema, occasional blistering
- Gastrointestinal—vomiting (Adamsite)

The eyes are the most immediate and severely effected of the target organs. The intense pain and blepharospasm incapacitates the victim. Severe lacrimation, conjunctival injection, and periorbital edema are also noted. The symptoms appear within seconds for pepper spray and within a minute for CS (32). Of the agents discussed, CN is the most potentially harmful, while CS and pepper spray are much safer. They all cause a conjunctivitis, but CN has been shown to cause corneal edema, corneal opacification, and glaucoma in animal models (35). There are reports of CN powder lodging in the stroma of the cornea. Much of the damage from CN was believed to be due to the traumatic effect of the propellants used as well as the proximity of the blast (36,37). The effects from CS and pepper spray typically resolve within 30 minutes, while that of CN may be more prolonged.

The upper respiratory tract is uniformly irritated with all harassing agents, with pepper spray having the fastest onset on action. The effects include pain and stinging in the nose and mouth, sneezing, increased secretions, and rhinorrhea. At usual concentrations and limited exposure, lower respiratory tract manifestations include coughing, chest tightness, and shortness of breath. The cilia function to clear the airways of the irritants and protect the alveoli from further damage. At high enough concentrations and prolonged exposures, this protective effect is lost, and there can be lower airway exposure and damage (38). Bronchospasm is relatively common, especially in those with underlying reactive airway disease, and can be potentially serious. Rare cases of pulmonary edema have been reported for CS (39). Capsaicin is especially concerning in this regard and has been implicated in several deaths attributed to severe bronchospasm (31,40). Animal models with prolonged and fatal exposure showed edema and inflammatory cell infiltration in the alveoli.

Dermatological effects manifest initially as pain and irritation. Erythema followed by blistering and burning can occur at higher doses. Usually these effects are minimal and transient. The concentration, duration of exposure, and even humidity appear to affect the severity of the burns when they occur (35). Higher humidity and moisture have been reported to worsen the effect. An acute and delayed allergic contact dermatitis is well described with CN and CS, although CN is a much more potent sensitizer. These effects are seen in target victims and especially those involved in the manufacture of these chemicals (41). DM and capsicum both cause erythema and pain, and DM may cause skin necrosis (31).

MEDICAL MANAGEMENT

In general, riot control agents cause little in the way of serious morbidity or mortality. The obvious exceptions include those exposed to higher concentrations, especially in an enclosed space, for a longer period of time. Those with underlying respiratory disease or decreased physiologic reserve may be more susceptible as well. Treatment is mainly supportive. Patients should be disrobed and washed with copious amounts of cold water. Soap and water may be more efficacious but may cause a transient increase in the patient's symptoms (37). The patient's clothing should be sealed in a plastic container until it can be washed in a cold solution for decontamination.

Most cases of capsaicin, CN, or CS exposure resolve spontaneously within 30 minutes of exposure, and do not require treatment. More severe ophthalmologic exposures may be treated as with other chemical eye exposures. Contact lenses should be removed and topical anesthetics can be used liberally for pain control, and irrigation with isotonic saline or lactated ringers is beneficial (35). Others have recommended eye exposures be treated by blowing dry air over them with a cold hair dryer or a fan (32,36,37). The eye should be examined in all cases for the presence of foreign bodies or more extensive eye injury. Referral to an ophthalmologist may be prudent, particularly for cases of more severe ocular trauma or iritis.

Upper respiratory symptoms are generally transient and should resolve without treatment. Occasionally lower tract toxicity may occur in patients with prolonged exposures. Patients with dyspnea can be treated with humidified oxygen, and those with bronchospasm or underlying reactive airway disease may benefit from β-2 agonist. Patients with prolonged dyspnea or chest tightness after a period of observation should be admitted and observed (31,32,35). Corticosteroids are of no proven benefit but may be considered for use in patients with moderate or severe toxicity. Accidental exposures in infants and neonates are potentially much more serious probably due to decreased protective reflexes and should be managed conservatively. Billmire et al. reported a case of an accidental exposure to pepper spray-induced respiratory failure in a 4 week old that was successfully treated with extracorporeal membrane oxygenation (ECMO) (42).

Dermal contamination should be treated similarly to other chemical burns with copious irrigation. An alkaline solution containing 6% sodium bicarbonate can hydrolyze CS and may be used as a decontaminating solution. Diluted Burrow's solution applied with moist dressings may be of some symptomatic relief. Cold silver nitrate has also been recommended (35). Allergic contact dermatitis should be treated with topical corticosteroids (31,41).

TRIAGE CONSIDERATIONS

A rapid priority in treating patients exposed to riot control agents is the safety of hospital staff and other victims. These patients should be taken to a well-ventilated area for decontamination as soon as possible to prevent secondary harm to staff or other patients.

PERSONAL PROTECTION

Standard universal precautions should be employed. Long sleeve gowns, rubber gloves, eye protection, and a well-fitted respiratory mask should be worn until the clothing has been removed and the patient has been properly decontaminated. A decontamination suite or a room with good ventilation should be used if possible to protect emergency personnel.

Riot Control Agents Summary

- All riot control agents may cause irritation to the skin and respiratory system.
- These agents are commonly used in police actions.
- In general, these agents have low morbidity and mortality, and the effects are short lived.
- Rapid decontamination is the removal and sealing of clothes.
- Wear protective clothing, and use a well-ventilated area.
- Thoroughly irrigate the eyes and skin.
- Humidified oxygen and beta-2 agonists may be beneficial in patients with severe respiratory symptoms.
- Skin exposures may benefit from dilute Burrow's solution compresses or corticosteroids for allergic contact dermatitis.
- Admit patients with prolonged respiratory symptoms and all infants with exposures.

OTHER AGENTS

LSD, THC, and phenothiazines have been tested in the past by the U.S. military and could theoretically be used as incapacitating agents (2). However, military experimentation has generally been considered unsuccessful. As a class, these common drugs are difficult to weaponize and can lead to unpredictable effects.

RESOURCES

1. Centers for Disease Control and Prevention
   http://www.bt.cdc.gov
2. National Library of Medicine and National Institute of Health Medlineplus
   http://www.nlm.nih.gov/medlineplus
   /biodefenseandbioterrorism.html
3. World Health Organization
   http://www.who.int
4. National Institute for Occupational Safety and Health
   http://www.cdc.gov/niosh/homepage.html

5. Agency for Toxic Substances and Disease Registry
   http://www.atsdr.cdc.gov/atsdrhome.html

QUESTIONS AND ANSWERS

1. **You are treating a 19-year-old police officer who responded to a crime scene and was exposed to an unknown aerosolized chemical agent one hour prior to presentation. He is one of several members in the unit who was not wearing a protective gas mask prior to the exposure. Your patient is disoriented, intermittently agitated, at times sedated, and exhibiting occasional random picking movements at his skin. His heart rate is 132 and his temperature is 41°C. During the exam, you note that his pupils are 4 mm, that his skin is somewhat warm to the touch, and that his axilla exhibits a lack of perspiration. His mucous membranes appear rather dry also. What is the most important initial therapeutic treatment for this patient?**
   A. Immediately administer atropine 2 mg IM, followed by haloperidol 5 mg IM, and then restrain the patient with a heavy bed sheet.
   B. The patient should be undressed, apply fans and misting to cool the patient off. Start IV fluids and administer benzodiazepines as needed for restraint and sedation. Physostigmine may then be given.
   C. One dose of physostigmine 2 mg IM is the only treatment needed.
   D. Give the patient a trial dose of naloxone and 1 g acetaminophen and then observe.
   E. Cover the patient with ice packs and bolus 2 liters of normal saline.

2. **The patient in the first question has responded well to the antidote and is now alert and oriented. The officer in charge would like to know whether he can take the officer back now that he has been treated. You tell him:**
   A. The patient is free to go, but must be watched closely and should return if the symptoms reoccur.
   B. The patient must be monitored in the hospital and treated with high-dose haloperidol as needed.
   C. The agent the patient was exposed to can last up to 3 days, and the symptoms will likely return so that the patient will need repeated doses of the antidote.
   D. The patient may now return to active duty, but he is to try and stay out of the heat.
   E. The patient needs to be observed in the ER for 6 more hours, if his symptoms do not return, he then is free to go.

3. **Which of the following lessons learned from the Chechnyan rebel hostage crisis is most valid?**
   A. Naloxone is a critical antidote that should not be overlooked when preparing hospitals for readiness against possible use of incapacitating agents.
   B. Sedative opiates, if not properly disseminated, can be associated with a high mortalilty rate.
   C. Consideration of proper ventilation in the target area should be done before using a calmative agent.

D. The therapeutic indices of 4-*n*-substituted fentanyl derivatives are in actuality high.

E. All of the above are correct.

4. A 42-year-old armed burglary suspect was subdued using oleoresin capsaicin. The police bring him in for evaluation of his complaints of shortness of breath. He complained earlier of stinging in the eyes, but he no longer has any visual complaints. He has a history significant for mild asthma. His vital signs are HR 112, RR 16, T 99.2°F, and O$_2$ sat of 98% on room air. On examination, he is anxious, and you auscultate a few faint wheezes, but his air exchange is good. You would do which of the following:

A. Order a chest X-ray, an arterial blood gas, and start him on oxygen, inhaled beta-2 agonist and administer a dose of physostigmine 2 mg IV.

B. After appropriate workup and treatment, call the hospitalist and get him admitted for observation.

C. Administer humidified oxygen, give one dose of a beta-2 agonist, and then reassess. If his condition improves, discharge the patient to the custody of the police.

D. After your exam, discharge the patient immediately since the ED is busy and this patient is obviously not very sick.

E. Order a 3% bicarbonate nebulized solution and then reassess the patient's symptoms in 20 minutes.

ANSWERS

1: *B.* *The patient in the first question was exposed to BZ. Initial treatment should be supportive. Hyperthermia from an anticholinergic should be treated aggressively with evaporation. Ice packs are not recommended. While physostigmine is the antidote of choice and would be indicated in this case, supportive care comes first. The correct dose of physostigmine is 1 to 2 mg IV/IM. Haloperidol may exacerbate the patient's hyperthermia and lower the seizure threshold and would be contraindicated for sedation. The patient does not exhibit signs of opioid intoxication and would not be expected to respond to naloxone.*

2: *C.* *BZ can last anywhere from 24 hours to about 3 days. Physostigmine is safe when used for BZ or any pure anticholinergic agent. The beneficial effects, however, do wear off, and the patient should be redosed every 6 hours to prevent relapse. Discharge after the patient recovers from the first dose would not be appropriate.*

3: *E.* *The rather novel use of what is thought to be carfentanil in Moscow raises awareness of the possibility of a sedative or calmative agents being used as an incapacitating agent. Many hospitals have inadequate doses to respond to an event like the one described above. Fentanyl derivatives have high safety margins; however, other problems such as ventilation and dispersal of equipotent doses as well as use of a second anesthetic gas may have been contributing factors in the tragic consequences.*

4: *C.* *Most exposures to riot control agents are benign, with the effects only lasting around 30 minutes. Exceptions do occur with the older agents that may still be around, such as corneal toxicity with Mace. People with underlying respiratory illnesses may be particularly susceptible to OC if exposed long enough, and a few deaths have occurred.*

Neonates and infants exposed are also at high risk and should be admitted for observation and treatment. The patient in our scenario does not manifest serious signs of pulmonary toxicity and should respond well to supportive treatment with beta-2 agonist and humidified oxygen. If symptoms were to persist, a period of inpatient observation is reasonable.

REFERENCES

1. Fitzgerald GM, Sole DP. CBRNE—incapacitating agents, Agent 15. In: White S, Talavera F, Darling RG, et al. eds. eMedicine.com, Inc.; 2001;2(10).

2. Carter M. Flying high for the US Army. New Sci. 1976;71 (1015):451.

3. Ketchum JS, Sidell RS. Incapacitating agents. In: Textbook of military medicine: medical aspects of chemical and biological warfare. Zajtchuck R, Bellamy RF, eds. Washington DC: Office of the Surgeon General, Department of the Army, USA, 1997. (www.vnh.org/MedAspChemBioWar)

4. Frontinu SJ, Bennet CH trans. The stategems. London: William Heineman; 1925. Cited in: Goodman E. The descriptive toxicology of atropine. Edgewood Arsenal, MD. Unpublished manuscript, 1961, and Zajtchuck R, Bellamy RF eds.Textbook of military medicine. Washington DC: Office of the Surgeon General; 1997.

5. Schultes R. Lecture 29—medicinal plants. In: BSCI 124 lecture notes. Undergraduate program in plant biology. University of Maryland, Oct. 16, 1998. (www.life.und.edu/classroom/bsci124/lec29.html)

6. Lewin, L. Die Gifte in der Weltgeschichte [Poisons in world history]. Berlin: Springer; 1920. Cited in: Goodman E. The descriptive toxicology of atropine. Edgewood Arsenal, MD. Unpublished manuscript, 1961, and Zajtchuck R, Bellamy RF, eds. Textbook of military medicine. Washington DC: Office of the Surgeon General; 1997.

7. Hay A. Surviving the impossible: the long march from Srebrenica: an investigation of the possible use of chemical warfare agents. Med Confl Surviv. 1998;14(2):120-55.

8. Suchard JR. Chemical and biologic weapons. In: Goldfrank L, Flomenbaum N, Lewin N, et al., eds. Goldfrank's toxicologic emergencies, 7th ed. New York: McGraw-Hill; 2002.

9. Burns M, Lindens C, Graudins A, Brown RM, Fletcher KE. A comparison of physostigmine and benzodiazepines for the treatment of anticholinergic poisoning. Ann Emerg Med. 2000;35(4):374-81.

10. Shannon M. Toxicology reviews: physostigmine. Pediat Emerg Care. 1998;14(3):224-25.

11. Daunderer M. Physostigmine salicylate as an antidote. Int J Clin Pharmacol Ther Toxicol. 1980;18(12):523-35.

12. Pentel P, Peterson CD. Asystole complicating physostigmine treatment of tricyclic antidepressant overdose. Ann Emerg Med. 1980;9(11):588-90.

13. Goldfrank L, Flomenbaum N, Lewin N. Anticholinergic poisoning. J Clin Toxicol. 1982;19(1):17-25.

14. Enserink M, Stone R. Questions swirl over knockout gas used in hostage crises. Science. November 8, 2002:1150-51.

15. Wax PM, Becker CE, Curry SC. Unexpected "gas" casualties in Moscow: a medical toxicology perspective. Ann Emerg Med. 2003;41(5):700-5.

16. National Journal Group. Russia: Theater gas was fentanyl, hostage death toll rises. NTI: Global Security Newswire. October 30, 2002.

17. Zilker T, Pfab R, Eyer F, von Meyer L. The mystery about the gas used for the release of the hostages in the Moscow musical theatre. J Toxicol Clin Tox. 2003;41(5): 661 (Abstract).

18. Borel JD. New narcotics in anesthesia. Contemp Anesth Pract. 1983;7:1-18.
19. Van Bever WFM, Niemegeers KHL, Janssen PAJ. N-4 Substituted 1-(2-Aryethel)-4-piperidinyl-*N*-phenylpropanamides. Arzneim-Forsch. 1976;26:1548-50.
20. Higgins M. Inhaled nebulised fentanyl for postoperative analgesia. Anaesthesia. 1991;46:973-6.
21. Worsley MH, Clark C. Inhaled fentanyl as a method of analgesia. Anaesthesia. 1990;45:449-51.
22. Haigh JC, Gates CC. Capture of wood bison (Bison bison athabascae) using carfentanil-based mixtures. J Wildl Dis. 1995;31(1):37-42.
23. Haigh JC, Lee LJ, Schweinsburg RE. Immobilization of polar bears with carfentanil. J Wildl Dis. 1983;19(2):140-4.
24. Jenkins SH. Carfentanil, bison, and statistics: the last word? J Wildl Dis. 1995;31(1):104-5.
25. Shaw M, Carpenter J, Leith D. Complications with the use of carfentanil citrate and xylazine hydrochloride to immobilize domestic horses. J Am Vet Med Assoc. 1995;206(6):833-6.
26. Hurlburt KM. Inhalational anesthetics. In: Dart RC, ed. Medical toxicology, 3rd ed. Philadelphia: Lippincott Williams & Wilkins; 2004, p 785.
27. Halothane. In: Poisindex, healthcare series, vol 120. Greenwood Village, CO: Thomson—Micromedex; 2004.
28. Miller M, Wild M, Lance W. Efficacy and safety of naltrexone hydrochloride for antagonizing carfentanil citrate immobilization in captive Rocky Mountain elk. J Wildl Dis. 1996;32(2):234-9.
29. SIPRI (Stockholm International Peace Research Institute). CB weapons today vol II—the problem of chemical and biological warfare: a study of the historical, technical, military, legal and political aspects of CBW, and possible disarmament measures. Almquist & Wiksell International, Stockholm, Sweden; 1973.
30. Beswick FW. Chemical agents used in riot control and warfare. Hum Toxicol. 1983;2(2):247-56.
31. Olajos EJ, Salem H. Riot control agents: pharmacology, toxicology, biochemistry and chemistry. J Appl Toxicol. 2001;21(5):355-91.
32. Smith J, Greaves I. The use of chemical incapacitant sprays: a review. J Trauma. 2002;52(3):595-600.
33. Loonam TM, Noailles PA, Yu J, et al. Substance P and cholecystokinin regulate neurochemical responses to cocaine and methamphetamine in the striatum. Life Sci. 2003;73(6):727-39.
34. Ulrich-Lai YM, Fraticelli AI, Engeland WC. Capsaicin-sensitive nerve fibers: a potential extra-ACTH mechanism participating in adrenal regeneration in rats. Microsc Res Technique. 2003;61(3):252-8.
35. Sidell FR. Riot control agents. In: Zajtchuk R, Bellamy RF, eds. Textbook of military medicine. Office of the Surgeon General, Department of the Army, USA, Washington, DC. 1997. (www.vnh.org/MedAspChemBioWar)
36. Scott RA. Treating CS gas injuries to the eye: illegal "mace" contains more toxic CN particles. Br Med J. 1995;311 (7009):871.
37. Gray P. Treating CS gas injuries to the eyes. Br Med J. 1995;311:871.
38. Delamanche S, Desforges P, Morio S, et al. Effect of oleoresin capsicum (OC) and ortho-chlorobenzylidene malononitrile (CS) on ciliary beat frequency. Toxicology. 2001;165 (2-3):79-85.
39. Vaca FE, Myers JH, Langdorf M. Delayed pulmonary edema and bronchospasm after accidental lacrimator exposure. Am J Emerg Med. 14(4):402-5, 1996.
40. Steffee CH, Lantz PE, Flannagan LM, et al. Oleoresin capsicum and "in custody deaths." Am J Forensic Med Pathol. 1995;16:185-92.
41. Goh CL. Allergic contact dermatitis to mace tear gas. Australas J Dermatol. 1987;28(3):115-6.
42. Billmire DF, Vinocur C, Ginda M, et al. Pepper-spray-induced respiratory failure treated with extracorporeal membrane oxygenation. Pediatrics. 1996;98(5):961-3.

Biological Agents

6

Anthrax

Anthony J. Carbone

NAME OF AGENT

Disease: Anthrax; Organism: *Bacillus anthracis*.

THEORETICAL AND SCIENTIFIC BACKGROUND

Anthrax is a zoonotic disease caused by the bacterium *Bacillus anthracis*. Its name is derived from a Greek word for coal, *anthrakis*, because the disease causes coal-like skin lesions in humans (Fig. 6-1) (1). The disease has been described since antiquity. The biblical fifth plague of ancient Egypt (circa 1500 B.C.) is believed to have been caused by anthrax (2). Virgil recorded a description of anthrax in 25 B.C. (3), and the disease was known as the "Black Bane" during the Middle Ages (4). Robert Koch used anthrax to demonstrate the microbial origin of disease in 1876 (5). Soon after, John Bell recognized *Bacillus anthracis* as the cause of woolsorter's disease (inhalational anthrax) and was instrumental in establishing wool disinfection procedures, dramatically reducing the incidence of occupational disease (6). Anthrax is also the first disease after smallpox for which an effective vaccine was developed [by William Greenfield in 1880 (7), followed by Louis Pasteur's heat-cured vaccine in 1881 (8)].

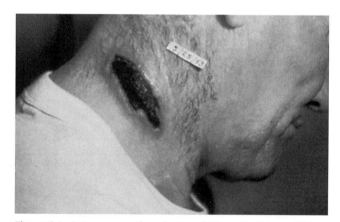

Figure 6-1. Cutaneous anthrax lesion of the neck. Source: CDC-PHIL, date unknown.

EPIDEMIOLOGY OF NATURALLY OCCURRING ANTHRAX

Anthrax is a naturally occurring disease that affects herbivores (primarily cattle, sheep, and goats) that become infected after grazing on soil contaminated with *B. anthracis* spores (9). The animals develop gastrointestinal anthrax followed by systemic dissemination and death (1). Humans generally acquire the disease following contact with anthrax-infected animals or contaminated animal products. Human-to-human transmission has not been described (2,9,10,12).

Anthrax occurs globally and is most common in agricultural regions with inadequate anthrax control programs for livestock. The disease has been reported in over 80 countries. Human cases are rare, but they have been reported in Africa, the Middle East, Asia, Southern and Eastern Europe, the Caribbean, and the Americas (13,14). Cutaneous anthrax is the most common naturally occurring form of anthrax with an estimated 2,000 cases annually worldwide (11). Turkey reports over 400 human cases annually, mostly in the form of cutaneous anthrax (15). The United States experiences rare outbreaks in cattle along the "anthrax belt" of the Great Plains and reported only six human cases between 1988 and 2001 (16,17). Inhalational anthrax is rare with only 18 cases reported in the United States during the 20th century; most of these cases were attributed to occupational exposure among goat hair mill and wool or tannery workers (18,19). The largest reported epidemic of human anthrax occurred in Zimbabwe with over 6,000 cases, virtually all cutaneous, with approximately 100 fatalities reported between 1978 and 1980. The outbreak was attributed to a lapse of established public health and veterinary practices during the Rhodesian Civil War (12,20). Gastrointestinal anthrax is uncommon, but probably underreported. Outbreaks of gastrointestinal anthrax are continually reported in Africa and Asia following ingestion of insufficiently cooked contaminated meat (2).

Deliberate Transmission

Anthrax has long been recognized as a potential biological weapon. The Japanese Imperial Army experimented with anthrax on prisoners of war and Chinese civilians during World War II (21,22). The U.S. military weaponized anthrax spores in the 1950s and 1960s before its offensive biological weapons program was terminated (23). The Soviet Union produced and stockpiled thousands of tons of weaponized anthrax beginning in 1973 and continuing until the fall of the Soviet Union in 1991 (24). One Soviet biological weapons factory, located in Sverdlovsk, USSR (present day Ekaterinburg, Russia), accidentally released a small amount of militarized anthrax spores in 1979, resulting in 68 reported fatalities. Soviet officials claimed the fatalities were due to gastrointestinal anthrax from tainted meat; however, local pathologists identified the causes of death as inhalational anthrax on autopsy (25–29). In 1995, Iraq admitted to having produced 8,500 liters of anthrax but declared that they destroyed all biological weapons shortly after the start of the Persian Gulf War in 1991 (30,31). The Japanese cult Aum Shinrikyo sprayed anthrax from the rooftop of their Tokyo headquarters in 1993 in an act of terrorism, which failed because the group unwittingly used a benign vaccine strain (32,33). In September 2001, an unknown terrorist mailed threatening letters containing anthrax spores to television news anchor Tom Brokaw, and U.S. Senators Tom Daschle and Patrick Leahy, through the U.S. Postal Service. When it was over, 23 individuals had contracted anthrax—10 with inhalational anthrax and the remainder with cutaneous anthrax. Five of the 23 (22%) victims died as a result of the anthrax infection; all five had been diagnosed with inhalational anthrax (34–37).

Microbiology

Bacillus anthracis is an aerobic, spore-forming, nonmotile, encapsulated, gram-positive rod (Fig. 6-2). The natural reservoir for *B. anthracis* is the soil in the spore form of the organism. Anthrax spores germinate into vegetative bacilli when they enter an environment that is rich in amino acids, nucleoside, and glucose, as is found in the blood and tissues of hosts. The vegetative bacilli will form spores when nutrients have been exhausted or when the environment is exposed to ambient air (38,39). Vegetative bacteria cannot survive outside of an animal or human host, whereas the *B. anthracis* spore is extremely hardy and has been known to survive in soil for decades (40). The vegetative cell is large, measuring 1 to 10 μm by 1 to 1.5 μm. Anthrax spores measure approximately 1 μm (Fig. 6-3). *B. anthracis* readily grows aerobically on sheep blood agar and is nonhemolytic under these conditions (2). The colonies are large (4 to 5 mm), rough, grayish-white, with a swirling "comet-tail" or "curled-hair" appearance (Fig. 6-4). Several laboratory tests are used to differentiate virulent *B. anthracis* strains from other innocuous *Bacillus* species. Unlike other *Bacillus* species (*B. subtillus* and *B. cereus,*) *B. anthracis* is characterized by the absence of hemolysis, motility, growth on phenylethyl alcohol blood agar, gelatin hydrolysis, and salicin fermentation (1,9,48). Microbiologists should be warned of the possibility of *B. anthracis* in order to run special tests on *Bacillus* species to rule

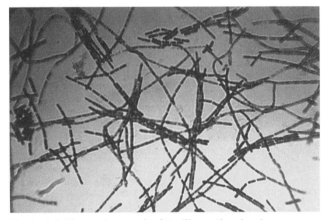

Figure 6–2. Photomicrograph of *Bacillus anthracis* using Gram stain technique. Source: CDC-PHIL, date unknown.

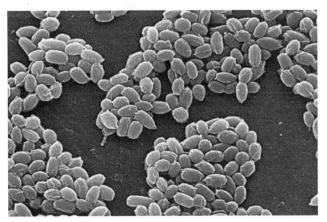

Figure 6–3. An electron micrograph of spores from the Sterne strain of *Bacillus anthracis* bacteria. Source: CDC-PHIL, 2002.

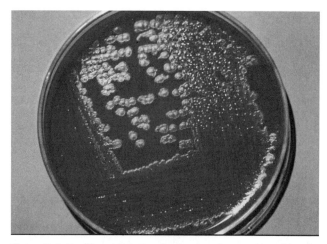

Figure 6–4. *Bacillus anthracis* colonies growing on sheep blood agar. Note that some colonies demonstrate the classic "comet-tailed" swirled appearance. Source: CDC-PHIL, date unknown.

out anthrax and to ensure that tests are processed under Biosafety Level 2 (BSL2) conditions.

Pathogenesis

Anthrax infections are nearly always fatal in animals, but they are not always fatal in humans. Anthrax spores enter the body by inhalation, ingestion, or breaks in the skin where they are phagocytosed by macrophages and carried via lymphatics to regional lymph nodes. The endospores germinate inside the macrophages and become vegetative bacteria. Vegetative bacteria are then released from the macrophages where they multiply in the lymphatic system and enter the bloodstream resulting in massive septicemia (41). The vegetative bacilli express virulence factors that lead to death of the host. The principle virulence factors for *B. anthracis* are encoded on two plasmids—one involved in the synthesis of an antiphagocytic polypeptide capsule, and the other containing the genes for the synthesis of three proteins it secretes: Protective Antigen (PA), Edema Factor (EF), and Lethal Factor (LF) (1,41,42). Individually these proteins are not cytotoxic; however the combination of PA with LF or EF results in formation of the binary cytotoxins, lethal toxin, and edema toxin, respectively. The PA permits the binding of lethal toxin and edema toxin to the host cell membrane and facilitates their transport across the cell membrane (43). Edema toxin inhibits the neutrophil function and is responsible for the formation of the prominent edema found in anthrax lesions (44,45). Lethal toxin attacks macrophages resulting in the production of reactive oxygen species and the release of the cytokines, tumor necrosis factor-α and interleukin-1α, which lead to shock and sudden death in appropriate concentrations (1,46–48).

Clinical forms of anthrax

Anthrax manifests itself in three major clinical forms depending upon the route of exposure: cutaneous, gastrointestinal, and inhalational anthrax. Ninety-five percent of human cases of anthrax are reported as cutaneous (1,2,48). The remaining cases tend to be inhalational from occupational exposure to contaminated animals and animal products. Gastrointestinal anthrax is rare, and no cases have been reported in the United States (49). Symptoms and incubation periods vary depending on the route of transmission and the size of the inoculum. In general, symptoms appear within 1 to 7 days of exposure but may develop within hours following a large inoculum; however, it could be as long as 60 days (1,41).

Cutaneous Anthrax. Cutaneous anthrax results from handling contaminated animal tissue or products. Anthrax spores enter the skin through small cuts and abrasions, germinate to the bacillary form, and multiply. Germination takes place in macrophages, and toxins release results in edema and tissue necrosis, with little or no purulence (1). Cutaneous anthrax usually remains local, although if untreated, the disease enters the lymphatics and becomes systemic in 5% to 20% of cases (50). Cutaneous anthrax has a mortality rate of 10% to 20% for untreated cases and is usually less than 1% with treatment (1,2).

Gastrointestinal Anthrax. Gastrointestinal anthrax is the least common, or more likely, the least reported of the three clinical forms of anthrax. Gastrointestinal anthrax is contracted after eating meat contaminated with *B. anthracis* spores. The spores can infect the system anywhere along the gastrointestinal tract and cause two distinct syndromes based upon the primary site of infection: abdominal and oropharyngeal anthrax. Autopsies suggest that the initial site of infection is most commonly the terminal ileum or cecum (28). The spores germinate into the vegetative form and migrate to the mesenteric and other regional lymph nodes. The bacilli multiply in the lymph nodes resulting in bacteremia and death. The case fatality rate for gastrointestinal anthrax is not precisely known, but it is estimated to be 25% to 60% (9,51). Gastrointestinal anthrax could potentially be the result of an act of bioterrorism. The Japanese Imperial Army's secret biological warfare program attempted to poison children with chocolate tainted with anthrax spores during World War II (52). The apartheid government of South Africa was found to have developed biological weapons and attempted to poison children with anthrax-containing chocolate (53).

Inhalational Anthrax. Inhalational anthrax develops after the deposition of spore-bearing particles, measuring 1 to 5 μm, into alveolar spaces. The minimum infectious inhaled dose for anthrax is not known for humans, but in nonhuman primate studies it has ranged from 2,500 to 80,000 spores (18,54,55). Inhaled spores are ingested by pulmonary macrophages and are carried to hilar and mediastinal lymph nodes where they germinate and multiply. Although the lung is the initial site of deposition of spores, typical bronchopneumonia does not occur with inhalational anthrax. Instead, multiplying bacilli in the hilar and mediastinal lymph nodes release toxins producing hemorrhagic mediastinitis (27,41). Systemic disease results when bacilli release toxins into the bloodstream causing systemic hemorrhage, edema, and necrosis. The mortality rate for untreated inhalational anthrax reaches 100%. The mortality rate can be reduced if appropriate antibiotic therapy is initiated within 48 hours of exposure, but it may still be as high as 90% (1,2,23,48). The mortality rate for the 2001 anthrax attack was 45% with therapy (10,36).

SIGNS AND SYMPTOMS

Cutaneous Anthrax. Cutaneous anthrax is painless, does not involve a disseminated rash, and results in a localized black eschar that gives the disease its name. Cutaneous anthrax usually occurs following the deposition of spores into skin with previous cuts or abrasions (9,11,56). Areas of exposed skin, such as the hands, arms, face, and neck, are the most frequently affected. Of the victims of the 2001 anthrax attacks who contracted cutaneous anthrax, skin trauma was not noted (57). The incubation period for cutaneous anthrax ranges from 1 to 12 days, but it usually develops within a day (2,11,26). The primary lesion is a painless, pruritic macule or papule resembling an insect bite that develops at the site of infiltration. The lesions enlarge, vesiculate, and often become hemorrhagic. By the second day, the vesicle usually ruptures to form a round, depressed ulcer. Within 1 to 2 days, smaller (1- to 3-mm) satellite vesicular lesions often surround the papule. These lesions are nonpurulent and contain clear or serosanguinous fluid that reveals numerous large bacilli on Gram stain. A painless, depressed, black eschar forms over the lesion and is often associated with significant localized, gelatinous, nonpitting edema. The edema may become massive, especially with lesions involving the face and neck. The eschar dries and falls off within the next 1 to 2 weeks, often without leaving a permanent scar. Lymphangitis and painful lymphadenopathy are often present with associated systemic symptoms. Antibiotic therapy does not appear to change the development of the skin lesion and eventual eschar, but it does decrease the incidence of systemic disease (11). The mortality rate without antibiotics is as high as 20% due to systemic complications. Death with appropriate antibiotic therapy is rare. The differential diagnosis of ulceroglandular lesions includes anti-phospholipid antibody syndrome, brown recluse spider bite, coumadin/heparin necrosis, cutaneous leishmaniasis, cutaneous tuberculosis, ecthyma gangrenosum, glanders, leprosy, mucormycosis, orf, plague, rat bite fever, rickettsial pox, staphylococcal/streptococcal ecthyma, tropical ulcer, tularemia, and typhus. The differential diagnosis for ulceroglandular syndromes includes cat scratch fever, chancroid, glanders, herpes simplex infection, lymphogranuloma venereum, melioidosis, plague, staphylococcal and streptococcal adenitis, tuberculosis, and tularemia (58).

Gastrointestinal Anthrax. Gastrointestinal anthrax develops after eating insufficiently cooked meat contaminated with large numbers of vegetative anthrax bacilli or spores and includes two distinct syndromes: abdominal and oropharyngeal anthrax (11). The symptoms of gastrointestinal anthrax appear 1 to 7 days after ingesting contaminated food and depend upon the site of infection along the alimentary canal.

Abdominal anthrax. The disease usually presents with fever, malaise, nausea, vomiting, and anorexia. The disease rapidly progresses to severe, bloody diarrhea and signs suggestive of acute abdomen and/or sepsis (1,48,56,59–61). The primary intestinal lesions are ulcerative and usually occur in the terminal ileum or cecum (62). Gastric ulcers may be associated with hematemesis or coffee-ground emesis (48). Constipation and diarrhea have both been described, and

stools are usually melenic or blood-tinged (41). Hemorrhagic mesenteric lymphadenitis and massive ascites are often present (60). Advanced disease may be similar to the sepsis syndrome occurring in late inhalational and cutaneous anthrax. Morbidity is due to blood loss, fluid and electrolyte imbalances, or subsequent shock. Death from intestinal perforation or toxemia occurs 2 to 5 days after the onset of disease (41). Early diagnosis of gastrointestinal anthrax is difficult and mortality may be greater than 50% (62).

Oropharyngeal anthrax. Deposition and germination of spores in the oropharynx result in a subset of gastrointestinal anthrax known as oropharyngeal anthrax. Patients present complaining of a severe sore throat, fever, dysphagia, and occasionally respiratory distress (21,48). Other clinical features include toxemia, inflammatory lesions of the oral cavity or oropharynx, and marked cervical lymphadenopathy with edema of the soft tissues of the cervical area (62). Swelling may be severe enough to compromise the airway. In an outbreak of anthrax in April 1982 in northern Thailand, 24 cases of oropharyngeal anthrax were reported (63). All of the afflicted had recently eaten water buffalo meat. All but one required hospitalization, and three of the 24 (12.4%) patients died despite hospitalization and antibiotic therapy (64). All of the patients sought medical attention because of painful neck swelling, and all but one complained of fever. Other common symptoms included sore throat, dysphagia, and hoarseness. The neck swelling was due to marked cervical lymphadenopathy and soft tissue edema. Early lesions are edematous. Within 7 days, central necrosis and ulceration develop and form whitish patches. By the second week, the patch develop into a pseudomembrane covering the ulcer similar to diphtheria (62).

Inhalational Anthrax. The classic clinical course of inhalational anthrax is one of a biphasic illness. The incubation period for inhalational anthrax typically ranges from 1 to 7 days, but may develop as quickly as hours or as long as 60 days following exposure depending upon the size of the inoculum (1,2,11,27,41). The initial phase begins with a nonspecific illness characterized by fever, chills, headache, malaise, myalgias, weakness, nonproductive cough, and some chest and/or abdominal discomfort and may last from hours to a few days (2,11,18,57,65). The initial phase may be followed by a short latent period lasting hours to a few days. The second phase manifests abruptly with sudden high fever, diaphoresis, acute dyspnea, cyanosis, chest discomfort, and shock (1,2,26–28,41). Stridor may be present due to extrinsic obstruction of the trachea by lymphadenopathy, mediastinal widening, and subcutaneous edema of the chest and neck (11). The disease progresses rapidly with hypotension, hypothermia, shock, and death occurring within 24 to 36 hours. The differential diagnosis for inhalational anthrax includes influenza and influenza-like illnesses from other causes. The CDC has published the results of a study comparing signs and symptoms of patients diagnosed with inhalational anthrax, laboratory-confirmed influenza, and influenza-like illnesses from other causes (66). In this study, sore throat and rhinorrhea were common in influenza and influenza-like illnesses, whereas they were rare in inhalational anthrax (sore throat—20%, rhinorrhea—10%). Shortness of breath was prevalent in the patients with inhalational anthrax (80%) compared to only 8% in influenza, and 6% for influenza-like illnesses from other causes. Chest discomfort or pleuritic chest pain was present in 80% of the anthrax patients and 35% of the influenza patients but only 23% of those suffering from influenza-like illnesses other than influenza (66).

Anthrax Meningitis. Hemorrhagic meningitis occurs in approximately 50% of inhalational anthrax cases and is believed to develop as a result of the frank bacteremia (1,2,11, 26–28,41). Patients with anthrax meningitis are indistinguishable from other forms of meningitis with patients exhibiting meningismus, delirium, and obtundation (1,2,11, 26–28,41). The cerebrospinal fluid is hemorrhagic in most cases, and polymorphonuclear pleocytosis is present. Numerous large, encapsulated, gram-positive bacilli are seen under microscopy. Anthrax meningitis is almost always fatal, despite intensive antibiotic therapy, with death occurring 1 to 6 days after onset of illness (41).

LABORATORY STUDIES

Routine blood studies are nonspecific and do not aid the diagnosis. Physiologic sequelae of severe anthrax infection in animal studies include profound hypoglycemia, hypocalcemia, hyperkalemia, respiratory acidosis, and terminal acidosis (11). One of the more useful diagnostic tests is the standard aerobic blood culture, which should grow in 6 to 24 hours (67). If laboratory personnel have been notified of the suspicion of anthrax, biochemical testing and colony morphology should provide a preliminary diagnosis in 12 to 24 hours (11). If cutaneous anthrax is suspected, a Gram stain and culture of vesicular fluid should confirm the diagnosis (11). Sputum Gram stain and culture are not likely to be diagnostic given the lack of a pneumonic process with inhalational anthrax (40). A peripheral blood smear should reveal gram-positive bacilli with systemic anthrax if antibiotic therapy has not been initiated. Immunohistochemical examination of fluid or tissue specimens with direct fluorescence assay (DFA) staining for the polysaccharide cell wall and capsule of *B. anthracis* will confirm the diagnosis (Fig. 6-5) (11). Various advanced detection methodologies, such as time-resolved fluorescence (TRF) and polymerase chain reaction (PCR) are available at designated Laboratory Response Network (LRN) reference laboratories. Table 6-1 below was published by the Centers for Disease Control and Prevention to clarify which diagnostic tests for anthrax are available at various levels of the LRN (68).

Radiographic studies

Radiographic studies should prove quite useful in diagnosing inhalational anthrax, although signs often appear late in active disease. The appearance of a widened mediastinum in a previously healthy patient with fever, myalgias, or dyspnea should suggest the diagnosis of inhalation anthrax (Fig. 6-6) (69,70). Some patients present with the additional finding of (hemorrhagic) pleural effusions, air bronchograms, and/or consolidation (57). The differential diagnosis of mediastinal widening includes normal variant (fat or tortuous vessel), aneurysm, histoplasmosis, sarcoidosis, tuberculosis, and lymphoma (11). In the anthrax attacks of 2001, radiographic studies were key in making the diagnosis of inhalational anthrax. Each of the first ten patients had abnormal chest x-rays, and the eight patients who received chest computed tomographs (CTs) had abnormal results. CT imaging may reveal hy-

perdense hilar and mediastinal adenopathy, mediastinal edema, infiltrates, and pleural effusion (11).

Postmortem examination

A diagnosis of inhalational anthrax may be made on postmortem examination if hemorrhagic necrotizing thoracic lymphadenitis or mediastinitis are found in a previously healthy

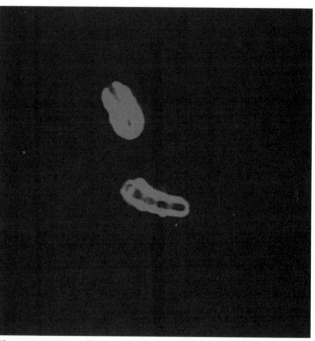

Figure 6–5. Direct fluorescent antibody (DFA) stain of *B. anthracis* capsule at 1,000X magnification. Source: CDC-PHIL, 2002.

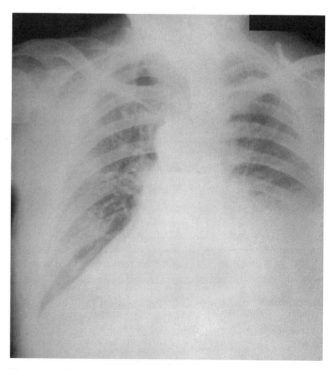

Figure 6–6. Posteroanterior chest radiograph of inhalational anthrax patient showing widened mediastinum on the 4th day of illness. Source: CDC-PHIL, 1966.

TABLE 6-1 Approved Tests for the Detection of *Bacillus antracis* in the Laboratory Response Network

	LABORATORY LEVEL			
TEST PROCEDURE	**A**	**B**	**C**	**D**
Gram stain (micromorphology)	X	x	X	x
Capsule (microscopic observation)	X	x	X	x
Routine culture:				
1. Colonial morphology	X	x	X	x
2. Hemolysis	X	x	X	x
3. Motility	X	x	X	x
4. Sporulation (microscopic observation)	X	x	X	x
Confirmatory tests:				
1. Lysis by gamma-phage	○	x	X	x
2. Direct fluorescence assay (polysaccharide cell wall and capsule)	○	x	X	x
3. Antimicrobial susceptibility testing	○	○	X	x
4. Advanced technology (e.g., time-resolved fluorescence testing, polymerase chain reaction testing)	○	○	X	x
5. Molecular characterization	○	○	○	x

Gram stain
Routine staining procedure for observation of bacterial micromorphology.

Capsule
In Level A laboratories, *India ink* may be used to visualize encapsulated *B. anthracis* in clinical specimens by direct examination of peripheral blood, cerebrospinal fluid, or cells grown on media supplemented with sodium bicarbonate. *M'Fadyean stain* (Level B) and *DFA for capsular antigen* (Level B) may also be employed. Note that some avirulent strains, such as the veterinary vaccine Sterne strain, do not produce the capsule.

Routine culture
Standard 5% sheep blood agar (SBA) and chocolate agar will support growth. *B. anthracis* will not grow on MacConkey agar.

Colonial morphology
On SBA, after 15 to 24 hours incubation at 35° to 37°C, well-isolated colonies are 2 to 5 mm in diameter. The flat or slightly convex colonies are irregularly round, with edges that are slightly undulate (irregular, wavy border), and have a *ground-glass appearance*. Colonies typically have a tenacious consistency; that is, teasing with an inoculating loop causes colony to "stand up" like beaten egg white.

Hemolysis
Colonies of *B. anthracis* are *nonhemolytic*. However, weak hemolysis may be observed under areas of confluent growth in aging cultures and should not be confused with beta-hemolysis.

Motility
B. anthracis is nonmotile. Working in a biological safety cabinet (BSC) with gloves, prepare routine *wet mount* and observe microscopically. Alternatively, *motility test medium* may be used.

Sporulation
Spores will appear in a growing culture after 18 to 24 hours of incubation at 35° to 37° C in a non-CO$_2$, atmosphere. *Oval, central to sub-terminal* spores that do not appreciably swell may be observed by *Gram stain* (Level A), *wet mount* (Level B), or *malachite green stain* (Level B).

Lysis by gamma-phage
Highly specific for *B. anthracis*, and when demonstrated concomitantly with the presence of a *capsule*, provides confirmatory identification.

Direct fluorescence assay
Used to detect the galactose/*N*-acetylglucosamaine cell-wall-associated polysaccharide and capsule produced by vegetative cells of *B. anthracis* strains. *Concomitant* demonstration of both antigens provides confirmatory identification.

Antimicrobial susceptibility testing
An array of selected antimicrobics is used to determine their respective minimum inhibitory concentrations using standardized methods against *B. anthracis*.

Advanced technology
Various advanced detection methodologies include time-resolved fluorescence (TRF), polymerase chain reaction (PCR), etc. These may have future applications within the LRN laboratories.

Molecular characterization
Various tests to determine the molecular characteristics of isolates are done. These include molecular subtyping using multi-locus variable-number tandem repeat analysis (MLVA), sequencing of genes coding for 16S ribosomal RNA.

Serologic tests for potential exposure to *B. anthracis* are currently being validated and at this time their clinical utility is not known.

From U.S. Centers for Disease Control and Prevention web site. Approved tests for the detection of *Bacillus anthracis* in the Laboratory Response Network (LRN). Available at: http://www.bt.cdc.gov/documentsapp/Anthrax/ApprovedLRNTests.asp. Last accessed on January 6, 2004.

adult (27). Hemorrhagic meningitis should also raise strong suspicions of systemic anthrax infection (2,27,71). DFA staining of infected tissues should be diagnostic for the polysaccharide cell wall and capsule of *B. anthracis* (11).

MEDICAL MANAGEMENT

NOTIFICATION

The U.S. Public Health Service requires that all suspected cases of anthrax be reported to local and state health departments, and that the diagnosis be confirmed by the Centers for Disease Control and Prevention or other LRN reference laboratories (11). If available, consult with hospital infectious disease and infection control services for the latest recommendations on the care of patients with anthrax.

ISOLATION

Isolation is *not required* for patients suspected of having an anthrax infection because there is no data to suggest the disease is contagious (1,2,11,23,26,41).

LABORATORY SPECIMENS

Blood, sputum, cerebral spinal fluid, pleural effusion, and stool or wound specimens should be taken for laboratory study as indicated by the clinical presentation *before* initiating antibiotic therapy. Nasal swab testing for anthrax spores may be used for epidemiological data but should not be used to rule out disease or exposure (11,36). Laboratory personnel should be notified of the possibility of *B. anthracis* so that steps are taken not to regard *Bacillus* species as benign and to ensure specimens are processed in a minimum of a BSL2 (72).

ANTIBIOTIC TREATMENT

Recommendations for antibiotic treatment of anthrax in this chapter are based on the comprehensive evaluation made by the Working Group on Civilian Biodefense as published in the *Journal of the American Medical Association* entitled, "Anthrax as a Biological Weapon: Medical and Public Health Management," commonly referred to as the JAMA Consensus Statement on Anthrax (10). The Working Group was comprised of experts on biological warfare from the Center for Civilian Biodefense Studies at Johns Hopkins, including Thomas V. Inglesby, D.A. Henderson, and Tara O'Toole; specialists such as David T. Dennis from the Centers for Disease Control and Prevention; and Edward Eitzen, Arthur M. Friedlander, and Gerald Parker from the U.S. Army Medical Research Institute of Infectious Diseases (USAMRIID) (10). The Working Group published an update of recommendations for management following the anthrax attacks of 2001 (11). The regimens stated here are based upon the recommendations of both consensus statements and the Centers for Disease Control and Prevention. Although these recommendations were based upon the evaluation of the most up-to-date studies available at the time, final selection of antibiotic therapy should be made based upon the clini-

cal situation and the most current medical information available. This author recommends verifying antibiotic selection with available local infectious disease specialists and public health authorities as well as those at the Centers for Disease Control and Prevention (CDC). Links to these sources are provided at the end of this chapter. Adjustments to antibiotic coverage should be made based upon antibiotic susceptibility testing of cultures taken from the patient prior to initiation of therapy (11).

The CDC recommendations for treatment of inhalational/ gastrointestinal and cutaneous anthrax are provided in Tables 6-2 and 6-3 (36). In general, the *treatment of choice for anthrax is ciprofloxacin or doxycycline for 60 days duration.* Note that distinctions have been made between *contained casualty* settings, *mass casualty settings,* and postexposure prophylaxis. A contained casualty setting is one in which a modest number of patients require treatment. In such a setting, parenteral antibiotic therapy is optimal. However, in the event of a deliberate act using aerosolized anthrax spores resulting in mass casualties, there will most likely be a shortage of intravenous antibiotics, equipment, and hospital beds. In such a setting, recommendations for oral antibiotic therapies are provided. It remains unclear whether the use of two or more antibiotics provides a survival advantage; however, combination therapy is a very reasonable treatment option in the face of life-threatening disease or when the possibility of a genetically engineered multidrug-resistant strain exists (10,11). When anthrax meningitis is suspected, infectious disease specialists recommend using intravenous ciprofloxacin augmented with chloramphenicol, rifampin, or penicillin (10,11). Doxycycline should not be used if meningitis is suspected because of its lack of adequate central nervous system penetration (57). Extended-spectrum cephalosporins and trimethoprim/sulfamethoxazole should not be used due to potential drug resistance.

PREGNANT WOMEN

The CDC and the Working Group recommend that pregnant women suspected of having anthrax be treated with the same regimen for nonpregnant adults—ciprofloxacin 400 mg IV bid in combination therapy for a contained attack, and 400 mg orally every 12 hours for mass casualty settings and postexposure prophylaxis (11,75). If susceptibility testing allows, amoxicillin 500 mg three times a day for 60 days may be substituted. Available data indicate that ciprofloxacin use during pregnancy is unlikely to be associated with high risk for fetal malformation or teratogenesis risk. Penicillins are generally considered safe for use during pregnancy and should be substituted if susceptibility testing indicates. The use of doxycycline during pregnancy poses risks of liver toxicity in pregnant women and fetal dental and bone defects and, therefore, should be reserved for situations where use of other antibiotics is not feasible (11,35).

BREASTFEEDING

Ciprofloxacin (and other fluoroquinolones), doxycycline (and other tetracyclines), and penicillin are secreted in breast milk. Therefore, a breastfeeding woman should be treated or receive prophylaxis using the same antibiotic recommended for her infant based on the current pediatric guidelines (11,76). Again, if susceptibility testing allows, switch breastfeeding mother to penicillin.

CHILDREN

Ciprofloxacin and other fluoroquinolones are generally avoided in children younger than 16 years because of a risk of permanent arthropathy in adolescent animals and transient arthropathy in a small number of children. However, given the risk of anthrax from a genetically engineered strain of *B. anthracis*, the Working Group recommends that ciprofloxacin be used as part of combination therapy in children with inhalational anthrax (10,11,76). The same holds true for doxycycline, which has been shown to retard skeletal growth in infants and to discolor teeth in infants and children. The Working Group recommends using doxycycline in children if antibiotic susceptibility testing, exhaustion of drug supplies, or adverse reactions preclude the use of ciprofloxacin (10,11,76). If susceptibility testing permits, amoxicillin should be used preferentially in children. The current anthrax vaccine is licensed for use in persons aged 18 to 65 years based on studies conducted on this age group (79). No similar studies exist in children; however, based on experiences with other inactivated vaccines, it is likely that the vaccine would be safe and effective in children (Tables 6-2 and 6-3) (10,11).

TABLE 6-2 Inhalational Anthrax Treatment Protocol[a,b] for Cases Associated with this Bioterrorism Attack

CATEGORY	INITIAL THERAPY (INTRAVENOUS)[c,d]	DURATION
Adults	Ciprofloxacin 400 mg every 12 h[a] **or** Doxycycline 100 mg every 12 h[f] **and** One or two additional antimicrobials[d]	IV treatment initially[e]. Switch to oral antimicrobial therapy when clinically appropriate: Ciprofloxacin 500 mg PO BID **or** Doxycycline 100 mg PO BID Continue for 60 days (IV and PO combined)[g]
Children	Ciprofloxacin 10–15 mg/kg every 12 h[h,i] **or** Doxycycline:[a,i] >8 yr and >45 kg: 100 mg every 12 h >8 yr and ≤45kg: 2.2 mg/kg every 12 h ≤8 yr: 2.2 mg/kg every 12 h **and** One or two additional antimicrobials[d]	IV treatment initially[e]. Switch to oral antimicrobial therapy when clinically appropriate: Ciprofloxacin 10–15 mg/kg PO every 12 h[i] **or** Doxycycline.[j] >8 yr and >45 kg: 100 mg PO BID >8 yr and ≤45 kg: 2.2 mg/kg PO BID ≤8 yr: 2.2 mg/kg PO BID Continue for 60 days (IV and PO combined)[g]
Pregnant Women[k]	Same for nonpregnant adults (the high death rate from the infection outweighs the risk posed by the antimicrobial agent)	IV treatment initially. Switch to oral antimicrobial therapy when clinically appropriate.[b] Oral therapy regimens same for nonpregnant adults.
Immunocompromised persons	Same for nonimmunocompromised persons and children	Same for nonimmunocompromised persons and children.

[a] For gastrointestinal and oropharyngeal anthrax, use regimens recommended for inhalational anthrax.

[b] Ciprofloxacin or doxycycline should be considered an essential part of first-line therapy for inhalational anthrax.

[c] Steroids may be considered as an adjunct therapy for patients with severe edema and for meningitis based on experience with bacterial meningitis of other etiologies.

[d] Other agents with in vitro activity include rifampin, vancomycin, penicillin, ampicillin, chloramphenicol, imipenem, clindamycin, and clarithromycin. Because of concerns of constitutive and inducible beta-lactamases in *Bacillus anthracis*, penicillin and ampicillin should not be used alone. Consultation with an infectious disease specialist is advised.

[e] Initial therapy may be altered based on clinical course of the patient; one or two antimicrobial agents (e.g., ciprofloxacin or doxycycline) may be adequate as the patient improves.

[f] If meningitis is suspected, doxycycline may be less optimal because of poor central nervous system penetration.

[g] Because of the potential persistence of spores after an aerosol exposure, antimicrobial therapy should be continued for 60 days.

[h] If intravenous ciprofloxacin is not available, oral ciprofloxacin may be acceptable because it is rapidly and well absorbed from the gastrointestinal tract with no substantial loss by first-pass metabolism. Maximum serum concentrations are attained 1–2 h after oral dosing, but may not be achieved if vomiting or ileus are present.

[i] In children, ciprofloxacin dosage should not exceed 1 g/day.

[j] The American Academy of Pediatrics recommends treatment of young children with tetracyclines for serious infections, (e.g,. Rocky Mountain spotted fever).

[k] Although tetracyclines are not recommended during pregnancy, their use may be indicated for life-threatening illness. Adverse effects on developing teeth and bones are dose related; therefore, doxycycline might be used for a short time (7–14 days) before 6 months of gestation.

From U.S. Centers for Disease Control and Prevention. Symptoms and signs of inhalational anthrax, laboratory-confirmed influenza, and influenza-like illness (ILI) from other causes. Notice to readers: considerations for distinguishing influenza-like illness from inhalational anthrax. MMWR. 9 November 2001:50(44);984–86.

TABLE 6-3 Cutaneous Anthrax Treatment Protocol[a] for Cases Associated with this Bioterrorism Attack

CATEGORY	INITIAL THERAPY (ORAL)[b]	DURATION
Adults[a]	Ciprofloxacin 500 mg BID **or** Doxycycline 100 mg BID	60 days[c]
Children[a]	Ciprofloxacin 10–15 mg/kg every 12 h (not to exceed 1 g/day)[b] **or** Doxycycline:[d] >8 yr and >45 kg: 100 mg every 12 h >8 yr and ≤45 kg: 2.2 mg/kg every 12 h ≤8 yr: 2.2 mg/kg every 12 h	60 days[c]
Pregnant Women[a,e]	Ciprofloxacin 500 mg BID **or** Doxycycline 100 mg BID	60 days[c]
Immunocompromised persons[a]	Same for nonimmunocompromised persons and children	60 days[c]

[a] Cutaneous anthrax with signs of systemic involvement, extensive edema, or lesions on the head or neck require intravenous therapy, and a multidrug approach is recommended.

[b] Ciprofloxacin or doxycycline should be considered first-line therapy. Amoxicillin 500 mg PO TID for adults or 80 mg/kg/day divided every 8 h for children is an option for completion of therapy after clinical improvement. Oral amoxicillin dose is based on the need to achieve appropriate minimum inhibitory concentration levels.

[c] Previous guidelines have suggested treating cutaneous anthrax for 7–10 days, but 60 days is recommended in the setting of this attack, given the likelihood of exposure to aerosolized *B. anthracis*.

[d] The American Academy of Pediatrics recommends treatment of young children with tetracyclines for serious infections (e.g., Rocky Mountain spotted fever).

[e] Although tetracyclines or ciprofloxacin are not recommended during pregnancy, their use may be indicated for life-threatening illness. Adverse effects on developing teeth and bones are dose related; therefore, doxycycline might be used for a short time (7–14 days) before 6 months of gestation.

From U.S. Centers for Disease Control and Prevention. Update: investigation of bioterrorism-related anthrax and interim guidelines for exposure management and antimicrobial therapy. MMWR. 26 October 2001; 50(42): 909–919.

SUPPORTIVE THERAPY

Toxin-mediated morbidity is a major complication of systemic anthrax. Corticosteroids have been suggested as adjunct therapy for inhalation anthrax associated with extensive mediastinal edema, respiratory compromise, and meningitis (36,41). If significant pleural effusions exist, they should be drained, often leading to significant clinical improvement (11). Pleural effusions are usually recurrent and hemorrhagic so chest tubes should be left in place. A rational case could be made for the use of passive immunization with anthrax antitoxin in addition to antibiotics therapy with serious cases of anthrax, but no appropriate antitoxin is commercially available (1). Finally, the correction of electrolyte and acid-base imbalances, glucose infusion, vasopressor administration, and early mechanical ventilation may prove helpful (11).

POSTEXPOSURE PROPHYLAXIS

Prophylaxis is indicated for persons exposed to an airspace contaminated with aerosolized *B. anthracis*. Prophylaxis is not indicated for patient contacts (household contacts, friends, coworkers) unless it has been determined that they have been similarly exposed to anthrax spores. Prophylaxis is not indicated for health care and mortuary workers who attend to patients or corpses using standard precautions, or for the prevention of cutaneous anthrax (10). The U.S. Food and Drug Administration (FDA) has approved three antibiotics for use in reducing the incidence or progression of anthrax after exposure to aerosolized *B. anthracis*: ciprofloxacin, doxycycline, and amoxicillin (73,74). Ciprofloxacin or doxycycline are the drugs of choice (11); amoxicillin is an option for children and pregnant or lactating women exposed to strains of *B. anthracis* that are susceptible to penicillin to avoid potential toxicity of quinolones and tetracyclines (36,75,76). The Advisory Committee on Immunization Practices (ACIP) recommends that the duration of postexposure antimicrobial prophylaxis should be 60 days if used alone in unvaccinated persons (74). After the anthrax attacks of 2001, the U.S. Department of Health and Human Services announced additional options for prophylaxis of inhalational anthrax for individuals who wish to take extra precautions, especially those with high levels of exposure (77). Three options are now offered: (a) 60 days of antibiotic prophylaxis, (b) 100 days of antibiotic prophylaxis, or (c) 100 days of antibiotic prophylaxis, plus the anthrax vaccine as an investigational new drug (IND) given in three doses over 4 weeks (76,78).

ANTHRAX VACCINE

Anthrax Vaccine Absorbed (AVA), manufactured under the trademark BioThrax by BioPort Corporation in Lansing, Michigan, is the only licensed human anthrax vaccine in the United States (74). The vaccine is derived from sterile culture fluid supernatant taken from an attenuated strain of *B. anthracis* (79). The filtrate contains a mix of cellular products including all three toxin components— PA, EF, and LF—and does not contain live or dead organism (80,81). The vaccine series consists of six 0.5-mL doses given subcutaneously at 0, 2, and 4 weeks, with three booster vaccinations given at 6, 12, and 18 months. The duration of efficacy of AVA in humans is unknown, so the manufacturer recommends an annual booster in order to maintain immunity (79). Contraindications to vaccination include a previous anthrax infection or an anaphylactic reaction following a previous dose of AVA or any of the vaccine components (74). The vaccine is currently available to members of the military, hazmat or decontamination team members, and veterinarians, laboratory workers, and livestock handlers whose work place them at high risk for contact with anthrax. The ACIP also recommends BioThrax for postexposure prophylaxis in a three-dose regimen (0, 2, 4 weeks) in combination with antimicrobial postexposure prophylaxis under an IND application with the FDA for unvaccinated persons at risk for inhalational anthrax (11,82,83).

TRIAGE CONSIDERATIONS

■ *Who gets seen first?* The decision should be based on established emergency department protocols. Generally, those patients with signs or symptoms of inhalational or gastrointestinal anthrax should be seen ahead of stable patients with cutaneous anthrax.

■ *Who needs isolation?* Anthrax is not contagious and patients do not require isolation. Patients with suspected or diagnosed anthrax should be handled with standard (universal) precautions.

■ *Who gets antibiotics?* Any patient suspected or confirmed to have infection with anthrax will need to be treated with antibiotics. Those patients believed to have inhalational, gastrointestinal, or serious cutaneous anthrax should be treated with intravenous ciprofloxacin if available. Those individuals believed to have had contact with anthrax spores should receiveprophylactic antibiotic therapy.

■ *Who needs admitting?* Patients with inhalational or gastrointestinal anthrax will need hospitalization. Those with cutaneous anthrax should be admitted based upon the seriousness of their condition and the availability of hospital beds in the event of a major outbreak or biological attack. Individuals exposed to anthrax spores, but in stable condition, should be able to be discharged with appropriate oral antibiotic therapy with close follow-up.

PERSONAL PROTECTION

INFECTION CONTROL AND DECONTAMINATION

Standard (Universal) Precautions. All persons who come in close contact with suspected or confirmed cases of anthrax should use the CDC Guidelines for Standard (Universal) Precautions (84,85). Exposure to the source of anthrax spores requires specialized protection. Both OSHA and the CDC recommend a NIOSH-certified Class-95 respirator or better. Refer to OSHA, NIOSH, or the CDC before selecting a respirator for potential occupational exposure.

Laboratory Biosafety. A minimum of BSL2 practices, containment equipment, and facilities are recommended for activities using clinical materials and diagnostic quantities of anthrax (86).

Post Mortem. Bodies of patients who have died from anthrax infection should be handled with routine strict precautions by trained personnel. Safety precautions for the transport of the dead for burial should be the same as those when transporting ill patients. Postmortem aerosol-producing procedures (e.g., sawing bone) are not recommended, but when necessary, they should be carried out using high-efficiency particulate filtered masks and negative-pressure rooms as is customary when dealing with *Mycobacterium tuberculosis* or similar microbes. If autopsies are performed, all instruments and materials should be autoclaved or incinerated. Embalming of bodies is potentially associated with special risks, and consideration should be given to cremation (11).

Decontamination. Hospital rooms, emergency department examination areas, reusable instruments, clothing, and linens should undergo terminal cleaning after being used by a suspected or confirmed anthrax patient, in accordance with standard precautions and hospital protocol (11). See CDC Guidelines for Environmental Infection Control in Health-Care Facilities for specifics (87). Decontamination may be accomplished using any Environmental Protection Agency (EPA)-approved hospital disinfectant; however, anthrax spores are extremely hardy and complete sterilization often requires specialized materials and expertise. Iodine can be used, but it must be used at disinfectant strengths, as antiseptic-strength iodophors are not usually sporicidal (23). Hypochlorite solution has been used successfully as a sporicidal agent, and boiling water for 10 minutes can reduce spore counts by at least 10^6-fold (88).

SUMMARY

Disease: ANTHRAX: cutaneous, gastrointestinal, and inhalational.

Organism: Spore-forming bacterium, *Bacillus anthracis.*

Reservoir: Spores in the soil with near worldwide distribution.

Transmission: Anthrax is not *contagious*; human-to-human transmission has not been documented. Transmission to humans occurs following contact with anthrax spores. Cutaneous anthrax develops from contact with infected animals and contaminated animal products (to include hides, wool, or bone-meal fertilizer). Gastrointestinal anthrax develops after eating uncooked meat contaminated with anthrax spores. Inhalational anthrax historically was transmitted after breathing an appropriate inoculum of anthrax spores in the air, often disseminated from contaminated animal furs. Deliberate transmission of anthrax is possible using spores and could be used to inflict all three types of anthrax.

Incidence of naturally occurring anthrax: Naturally occurring anthrax occurs infrequently in the United States. There is usually one or fewer cases of human anthrax a year in the United States, typically along the Cattle Belt of the Great Plains, which results in a case of cutaneous anthrax. Therefore, hospital and public health authorities should be notified immediately of any suspected or confirmed cases of anthrax.

Mortality rate: The mortality rate for untreated inhalational anthrax approaches 100%. The mortality rate can be reduced if appropriate antibiotic therapy is initiated within 48 hours of exposure, but it may still be as high as 90% (1,2,23,48). The mortality rate for the 2001 anthrax attack was 50% with therapy (10,34). The case fatality rate for gastrointestinal anthrax is unknown, but it is estimated to be 25% to 60%. Cutaneous anthrax is the least severe with a mortality rate of 10% to 20% for untreated cases, and it should be less than 1% with treatment. Anthrax meningitis has been invariably fatal.

Incubation period: The incubation period for anthrax depends upon the route of exposure and the size of the inoculum, typically in the range of 1 to 7 days following exposure to spores. However, development of inhalational anthrax has occurred as early as a few hours and as late as 2 months following exposure. Most inhalational anthrax cases present within 48 hours following exposure (25–28,85).

Major signs and symptoms:

- *All:* Fever, malaise, headache, myalgias, and weakness.
- *Cutaneous:* Painless, pruritic papule that becomes vesicular, ruptures, ulcerates, and forms a depressed, black eschar. Surrounding edema may be quite prominent.
- *Gastrointestinal:* Nausea, vomiting, bloody diarrhea, and abdominal pain. Oropharyngeal anthrax presents with sore throat, neck swelling, dysphagia, and occasionally respiratory distress.
- *Inhalational:* Nonproductive cough, dyspnea, chest pain, hemoptysis, with rapidly progressive respiratory failure.

- *Diagnosis:* Physical findings are nonspecific, and routine blood or urine studies are not helpful. The organism is detectable by Gram stain and culture of the blood, CSF, pleural fluid or wound aspirate prior to the administration of antibiotic therapy. Radiographic studies are quite helpful with the diagnosis of inhalational anthrax. A widened mediastinum may be seen on CXR in later stages of illness. Definitive diagnosis is made via demonstration of lyses by gamma-phage, DFA of the polysaccharide cell wall and capsule, time-resolved fluorescence, polymerase chain reaction, and molecular characterization at upper level laboratories within the LRN.

- *Treatment:* Notify public health authorities as soon as anthrax is suspected. Early administration of antibiotic therapy (after collection of laboratory specimens) is crucial. *The drugs of choice for inhalation anthrax are ciprofloxacin 400 mg or doxycycline 100 mg IV every 12 hours* in a contained casualty setting (10,11). The duration of treatment with antibiotics should be for a *minimum of 60 days.* If the strain is shown to be susceptible, Penicillin-G IV may be substituted. In mass casualty situations where intravenous therapy is not feasible, oral ciprofloxacin may be prescribed. Children generally receive the same medications as adults (ciprofloxacin 20 to 40 mg/kg/day divided into two daily doses not to exceed 1 g/day); doxycycline is not generally recommended for children or pregnant or lactating women.

- *Prophylaxis:* Prophylactic antibiotic treatment is recommended for individuals with a history of exposure to anthrax spores. The preferred regimen is ciprofloxacin twice daily for 60 days. The anthrax vaccine may be available for concomitant prophylactic therapy in a three-dose regimen under IND application with the FDA.

- *Personal protection:* When possible, decontaminate the patient outside the treatment facility according to accepted hazmat standard operating procedures. Once decontaminated, use CDC-recommended standard universal precautions for all suspected or confirmed cases of anthrax.

- *Isolation and decontamination:* Health care workers should use standard precautions when contact with a potentially infected patient exists. After an invasive procedure or autopsy is performed, the area used should be thoroughly disinfected with a sporicidal agent such as hypochlorite solution, and instruments should be autoclaved to kill spores completely.

- *Vaccine:* AVA, a cell-free anthrax vaccine licensed under the trade name BioThrax, is available to members of the military, laboratory workers, and livestock workers who are at significant risk of exposure to anthrax. The vaccine is given in six doses at 0, 2, 4 weeks and 6, 12, 18 months. BioThrax is also recommended as postexposure prophylaxis, in conjunction with appropriate antibiotic therapy, as an emergency IND (82). The vaccine is available in a three-dose regimen (0, 2, 4 weeks) with postexposure prophylactic antibiotic therapy; use of the anthrax vaccine alone is not recommended for postexposure prophylaxis.

RESOURCES

1. JAMA Consensus Statement on Anthrax. Inglesby TV, Dennis DT, Henderson DA, et al. Anthrax as a biological weapon: medical and public health management. JAMA. 1999;1735-45. Available at: http://www.bt.cdc.gov /Agent/Anthrax/Consensus.pdf. Accessed January 6, 2004.

2. JAMA Consensus Statement on Anthrax, 2002 Update on Management. Inglesby TV, Dennis DT, Henderson DA, et al. Anthrax as a biological weapon, 2002: update recommendations for management. JAMA. May 2002;1:287(17)2236-52.

3. CDC Anthrax Home Page. U.S. Centers for Disease Control and Prevention, Emergency Preparedness and Response web site on anthrax. Available at: http://www.bt.cdc.gov/agent/anthrax/index.asp. Accessed January 6, 2004.

4. MEDLINEplus Health Information Anthrax Web Site. A service of the U.S. National Library of Medicine and the National Institutes of Health. Available at: http://www.nlm.nih.gov/medlineplus/anthrax.html. Accessed January 6, 2004.

5. USAMRIID's Medical Management of Biological Casualties Handbook. 4th ed. Kortepter M, Christopher G, Cieslak T, et al., eds. Fort Detrick MD: U.S. Army Medical Research Institute of Infectious Diseases; 2001. Available at: http://www.usamriid. army.mil/education/bluebook.html. Accessed January 6, 2004.

6. Military Textbook of Medical Aspects of Chemical and Biological Warfare. Friedlander AM. Anthrax. In: Zatjtchuk R, Bellamy RF eds. Medical aspects of chemical and biological warfare. Bethesda, MD: Office of the Surgeon General; 1997. Available at: http://www.nbc-med.org/SiteContent/HomePage/WhatsNew/MedAspects/Ch-22electrv699.pdf. Accessed January 6, 2004.

7. Harrison's Principles of Internal Medicine, Chapter 141: Diphtheria, Corynebacterium Infections, and Anthrax. Holmes RK. In: Fauci AS, Braunwald E, Isselbacher KJ, Isselbacher KJ, Wilson JD, Martin JB, Kasper DL, et al., eds. Harrison's principles of internal medicine, 15th ed. New York: McGraw-Hill; 2001. p. 914–5. Available at: http://www.mheducation.com /HOL2_chapters/HOL_chapters/chapter141.htm. Accessed January 6, 2004.

8. The U.S. Centers for Disease Control and Prevention Emergency Operations Center. Toll-free telephone number: 1-770-488-7100.

9. The U.S. Army Medical Research Infectious Disease (USAMRIID) Emergency Response Line. Toll-free telephone number: 1-888-872-7443.

QUESTIONS AND ANSWERS

1. Anthrax occurs endemically in all of the following populated continents EXCEPT:
   A. Europe
   B. North America
   C. South America
   D. Australia
   E. Asia

2. What is the most common clinical form of anthrax?
   A. Meningitic
   B. Gastrointestinal
   C. Inhalational
   D. Cutaneous
   E. Oropharyngeal

3. Each of the following statements regarding inhalational anthrax is true EXCEPT:
   A. Gastrointestinal symptoms may be present.
   B. Patients usually present within 48 hours of exposure.
   C. A true pneumonia is not usually present.
   D. Mediastinal widening is noted on chest radiograph in late stage disease.
   E. It is often transmitted from person to person.

4. According to the Working Group on Civilian Biodefense (JAMA Consensus Statement on Anthrax), what is the drug of choice for initially treating an isolated case of inhalation anthrax in an adult?
   A. Erythromycin
   B. Trimethoprim-Sulfamethoxazole
   C. Ciprofloxacin
   D. Amoxicillin
   E. Streptomycin

ANSWERS

1: *D. Australia*
2: *D. Cutaneous*
3: *C. A true pneumonia is not usually present.*
4: *C. Ciprofloxacin*

REFERENCES

1. Holmes R. Diptheria, other corynebacterial infections, and anthrax. In: Braunwald E, Fauci AS, Kasper DL, et al. eds. Harrison's principles of internal medicine, 15th ed. New York: McGraw-Hill; 2001.
2. Friedlander AM. Anthrax. In: Zajtchuk R, Bellamy RF, eds. Textbook of military medicine: medical aspects of chemical and biological warfare. Washington, DC: Office of the Surgeon General; 1997:467-78.
3. Dirckx JH. Virgil on anthrax. Am J Dermatopathol. 1981;3:191-5.
4. Turnbull PCB. Bacillus. In: Baron S ed. Medical microbiology, 3rd ed. New York: Churchill Livingstone Inc; 1991:249-62.
5. Koch R. Die Aetiologie der Milzbrand-Krankheit, begründet auf die Entwicklungsgeschicte des *Bacillus anthracis*. Beiträge zur Biologie der Pflanzen. 1876;2:277-310.
6. Eurich FW. The history of anthrax in the wool industry of Bradford, and of its control. Lancet. 1926;57-8.

7. Tigertt WD. Anthrax: William Smith Greenfield, MD, FRCP, professor superintendent, the Brown Animal Sanatory Institution (1878–1881)—concerning the priority due to him for the production of the first vaccine against anthrax. J Hyg (London). 1980;85:415-20.

8. Pasteur L, Chamberland, R. Compte rendu sommaire des expériences faites à Pouilly—'le-Fort, prés Melun, sur la vaccination charbonneuse. Comptes Rendus des séances De L'Acamémie des Sciences. 1881;92:1378-83.

9. Pile JC, Malone JD, Eitzen EM, Friedlander AM. Anthrax as a potential biological warfare agent. Arch Intern Med. 1998;158: 429-34.

10. Inglesby TV, O'Toole T, Henderson DA, et al. Anthrax as a biological weapon, 2002: updated recommendations for management. JAMA. 1 May 2002;287(17):2236-52.

11. Inglesby TV, O'Toole T, Henderson DA, et al. Anthrax as a biological weapon, 2002: updated recommendations for management. JAMA. 1 May 2002;287(17):2236-52.

12. Davies JCA. A major epidemic of anthrax in Zimbabwe, part III. Cent Afr J Med. 1985;31:176-9.

13. Fujikura T. Current occurrence of anthrax in man and animals. Salisbury Med Bull Suppl. 1990;68:1.

14. Turnbull PCB. Guidelines for the surveillance and control of anthrax in humans and animals, 3rd ed. Geneva: World Health Organization; 1998.

15. World Anthrax Data Site, A service of the World Health Organization Center for Remote Sensing and Geographic Information Systems for Public Health available at: http://www. vetmed.lsu.edu/whocc/mp_world.htm. Last accessed December 31, 2003.

16. Last major outbreak of naturally occurring anthrax in the United States occurred in August 2000 with 248 cattle infected in Nevada, Minnesota, North Dakota, and South Dakota. World Anthrax Data Site, A service of the World Health Organization Center for Remote Sensing and Geographic Information Systems for Public Health available at: http://www. vetmed.lsu.edu/whocc/mp_world.htm. Last accessed December 31, 2003.

17. Brachman PS, Friedlander AM. Anthrax. In: Plotkin SA, Mortimer EA, eds. Vaccines, 2nd ed. Philadelphia: WB Saunders Co; 1994.

18. Brachman PS. Inhalation anthrax. Ann NY Acad Sci. 1980;353:83-93.

19. LaForce FM. Woolsorters' disease in England. Bull NY Acad Med. 1978;54:956-63.

20. Turner M. Anthrax in humans in Zimbabwe. Cent Afr J Med. 1980;26:160-1.

21. Harris SH. Factories of death: Japanese biological warfare, 1932-45 and the American cover-up. New York: Rutledge; 2002.

22. Gold H. Unit 731-testimony: Japan's wartime human experimentation program. Boston: Charles E Tuttle Co; 1996.

23. Kortepter M, Christopher G, Cieslak T, et al., eds. USAMRIID's medical management of biological casualties handbook, 4th ed. Fort Detrick, MD: U.S. Army Medical Research Institute of Infectious Diseases; 2001.

24. Alibek K, Handelman S. Biohazard: the chilling story of the largest covert biological weapons program in the world—told from the inside by the man who ran it. New York: Random House; 1998.

25. Guillemin J. Anthrax: the investigation of a deadly outbreak. Berkeley: University of California Press; 1999.

26. Meselson M, Guilleman J, Hugh-Jones M, et al. The Sverdlovsk anthrax outbreak of 1979. Science. 18 November 1994; 266 (5188):1202-8.

27. Abramova FA, Grinberg LM, Yampolskaya OV, Walker DH. Pathology of inhalational anthrax in 42 cases from the Sverdlovsk outbreak of 1979. Proc Natl Acad Sci USA. 1993;90:2291-4.

28. Walker DH, Yampolska L, Grinberg LM. Death at Sverdlovsk: what have we learned? Am J Pathol. 1994;144:1135-41.

29. Wade N. Death at Sverdlovsk: a critical diagnosis. Science. 1980;209:1501-2.

30. United Nations Security Council. Fifteenth quarterly report on the activities of the United Nations Monitoring, Verification and Inspection Commission in accordance with paragraph 12 of Security Council resolution 1284 (1999), 26 November 2003.

31. Zilinskas RA. Iraq's biological weapons: the past as future? JAMA. 1997;278:418-24.

32. Ballard T, Pate J, Ackerman G, et al. Chronology of Aum Shinrikyo CBW activities. Center for Non-proliferation Studies Report. Monterey, California: Monterey Institute of International Studies; March 2001.

33. Choy S. In the spotlight: Aum Shinrikyo. Washington DC: Center for Defense Information; 23 July 2002.

34. U.S. Centers for Disease Control and Prevention. Update: investigation of bioterrorism-related anthrax and adverse events from anti-microbial prophylaxis. MMWR. 9 November 2001;50:973-6.

35. U.S. Centers for Disease Control and Prevention. Update: investigation of bioterrorism-related anthrax and interim guidelines for clinical evaluation of persons with possible anthrax. MMWR. 2 November 2001;50:941-8.

36. U.S. Centers for Disease Control and Prevention. Update: investigation of bioterrorism-related anthrax and interim guidelines for exposure management and antimicrobial therapy. MMWR. October 2001; 50:909-19.

37. U.S. Centers for Disease Control and Prevention. Update: investigation of anthrax associated with intentional exposure and interim public health guidelines. MMWR. October 2001;50: 889-93.

38. Dragon DC, Rennie RP. The ecology of anthrax spores. Can Vet J. 1995;36:295-301.

39. Titball RW, Turnbull BC, Hutson RA. The monitoring and detection of *Bacillus anthracis* in the environment. J Appl Bacteriol. 1991;70(suppl):9S-18S.

40. Williams RP. Bacillus anthracis and other spore forming bacilli. In: Braude AI, Davis LE, Fierer J eds. Infectious disease and medical microbiology. Philadelphia: WB Saunders Co; 1986.

41. Dixon TC, Meselson M, Guillemin J, Hanna PC. Anthrax. N Engl J Med. 1999;341:815-26.

42. Duesbery NS, Vande Woude GF. Anthrax toxins. Cell Mol Life Sci. 1999;55:1599.

43. Leppla SH, Friedlander AM, Singh Y, et al. A model for anthrax toxic action at the cellular level. Salisbury Med Bull Suppl. 1990;68:41-3.

44. O'Brien J, Friedlander AM, Dreier T, et al. Effects of anthrax toxin components on human neutrophils. Infect Immunol. 1985;47:306-10.

45. Leppa SH. Anthrax toxin edema factor: a bacterial adenylate cyclase that increases cyclic AMP concentrations in eukaryotic cells. Proc Natl Acad Sci USA. 1982;79:2162-6.

46. Hanna PC. Anthrax pathogenesis and host response. Curr Top Microbiol Immunol. 1998;225:13-35.

47. Hanna PC, Acosta D, Collier RJ. On the role of macrophages in anthrax. Proc Natl Acad Sci USA. 1993;90:10198-201.

48. Swartz MN. Recognition and management of anthrax: an update. N Eng J Med. 2001;345:1621-6.

49. U.S. Centers for Disease Control and Prevention. Use of anthrax vaccine in the United States: recommendations of the Advisory Committee on Immunization Practices (ACIP). MMWR. 15 December 2000;49(RR-15):1-14.

50. Longfield R. Anthrax. In: Stickland GT, ed. Hunter's tropical medicine, 7th ed. Philadelphia: WB Saunders Co; 1991.

51. Onerci M, Ergin NT. Oropharyngealer Milzbrand [Oropharyngeal anthrax]. Laryngorhinootologie. 1993;72:350-1.

52. Harris S. Japanese biological warfare research on humans: a case study of microbiology and ethics. Ann NY Acad Sci. 1992;666: 21–49.

53. Daley S. In support of apartheid: poison whisky and sterilization. New York Times, June 11, 1998, section A, page 3.
54. Watson A, Keir D. Information on which to base assessments of risk from environments contaminated with anthrax spores. Epidemiol Infect. 1994;113:479-90.
55. Albrink WS, Goodlow RJ. Experimental inhalation anthrax in chimpanzee. Am J Pathol. 1959;35:1055-65.
56. Myenye KS, Siziya S, Peterson D. Factors associated with human anthrax outbreak in the Chikupo and Ngandu villages of Murewa district in Mashonaland East Province, Zimbabwe. Cent Afr J Med. 1996;42:312-5.
57. Conference summary: clinical issues in the prophylaxis, diagnosis, and treatment of anthrax. Emerg Inf Dis. February 2002;8(2):222-5.
58. American Academy of Dermatology web site. Cutaneous anthrax management algorithm. Available at: http://www.aad.org/BioInfo/Biomessage2.html. Accessed January 6, 2004.
59. Tekin A, Bulut N, Unal T. Acute abdomen due to anthrax. Br J Surg. 1997;84:813.
60. Dulz W, Saidi F, Kouhout E. Gastric anthrax with massive ascites. Gut. 1970;11:352-4.
61. Nalin DR, Sultana B, Sahunja R, et al. Survival of a patient with intestinal anthrax. Am J Med. 1977;62:130-2.
62. Sirisanthana T, Brown AE. Anthrax of the gastrointestinal tract. Emerg Infect Dis. July 2002;8(7):649-51.
63. Kunanusont C, Limpakarnjanarat K, Foy JM. Outbreak of anthrax in Thailand. Ann Trop Med Parasitol. 1990;84:507-12.
64. Sirisanthana T, Navacharoen N, Tharavichitkul P, et al. Outbreak of oral-pharyngeal anthrax: an unusual manifestation of human infection with Bacillus anthracis. Am J Trop Med Hyg. 1984;33:144-50.
65. Albrink WS, Brooks SM, Biron RE, Kopel M. Human inhalation anthrax. Am J Pathol. 1960;36:457-1.
66. U.S. Centers for Disease Control and Prevention. Symptoms and signs of inhalational anthrax, laboratory-confirmed influenza, and influenza-like illness (ILI) from other causes. Notice to readers: considerations for distinguishing influenza-like illness from inhalational anthrax. MMWR 9 November 2001;50(44):984-6.
67. Refer to: Level A laboratory procedures for the identification of Bacillus anthracis. Laboratory Response Network, 24 March 2003. Available at: http://www.bt.cdc.gov/Agent/anthrax/LevelAProtocol/anthraxlabprotocol.pdf. Last accessed on January 6, 2004.
68. U.S. Centers for Disease Control and Prevention web site. Approved tests for the detection of Bacillus anthracis in the Laboratory Response Network (LRN). Available at: http://www.bt.cdc.gov/documentsapp/Anthrax/ApprovedLRNTests.asp. Last accessed on January 6, 2004.
69. Vessal K, Yeganehdoust J, Dutz W, Kohout E. Radiologic changes in inhalation anthrax. Clin Radiol. 1975;26:471-4.
70. American College of Physicians web site on bioterrorism. Inhalation anthrax chest x-ray. Available at http://www.acponline.org/bioterro/chest_xray.htm. Accessed December 31, 2003.
71. Brachman PS. Anthrax. In: Hoeprich PD, Jordan MC, Ronald AR, eds. Infectious diseases. Philadelphia: JB Lippincott; 1994:1003-8.
72. U.S. Centers for Disease Control and Prevention and National Institutes of Health. Biosafety in microbiological and biomedical laboratories, 4th ed. Washington DC: Government Printing Office; May 1999. Available at: http://www.cdc.gov/od/ohs/biosfty/bmbl4/bmbl4s7a.htm.
73. U.S. Food and Drug Administration. Prescription drug products; doxycycline and penicillin G procaine administration.
74. U.S. Centers for Disease Control and Prevention. Use of anthrax vaccine in the United States: recommendations of the Advisory Committee on Immunization Practices (ACIP). MMWR. 15 December 2000;49(RR-15):12-4.
75. U.S. Centers for Disease Control and Prevention. Updated recommendations for antimicrobial prophylaxis among asymptomatic pregnant women after exposure to Bacillus anthracis, October 2001. MMWR. October 2001;50:960.
76. U.S. Centers for Disease Control and Prevention. Update: interim recommendations for antimicrobial prophylaxis for children and breastfeeding mothers and treatment of children with anthrax, October 2001. MMWR. October 2001;50:1014-6.
77. U.S. Department of Health and Human Services. Statement by the Department of Health and Human Services regarding additional options for preventive treatment for those exposed to inhalational anthrax. Washington DC: HHS News, 18 December 2001.
78. U.S. Centers for Disease Control and Prevention. Additional options for preventive treatment for persons exposed to inhalational anthrax. MMWR. 2001;50:1142-51.
79. BioThrax [package insert]. Lansing, MI: BioPort Corp; 31 Jan 2002.
80. U.S. Centers for Disease Control and Prevention. Recommendations of the Advisory Committee on Immunization Practices (ACIP): adult immunization. MMWR. 1984;33(15):33-4.
81. Turnbull PCB, Broster MG, Carman JA, et al. Development of antibodies to protective antigen and lethal factor components of anthrax toxin in humans and guinea pigs and their relevance to protective immunity. Infect Immun. 1986;52:356-63.
82. U.S. Centers for Disease Control and Prevention. Notice to readers: use of anthrax vaccine in response to terrorism: supplemental recommendations of the Advisory Committee on Immunization Practices (ACIP). MMWR. 2002;51(45): 1024–26.
83. U.S. Food & Drug Administration. Guidance for institutional review boards and clinical investigators, 1998 update: emergency use of an investigational drug or biologic. Available at: http://www.fda.gov/oc/ohrt/irbs/drugsbiologics.html#emergency. Accessed January 6, 2004.
84. Garner JS, Hospital Infection Control Practices Advisory Committee. Guideline for isolation precautions in hospitals. Infect Control Hosp Epidemiol. 1996;17:53-80, and Am J Infect Control. 1996;24:24-52. Available at the CDC's Division of Healthcare Quality Promotion web site: http://www.cdc.gov /ncidod/hip/ISOLAT/Isolat.htm.
85. U.S. Army Field Manual 8-284/U.S. Navy NAVMED P-5042/U.S. Air Force AFMAN (I)44-156/U.S. Marine Corps MCRP 4-11.1C. Treatment of biological warfare agent casualties. Headquarters, Departments of the Army, the Navy, and Air Force, and Commandant, Marine Corps; 17 July 2000.
86. U.S. Centers for Disease Control and Prevention and National Institutes of Health. Biosafety in microbiological and biomedical laboratories, 4th ed. Washington DC: Government Printing Office; May 1999. Available at: http://www.cdc.gov/od/ohs/biosfty/bmbl4/bmbl4s7a.htm.
87. U.S. Centers for Disease Control and Prevention. Guidelines for environmental infection control in health-care facilities: recommendations of the CDC and the Healthcare Infection Control Practices Advisory Committee (HICPAC). Bethesda, MD: U.S. Department of Health and Human Services, Centers for Disease Control and Prevention; 2003. Available at: http://www.cdc.gov/ncidod/hip/enviro/Enviro_guide_03.pdf. Accessed January 6, 2004.
88. Whitney EA, Beatty ME, Taylor TH, et al. Inactivation of Bacillus anthracis spores. Emerging Infec Dis, June 2003;9 (6):623-7.

7

Plague

Anthony J. Carbone

NAME OF AGENT

Disease: Plague; Organism: *Yersinia pestis.*

MICROBIOLOGY

The disease known as plague is caused by *Yersinia pestis*, a bacterium of the Enterobacteriaceae family. The plague bacillus is a small, ovoid, nonmotile, nonspore-forming, nonlactose-fermenting, gram-negative, rod-shaped bacterium. Bipolar uptake occurs when using Wayson, Wright, Giemsa, methylene blue, and occasionally gram-stained preparations, revealing the classic "safety pin"-shaped coccobacilli under magnification (Fig. 7-1) (1,2)

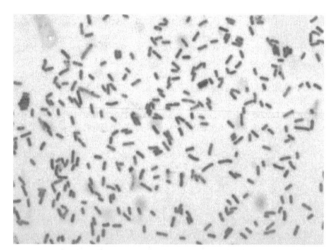

Figure 7–1. Gram stain. *Yersinia pestis*, gram-negative bacillus at 1,000X. (From Centers for Disease Control-PHIL; Date: 2002.)

THEORETICAL AND SCIENTIFIC BACKGROUND

BRIEF HISTORY

Plague is a zoonotic disease (animal disease that is naturally communicable to humans) caused by the bacterium *Yersinia pestis*. Plague has been responsible for three great pandemics of human disease occurring in the 6th, 14th, and 20th centuries of the modern era, resulting in the deaths of millions and changing the course of history (3).

The first pandemic, known as the Justinian Plague, began in the port cities of Egypt in 541 A.D. and spread throughout the Mediterranean basin, the Middle East, and Europe, killing an estimated 50% to 60% of the population before it ran its course in 545 A.D. and decimated the Eastern Roman Empire (4).

The second plague pandemic, known as the Black Death, is believed to have originated in Mongolia around 1320 and spread throughout the occupied world over the next 130 years killing approximately one-third of the world's population at the time (5–7).

The third plague pandemic erupted in China in 1855, killing 12 million people in China and India alone, before reaching San Francisco's Chinatown in 1900 (8). During the next 4 years 121 people in California were infected, killing all but three. A secondary plague epidemic erupted in San Francisco in 1907 with 160 cases and 77 deaths (9). Since the San Francisco epidemics, plague has been endemic in the United States, predominantly in the southwestern states.

Because of plague's legacy of death, devastation, and fear, armies throughout the centuries have tried to exploit *Yersinia pestis* as a weapon of war. The first documented use of plague as a military weapon was during the siege of Kaffa, a Crimean port city on the Black Sea, during the year 1346. The besieging Tartars catapulted the corpses of their own plague victims into the city. The Genoese fled Kaffa and returned to Italy bringing plague along with them and very likely starting the Black Death in Europe (10–13). This practice was repeated as late as late as 1710 when the Russians used the same tactic against the Swedes in the Russian-Swedish War of 1700–1725 during the Siege of Revel (14).

During the 1930s and 1940s, the Japanese Imperial Army experimented with plague within its secret biological weapons program in occupied Manchuria. Approximately 3,000 scientists under the direction of Japanese General Ishii Shiro, a military physician and microbiologist who was fascinated with plague, worked to weaponize *Yersinia pestis*. Japanese Unit 731 operated a plague flea factory in Manchuria with 4,500 breeding machines, producing about 100 million plague-infected fleas every few days. The Japanese Unit 100 reportedly dropped plague-infected fleas over China resulting in a number of plague outbreaks where none had previously occurred (15–17).

The United States studied plague as a potential weapon in the 1950s before its offensive program was terminated by President Richard Nixon in 1969 (18). In 1972 the United States, the Soviet Union, and one hundred other countries signed the Biological Weapons Convention (19). Shortly after the treaty was signed, the Soviet government initiated a massive clandestine offensive biological weapons program under the name *Biopreparat* that researched, weaponized, tested, produced, and stockpiled tons of deadly biological agents, including a multidrug-resistant weaponized form of plague that could be easily aerosolized (20,21).

EPIDEMIOLOGY OF NATURALLY OCCURRING PLAGUE

Naturally occurring plague is primarily a disease of rodents, which is transmitted to humans in sporadic cases and epidemics. Natural infestation occurs in a variety of susceptible host rodents such as the infamous *Rattus rattus* (22), the black house and ship rat, and other animals including ground and tree squirrels, prairie dogs, and carnivores such as coyotes, bobcats, dogs, and cats (23). Plague is a naturally occurring enzootic infection of rats, prairie dogs, and other rodents on every populated continent except Australia (24). On average, there have been approximately 1,700 cases a year reported worldwide in the past 50 years (25). India experienced a major plague outbreak in 1994 in the industrial city of Surat following a severe earthquake. When it was over, 56 people were reported to have died from plague, while some 6,500 individuals were treated with antibiotics (Fig. 7-2) (26).

Plague has been endemic within the continental United States since it was first observed in California in 1907 (27,28). The last major outbreak of plague in the United

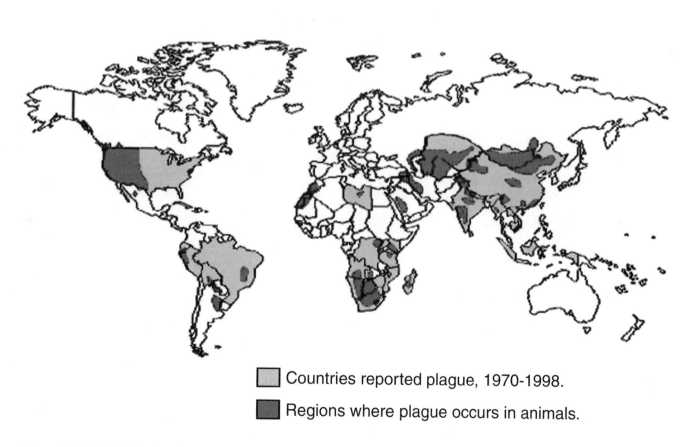

Countries reported plague, 1970-1998.

Regions where plague occurs in animals.

Figure 7–2. World distribution of plague, 1998. (From CDC plague web site, Division of Vector-Borne Infectious Diseases, Centers for Disease Control and Prevention, Atlanta, GA. Available at: http://www.cdc.gov/ncidod/dvbid/plague/epi.htm.)

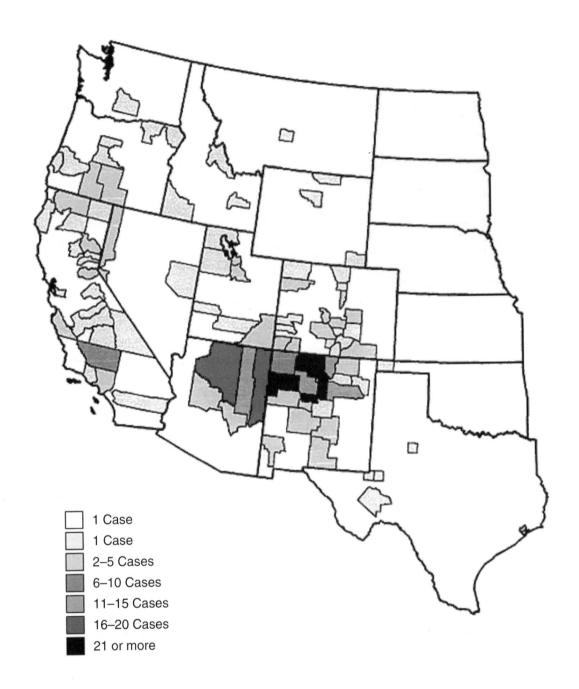

Figure 7–3. Reported human plague cases by county: United States, 1979–1997. (From CDC plague web site, Division of Vector-Borne Infectious Diseases, Centers for Disease Control and Prevention, Atlanta, GA. Available at: http://www.cdc.gov/ncidod/dvbid/plague/epi.htm.)

States occurred in Los Angeles in 1924–1925 when 40 people were infected and only two survived (29). The Centers for Disease Control and Prevention (CDC) report an average of 13 cases of plague annually with the majority of cases occurring within the four southwestern states of New Mexico, Arizona, Colorado, and California (Fig. 7-2). In a 1997 study published by the CDC, 390 cases of plague were reported in the United States from 1947 to 1996. Of these

cases, 84% were reported as bubonic, 13% were septicemic, and 2% were pneumonic plague; case fatality rates were 14%, 22%, and 57%, respectively (30).

Most cases of plague in humans occur in the summer months when the risk for exposure to infected fleas is greatest (31). Most cases of plague in the United States have been in men younger than 20 years old (32), and occurred within a 1-mile radius of their homes (Fig. 7-3) (33).

TRANSMISSION

Infected Fleas

Although plague bacilli can be found in the feces and urine of infected animals, and one can become infected by feeding upon or even handling the flesh of infected animals, human plague is most commonly transmitted by infected fleas (34–36). Historically, the oriental rat flea, *Xenopsylla cheopis*, is believed to have been largely responsible for the spread of bubonic plague (37); however, some 200 species of animals and 80 species of fleas have been associated with plague transmission worldwide (38). The most important vector of human plague in the United States is the flea *Diamanus montanus*, the most common flea on rock squirrels and California ground squirrels (39). Plague vector fleas prefer the blood of their rodent hosts, but if the rodent population begins to thin, the fleas will switch to human hosts for survival. Large numbers of rodents usually die off prior to human epidemics, precipitating the transfer of the flea population from its natural rat reservoir to humans (Fig. 7-4) (40).

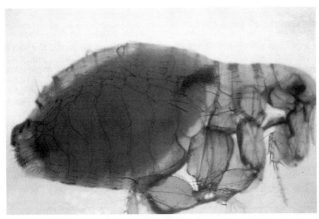

Figure 7–4. The oriental rat flea, *Xenopsylla cheopis*, is one of the major vectors responsible for transmitting plague between animals and man. (From Centers for Disease Control-PHIL; date unknown.)

Direct Contact

Plague can be transmitted directly to humans by handling an infected animal, dead or alive, or by stumbling into an infected animal's nest while walking. Rock squirrels and California ground squirrels are known to infect man via direct contact and fleas. Fur trappers often develop plague via direct contact while skinning infected animals (41–44).

Human-to-Human Transmission

Human-to-human transmission of plague is rare, but it can occur from close contact with patients coughing from pneumonic plague. Respiratory transmission is thought to occur more efficiently via larger droplets or fomites rather than from small-particle aerosols (45). The last case of human-to-human transmission of plague in the United States occurred during the Los Angeles epidemic of 1924 (46).

Deliberate Aerosol Attack

The deadliest method of transmission would be via a deliberate attack using aerosolized plague over a large area. Japanese General Ishii Shiro attempted to initiate plague outbreak over China during World War II using ceramic bombs filled with plague-infected human fleas, *Pulex irritans*, to target humans directly with the hope of creating a plague outbreak (47–50). During the 1970s and 1980s, the Soviet Union's secret biological weapons (BW) program perfected the methodology by first developing a multidrug-resistant plague bacillus and then weaponizing the agent so that it could be preserved and stored into a variety of warheads and aerosolized easily when over a target area (51,52). Despite the fall of the Soviet Union, and the reported dismantling of the BW program, this method of aerosol transmission poses the greatest threat to mass casualties of pneumonic plague today.

PATHOGENESIS IN NATURALLY OCCURRING PLAGUE

In the majority of cases of naturally occurring plague, a flea such as *Xenopsylla cheopis* survives by living off of a host rodent like the ground squirrel. If the rodent is infected with plague, the flea draws viable *Yersinia pestis* organisms into its esophagus during a feed. The bacteria then multiply in the flea's stomach. If the host rodent dies, it looks for new hosts and this is when man is most likely to be bitten by an infected flea. When the flea bites the skin of a person and begins to feed, plague bacilli are mixed with the blood drawn from the host and regurgitated into the bite. The flea may also discharge infected feces into the bite wound (53).

The flea's bite leads to an inoculation of up to thousands of plague bacilli into the victim's skin. [As few as 1 to 10 *Yersinia pestis* organisms are sufficient to infect rodents and primates via oral, subcutaneous, intradermal, and intravenous routes (54).] The bacteria infiltrate through the cutaneous tissue into the cutaneous lymphatic vessels and deposit into regional lymph nodes where they are phagocytosed but resist destruction. During the incubation period, lasting 2 to 8 days, the bacteria multiply rapidly causing suppurative lymphadenitis, which manifests as the characteristic bubo.

Without treatment, the lymph node architecture is destroyed resulting in bacteremia and septicemia spreading plague to other organs (55,56). The tissues most commonly infected include the spleen, liver, lungs, skin, and mucous membranes (57). The endotoxin of *Yersinia pestis* contributes to the development of septic shock in a manner similar to other forms of gram-negative sepsis leading to disseminated intravascular coagulation, shock, and coma (58,59).

Much less is understood about the pathogenesis of pneumonic plague. Estimates of infectivity via the respiratory route are in the range of 100 to 500 organisms for primary pneumonic plague (60,61). Secondary pneumonic plague occurs in untreated cases of bubonic plague that lead to septicemia and seeding of pulmonary tissue.

CLINICAL FORMS OF PLAGUE

1. *Bubonic Plague:* In the United States, most patients (approximately 85%) with human plague present clinically with the bubonic form. Bubonic plague arises from the bite of an infected flea and the bacteria become localized in an inflamed lymph node (femoral, inguinal, or axillary depending upon the site of the bite) where the bacteria replicates.

2. *Septicemic Plague:* A smaller number of patients (approximately 15%) will develop gram-negative sepsis without evidence of a bubo in what is termed "primary septicemic plague."

3. *Pneumonic Plague:* Primary pneumonic plague occurs from the inhalation of *Yersinia pestis* bacteria passed from humans or cats suffering with pneumonic plague (approximately 2% of all cases). This is the form of plague that would be expected following a deliberate attack using aerosolized *Yersinia pestis* and is nearly always fatal if not treated quickly. Secondary pneumonic plague arises from poorly treated bubonic or septicemic plague when *Yersinia pestis* bacteremia seeds pulmonary tissues.

4. *Plague Meningitis:* Plague meningitis is seen in 6% to 7% of all cases of plague, usually in children following ineffective treatment. Symptoms are similar to other forms of acute bacterial meningitis.

5. *Pharyngeal Plague:* On extremely rare occasions, individuals may develop a plague pharyngitis following the inhalation or ingestion of plague bacilli. Pharyngeal plague mimics tonsillitis associated with cervical lymphadenopathy (the cervical bubo).

INCUBATION PERIODS

The incubation period for bubonic plague from flea bites is 2 to 8 days before symptoms develop. The incubation period for septicemic plague can be shorter at 1 to 7 days. The incubation period for pneumonic plague following respiratory exposure to an aerosol is usually 2 to 4 days (62).

MORTALITY RATES

The mortality rate of plague varies based upon a variety of factors including the mode of inoculation, the amount of bacterial inoculation, the age and health of the infected person, and whether or not the agent is natural or has been genetically engineered (63,64). The historical mortality rate of *untreated* bubonic plague is approximately 60%, with death occurring within 10 days of onset (65,66). The mortality rate for bubonic plague drops to less than 5% with early appropriate antibiotic therapy (67), whereas *untreated* septicemic and pneumonic plague have mortality rates of nearly 100%. In fact, even with modern antibiotic therapy, survival is unlikely if treatment is delayed more than 18 hours following respiratory exposure (68).

PLAGUE FOLLOWING DELIBERATE USE AS A BIOLOGICAL WEAPON

Clinicians and public health officials need to realize that the epidemiology of disease for a deliberate attack using plague as a biological weapon would differ substantially from a naturally occurring outbreak of plague. Intentional dissemination of plague will most likely involve the use of an aerosol of *Yersinia pestis* in order to inflict large numbers of casualties with deadly pneumonic plague. Victims of such an attack would present with symptoms resembling a host of other severe respiratory diseases making the initial diagnosis of plague difficult.

The indications that plague had been intentionally disseminated would include (a) the presence of plague in areas not known to have endemic enzootic infection, (b) the absence of prior rodent deaths, and (c) severe rapidly progressive respiratory disease in a number of previously healthy individuals, suggestive of pneumonic plague.

SIGNS AND SYMPTOMS

BUBONIC PLAGUE

The pathognomic sign of bubonic plague is a very painful, swollen, warm-to-touch, lymph node called a *bubo*. This sign accompanied with fever, malaise, exhaustion, and a history of possible exposure to rodents, fleas, wild rabbits, or sick or dead carnivores should lead to the suspicion of plague.

Patients typically develop symptoms of bubonic plague 2 to 8 days following the bite from an infected flea. There is usually sudden onset of fever, chills, and weakness, followed by the formation of the tell-tale bubo up to one day later (69). Since fleas usually bite a person on the lower extremities, femoral and inguinal buboes are most common. Infections from skinning infected animals usually produce axillary buboes.

Buboes can grow from 1 to 10 cm in size and can be so painful that they prevent the patient from moving the effected site (70). The overlying skin is erythematous, warm, and extremely tender. There is often a considerable amount of surrounding edema, but rarely lymphangitis. The buboes are usually nonfluctuant, but may point, ulcerate, and drain spontaneously. Rarely, necrosis is present at which point the bubo will require incision and drainage (71,72). Approximately 4% to 10% of bubonic plague patients are reported to have a visible ulcer or pustule at the flea inoculation site (73,74). Buboes usually recede in 10 to 14 days if treated appropriately with antibiotics and generally do not require incision and drainage beyond diagnostic aspiration (Figs. 7-5 to 7-7) (75).

SEPTICEMIC PLAGUE

A small portion of patients who have been bitten by an infected flea develop *Yersinia pestis* septicemia without a discernable bubo in the form of the disease known as primary septicemic plague (76). Septicemia can also develop secondary to bubonic plague in what is termed secondary septicemic plague (77).

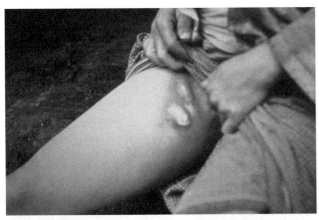

Figure 7–5. Femoral bubo. This plague patient is displaying a swollen, ruptured inguinal lymph node, or bubo. (From Centers for Disease Control-PHIL; Date: 1993.)

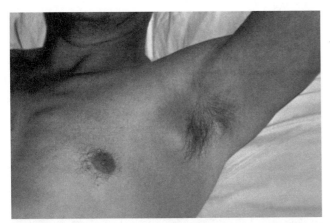

Figure 7–6. Axillary bubo. An axillary bubo and edema exhibited by a plague patient. (From Centers for Disease Control-PHIL; Date: 1962.)

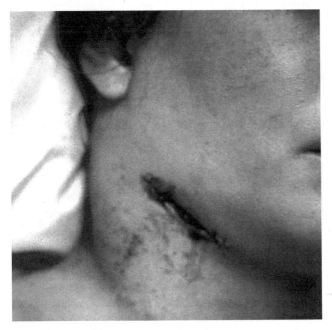

Figure 7–7. Cervical bubo. Plague patient whose symptoms include this swollen, ulcerated cervical lymph node. (From Centers for Disease Control-PHIL; Date: 1993.)

Frequently, the plague infection spreads hematogenously resulting in capillary fragility and causing cutaneous petechiae and ecchymoses, which can mimic meningococcemia (78). Plague septicemia can produce small artery thromboses in the acral vessels of the nose and digits, resulting in gangrene and complete necrosis (79). Black necrotic appendages and more proximal purpuric lesions caused by endotoxemia are often present (80). These signs are believed to be responsible for the term "black death" during the second plague pandemic (81). Unfortunately, the late finding of acral gangrene will not be helpful in the early diagnosis of plague when life-saving antibiotics should be given (Figs. 7-8 and 7-9) (82).

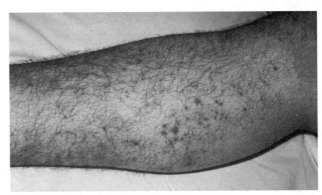

Figure 7–8. Petechiae and purpura. Capillary fragility is one of the manifestations of a plague infection, evident here on the leg of an infected patient. (From Centers for Disease Control-PHL; Date: 1954.)

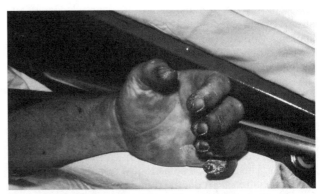

Figure 7–9. Acral gangrene. This patient presented with symptoms of plague that included gangrene of the right hand causing necrosis of the fingers. (From Centers for Disease Control-PHL; Date: 1975.)

PNEUMONIC PLAGUE

Symptoms of pneumonic plague begin after an incubation period of 1 to 6 days (average of 2 to 4 days) and include sudden-onset of high fever, chills, headache, malaise followed by cough, often with hemoptysis, chest pain, and dyspnea (83–85). Patients develop progressive dyspnea, stridor, and cyanosis. Patients with terminal pneumonic or septic plague develop livid cyanosis (86,87). Death results from respiratory failure, circulatory collapse, and bleeding diathesis if the condition was not diagnosed early and treated properly (88). During pre-antibiotic era epidemics, the average time from respiratory exposure to death from pneumonic plague in humans is reported to be from 2 to 4 days (89).

Primary pneumonic plague rarely occurs in the United States. There have been two such cases in the United States in the past 20 years, both occurring after handling domestic cats with pneumonic plague. Both patients complained of typical pneumonic symptoms, but they also complained of prominent gastrointestinal symptoms of nausea, vomiting, abdominal pain, and diarrhea. Diagnosis was delayed more than 24 hours after symptom development in both cases, and both patients died (90,91).

PLAGUE MENINGITIS

Plague bacilli can spread hematogenously to the central nervous system if appropriate antibiotic therapy is not initiated soon enough. The resulting plague meningitis with fever, meningismus, and other meningeal signs is indistinguishable from meningococcemia (92). Plague meningitis occurs in approximately 6% of septicemic and pneumonic cases (93).

DIFFERENTIAL DIAGNOSIS

Diagnosis of plague is based primarily on clinical suspicion. An acutely ill patient complaining of sudden onset of fever, headache, malaise, and a painful, enlarged mass in the groin or axilla (especially if in an endemic area or following exposure to rodents, rabbits, or fleas) should lead to the presumptive diagnosis of bubonic plague. The differential diagnosis for bubonic plague includes tularemia, cat scratch fever, lymphogranuloma venereum, chancroid, scrub typhus, and other staphylococcal and streptococcal infections. Diagnosis can be aided by Gram staining aspirate from the bubo.

The differential diagnosis of septicemic plague should include meningococcemia, other gram-negative sepsis, and the rickettsioses.

The diagnosis of pneumonic plague is usually much more complicated because a plague aerosol is colorless, odorless, and tasteless. There will not have been an explosion or gas cloud to announce the presence of lethal agent in the air. And the development of symptoms would not occur for 1 to 3 days. The patient who presents with systemic toxicity, a productive cough with bloody sputum can lead to a large differential. However, the sudden appearance of large numbers of previously healthy patients with severe, rapidly progressive pneumonia with hemoptysis should strongly suggest pneumonic plague and a deliberate bioterrorist attack (94). Demonstration of gram-negative rods in the patient's sputum should readily suggest pneumonic plague because *Yersinia pestis* is the only gram-negative bacterium that can cause extensive, fulminate pneumonia with bloody sputum in an otherwise healthy, immunocompetent patient (95).

LABORATORY STUDIES

Routine Blood Studies

Routine blood studies are marginally helpful but will not provide a definitive diagnosis. Complete blood count (CBC) with differential should reveal leukocytosis with a total white blood cell count up to 20,000 cells with a "left

shift" of increased bands, and greater than 80% polymorphonuclear cells (96). One often finds increased fibrin-split products indicative of low-grade disseminated intravascular coagulation (DIC). Serum blood urea nitrogen (BUN), creatinine, alanine amniotransferase (ALT), aspartate amniotransferase (AST), and bilirubin may also be elevated, indicative of multiorgan failure (97,98).

Microscopy Studies

A presumptive diagnosis of plague can be made microscopically by identifying the classic coccobacilli of *Yersinia pestis* using Gram (Fig. 7-10), Wright, Giemsa (Fig. 7-11), or Wayson's stained smears of lymph node needle aspirate, sputum, blood, or cerebrospinal fluid specimens. Direct fluorescent antibody (DFA) staining is quite useful when available due to the DFA stain's affinity for the F_1 capsular antigen of *Yersinia pestis* (Figs. 7-10 to 7-12).

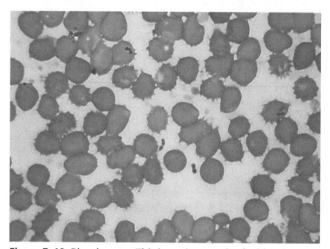

Figure 7–10. Blood smear. This is a micrograph of a blood smear containing *Yersinia pestis* plague bacteria. (From Centers for Disease Control-PHIL; Date: 1975.)

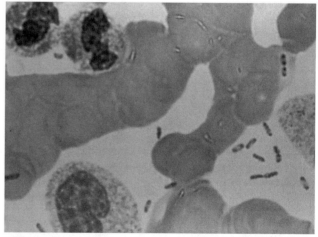

Figure 7–11. Wright's stain. Dark stained bipolar ends of *Yersinia pestis* can clearly be seen in this Wright's stain of blood from a plague victim. (From Centers for Disease Control-PHIL; Date: 1993.)

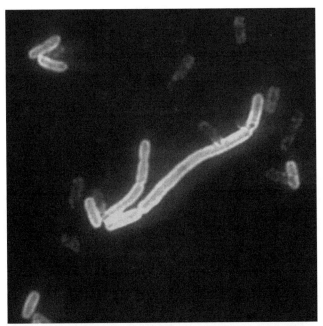

Figure 7–12. Immunofluorescent study. DFA study revealing *Yersinia pestis* at 200X. (From Centers for Disease Control-PHIL; Date: 2002.)

Bacterial Cultures

Bacterial cultures of blood, bubo aspirate, sputum, and cerebrospinal fluid (CSF) (if indicated) should be performed. *Yersinia pestis* grows best aerobically at 28°C on sheep blood or MacConkey agar media. Growth is usually demonstrated in 24 to 48 hours, revealing tiny 1 to 3 mm "beaten-copper" colonies at 48 hours. At 72 hours, "fried-egg" colonies may be identified. Laboratory personnel need to be warned of suspected plague because automated bacterial identification systems may misdiagnose *Yersinia pestis*, or take up to 6 days to identify (Fig. 7-13).

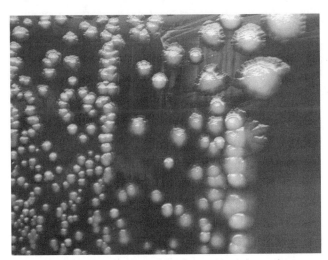

Figure 7–13. Culture on sheep blood agar. *Yersinia pestis* grows well on most standard laboratory media. After 48 to 72 hours, gray-white to slightly yellow opaque raised, irregular "fried egg" morphology; alternatively, colonies may have a "hammered copper" shiny surface. (From Centers for Disease Control-PHIL; Date: 2002.)

Radiographic Studies

Radiographic findings of the chest are variable in pneumonic plague but usually reveal bilateral infiltrates, which may be patchy or a consolidated bronchopneumonia (Fig. 7-14) (99,100).

The CDC's Laboratory Test Criteria for Diagnosis of Plague helps health care workers determine if clinical and laboratory results make the diagnosis of plague *suspected*, *presumptive*, or *confirmed* (Table 7-1).

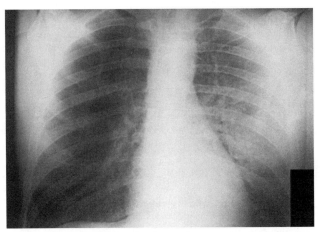

Figure 7–14. CXR pneumonic plague. Anteroposterior chest radiograph of plague patient showing bilateral pulmonary infiltrates. (From Centers for Disease Control-PHIL; Date: 1975.)

MEDICAL MANAGEMENT

NOTIFICATION

It is a U.S. Public Health Service requirement that all suspected cases of plague be reported to local and state health departments, and that the diagnosis be confirmed by the Centers for Disease Control and Prevention (101).

ISOLATION

Any patient suspected or confirmed to have pneumonic plague should remain isolated during the first 48 hours of antibiotic treatment, and until clinical improvement results (102–104). If large numbers of patients with pneumonic plague exist, they may be cohorted while undergoing antibiotic therapy. Standard Universal Precautions should be used whenever handling patients with suspected or confirmed infections or contact with plague; Respiratory Droplet Precautions should be added for suspected or confirmed pneumonic plague (105). In large pneumonic plague epidemics during the past century, human-to-human transmission was prevented by simply wearing masks (106–109). Therefore, existing national guidelines recommend the use of disposable surgical masks to prevent transmission of pneumonic plague (110). The use of masks is recommended for patients and health care professionals, as well as others who may come within close contact (defined as 2 meters) (111,112) of a patient with suspected pneumonic plague. Patients being transported should be wearing surgical masks (113).

TABLE 7-1	CDC's Laboratory Criteria for Diagnosis of Plague

SUSPECTED PLAGUE SHOULD BE CONSIDERED IF THE FOLLOWING CONDITIONS ARE MET:

1. Clinical symptoms are compatible with plague (i.e., fever and lymphadenopathy in a person who resides in or recently traveled to a plague-endemic area).
2. Small gram-negative and/or bipolar-staining coccobacilli are seen on a smear taken from such affected tissues as
   • Bubo (bubonic plague)
   • Blood (septicemic plague)
   • Tracheal/lung aspirate (pneumonic plague)

PRESUMPTIVE PLAGUE SHOULD BE CONSIDERED WHEN *ONE OR BOTH* OF THE FOLLOWING CONDITIONS ARE MET:

1. If immunofluorescence stain of smear or material is positive for the presence of *Yersinia pestis* F1 antigen.
2. If only a single serum specimen is tested and the anti-F1 antigen titer by agglutination is >1:10.*

CONFIRMED PLAGUE IS DIAGNOSED IF *ONE* OF THE FOLLOWING CONDITIONS IS MET:

1. If a culture isolated is lysed by specific bacteriophage.
2. If two serum specimens demonstrate a fourfold anti-F1 antigen titer difference by agglutination testing.*
3. If a single serum specimen tested by agglutination has a titer of >1:128 and the patient has no known previous plague exposure or vaccination history.*

*Agglutination testing must be shown to be specific to *Y. pestis* F1 antigen by hemagglutination inhibition.

Laboratory Test Criteria for Diagnosis of Plague. Taken from the CDC's plague web site, Division of Vector-Borne Infectious Diseases, Centers for Disease Control and Prevention, Atlanta, GA. Available at: http://www.cdc.gov/ncidod/dvbid/plague/lab-test-criteria.htm. Last accessed October 1, 2003.

LABORATORY SPECIMENS

Blood, sputum, bronchial washing, CSF, or lymph node aspirates should be taken for laboratory study as indicated by the clinical presentation, as soon as possible *before* initiating antibiotic therapy.

ANTIBIOTIC TREATMENT

Recommendations for antibiotic treatment of plague in this chapter are based here on the comprehensive evaluation made by the Working Group on Civilian Biodefense as published in the *Journal of the American Medical Association* entitled, "Plague as a Biological Weapon: Medical and Public Health Management," commonly referred to as the JAMA Consensus Statement on Plague (114). The Working Group was comprised of experts on biological warfare from the Center for Civilian Biodefense Studies at Johns Hopkins, including Thomas V. Inglesby, D.A. Henderson, and Tara O'Toole; specialists such as David T. Dennis from the Centers for Disease Control and Prevention; and Edward Eitzen, Arthur M. Friedlander, and Gerald Parker from the U.S. Army Medical Research Institute of Infectious Diseases (115).

Although the recommendations made by the Working Group published in the JAMA Consensus Statement were made based upon the evaluation of the most up-to-date studies available at the time, and their recommendations are still valid at the time of this publication, final selection of antibiotic therapy should be made based upon the clinical situation and the most current medical information available. This author recommends verifying antibiotic selection with available infectious disease specialists and public health authorities within your state and at the Centers for Disease Control and Prevention. Links to these sources are provided at the end of this chapter. Adjustments to antibiotic coverage should be made based upon antibiotic susceptibility testing of cultures taken from the patient prior to initiation of therapy (116).

The Working Group's recommendations for antibiotic therapy are provided in Table 7-2. Note that the Working Group makes a distinction between *contained casualty* settings and *mass casualty settings* and postexposure prophylaxis. A contained casualty setting is one in which a modest number of patients require treatment. In such a setting, parenteral antibiotic therapy is optimal. However, in the event of a deliberate act of bioterrorism using aerosolized plague agent resulting in mass casualties, there will most likely be a shortage of intravenous antibiotics, equipment, and possibly hospital beds. In such a setting, recommendations for oral antibiotic therapies are provided (117).

Streptomycin has been recognized as the treatment of choice for bubonic, septicemic, and pneumonic plague since 1948 and remains the drug of choice for adults and children in the contained casualty setting (118,119). *Chloramphenicol is the drug of choice for plague meningitis* for adults and children in both the contained and the mass casualty setting, with IV therapy if available, otherwise supplanted by oral preparations (120). If streptomycin is unavailable, gentamicin may be substituted. Alternative therapies in the contained casualty setting include intravenous doxycycline or ciprofloxacin (Table 7-2).

In mass casualty situations where intravenous therapy may not be feasible, oral doxycycline, ciprofloxacin, or chloramphenicol therapy may be substituted (Table 7-2) (121).

TABLE 7-2 JADA Consensus Statement Treatment of Pneumonic Plague Table[*]

PATIENT CATEGORY	RECOMMENDED THERAPY
	CONTAINED CASUALTY SETTING
Adults	Preferred choices
	Streptomycin, 1 g IM twice daily
	Gentamicin, 5 mg/kg IM or IV once dialy or 2 mg/kg loading dose followed by 1.7 mg/kg IM or IV 3 times daily[#]
	Alternative choices
	Doxycycline, 100 mg IV twice daily or 200 mg IV once daily
	Ciprofloxacin, 400 mg IV twice daily[¶]
	Chloramphenicol, 25 mg/kg IV 4 times daily[§]
Children[***]	Preferred choices
	Streptomycin, 15 mg/kg IM twice daily (maximum daily dose, 2 g)
	Gentamicin, 2.5 mg/kg IM or IV 3 times daily[†]
	Alternative choices
	Doxycycline,
	If ≥45 kg, give adult dosage
	If <45 kg, give 2.2 mg/kg IV twice daily (maximum, 200 mg/d)
	Ciprofloxacin, 15 mg/kg IV twice daily[¶]
	Chloramphenicol, 25 mg/kg IV 4 times daily[§]
Pregnant Women[†††]	Preferred choices
	Gentamicin, 5 mg/kg IM or IV once daily or 2 mg/kg loading dose folowed by 1.7 mg/kg IM or IV 3 times daily[†]
	Alternative choices
	Doxycycline, 100 mg IV twice daily or 200 mg IV once daily
	Ciprofloxacin, 500 mg twice daily[†]
	MASS CASUALTY SETTING AND POSTEXPOSURE PROPHYLAXIS[#]
Adults	Preferred choices
	Doxycycline, 100 mg orally twice daily [††]
	Ciprofloxacin, 400 mg IV twice daily[¶]
	Alternative choices
	Chloramphenicol, 25 mg/kg orally 4 times daily[§**]
Children	Preferred choices
	Doxycycline, [††]
	If ≥45 kg, give adult dosage
	If <45 kg, then give 2.2 mg/kg orally twice daily
	Ciprofloxacin, 20 mg/kg orally twice daily
	Alternative choices
	Chloramphenicol, 25 mg/kg orally 4 times daily[§**]
Pregnant Women	Preferred choices
	Doxycycline, 100 mg orally twice daily[††]
	Ciprofloxacin, 500 mg/kg orally twice daily
	Alternative choices
	Chloramphenicol, 25 mg/kg orally 4 times daily[§**]

TABLE 7-2 JAMA Consensus Statement Treatment of Pneumonic Plague Table* *(continued)*

* These are consensus recommendations of the Working Group on Civilian Biodefense and are not necessarily approved by the Food and Drug Administration. See "Therapy" section for explanations. One antimicrobial agent should be selected. Therapy should be continued for 10 days. Oral therapy should be substituted when patient's condition improves. IM indicates intramuscularly; IV, intravenously.

† Aminoglycosides must be adjusted according to renal function. Evidence suggests that gentamicin, 5 mg/kg IM or once daily, would be efficacious in children, although this is not yet widely accepted in clinical practice. Neonates up to 1 week of age and premature infants should receive gentamicin, 2.5 mg/kg IV twice daily.

¶ Other fluoroquinolones can be substituted at doses appropriate for age. Ciprofloxacin dosage should not exceed g/d in children.

§ Concentration should be maintained between 5 and 20 µg/ml. Concentrations greater than 25 µg/ml can cause reversible bone marrow suppression (35,62).

*** Refer to "Management of Special Groups" for details. In children, ciprofloxacin dose should not exceed 1 g/d, chloramphenicol should not exceed 4 g/d. Children younger than 2 years should not receive chloramphenicol.

††† Refer to "Management of Special Groups" for details and for discussion of breastfeeding women. In neonates, entamicin loading dose of 4 mg/kg should be given initially.

\# Duration of treatment of plague in mass casualty setting is 10 days. Duration of postexposure prophylaxis to prevent plague infection is 7 days.

** Children younger than 2 years should not receive chloramphenicol. Oral formulation available only outside the United States.

†† Tetracycline could be substituted for doxycycline.

From Working Group Recommendations for Treatment of Patients with Pneumonic Plague in the Contained and Mass Casualty Settings and for Postexposure Prophylaxis. Inglesby TV, Dennis DT, Henderson DA, et al. Plague as a biological weapon: medical and public health management. JAMA. 3 May 2000;283(17):2287.

In all cases of plague, a single antibiotic is recommended for a minimum of 10 days, or until clinical improvement results. Again, adjustments to antibiotic therapy should be made based upon antibiotic susceptibility testing of cultures taken from the patient prior to initiation of therapy (122).

PREGNANT WOMEN

In general, aminoglycosides are to be avoided in pregnant women if possible, unless severe illness warrants (123,124). However, in the setting of pneumonic plague, there is no more efficacious alternative. In the contained casualty setting, *gentamicin is the preferred aminoglycosides for pregnant women* with pneumonic plague since streptomycin has been associated with rare reports of irreversible deafness in children following fetal exposure (125). In the mass casualty setting, doxycycline should be used if parenteral gentamicin is unavailable (Table 7-2) (126).

BREASTFEEDING

The Working Group recommends that the best treatment for breastfeeding women with plague is to provide the mother and infant with the same antibiotic based upon the best antibiotic for the infant: IV gentamicin in the contained setting and oral doxycycline in the mass casualty setting (Table 7-2) (127).

POSTEXPOSURE PROPHYLAXIS

The Working Group recommends that in a community experiencing a pneumonic plague outbreak, all persons developing a new cough or a temperature of 38.5°C or higher should be promptly treated with parenteral antibiotics according to Table 7-2. In mass casualty settings or when resources will

not allow for parenteral antibiotics, then oral therapy should be initiated according to Table 7-2. For infants, tachypnea would also be an indication for immediate therapy (128,129).

Asymptomatic persons having household, hospital, or close contact (less than 2 meters/6.5 feet) with a patient with untreated pneumonic plague should receive postexposure prophylaxis for seven days (130), while watching for the development of fever and cough based on the recommendations in Table 7-2 (131).

SUPPORTIVE THERAPY

Patients with pneumonic or septicemic plague will require advanced medical supportive care in addition to antibiotic therapy (132). Complications of gram-negative sepsis, such as adult respiratory distress syndrome, DIC, shock, and multiorgan failure, should be expected (133).

TRIAGE CONSIDERATIONS

WHO GETS SEEN FIRST?

Based on standard emergency department protocols, those with septicemic and pneumonic plague will most likely need to be seen ahead of stable patients with bubonic plague.

WHO NEEDS ISOLATION?

Any patient suspected or confirmed to have pneumonic plague needs respiratory isolation. Those with bubonic or septicemic plague should be handled with standard (universal) precautions.

WHO GETS ANTIBIOTICS?

Any patient suspected or confirmed to have infection with plague will need to be treated with antibiotics. Those patients believed to have pneumonic or septicemic plague should be treated with intravenous streptomycin (or gentamicin) if available.

WHO NEEDS ADMITTING?

Patients with pneumonic or septicemic plague will need admitting. Those with bubonic plague should be admitted based upon their condition and the availability of hospital beds in the event of a major outbreak or biological attack.

PERSONAL PROTECTION

INFECTION CONTROL AND DECONTAMINATION

Standard (Universal) Precautions

All persons who come in close contact with suspected or confirmed cases of plague should use the Centers for Disease Control and Prevention Guidelines for Standard (Universal) Precautions (134,135). Hospitals are required to follow Occupational Safety and Health Administration (OSHA) Bloodborne Pathogens regulations, which also serve to protect health care workers from transmission (136). CDC-recommended Transmission-Based Droplet Precautions are to be added for suspected or confirmed cases of pneumonic plague (137). As a general rule, pneumonic plague should be handled with the same precautions used to protect against the more common respiratory disease, tuberculosis (138). Transmission-Based Contact Precautions should be used for draining buboes.

Laboratory Biosafety

Simple laboratory work with the plague bacillus, such as handling clinical material or cultures, should be handled using Biosafety Level 2 conditions. Biosafety Level 3 precautions are required when performing activities (e.g., centrifuging, vigorous shaking, grinding, or cutting bone) involving high risk for aerosol or droplet production (139,140).

Post Mortem

Bodies of patients who have died from plague infection should be handled with routine strict precautions by trained personnel. Safety precautions for the transport of the dead for burial should be the same as those when transporting ill patients (141). Postmortem aerosol-producing procedures (e.g., sawing bone) are not recommended, but when necessary, they should be carried out using high-efficiency particulate-filtered masks and negative-pressure rooms as is customary when dealing with *Mycobacterium tuberculosis* (142).

Decontamination

Hospital rooms, emergency department examination areas, reusable instruments, clothing, and linens should undergo terminal cleaning, after being used by a suspected or confirmed plague patient, in accordance with standard precautions and hospital protocol (143). Decontamination may be accomplished using any Environmental Protection Agency (EPA) hospital-approved disinfectant, or a hypochlorite solution (one part household bleach with nine parts water). Aerosolized plague is believed be susceptible to sunlight and is expected to survive for only about 1 hour outdoors.

Environmental Decontamination

The plague bacillus does not pose a significant environmental threat to the population following an aerosol attack because *Yersinia pestis* is very sensitive to light and heat and does not survive long. A World Health Organization (WHO) study conducted in 1970 estimated that a plague aerosol would remain infectious for only 1 hour after an outdoor release (144). The bacillus would be expected to survive longer if indoors and protected from sunlight and heat. On the other hand, plague fleas are relatively hardy and can survive outdoors without a host for at least 6 months (145), and cleanup of susceptible rodents should be a public health priority in the event of a bubonic plague outbreak.

Vaccines

Plague vaccines using dead or inactivated *Yersinia pestis* have been around since the first killed whole-cell vaccine was developed by Russian physician Waldemar Haffkine in 1896 (146). The United States licensed a Formalin-killed, phenol-preserved whole-cell, injected vaccine that was available in the United States from 1946 until 1999 when it was withdrawn from the market by the manufacturer (147). The vaccine offered protection against bubonic plague, but it did not prevent or ameliorate the development of primary pneumonic plague when exposure to aerosolized plague bacteria (148–150). Live-attenuated vaccines have been unsuccessful because they are much more reactogenic than the killed vaccine (151). Research is ongoing in the pursuit of a vaccine that protects against primary pneumonic plague (152,153), and the National Institute of Allergy and Infectious Diseases (NIAID) is currently accepting research proposals for new plague vaccine for the general public.

SUMMARY

Disease: PLAGUE: Bubonic, pneumonic, septicemic, and rarely meningitic.

Organism: bacterium *Yersinia pestis.*

Transmission:

- Flea bites from infected rodents.
- Direct contact with infected tissues or body fluids from handling sick or dead animals.
- Respiratory droplets from cats and humans with pneumonic plague.
- Intentional aerosolized weaponized agent.

Incidence of naturally occurring plague: An average of 13 cases a year (range of 5 to 15) in the United States, usually in one of the southwestern states (New Mexico, Arizona, Colorado, and California). Plague may occur anytime during the year.

Mortality rate: The mortality rate for untreated pneumonic and septicemic plague is 100%; it is 60% for untreated bubonic plague.

Incubation period: Bubonic plague: 2 to 6 days; primary pneumonic plague: 1 to 3 days.

Major signs and symptoms:

- *All:* fever, malaise, headache, myalgias, dyspepsia, vomiting, and diarrhea.
- *Bubonic:* fever, malaise, headache, myalgias, tender lymphadenopathy (femoral, inguinal, axillary, and cervical), high fever.
- *Septicemic:* absence of tender lymphadenopathy, severe fever, and rapid progression to sepsis with multiorgan failure. Patients often complain of abdominal pain.
- *Pneumonic:* fever, malaise, headache, myalgias, cough, dyspnea, chest pain, hemoptysis, with rapidly progressive respiratory failure. Patients often complain of dyspepsia, abdominal pain, nausea, vomiting, and diarrhea.

Diagnosis:

- *Suspected:* Suspect plague if large numbers of previously healthy individuals present with rapidly progressive gram-negative pneumonia, especially with hemoptysis.

- *Presumptive:* Diagnosis can be made by Gram, Wright, Giemsa, or Wayson stain of blood, sputum, CSF, or lymph node aspirates. DFA studies can be helpful.

- *Definitive:* Requires a positive culture of *Yersinia pestis.* PCR can be used if available.

Treatment: Isolate the patient and notify public health authorities as soon as plague is suspected. Early administration of antibiotic therapy (following laboratory specimens) is crucial. The *drug of choice for pneumonic plague is streptomycin,* 1 g IM twice daily. If streptomycin is unavailable, use gentamicin IM, followed by doxycycline or ciprofloxacin IV. *Chloramphenicol is the drug of choice for plague meningitis.* In mass casualty situations where intravenous therapy is not feasible, oral doxycycline, ciprofloxacin, or chloramphenicol may be substituted (154).

Prophylaxis: Prophylaxis is recommended for individuals with a history of exposure to plague or infected fleas. The preferred antibiotics include the tetracyclines, chloramphenicol, or one of the effective sulfonamides.

Personal protection: Use standard universal precautions for all suspected or confirmed cases of plague. Add Respiratory Droplet Precautions for suspected or confirmed cases of pneumonic plague.

Decontamination: Decontamination may be accomplished using any EPA hospital-approved disinfectant or a hypochlorite solution (or one part household bleach with nine parts water), which work best if left on contaminated areas for 30 minutes before proceeding with usual cleaning. Decontamination of clothing and fomites should be conducted. Aerosolized plague is believed to survive for about 1 hour.

Vaccine: Vaccine is no longer commercially available in the United States. The injected, Formalin-killed, whole-cell vaccine made many years ago does not protect against inhaled exposure to plague bacteria and was withdrawn from the market by the manufacturer in 1999. NIAID is currently accepting research proposals for new plague vaccine for the general public.

RESOURCES

1. JAMA Consensus Statement on Plague. Inglesby TV, Dennis DT, Henderson DA, et al. Plague as a biological weapon: medical and public health management. JAMA. 2000;2281–90. Available at: http://www.bt.cdc.gov/Agent/Plague/Consensus.pdf. Accessed October 1, 2003.

2. CDC Plague Home Page. Division of Vector-Borne Diseases Infectious Diseases, Center for Disease Control and Prevention, web site on plague. Available at: http://www.cdc.gov/ncidod/dvbid/plague/. Accessed October 1, 2003.

3. WHO Plague Web Site. Communicable disease surveillance and response, World Health Organization. Available at: http://www.who.int/csr/disease/plague /en/. Accessed October 1, 2003.

4. MEDLINEplus Health Information Plague Web Site. A service of the U.S. National Library of Medicine and the National Institutes of Health. Available at: http://www.nlm.nih.gov/medlineplus/plague.html. Accessed October 1, 2003.

5. USAMRIID's Medical Management of Biological Casualties Handbook. 4th ed. Kortepter M, Christopher G, Cieslak T, et al., editors. Fort Detrick, MD: U.S. Army Medical Research Institute of Infectious Diseases; 2001. Available at: http://www.usamriid.army.mil/education/bluebook.html. Accessed October 1, 2003.

6. Military Textbook of Medicine: Medical Aspects of Chemical and Biological Warfare. McGovern TW, Friedlander AM. Plague. In: Zatjtchuk R, Bellamy RF, editors. Medical aspects of chemical and biological warfare. Bethesda, MD: Office of the Surgeon General; 1997. Available at: http://www.nbc-med.org/SiteContent/HomePage/WhatsNew/MedAspects/contents.html.

7. Harrison's Principles of Internal Medicine Plague Chapter. Campbell GL, Dennis DT. Plague and other Yersinia infections. In: Fauci AS, Braunwald E, Isselbacher KJ, et al., editors. Harrison's principles of internal medicine, 14th ed. New York: McGraw-Hill, Health Professions Division; 1998.

QUESTIONS AND ANSWERS

1. Plague occurs endemically in all of the following populated continents EXCEPT:
   A. Europe
   B. North America
   C. South America
   D. Australia
   E. Asia

2. What is the most common clinical form of plague?
   A. Meningitic
   B. Bubonic
   C. Pneumonic
   D. Septicemic
   E. Pharyngitic

3. Each of the following statements regarding the clinical presentation of pneumonic plague is true EXCEPT:
   A. Gastrointestinal symptoms may be present.
   B. It has a several-week course of development.
   C. It is the most likely form of plague expected from a terrorist attack.
   D. A cervical bubo is sometimes present.
   E. It may be transmitted to humans from cats.

4. According to the Working Group on Civilian Biodefense (JAMA Consensus Statement on Plague), what is the drug of choice for treating an isolated case of pneumonic plague in an adult?
   A. Erythromycin
   B. Trimethoprim-Sulfamethoxazole
   C. Amoxicillin
   D. Tetracycline
   E. Streptomycin

ANSWERS

1: *D. Australia*
2: *B. Bubonic*
3: *B. It has a several-week course of development.*
4: *E. Streptomycin*

REFERENCES

1. Freeman BA, ed. Burrows textbook of microbiology, 22nd ed. Philadelphia: WB Saunders Company; 1985: 513-22.

2. Aleksic S, Bockemuhl J. *Yersinia* and other enterobacterieaceae. In: Murray P, ed. Manual of clinical microbiology. Washington DC: American Society for Microbiology; 1999: 483-96.

3. McGovern TW, Friedlander AM. Plague. In: Zatjtchuk R, Bellamy RF eds. Medical aspects of chemical and biological warfare. Bethesda, MD: Office of the Surgeon General; 1997:479-502.

4. Bray RS. Armies of pestilence: the effects of pandemics on history. Cambridge, UK: Lutterworthy Press; 1998.

5. Bray RS. Armies of pestilence: the effects of pandemics on history. Cambridge, UK: Lutterworthy Press; 1998.

6. Herlihy D, Cohn SK, eds. The black death and the transformation of the west. Cambridge, MA: Harvard University Press; 1997.

7. Porter S. The great plague. Gloucestershire, UK: Sutton Publishing Company; 2000.

8. Risse GB. A long pull, a strong pull and all together: San Francisco and bubonic plague, 1907–1908. Bull Hist Med. 1992;66(2):260-86.

9. Chase M. The Barbary plague: the black death in Victorian San Francisco. New York: Random House; 2003.

10. Mee C. How a mysterious disease laid low Europe's masses. Smithsonian. February 1990;20:66-79.

11. DeMussis G. Historica de Morbo s. Mortalitate quae fuit Anno Dni MCCCXLVIII. Cite in: De Mussis and the great plague of 1348: a forgotten episode of bacteriological warfare. MAMA. 1966;196(1):179-82.

12. Derbes VJ. De Mussis and the great plague of 1348: a forgotten episode of bacteriological warfare. JAMA. 1966;196(1):59-62.

13. Geissler E, ed. Biological and toxin weapons today. Oxford UK: Oxford University Press, Stockholm International Peace Research Institute; 1986.

14. Stockholm International Peace Research Institute (SIPRI). The rise of chemical-biological weapons, vol 1. In: The problem of chemical and biological warfare. New York: Humanities Press; 1971.

15. Harris SH. Factories of death. New York: Routledge; 1994.

16. Tomilin VV, Bereznhai RV. Exposure of criminal activity of the Japanese military authorities regarding preparation for bacteriological warfare. Voen Med Zh. 1985;8:26-69.

17. Gold H. Unit 731 testimony. Tokyo: Charles E. Tuttle Company; 1996.

18. Cavanough DC, Cadigan FC, Williams JE, Marshall JD. Plague. In: Ognibene AJ, Barrett O, eds. General medicine and infectious diseases, vol 2: internal medicine in Vietnam. Washington DC: Office of the Surgeon General and the Center of Military History; 1982: chapter 8, section 1.

19. The Biological and Toxin Weapons Convention. The Convention on the prohibition of the development, production and stockpiling of bacteriological (biological) and toxin weapons and on their destruction. Signed in Moscow, Washington, and London on April 10, 1972 and entered into force March 26, 1975.

20. Alibek K, Handelman S. Biohazard: the chilling true story of the largest covert biological weapons program in the world-told from inside by the man who ran it. New York: Random House; 1999.

21. Bozheyeva G, Kunakbayev Y, Yeleukenov D. Former Soviet biological weapons facilities in Kazakhstan: past, present, and future. Occasional paper no.1. Center for nonproliferation studies. Monterey, CA: Monterey Institute of International Studies; 1999.

22. Nowalk RM. Walkers mammals of the world, vol 2, 5th ed. Baltimore: Johns Hopkins University Press; 1991.

23. Freeman BA, ed. Burrows textbook of microbiology, 22nd ed. Philadelphia: WB Saunders Company; 1985; 513-22.

24. Perry RD, Fetherston JD. Yersinia pestis: etiologic agent of plague. Clin Microbiol Rev. 1997;10:35-66.

25. Perry RE, Fetherston JD. Yersinia pestis: etiologic agent of plague. Clin Microbiol Rev. 1997;10:35-66.

26. Centers for Disease Control and Prevention. Update: human plague—India, 1994. MMWR. 1994;43(41):761.

27. Catan JL, Kartman L. Human plague in the United States: 1900–1966. JAMA. 1968;205(6):81-4.

28. Cavanaugh DC. KF Meyer's work on plague. J Infect Dis. 1974;129(suppl):S10-12.

29. Kellog WH. An epidemic of pneumonic plague. Am J Public Health. 1920;10:599–605.

30. Centers for Disease Control and Prevention. Fatal human plague. MMWR. 1997;278:380-2.

31. Centers for Disease Control and Prevention. Prevention of plague. MMWR. 1996;45(RR-14):1-15.

32. Harrison FJ. Prevention and control of plague. Aurora, CO: US Army Center for Health Promotion and Preventative Medicine, Fitzsimons Army Medical Center; September 1995. Technical guide 103.

33. Caten JL, Kartman L. Human plague in the United States: 1900-1966. JAMA. 1968;205(6):81-4.

34. Freeman BA, ed. Burrows textbook of microbiology, 22nd ed. Philadelphia: WB Saunders Company; 1985: 513-22.

35. McGovern TW, Friedlander AM. Plague. In: Zatjtchuk R, Bellamy RF, eds. Medical aspects of chemical and biological warfare. Bethesda, MD: Office of the Surgeon General; 1997: 479-502.

36. Inglesby TV, Dennis DT, Henderson DA, et al. Plague as a biological weapon: medical and public health management. JAMA. 3 May 2000;283(17):2281-90.

37. Perry RE, Fetherston JD. Yersinia pestis: etiologic agent of plague. Clin Microbiol Rev. 1997;10:35-66.

38. McGovern TW, Friedlander AM. Plague. In: Zatjtchuk R, Bellamy RF, eds. Medical aspects of chemical and biological warfare. Bethesda, MD: Office of the Surgeon General; 1997: 479-502.

39. Harrison FJ. Prevention and control of plague. Aurora, CO: US Army Center for Health Promotion and Preventative Medicine, Fitzsimons Army Medical Center; September 1995. Technical guide 103.

40. Inglesby TV, Dennis DT, Henderson DA, et al. Plague as a biological weapon: medical and public health management. JAMA. 3 May 2000;283(17):2281-90.

41. Bayliss JH. The extinction of bubonic plague in Britain. Endeavour. 1980;4(2):58-66.

42. Harrison FJ. Prevention and control of plague. Aurora, CO: US Army Center for Health Promotion and Preventative Medicine, Fitzsimons Army Medical Center; September 1995. Technical guide 103.

43. Craven RB, Maupin GO, Beard ML, et al. Reported cases of human plague infections in the United States, 1970–1991. J Med Entolmol. 1993;30(4):758-61.

44. Gage KL, Lance SE, Dennis DT, Montenieri JA. Human plague in the United States: a review of cases from 1988–1992 with comments on the likelihood of increased plague activity. Border Epidemiol Bull. 1992;19(6):1-10.

45. Cavanough DC, Williams JE. Plague: some ecological interrelationships. In: Trauber, Starcke H, eds. Fleas. Rotterdam: A.A.Balkema; 1980: 245-56.

46. Kellog WH. An epidemic of pneumonic plague. Am J Public Health. 1920;10:599–605.

47. McGovern TW, Friedlander AM. Plague. In: Zatjtchuk R, Bellamy RF, eds. Medical aspects of chemical and biological warfare. Bethesda, MD: Office of the Surgeon General; 1997:479-502.

48. Harris SH. Factories of death. New York: Routledge; 1994.

49. Tomilin VV, Berezhnai RV. Exposure of criminal activity of the Japanese military authorities regarding preparation for bacteriological warfare. Voen Med Zh. 1985;8:26-69.

50. Gold H. Unit 731 testimony. Tokyo: Charles E. Tuttle Company; 1996.

51. Alibek K, Handelman S. Biohazard: the chilling true story of the largest covert biological weapons program in the world-told from inside by the man who ran it. New York: Random House; 1999.

52. Bozheyeva G, Kunakbayev Y, Yeleukenov D. Former Soviet biological weapons facilities in Kazakhstan: past, present, and future. Occasional paper no.1. Center for Nonproliferation Studies. Monterey, CA: Monterey Institute of International Studies; 1999.

53. Freeman BA, ed. Burrows textbook of microbiology, 22nd ed. Philadelphia: WB Saunders Company; 1985: 513-22.

54. Brubaker RR. Factors promoting acute and chronic diseases caused by Yersinia. Clin Microbiol Rev. 1991;4(3):309-24.

55. Inglesby TV, Dennis DT, Henderson DA, et al. Plague as a biological weapon: medical and public health management. JAMA. 3 May 2000;283(17):2281-90.

56. Butler T. Yersinia species (including plague). In: Mandell GL, Bennett JE, Dolin R, eds. Principles and practice of infectious diseases. New York: Churchill Livingstone; 1995:2070-78.

57. McGovern TW, Friedlander AM. Plague. In: Zatjtchuk R, Bellamy RF, eds. Medical aspects of chemical and biological warfare. Bethesda, MD: Office of the Surgeon General; 1997:479-502.

58. McGovern TW, Friedlander AM. Plague. In: Zatjtchuk R, Bellamy RF, eds. Medical aspects of chemical and biological warfare. Bethesda, MD: Office of the Surgeon General; 1997:479-502.

59. Brubaker RR. Factors promoting acute and chronic diseases caused by Yersinia. Clin Microbiol Rev. 1991;4(3):309-24.

60. Ehrenkranz NF, Meyer KF. Studies on immunization against plague, VIII: study of three immunizing preparations in protecting primates against pneumonic plague. J Infect Dis. 1955;96:138-44.

61. Speck RS, Wolochow H. Studies on the experimental epidemiology of respiratory infections, experimental pneumonic plague in *Macacus rhesus*. J Infect Dis. 1957;100:58-68.

62. Campbell GL, Dennis DT. Plague and other Yersinia infections. In: Fauci AS, Braunwald E, Isselbacher KJ, et al, eds. Harrison's principles of internal medicine, 14th ed. New York: McGraw-Hill, Health Professions Division; 1998: 975-83.

63. Inglesby TV, Dennis DT, Henderson DA, et al. Plague as a biological weapon: medical and public health management. JAMA. 3 May 2000;283(17):2281-90.

64. McGovern TW, Friedlander AM. Plague. In: Zatjtchuk R, Bellamy RF, eds. Medical aspects of chemical and biological warfare. Bethesda, MD: Office of the Surgeon General; 1997:479-502.

65. Freeman BA, ed. Burrows textbook of microbiology, 22nd ed. Philadelphia: WB Saunders Company; 1985: 513-22.

66. Inglesby TV, Dennis DT, Henderson DA, et al. Plague as a biological weapon: medical and public health management. JAMA. 3 May 2000;283(17):2281-90.

67. Kortepter M, Christopher G, Cieslak T, et al., eds. USAMRIID's medical management of biological casualties handbook, 4th ed. Fort Detrick, MD: U.S. Army Medical Research Institute of Infectious Diseases; 2001: 35-9.

68. Kortepter M, Christopher G, Cieslak T, et al., eds. USAMRIID's medical management of biological casualties handbook. 4th ed. Fort Detrick, MD: U.S. Army Medical Research Institute of Infectious Diseases; 2001: 35-9.

69. Campbell GL, Dennis DT. Plague and other Yersinia infections. In: Fauci AS, Braunwald E, Isselbacher KJ, et al., eds. Harrison's principles of internal medicine, 14th ed. New York: McGraw-Hill, Health Professions Division; 1998: 975-83.

70. Butler T. Yersinia species (including plague). In: Mandell GL, Bennett JE, Dolin R, eds. Principles and practice of infectious diseases. New York: Churchill Livingstone; 1995:2070-8.

71. McGovern TW, Friedlander AM. Plague. In: Zatjtchuk R, Bellamy RF, eds. Medical aspects of chemical and biological warfare. Bethesda, MD: Office of the Surgeon General; 1997: 479-502.

72. Legter LJ, Cottingham AJ Jr, Hunter DH. Clinical and epidemiological notes on a defined outbreak of plague in Vietnam. Am J Trop Med Hyg. 1970;19:639-52.

73. Welty TK. Plague. Am Fam Phys. 1986;33(6):159–64.

74. Crook LD, Tempest B. Plague: a clinical review of 27 cases. Arch Intern Med. June 1992;152:1253-6.

75. McGovern TW, Friedlander AM. Plague. In: Zatjtchuk R, Bellamy RF, eds. Medical aspects of chemical and biological warfare. Bethesda, MD: Office of the Surgeon General; 1997:479-502.

76. Campbell GL, Dennis DT. Plague and other *Yersinia* infections. In: Fauci AS, Braunwald E, Isselbacher KJ, et al. eds. Harrison's principles of internal medicine, 14th ed. New York: McGraw-Hill, Health Professions Division; 1998: 975-83.

77. Campbell GL, Dennis DT. Plague and other Yersinia infections. In: Fauci AS, Braunwald E, Isselbacher KJ, et al. eds. Harrison's principles of internal medicine, 14th ed. New York: McGraw-Hill, Health Professions Division; 1998: 975-83.

78. McGovern TW, Christopher GW, Eizen EM. Cutaneous manifestations of biological warfare and related threat agents. Arch Dermatol. March 1999;135:311-22.

79. Conrad FB, LeCocq FR, Krain R. A recent epidemic of plague in Vietnam. Arch Intern Med. 1968;122:193-8.

80. Kortepter M, Christopher G, Cieslak T, et al., eds. USAMRIID's medical management of biological casualties handbook, 4th ed. Fort Detrick, MD: U.S. Army Medical Research Institute of Infectious Diseases; 2001.

81. Butler T. Yersinia species (including plague). In: Mandell GL, Bennett JE, Dolin R, eds. Principles and practice of infectious diseases. New York: Churchill Livingstone; 1995: 2070-8.

82. Inglesby TV, Dennis DT, Henderson DA, et al. Plague as a biological weapon: medical and public health management. JAMA. 3 May 2000;283(17):2281-90.

83. Franz DR, Jahrling PB, Friedlander AM, et al. Clinical recognition and management of patients exposed to biological warfare agents. JAMA. 6 Aug 1997;278(5):399-411.

84. Wu L-T. A treatise on pneumonic plague. Geneva, Switzerland: League of Nations Health Organization; 1926.

85. Butler T. Yersinia species (including plague). In: Mandell GL, Bennett JE, Dolin R, eds. Priniciples and practice of infectious diseases. New York: Churchill Livingstone; 1995;2070-8.

86. McGovern TW, Christopher GW, Eizen EM. Cutaneous manifestations of biological warfare and related threat agents. Arch Dermatol. Mar 1999;135:311-22.

87. Cavanaugh DC, Cadigan FC, Williams JE, Marshall JD. Plague. In: Ognibene AJ, Barrett ON, eds. General medicine and infectious diseases. Washington DC: Office of the Surgeon General and Center of Military History; 1982.

88. Kortepter M, Christopher G, Cieslak T, et al., eds. USAMRIID's medical management of biological casualties handbook, 4th ed. Fort Detrick, MD: U.S. Army Medical Research Institute of Infectious Diseases; 2001: 35.

89. Wu L-T. A treatise on pneumonic plague. Geneva, Switzerland: League of Nations Health Organization; 1926.

90. Centers for Disease Control and Prevention. Pneumonic plague—Arizona. MMWR. 1992;41:737-9.

91. Werner SB, Weidmer CE, Nelson BC, et al. Primary plague pneumonia contracted from a domestic cat in South Lake Tahoe, California. JAMA. 1984;251:929-31.

92. Becker TM, Poland JD, Quan TJ, et al. Plague meningitis—a retrospective analysis of cases reported in the United States, 1970–1979. West J Med. 1987;147:554-7.

93. Kortepter M, Christopher G, Cieslak T, et al., eds. USAMRIID's medical management of biological casualties hand-

book, 4th ed. Fort Detrick, MD: U.S. Army Medical Research Institute of Infectious Diseases; 2001.

94. Centers for Disease Control and Prevention. Recognition of illnesses associated with the intentional release of a biological agent. MMWR. 19 Oct 2001;50(41):893-7.

95. McGovern TW, Friedlander AM. Plague. In: Zatjtchuk R, Bellamy RF, eds. Medical aspects of chemical and biological warfare. Bethesda, MD: Office of the Surgeon General; 1997: 479-502.

96. McGovern TW, Friedlander AM. Plague. In: Zatjtchuk R, Bellamy RF, eds. Medical aspects of chemical and biological warfare. Bethesda, MD: Office of the Surgeon General; 1997: 479-502.

97. Kortepter M, Christopher G, Cieslak T, et al., eds. USAMRIID's medical management of biological casualties handbook, 4th ed. Fort Detrick, MD: U.S. Army Medical Research Institute of Infectious Diseases; 2001.

98. Dennis D, Meier F. Plague. In: Horsburgh CR, Nelson AM, eds. Pathology of emerging infections. Washington DC: ASM Press; 1997: 21-47.

99. Alsofrom DJ, Mettler FA Jr, Mann JM. Radiographic manifestations of plague in New Mexico, 1975–1980: a review of 42 proved cases. Radiology. 1981;139:561-5.

100. Crook LD, Tempest B. Plague: a clinical review of 27 cases. Arch Intern Med. June 1992;152:1253-6.

101. Inglesby TV, Dennis DT, Henderson DA, et al. Plague as a biological weapon: medical and public health management. JAMA. 3 May 2000;283(17):2281-90.

102. McGovern TW, Friedlander AM. Plague. In: Zatjtchuk R, Bellamy RF, eds. Medical aspects of chemical and biological warfare. Bethesda, MD: Office of the Surgeon General; 1997: 479-502.

103. American Public Health Association. Plague. In: Benenson AS, ed. Control of communicable diseases manual. Washington DC: American Public Health Association; 1995: 353-8.

104. World Health Organization. WHO Expert Committee on Plague: 3rd report. Geneva: World Health Organization; 1970: 1-25. Technical report series 447.

105. Kortepter M, Christopher G, Cieslak T, et al., eds. USAMRIID's medical management of biological casualties handbook, 4th ed. Fort Detrick, MD: U.S. Army Medical Research Institute of Infectious Diseases; 2001.

106. Meyer K. Pneumonic plague. Bacteriol Rev. 1961;25:249-61.

107. Kellog WM. An epidemic of pneumonic plague. Am J Public Health. 1920;10:599–605.

108. Wu L-T. A treatise on pneumonic plague. Geneva: League of Nations Health Organization; 1926.

109. Chernin E. Richard Pearson Strong and the Manchurian epidemic of pneumonic plague, 1910–1911. J Hist Med Allied Sci. 1989;44:296-319.

110. American Public Health Association. Plague. In: Benenson AS, ed. Control of communicable diseases manual. Washington DC: American Public Health Association; 1995: 353-8.

111. Wu L-T. A treatise on pneumonic plague. Geneva: League of Nations Health Organization; 1926.

112. Centers for Disease Control and Prevention. Prevention of plague: recommendations of the Advisory Committee on Immunization Practice (ACIP). MMWR. 1996;45(RR-14):1-15.

113. Inglesby TV, Dennis DT, Henderson DA, et al. Plague as a biological weapon: medical and public health management. JAMA. 2000 May 3;283(17):2281-90.

114. Inglesby TV, Dennis DT, Henderson DA, Bartlett JG, Ascher MS, Eitzen E, et al. Plague as a biological weapon: medical and public health management. JAMA. 3 May 2000;283(17): 2281-90.

115. Inglesby TV, Dennis DT, Henderson DA, et al. Plague as a biological weapon: medical and public health management. JAMA. 2000 May 3;283(17):2281-90.

116. Inglesby TV, Dennis DT, Henderson DA, et al. Plague as a biological weapon: medical and public health management. JAMA. 3 May 2000;283(17):2281-90.

117. Inglesby TV, Dennis DT, Henderson DA, et al. Plague as a biological weapon: medical and public health management. JAMA. 3 May 2000;283(17):2281-90.

118. McGovern TW, Friedlander AM. Plague. In: Zatjtchuk R, Bellamy RF, eds. Medical aspects of chemical and biological warfare. Bethesda, MD: Office of the Surgeon General; 1997:479-502.

119. Inglesby TV, Dennis DT, Henderson DA, et al. Plague as a biological weapon: medical and public health management. JAMA. 3 May 2000;283(17):2281-90.

120. Inglesby TV, Dennis DT, Henderson DA, et al. Plague as a biological weapon: medical and public health management. JAMA. 3 May 2000;283(17):2281-90.

121. Inglesby TV, Dennis DT, Henderson DA, et al. Plague as a biological weapon: medical and public health management. JAMA. 3 May 2000;283(17):2281-90.

122. Inglesby TV, Dennis DT, Henderson DA, et al. Plague as a biological weapon: medical and public health management. JAMA. 3 May2000;283(17):2281-90.

123. American Hospital Formulary Service. AHFS drug information. Bethesda, MD: American Society of Health System Pharmacists; 2000.

124. Sakala E. Obstetrics and gynecology. Baltimore, MD: Williams & Wilkens; 1997:945.

125. American Hospital Formulary Service. AHFS drug information. Bethesda, MD: American Society of Health System Pharmacists; 2000.

126. Inglesby TV, Dennis DT, Henderson DA, et al. Plague as a biological weapon: medical and public health management. JAMA. 3 May 2000;283(17):2281-90.

127. Inglesby TV, Dennis DT, Henderson DA, et al. Plague as a biological weapon: medical and public health management. JAMA. 3 May 2000;283(17):2281-90.

128. American Public Health Association. Plague. In: Benenson AS, ed. Control of communicable diseases manual. Washington DC: American Public Health Association; 1995: 353-8.

129. Inglesby TV, Dennis DT, Henderson DA, , et al. Plague as a biological weapon: medical and public health management. JAMA. 3 May 2000;283(17):2281-90.

130. American Public Health Association. Plague. In: Benenson AS, ed. Control of communicable diseases manual. Washington DC: American Public Health Association; 1995: 353-8.

131. Inglesby TV, Dennis DT, Henderson DA, et al. Plague as a biological weapon: medical and public health management. JAMA. 3 May 2000;283(17):2281-90.

132. Inglesby TV, Dennis DT, Henderson DA, et al. Plague as a biological weapon: medical and public health management. JAMA. 3 May 2000;283(17):2281-90.

133. Campbell GL, Dennis DT. Plague and other *Yersinia* infections. In: Fauci AS, Braunwald E, Isselbacher KJ, et al., eds. Harrison's principles of internal medicine, 14th ed. New York: McGraw-Hill, Health Professions Division; 1998: 975-83.

134. Centers for Disease Control. Update: universal precautions for prevention of transmission of human immunodeficiency virus, hepatitis B virus, and other bloodborne pathogens in health-care settings. MMWR. 1988;37:377-82, 387-8.

135. Centers for Disease Control. Guidelines for the prevention of transmission of human immunodeficiency virus and hepatitis B virus to healthcare and public safety workers. MMWR. 1989;38(S-6):1-36.

136. Occupational Safety & Health Administration. OSHA revised bloodborne pathogens 1010.1030. Occupational Safety & Health Administration, Department of Labor, 66 Federal Register 5325 January, 18, 2001.

137. Inglesby TV, Dennis DT, Henderson DA, et al. Plague as a biological weapon: medical and public health management. JAMA. 3 May 2000;283(17):2281-90.

138. Centers for Disease Control and Prevention. Guidelines for preventing the transmission of tuberculosis in health-care facilities, 1994. MMWR. 1994;43(RR-13):1-132, and Federal Register 1994;59(208):54242–303.

139. Inglesby TV, Dennis DT, Henderson DA, et al. Plague as a biological weapon: medical and public health management. JAMA. 3 May 2000;283(17):2281-90.

140. Morse S, McDade J. Recommendations for working with pathogenic bacteria. Meth Enzymol.1994;235:1-26.

141. World Health Organization. Safety measures for use in outbreaks in communicable disease outbreaks. Geneva: World Health Organization; 1986.

142. Gershon RR, Vlahov D, Cejudo JA, et al. Tuberculosis risk in funeral home employees. J Occup Environ Med. 1998;40: 497-503.

143. American Public Health Association. Plague. In: Benenson AS, ed. Control of communicable diseases manual. Washington DC: American Public Health Association; 1995: 353-8.

144. World Health Organization. Health aspects of chemical and biological weapons. Geneva: World Health Organization; 1970:98-109.

145. Harrison FJ. Prevention and control of plague. Aurora, CO: U.S. Army Center for Health Promotion and Preventative Medicine, Fitzsimons Army Medical Center; September 1995. Technical guide 103.

146. McGovern TW, Friedlander AM. Plague. In: Zatjtchuk R, Bellamy RF, eds. Medical aspects of chemical and biological warfare. Bethesda, MD: Office of the Surgeon General; 1997: 479-502.

147. Centers for Disease Control and Prevention. Prevention of plague; recommendations of the Advisory Committee on Immunization Practice (ACIP). MMWR. 1996;45(RR-14): 1-15.

148. Ehrenkranz NF, Meyer KF. Studies on immunization against plague, VIII: study of three immunizing preparations in protecting primates against pneumonic plague. J Infect Dis. 1955;96:138-44.

149. Speck RS, Wolochow H. Studies on the experimental epidemiology of respiratory infections, experimental pneumonic plague in *Macacus rhesus*. J Infect Dis. 1957;100:58-68.

150. Centers for Disease Control and Prevention. Prevention of plague; recommendations of the Advisory Committee on Immunization Practice (ACIP). MMWR. 1996;45(RR-14):1-15.

151. Meyer KF, Cavanaugh DC, Bartelloni PJ, Marshal JD Jr. Plague immunization, I: past and present trends. J Infect Dis. 1974;129(suppl):S13-S18.

152. Inglesby TV, Dennis DT, Henderson DA, et al. Plague as a biological weapon: medical and public health management. JAMA. 3 May 2000;283(17):2281-90.

153. Titball RW, Eley S, Williamson ED, Dennis DT. Plague. In: Plotkin S, Mortimer EA, eds. Vaccines. Philadelphia: WB Saunders; 1999: 734-42.

154. Inglesby TV, Dennis DT, Henderson DA, et al. Plague as a biological weapon: medical and public health management. JAMA. 3 May 2000;283(17):2281-90.

8

Smallpox

Lisa Rotz, Inger Damon, and Joanne Cono

NAME OF AGENT

Variola (Smallpox) Virus

MICROBIOLOGY

The etiological agent of smallpox is a double-stranded DNA virus, variola virus, which belongs to the family Poxviridae, genus orthopoxvirus. This genus includes several other related viruses, including vaccinia virus, which is used to produce smallpox vaccine because it induces cross-protective immunity to other orthopoxviruses. These viruses are brick-shaped on electron micrography and measure about 300 by 250 by 200 nm (1).

THEORETICAL AND SCIENTIFIC BACKGROUND

Prior to the eradication of smallpox, humans were the only known natural reservoir. The last known naturally occurring case of smallpox was in Somalia in 1977 (2). Routine vaccination against smallpox was discontinued worldwide in the early 1980s following elimination of the disease through a global eradication program led by the World Health Organization (WHO). Protection against smallpox following vaccination is not lifelong. High-level protection lasts for approximately 5 years, and waning but still substantial protection can persist for up to 10 years following initial vaccination with vaccinia virus, the related orthopoxvirus used in the live-virus vaccine for smallpox (3,4). Protection against death from the disease may persist even longer than protection against disease in vaccinated individuals and may be seen in persons vaccinated over two decades ago (5,6). All

children and most adults are now considered susceptible to the development of disease if exposed to variola virus, either because they were never vaccinated or were vaccinated more than 20 years ago and are no longer fully protected. Although the last case of smallpox occurred over 25 years ago, the specter of bioterrorism has raised concerns for the use of this virus as an agent of terrorism (7).

Human-to-human transmission of variola virus usually occurs by inhalation of virus-containing large airborne droplets of saliva from an infected person with subsequent deposition on the oropharyngeal region of the susceptible individual. Transmission usually requires prolonged close contact (face-to-face), although infrequently airborne transmission over greater distances has been described (8). Transmission via direct contact with material from the smallpox pustules or crusted scabs can also occur; however, scabs are much less infectious than respiratory secretions, presumably due to binding of the virions in the fibrin matrix of the scab. During the smallpox era, the overall average secondary attack rate was 58.4% in previously unvaccinated close household contacts and 3.8% in previously vaccinated household contacts (2). Higher attack rates that have been reported from some studies may have been associated with more favorable environmental conditions for transmission (e.g., low heat and low humidity). Because of the lack of natural and vaccine-induced immunity, it is difficult to predict the exact attack rates in today's population.

Following deposition on the mucous membranes, the virus passes into local lymph nodes with a brief period of viremia. Next, a latent period of up to 2 weeks occurs during which the virus multiplies in the reticuloendothelial system. The onset of initial symptoms (the prodromal phase) is preceded by another short viremic period. During the prodromal phase, the virus multiplies and invades the mucous membranes of the mouth and dermal layers of the skin. This leads to the development of the oropharyngeal and skin lesions that contain infectious viral particles (2). Transmission of the virus via large airborne droplets remains highest during the first 7 to 10 days following the onset of rash but decreases significantly during the later stages of the disease (9).

SIGNS AND SYMPTOMS

Notify public health officials immediately of any suspected smallpox patient. The three clinical forms of smallpox, ordinary, flat, or hemorrhagic, may occur in *unvaccinated or distantly vaccinated* individuals. During the smallpox era, ordinary smallpox generally accounted for about 90% of the cases. Flat and hemorrhagic clinical presentations accounted for a much lower percentage (7% and <3%, respectively) (1,10,11). An additional form, modified type, was seen in individuals with previous vaccination who were no longer fully protected. Although the case-fatality rate varied with the different clinical forms of smallpox, it was approximately 30% in unvaccinated individuals.

Differing clinical forms of disease are thought to be caused by the host's response to infection rather than different strains of virus. The clinical course of ordinary or typical smallpox begins with an asymptomatic incubation period following infection, which may last from 7 to 17 days (average 12 to 14 days). After the incubation period, the first symptoms begin with a prodromal phase and include fever, malaise, prostration, headache, and backache. During the prodromal phase, individuals often feel very ill, which may prompt them to remain at home or seek medical care. This nonspecific viral syndrome phase usually lasts from 2 to 4 days before the onset of the rash or exanthem phase. Virus transmissibility or infectiousness begins as the fever peaks at the end of the prodrome period and coincides with the onset of the rash. This rash begins as lesions on the buccal and pharyngeal mucosa, soon followed by the appearance of rash on the face, forearms, and hands (2,9). The rash spreads downward, and within a day or so, the trunk and lower limbs are involved, including the palms and soles. Usually the rash is evident on most parts of the body within 24 hours. Ultimately the distribution of the rash is centrifugal: most profuse on the face, and more abundant on the

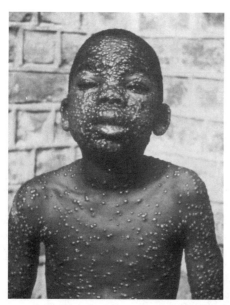

Figure 8–1. This photograph depicts an African child displaying the typical centrifugal rash distribution of smallpox on his face, chest, and arms. (From CDC, Public Health Images Library # 3268.)

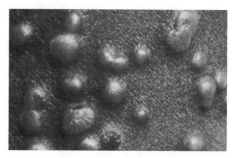

Figure 8–2. Closeup of smallpox pustules found on the thigh of a patient during day 6 of the rash. (From CDC/Dr. Paul B. Dean, Public Health Images Library # 2553.)

forearms than the upper arms, and on the lower legs than the thighs (Fig. 8-1).

The lesions of the rash begin as macules, which are small discolored skin patches. The macules progress to firm papules, then vesicles, which soon become opaque and pustular (Fig. 8-2). Progression of the rash is slower than varicella (chickenpox) with usually 1 to 2 days between each stage (macule to papule to pustule). In addition, the lesions tend to progress through stages together so lesions in any area of the body are all in the same stage of development. The pustules, which are considered the characteristic lesions of smallpox, are typically raised and firm to the touch, or "shotty," as if BB pellets were embedded in the skin. Approximately 8 to 9 days after onset of the rash, the pustules become pitlike and dimpled. Around day 14, the pustules dry up and become crusted. By about day 19, after onset of prodromal symptoms, most pustules begin to scab and separate, with those on the palms and soles separating last. Virus particles can be present in large numbers in the scabs but are generally not highly infectious because they are enclosed within the hard, dry scab.

Flat-type or malignant smallpox, a very rare manifestation of the disease, is believed to be associated with a deficient cellular immune response to variola virus (2). This form of the disease is characterized by a rapidly progressive septic state and is very rare in previously vaccinated individuals. The skin lesions develop slowly, become confluent, and remain flat and soft, never fully progressing to the pustular stage. They have been described as "velvety" to the touch, and sections of the skin where lesions have become confluent may slough off. The majority of flat-type smallpox cases are fatal (97% among unvaccinated individuals), but if the patient survives, the lesions gradually disappear without forming scabs.

Hemorrhagic-type smallpox, which is also rare, is associated with petechiae (minute hemorrhagic spots) in the skin and bleeding from the conjunctiva and mucous membranes. This type of smallpox maintains a higher level of prolonged viremia as opposed to the other clinical forms of the disease. Illness with severe prodromal symptoms that include high fever, severe headache, and abdominal pain begins after a sometimes shortened incubation period. Soon after illness onset, a dusky erythema develops, which is followed by petechiae and skin and mucosal hemorrhages. Death usually occurs within the first week of illness (1), often before lesions more characteristic of smallpox rash develop. The two forms of hemorrhagic-type smallpox, early and late, are differentiated by the occurrence of hemorrhages *after* the appearance of the rash in the late form. Hemorrhagic-type smallpox occurs among all ages and in both sexes but is more common in adults and almost universally fatal. Pregnant women also seem to be more susceptible to developing this form of smallpox than other adults. The underlying molecular biologic reasons for the severe toxemia and other effects of this form of smallpox are unclear.

A modified form of smallpox can occur in previously vaccinated individuals. The modification referred to in this form of smallpox relates to the character and development of the rash with more rapid progression and resolution of the lesions. In general, the prodrome stage with fever still occurs and may also consist of severe headache and backache, with a duration that may not be shortened. However, once the skin lesions appear, they generally evolve more quickly with crusting completed within 10 days. The lesions may be fewer in number and are more superficial than those seen in ordinary-type smallpox. Although a febrile prodrome generally still occurs, fever during the rash stage is usually absent with this modified form of smallpox.

In situations where smallpox was not expected, smallpox was at times confused with chickenpox. In contrast to chickenpox, all lesions on any one part of the body are at the same stage of development with smallpox. Distribution of the rash in chickenpox is uniform or centripetal; there may be more lesions on the trunk than on the face and distal limbs, and abdominal involvement is equivalent to back involvement. The rash of chickenpox manifests as uniloculated vesicles that do not umbilicate or dimple. The vesicles may also have irregular borders. There are usually no lesions on the palms and soles in chickenpox.

The Centers for Disease Control and Prevention (CDC) has developed several resources that can be used to assist clinicians in evaluating acute generalized vesicular or pustular rash illnesses for their likelihood of being smallpox in a nonoutbreak setting. These tools can be found on the CDC web site at http://www.bt.cdc.gov/agent/smallpox/diagnosis/evalposter.asp and include an interactive online version of the clinical evaluation algorithm.

A number of nucleic acid polymerase chain reaction (PCR) assays detect the presence of orthopoxvirus in clinical specimens. The speciation of orthopoxvirus is then facilitated by endonuclease restriction fragment length polymorphism (RFLP) analysis (12–14). The Laboratory Response Network (LRN), an affiliation of public health laboratories with the Association of Public Health Laboratories (APHL) and CDC, has a variety of real-time PCR assays that can be used for the detection of orthopoxviruses in clinical specimens. A subset of LRN laboratories with appropriate biocontainment capabalities, also has specific smallpox (variola) testing capacity. Electron microscopy, in facilities with well-trained personnel, is another sensitive method for evaluating rash specimens for the presence of poxvirus particles.

MEDICAL MANAGEMENT

There are no proven curative treatments for clinical smallpox. Medical management of a patient with smallpox is mainly *supportive* and consists of (a) isolation of the patient to prevent transmission of the smallpox (variola) virus to nonimmune persons, (b) monitoring and maintaining fluid and electrolyte balance, (c) skin care, and (d) monitoring for and treatment of complications. Recovery from smallpox results in prolonged immunity to reinfection with variola virus. Variola virus does not persist in the body after recovery.

Hospitalized suspected and confirmed smallpox patients should be isolated in a negative-pressure room, and strict airborne and contact precautions should be maintained at all times. These precautions include use of N-95 or greater respirators, gloves and gowns, and careful hand washing for all health care workers entering the patient's room. If possible, previously vaccinated personnel should be utilized to evaluate and care for suspected or confirmed cases of smallpox. If previously vaccinated personnel are unavailable, staff without contraindications to vaccination can provide care utilizing the appropriate airborne and contact personal protective equipment, with vaccination provided as soon as possible (15).

During the vesicular and pustular stages of smallpox, patients may experience significant fluid losses and become hypovolemic or develop shock. Fluid loss can result from (a) fever, (b) nausea and vomiting, (c) decreased fluid intake due to swallowing discomfort from pharyngeal lesions, (d) body fluid shifts from the vascular bed into the subcutaneous tissue, and (e) massive skin desquamation in patients with extensive confluent lesions. Electrolyte and protein loss may also occur in these patients. Fluid and electrolyte balance should be monitored in hospitalized patients with appropriate oral or intravenous correction of imbalances. Patients with less severe disease should be encouraged to maintain good oral intake of fluids.

Nausea and vomiting can occur in the earlier stages of smallpox, especially in the prodromal period before rash development, and should be treated symptomatically. Occasionally, diarrhea may occur in the prodromal period or in the second week of illness and should also be treated symptomatically. Acute dilation of the stomach rarely occurs and is more common in infants. In some severe cases of smallpox (especially flat-type), extensive viral infection of the intestinal mucosa occurs with sloughing of the mucosal membrane. Most of these cases are fatal.

Occasionally, bacterial superinfections may also occur and should be treated with appropriate antibiotic therapy. Bacterial superinfections can include abscesses of skin lesions, pneumonia, osteomyelitis, joint infections, and septicemia. Laboratory diagnostics (e.g., Gram stain, culture, and antibiotic susceptibility testing) should be performed to help guide antibiotic therapy.

Viral bronchitis and pneumonitis can be complications of severe smallpox. Treatment is symptomatic with measures to treat hypoxemia with supplemental oxygen and/or intubation/ventilation as indicated. Secondary bacterial pneumonia can occur and should be treated with appropriate antibiotics as guided by laboratory diagnostics (e.g., Gram stain, culture, and antibiotic susceptibility testing). Pulmonary edema is common in the more severe forms of smallpox (hemorrhagic and flat-type) and should be treated with careful monitoring of oxygenation, fluid status, blood pressure with supplemental oxygen, and diuretics administered as needed. Although cough is not usually a prominent symptom of clinical smallpox, patients with a cough during the first week of illness may transmit disease more readily than those without a cough because this is the period when oral secretions contain the largest amount of virus. A cough is more likely to produce small particle aerosols that can travel over greater distances. Patients that develop a cough later in the course of disease (after day 10), when viral counts in secretions are lower, are not as infectious as those that develop coughs earlier.

Corneal ulceration and/or keratitis, complications sometimes leading to blindness, occurred more frequently in hemorrhagic-type smallpox but were occasionally seen in the more typical ordinary-type smallpox. Occasionally, blindness can occur, but it generally is a result of an underlying condition such as malnutrition and/or an opportunistic ocular bacterial infection. The virus itself does not cause the corneal opacity that can lead to blindness. In one case series (10), corneal ulcers occurred in 1% of nonhemorrhagic-type smallpox cases, and keratitis occurred in about 0.25%. Corneal ulcerations can appear around the second week of illness and begin at the corneal margins. Ulcers can heal rapidly, leaving a minor opacity or, on occasion, may cause severe corneal scarring.

Encephalitis occurs in about 1 out of every 500 cases of smallpox. It usually appears between day 6 and day 10 of illness when the rash is still in the papular or vesicular stage. During the smallpox era, this complication was a minor contributor to the case-fatality rate of typical smallpox, the most common form of smallpox. Although sometimes slow, recovery was usually complete.

Multiple studies of antivirals during the smallpox eradication failed to show significant benefit in the treatment of smallpox (16,17). Cidofovir (Vistide, Gilead Sciences, Foster City, CA) has shown some in vitro and in vivo (animal studies) activity against orthopoxviruses (18–20). However, its true effectiveness for treating clinical smallpox or vaccine adverse events is not known (9). This medication is currently labeled for the treatment of cytomegalovirus (CMV) retinitis and has been associated with renal failure. Vaccinia human immunoglobulin (VIG), which is licensed to treat certain post–smallpox vaccination adverse effects, has shown no efficacy in the treatment of clinically established smallpox (15,21).

VACCINATION IN THE PREVENTION OF SMALLPOX SPREAD

The major public health tool in fighting a smallpox outbreak is vaccination of those exposed to the virus. Because a bioterrorist attack may be widespread and occult, large segments of the population may need to be vaccinated. This would require a large-scale effort by the medical and public health workforce, with significant assistance needed from all levels of government and society. In addition, the smallpox vaccine, because it is a live-virus vaccine, carries certain risks with it. In the event of an outbreak, the risks of vaccination are minuscule compared to the risks of the actual diseases, but medical care considerations in a smallpox outbreak are not limited to individuals with clinical smallpox. They also extend to treating complications that can be seen following smallpox vaccination. Serious complications are rare after primary vaccination and even less likely in previously vaccinated persons who are revaccinated. However, the following serious complications to vaccination can occur and may require medical intervention: progressive vaccinia, eczema vaccinatum, generalized vaccinia, postvaccination encephalomyelitis, inadvertent inoculation of vaccinia virus, fetal vaccinia, and myopericarditis.

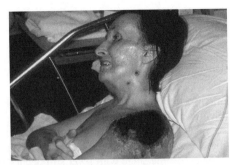

Figure 8–3. This patient presented with progressive vaccinia (also called vaccinia gangrenosum) after having been vaccinated for smallpox. (From CDC/California Department of Health Services, Public Health Images Library # 4590.)

Sequelae may follow recovery from smallpox. The most common are pockmarks, which may occur all over the body but usually are most profuse on the face. Lesion scars or pockmarks are caused mainly by destruction of infected sebaceous glands and most prominent on the face where these glands are larger and more numerous. In addition to the complications just listed, osteomyelitis can also occur as a complication of smallpox infection.

Progressive vaccinia (PV) is a rare and often fatal vaccine complication characterized by progressive, often painless, necrosis at the vaccination site, with or without metastases to skin at other body sites (22) (Fig. 8-3). In a national survey in 1968, five cases (including two deaths) of progressive vaccinia occurred among 6 million primary vaccinees (0.83 cases/million) and six cases (including two deaths) occurred among 8.6 million persons revaccinated with the licensed smallpox vaccines containing the New York City Board of Health (NYCBH) strain (0.7 cases/million) (23). PV is seen in persons with severe immunodeficiencies. Individuals with deficits of the cell-mediated immune system have a poorer prognosis than those with deficiencies of the humoral immune system. Congenital or acquired immunodeficiency diseases or other forms of immunosuppression (e.g., by medications such as high-dose steroids or chemotherapeutics) put an individual at risk for this complication. This diagnosis should be considered if the vaccination site lesion continues to progress and expand without apparent healing more than 15 days after vaccination (24). Initially, limited or no inflammation is present at the site and histopathological examination shows an absence of inflammatory cells (25). Individuals with PV can become viremic and develop vaccinial lesions at distant body sites. Management of progressive vaccinia includes aggressive therapy with vaccinia immune globulin (VIG), monitoring with supportive care, and contact infection control precautions to prevent secondary or nosocomial spread of the live virus contained in the lesions. Rarely, surgical debridement is used with varying success (22).

Eczema vaccinatum (EV) can occur in people with a history of atopic dermatitis (eczema), irrespective of disease severity or activity. This complication can occur following primary vaccination or contact with another person who has a nonscabbed vaccination site that contains live vaccinia virus. It is characterized by a localized or generalized papular, vesicular, or pustular rash (Fig. 8-4). The rash has a predilection for areas of previous eczematous lesions but can occur anywhere on the body. Individuals with EV are often systemically ill with fever, malaise, and lymphadenopathy accompanying the rash. Other nonatopic exfoliative skin conditions can also

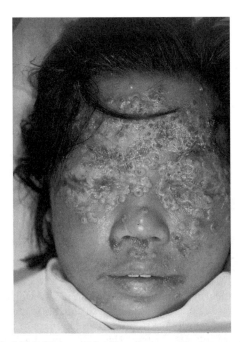

Figure 8–4. This 28-year-old with eczema vaccinatum contracted it from her vaccinated child. She had had a history of atopic dermatitis, but her dermatitis was inactive at the time of the child's vaccination. Treatment with vaccinia immune globulin (VIG), idoxuridine eye drops, and methisazone (Marboran) resulted in healed lesions with no scarring or lasting ocular damage. [From CDC/Allen W. Mathies, MD, John Leedom, MD/ California Emergency Preparedness Office (Calif/EPO), Immunization Branch, Public Health Images Library # 4621.]

place an individual at risk for EV, but generally, the illness is less severe than that seen in individuals with atopic dermatitis. No data exists to predict the absolute risk for these persons, but in the 1968 national survey there were 66 cases (no deaths) among 14.5 million vaccines (4.6 cases/million) and 60 cases (one death) among their several million contacts.

Treatment of EV includes the administration of VIG, hemodynamic support with fluid replacement and electrolyte monitoring, and careful skin care. Early VIG administration reduced the mortality from 40% to 30% in one study to 7% (26). Because large surface areas of skin can be compromised in EV, fluid and electrolyte losses can be significant. In addition, EV patients should be followed closely for signs or symptoms of infection or sepsis. Contact infection control precautions should be followed because the lesions of EV also contain live virus.

Generalized vaccinia (GV) is a generalized maculopapular or vesicular skin rash, sometimes covering the whole body, usually occurring within 6 to 9 days after primary vaccination. The rash is generally benign, self-limited, and has a very good prognosis, with most cases being managed on an outpatient basis. Systemic symptoms usually do not accompany GV, although fever occasionally may precede the rash. The course of the individual lesions resembles that of the lesion at the inoculation site; however, if the rash is profuse the lesions may vary greatly in size. This complication is estimated to occur in about 242 out of every one million primary vaccinations (27). In general, this complication of vaccination does not require the administration of VIG unless it is severe and the patient is systemically ill or the patient has an underlying immunocompromising condition. Treatment with nonsteroidal antiinflammatory agents (NSAIDs) or oral antipruritics may provide

symptomatic treatment. Because the lesions of GV may contain live virus, patients should be managed utilizing contact infection control precautions and advised to keep lesions covered as much as possible (22).

Postvaccination encephalomyelitis (PVEM) is a rare complication that can occur in primary vaccinees. The frequency of its occurrence differed widely from country to country and with the strain of vaccinia virus utilized in the vaccine. The incidence of PVEM was lower with the New York Board of Health (NYBOH) vaccinia virus strain utilized in the U.S. smallpox vaccines (2,23,28). PVEM typically affected persons ‡2 years, but could not otherwise be predicted based on preexisting medical conditions like other severe smallpox vaccine reactions (e.g., EV and PV). This postvaccination reaction typically occurs 11 to 15 days following vaccination and is thought to generally be the result of an autoimmune process, although the pathophysiology is unclear. Rarely has vaccinia virus been isolated from the cerebral spinal fluid (CSF) of PVEM or postvaccination encephalopathy (PVE) cases, and controlled trials have not been done to determine the true significance of this infrequent finding (23,29). Symptoms of PVEM include fever, headache, vomiting, confusion, delirium, disorientation, restlessness, drowsiness or lethargy, seizures, and coma. The CSF can demonstrate an elevated pressure but generally has a normal cell count and chemistry profile. The principal pathological lesions resembled those of other postinfectious encephalitides and includes perivenous inflammation and demyelination (2,30).

Infants less than 2 years old can also develop a rare PVE similar to PVEM. Acute onset of PVE occurs earlier in the postvaccination period (6 to 10 days postvaccination), presents with the same symptoms as PVEM, and may also include hemiplegia and aphasia. Generalized cerebral edema with a mild lymphocytic meningeal infiltration, widespread ganglion degenerative changes, and occasional perivascular hemorrhages are the associated pathological changes in this form of post–smallpox vaccination central nervous disease.

PVEM following vaccination has been reported in about 3 to 12 per million primary vaccines (28). The previously reported mortality rate for PVEM or PVE is 15% to 25% , and 25% of survivors were still left with some neurological deficits (23).

Diagnosis of PVE or PVEM is one of exclusion because there are no specific diagnostic tests to confirm the diagnosis of this complication and many other infectious and toxic etiologies that can result in similar clinical symptoms. No clinical criteria, laboratory tests, or CNS radiological studies are definite for the diagnosis of PVE or PVEM. There is no specific therapy for this complication other than supportive care that includes anticonvulsants and intensive care monitoring when required. Because this complication is not believed to be the result of viral proliferation, the role of modern antiviral medications is unclear. In addition, no previous studies with VIG have shown this intervention is effective in the treatment of PVEM or PVE (22).

Fetal vaccinia (FV) is an extremely rare complication that can occur following smallpox vaccination during pregnancy or shortly before conception. Fewer than 50 cases have been reported in the literature. Skin lesions and organ involvement are the usual manifestations of this complication, which often results in premature delivery or fetal or neonatal death. FV has been associated with vaccination in all three trimesters of pregnancy.

Accidental infection or inadvertent inoculation (AI) of vaccinia virus to some part of the body distant from the vaccination site or of another person can occur when live vaccinia virus, present at the site until it has healed, is inadvertently transferred from the vaccination site to another body site or individual. This condition most commonly occurs in children (22) and usually results in a lesion similar to the vaccination site. The body sites most commonly affected include the face, mouth, lips, genitalia, and eyelid. Accidental infections of distal body sites are usually not serious and do not require specific treatment. Accidental infections of other individuals is also usually not serious unless the individual has a preexisting condition (e.g., eczema or immune disorders) that makes them more susceptible to severe reactions to vaccinia.

Vaccinia infections involving the eye or eyelid (ocular implantations), however, can be more serious and even threaten sight if not evaluated and treated appropriately. Accidental implantation is the most common postvaccination complication, accounting for about one-half of all complications in individuals receiving smallpox vaccine. This complication can be prevented by careful attention to hand hygiene after touching the site, site dressings, or other materials that have come into contact with the vaccination site. In addition, scratching or unnecessary touching of the vaccine site should be avoided.

Ocular vaccinia implantations can result in blepharitis, conjunctivitis, keratitis, iritis, or a combination of these presentations. These complications should be managed in consultation with an ophthalmologist. Although controlled studies have not evaluated the usefulness of current topical optic antiviral solutions in the treatment of ocular vaccinia infections, their off-label use for this purpose has been recommended by some ophthalmologists (22). Both trifluridine (Viroptic, King Pharmaceuticals, Inc., Bristol, TN) and vidarabine (Vira-A, King Pharmaceuticals, Inc., Bristol, TN) have stated in vitro and in vivo activity against vaccinia virus in the product labeling, but neither have been approved by the Food and Drug Administration (FDA) specifically for treatment of ocular vaccinia disease. Under certain conditions, VIG may also be considered in the treatment of severe ocular disease. When keratitis is present, the potential benefit of VIG should be carefully evaluated because studies utilizing an animal model have indicated a possible increase in the risk of corneal scarring when VIG was used in the presence of this complication (31). However, if another sight-threatening complication is present with keratitis (e.g., vision-threatening lid malformation), VIG can be considered in limited doses. Use of VIG to treat other serious vaccine complications such as eczema vaccinatum is also indicated, regardless of the presence of keratitis. VIG is not recommended for the treatment of isolated keratitis.

Cardiac adverse events have also been described following smallpox vaccination. These events include myopericarditis, ischemia, and arrhythmias, although causality has not been established (32–35). Of the reported events, myopericarditis appears to have the strongest potential association with vaccinia vaccine (33,36,37). This postvaccination complication has been previously reported from Europe and Australia where non-NYCBOH strain was used (38,39), but it was not a previously well-described complication following vaccination with the New York Board of Health strain used in the United States.

In January 2003 a smallpox vaccination program for selected civilian public health and medical response teams was initiated as part of an overall effort to prepare the United States in the event of a terrorist attack using smallpox. The U.S. military initiated a similar smallpox vaccination program several months earlier. The rate of myo/pericarditis reported in the civilian program, including suspected and probable cases, was approximately 1:1,700 vaccinees, and the rate reported in the military program was approximately 1:12,000 vaccinees. This complication is generally manifested by chest pain and can also be associated with dyspnea, palpitations, electrocardiogram changes, and transient cardiac enzyme elevation. All patients with reported myopericarditis following smallpox vaccination in the current U.S. civilian responder and military vaccination programs recovered (36).

TRIAGE CONSIDERATIONS

All individuals presenting to a medical facility with an acute generalized vesicular or pustular rash should be immediately triaged to an appropriate respiratory isolation room within the facility for further evaluation. This triage procedure should be a routine part of medical facility protocols, regardless of the known or unknown presence of smallpox in a community. Other more common vesicular rash illnesses such as varicella and measles can be transmitted via the respiratory route and would present an infectious risk to nonimmune staff and other patients in the facility.

Smallpox patients admitted to a hospital where other nonsmallpox patients are present must be managed under strict airborne and contact isolation precautions in order to prevent the nosocomial spread of disease. Standard precautions should also be followed. In an outbreak situation where there may be many smallpox cases requiring treatment, designated smallpox evaluation and medical treatment facilities may be established in the community by public health authorities. If such facilities are established, suspected smallpox patients should be triaged to these facilities where they can be vaccinated, evaluated, and treated accordingly. Suspected smallpox patients who are isolated together should be vaccinated against smallpox to prevent against accidental exposure to the disease in someone who may have been clinically misdiagnosed as a case of smallpox while awaiting laboratory confirmation (40).

PERSONAL PROTECTION

Vaccination of an individual within 3 days of exposure to smallpox virus can prevent or significantly lessen the severity of smallpox symptoms in the vast majority of people (41). Vaccination up to a week after exposure likely offers some protection from disease or may modify the severity of disease (10,11). Although recent successful vaccination can provide a high level of immunity for health care personnel, appropriate airborne, contact, and standard infection control procedures should still be followed when caring for smallpox patients. Protective clothing including gowns, masks (properly fitted N95 or higher respirator masks), and gloves should be worn by all personnel who enter and leave an isolation room or area where smallpox patients are managed.

SUMMARY Key Features of Smallpox Disease

Incubation Period (Duration: 7 to 17 days) *Not contagious*	Exposure to the virus is followed by an incubation period during which people do not have any symptoms and may feel fine. This incubation period averages about 12 to 14 days but can range from 7 to 17 days. During this time, people are not contagious.
Initial Symptoms (*Prodrome*) (Duration: 2 to 4 days) *Sometimes contagious**	The first symptoms of smallpox include fever, malaise, head and body aches, and sometimes vomiting. The fever is usually high, in the range of 101° to 104°F. At this time, people are usually too sick to carry on their normal activities. This is called the *prodrome* phase and may last for 2 to 4 days.
Early Rash (Duration: about 4 days) *Most contagious*	A rash emerges first as small red spots on the tongue and in the mouth. These spots develop into sores that break open and spread large amounts of the virus into the mouth and throat. At this time, the person becomes most contagious. Around the time the sores in the mouth break down, a rash appears on the skin, starting on the face and spreading to the arms and legs and then to the hands and feet. Usually the rash spreads to all parts of the body within 24 hours. As the rash appears, the fever usually falls and the person may start to feel better. By the third day of the rash, the rash becomes raised bumps. By the fourth day, the bumps fill with a thick, opaque fluid and often have a depression in the center that looks like a belly button. (This is a major distinguishing characteristic of smallpox.) Fever often will rise again at this time and remain high until scabs form over the bumps.
Pustular Rash (Duration: about 5 days) *Contagious*	The bumps become pustules—sharply raised, usually round, and firm to the touch as if there is a small round object under the skin. People often say the bumps feel like BB pellets embedded in the skin.
Pustules and Scabs (Duration: about 5 days) *Contagious*	The pustules begin to form a crust and then scab. By the end of the second week after the rash appears, most of the sores have scabbed over.
Resolving Scabs (Duration: about 6 days) *Contagious*	The scabs begin to fall off, leaving marks on the skin that eventually become pitted scars. Most scabs will have fallen off 3 weeks after the rash appears. The person is contagious to others until all of the scabs have fallen off.
Scabs Resolved *Not contagious*	Scabs have fallen off. Person is no longer contagious.

* Smallpox may be contagious during the *prodrome* phase, but it is most infectious during the first 7 to 10 days following rash onset.

Source: CDC. Adapted from table http://www.bt.cdc.gov/agent/smallpox/overview/disease-facts.asp.

RESOURCES

1. CDC: Emergency Preparedness and Response Smallpox web site at http://www.bt.cdc.gov/agent/smallpox/index. asp. Comprehensive information about smallpox, smallpox vaccine, evaluation tool for suspected smallpox patients, diagnosis and treatment of vaccine adverse events, and general smallpox response planning.

2. Smallpox Vaccination Overview for Clinicians: A Guide to Resources on the CDC web site at http://www.bt.cdc. gov/agent/smallpox/vaccination/clinicians.asp. Informa-

tion for clinicians about normal and expected vaccine reactions and diagnosis and management of adverse vaccine events.

3. Bioterrorism Readiness Plan: A Template for Healthcare facilities APIC. Bioterrorism Taskforce and CDC Hospital Infections Program Bioterrorism Working Group, 1999 at http://www.cdc.gov/ncidod /hip/Bio/13apr99 APIC-CDCBioterrorism.PDF. General guidance for health care bioterrorism response planning, including smallpox.

4. World Health Organization at: http://www.who.int/csr/ disease/smallpox/en/. General smallpox information and teaching slide sets for smallpox.

QUESTIONS AND ANSWERS

1. Smallpox has which of the following clinical features?
   A. Meningitic prodrome
   B. Rash lesions in the same stage of development on any one area of the body
   C. Characteristic lesions are deep-seated, firm, well-circumscribed pustules
   D. Rash more prominent on trunk
   E. B and C

2. Individuals with smallpox are most infectious during which point of their illness?
   A. When all scabbed lesions have separated
   B. During the incubation period
   C. The first 7 to 10 days following the appearance of rash
   D. When the rash lesions have all progressed to pustules
   E. At the onset of fever

3. Which of the following infection control and personal protection measures should be followed when providing care for a person with smallpox or suspected smallpox?
   A. Airborne precautions with isolation in a negative-pressure room
   B. Contact and Standard precautions
   C. Turnout ("bunker") gear and self-contained air
   D. Vaccination with vaccinia (smallpox) vaccine
   E. A and D

4. Which of the following has the lowest risk of serious complications following smallpox vaccination?
   A. An individual with active eczema (atopic dermatitis)
   B. An individual with only a history of eczema (atopic dermatitis) as a child
   C. A individual taking immune suppressive medications following organ transplantation
   D. A 50-year-old male being revaccinated after receiving primary smallpox vaccination as a child
   E. All are at equal risk for serious complications following smallpox vaccination.

ANSWERS

1: *E.* *B and C*
2: *C.* *The first 7 to 10 days following the appearance of rash*
3: *E.* *A and D*
4: *D.* *A 50-year-old male being revaccinated after receiving primary smallpox vaccination as a child*

REFERENCES

1. Breman JG, Henderson DA. Diagnosis and management of smallpox. N Engl J Med 2002;346(17):1300-8.
2. Fenner F, Henderson DA, Arita I, et al. Smallpox and its eradication. Geneva, Switzerland: World Health Organization; 1988.
3. WHO Expert Committee on smallpox eradication. Second report. World Health Organ Tech Rep Ser 1972;493:5-64.
4. Public Health Service. Recommendations of the Public Health Service Advisory Committee on Immunization Practices: smallpox vaccination. Washington, DC: Public Health Service; 1972.
5. Mack TM. Smallpox in Europe, 1950-1971. J Infect Dis 1972;125(2):161-9.
6. Hanna W. Studies in small-pox and vaccination. Bristol: Wright; 1913.
7. Henderson DA. The looming threat of bioterrorism. Science 1999;283(5406):1279-82.
8. Gelfand HM, Posch J. The recent outbreak of smallpox in Meschede, West Germany. Am J Epidemiol 1971;93:234-7.
9. Henderson DA, Inglesby TV, Bartlett JG, et al. Smallpox as a biological weapon: medical and public health management. Working Group on Civilian Biodefense. JAMA 1999;281(22):2127-37.
10. Rao AR. Smallpox. Bombay, India: The Kothari Book Depot; 1972.
11. Dixon CW. Smallpox. London: J&A Churchill; 1962.
12. Ropp SL, Jin Q, Knight JC, et al. PCR strategy for identification and differentiation of small pox and other orthopoxviruses. J Clin Microbiol 1995;33(8):2069-76.
13. Meyer H, Ropp SL, Esposito JJ. Gene for A-type inclusion body protein is useful for a polymerase chain reaction assay to differentiate orthopoxviruses. J Virol Methods 1997;64(2):217-21.
14. Meyer H, Ropp SL, Esposito JJ. Poxviruses. In: Warnes J, Stephenson J, eds. Methods in molecular medicine: diagnostic virology protocols. Totowa: Humana Press; 1998:199-211.
15. CDC. Vaccinia (Smallpox) Vaccine. Recommendations of the Advisory Committee on Immunization Practices (ACIP), 2001. MMWR 2001;50(RR-10).
16. Koplan JP, Monsur KA, Foster SO, et al. Treatment of variola major with adenine arabinoside. J Infect Dis 1975; 131(1):34-9.
17. Monsur KA, Hossain MS, Huq F, et al. Treatment of variola major with cytosine arabinoside. J Infect Dis 1975;131(1):40-3.
18. Smee DF, Bailey KW, Wong MH, et al. Effects of cidofovir on the pathogenesis of a lethal vaccinia virus respiratory infection in mice. Antiviral Res 2001;52(1):55-62.
19. Bray M, Martinez M, Smee DF, et al. Cidofovir protects mice against lethal aerosol or intranasal cowpox virus challenge. J Infect Dis 2000;181(1):10-19.
20. De Clercq E. Acyclic nucleoside phosphonates in the chemotherapy of DNA virus and retrovirus infections. Intervirology 1997;40(5-6):295-303.
21. Koplan JP, Marton KI. Smallpox vaccination revisited: Some observations on the biology of vaccinia. Am J Trop Med Hyg 1975;24:656-63.
22. Cono J, Casey CG, Bell DM. Smallpox vaccination and adverse reactions. Guidance for clinicians. MMWR Recomm Rep 2003;52(RR-4):1-28.
23. Lane JM, Ruben FL, Neff JM, et al. Complications of smallpox vaccination, 1968: results of ten statewide surveys. J Infect Dis 1970;122(4):303-9.
24. Goldstein JA, Neff JM, Lane JM, et al. Smallpox vaccination reactions, prophylaxis, and therapy of complications. Pediatrics 1975;55(3):342-7.
25. Keidan SE, McCarthy K, Haworth J. Fatal generalized vaccinia with failure of antibody production and absence of serum gamma globulin. Arch Dis Child 1953;28(138):110-6.
26. Kempe CH. Studies on smallpox and complications of smallpox vaccination. Pediatrics 1960;26:176-89.
27. CDC. SMALLPOX FACT SHEET—Information for clinicians adverse reactions following smallpox vaccination. U.S. Department of Health and Human Services, CDC; 2003. Available from http://www.bt.cdc.gov/agent/smallpox/vaccination/reactions-vacc-clinic.asp.
28. Lane JM, Ruben FL, Neff JM, et al. Complications of smallpox vaccination, 1968. N Engl J Med 1969;281(22):1201-8.
29. Gurvich EB, Vilesova IS. Vaccinia virus in postvaccinal encephalitis. Acta Virol 1983;27(2):154-9.
30. De Vries E. Postvaccinial perivenous encephalitis. A pathological anatomical study on the place of postvaccinial perivenous encephalitis in the group encephalitides (the disease of Turn-

bull-Lucksch-Bastiaanse). Folia Psychiatr Neurol Jpn 1960; Suppl 5:1-181.

31. Fulginiti VA, Winograd LA, Jackson M, et al. Therapy of experimental vaccinal keratitis. Effect of idoxuridine and VIG. Arch Ophthalmol 1965;74(4):539-44.

32. CDC. Supplemental recommendations on adverse events following smallpox vaccine in the pre-event vaccination program: recommendations of the Advisory Committee on Immunization Practices. MMWR Morb Mortal Wkly Rep 2003; 52(13):282-4.

33. CDC. Cardiac adverse events following smallpox vaccination—United States, 2003. MMWR Morb Mortal Wkly Rep 2003;52(12):248-50.

34. MacAdam DB, Whitaker W. Cardiac complications after vaccination with smallpox. Br Med J 1962;5312:1099-1100.

35. Ahlborg B, Linroth K, Nordgren B. ECG-changes without subjective symptoms after smallpox vaccination of military personnel. Acta Med Scand Suppl 1966;464:127-34.

36. CDC. Update: cardiac-related events during the civilian smallpox vaccination program—United States, 2003. MMWR Morb Mortal Wkly Rep 2003;52(21):492-6.

37. Grabenstein JD, Winkenwerder W Jr. US military smallpox vaccination program experience. JAMA 2003;289(24):3278-82.

38. Karjalainen J, Heikkila J, Nieminen MS, et al. Etiology of mild acute infectious myocarditis. Relation to clinical features. Acta Med Scand 1983;213(1):65-73.

39. Helle EP, Koskenvuo K, Heikkila J, et al. Myocardial complications of immunisations. Ann Clin Res 1978;10(5):280-7.

40. CDC. Smallpox response plan and guidelines (Version 3.0). 2002. US Department of Health and Human Services, CDC. 2002. Available from http://www.bt.cdc.gov/agent/smallpox /response-plan/index.asp.

41. Dixon CW. Smallpox in Tripolitania, 1946: an epidemiological and clinical study of 500 cases, including trials of penicillin treatment. J Hyg 1948;46(4):351-77.

9

Viral Hemorrhagic Fevers

Erik J. Won and Anthony Carbone

NAME AND DESCRIPTION OF AGENTS

Viral hemorrhagic fever (VHF) has a variety of clinical manifestations and causative agents but is best characterized as an acute febrile illness with abnormalities of circulatory regulation and generalized signs of increased vascular permeability. Bleeding manifestations with fever in the presence of a bioterrorist threat should raise suspicions of VHF.

The etiology of VHF syndrome is represented by a diverse group of RNA viruses in four distinct families: (a) Arenaviridae, (b) Bunyaviridae, (c) Filoviridae, and (d) Flaviviridae. All of these viruses are enveloped with animal or insect reservoirs, although the natural host of the filoviruses (Ebola and Marburg) remains unknown. Viruses causing VHF are initially transmitted to humans via contact with the reservoir host or vector. Viruses carried by rodent reservoirs are transmitted to humans through contact with urine, feces, or carcasses of infected rodents. Arthropod vectors spread the virus by mosquito or tick bite. Humans are not the natural reservoir for any strains; however, some of these viruses can be spread from person to person by either direct contact or aerosolized particles.

THEORETICAL AND SCIENTIFIC BACKGROUND:

A consensus statement from an expert panel of 26 professionals (1) determined the VHF agents posing the most serious risk as biological weapons were Ebola and Marburg viruses (Filoviridae), Lassa fever and New World arenaviruses (Arenaviridae), Rift Valley Fever (Bunyaviridae), and yellow fever, Omsk hemorrhagic fever, and Kyasanur Forest disease (Flaviviridae). These agents met several criteria set forth by The Working Group on Civilian Biodefense for agents that pose particularly serious health risks as bioweapons. These criteria include: (a) high morbidity and mortality; (b) potential for person-to-person transmission; (c) low infective dose and highly infectious by aerosol dissemination, with a commensurate ability to cause large outbreaks; (d) effective vaccine unavailable or available only in limited supply; (e) potential to cause public and health

care worker anxiety; (f) availability of pathogen or toxin; (g) feasibility of large-scale production; (h) environmental stability; and (i) prior research and development as a biological weapon. The viruses excluded from this list had limitations in their potential use as weapons of mass destruction (some were difficult to produce in large amounts; others did not replicate to high enough concentrations in cell cultures to be weaponized).

FILOVIRIDAE (EBOLA AND MARBURG)

The filoviruses include Ebola and Marburg viruses. Both viruses are recognized as Category A, or high priority, by the National Institute for Allergy and Infectious Diseases (NIAID) (2) and Category A (Biosafety Level 4) agents by the Center for Disease Control and Prevention (CDC) (3,4).

The first recorded outbreak of Marburg occurred in Europe (Germany and Yugoslavia) in 1967 and remains the only outbreak to have occurred outside of Africa. This outbreak resulted from the unwitting importation of infected monkeys from Uganda. A total of 18 human outbreaks of Ebola and Marburg VHF have been reported with 10 outbreaks involving 30 or more victims.

The reservoir for Ebola and Marburg viruses is currently unknown. Isolating the wild reservoir has proven to be an arduous and daunting task. During the 1995 outbreak in Kikwit, Zaire, 3,000 vertebrates of multiple species and 30,000 arthropods were sampled without any trace of Ebola detected (5). As such, there have been no confirmatory studies to evaluate how virus is transmitted from host to human. The primary mode of person-to-person transmission is through direct contact with blood, secretions, and infected tissue. Experiments in nonhuman primates have documented transmission of infection after direct administration of Marburg virus into the mouths and noses of experimental animals (6). Several human infections have also occurred through contact of contaminated fingers with oral mucosa and conjunctiva (7). Percutaneous needlestick injuries are thought to be a particularly lethal mode of transmission. Eighty-five of 318 cases (26.7%) in a 1976 Ebola epidemic in Zaire occurred from individuals injected with contaminated syringes, and all cases acquired by injection resulted in death (8). Evidence suggests that percutaneous exposure to very low concentrations of virus can result in infection (9).

It is unclear whether disease transmission can occur from touching an infected patient or corpse through intact skin. A review of the Ebola outbreak in 1995 (Kikwit, Democratic Republic of the Congo) revealed infection in several subjects who prepared bodies for burial (10,11). Local customs and burial practices involve washing the body and trimming hair and nails, both of which pose a significant contact exposure to the subjects (12). Animal studies using guinea pigs were unable to demonstrate Marburg virus transmission through intact skin; however, infection through open skin lesions did occur (4).

Some animal studies have raised concerns about person-to-person transmission through aerosolized particles (5,13). Epidemiologic data suggests this is an unlikely route of human transmission, but it cannot be completely ruled out. In 1995 in the Democratic Republic of the Congo, 316 subjects were infected with Ebola. Only three health care workers became infected: one had a needlestick injury, one was nonadherent to barrier precautions, and one who always used barrier precautions is believed to have accidentally rubbed her eyes with a contaminated glove (14). Seventy-eight household members, without direct physical contact, were disease-free. However, in this outbreak, the only risk factor identified for five patients was visiting an infected patient in the absence of physical contact. These cases led researchers to conclude that airborne transmission could not be ruled out (15) but seemed, at most, a secondary mode of transmission. In 2000 in Uganda, 224 people died in an outbreak of Ebola. Of the medical personnel who became ill, 64% were infected after isolation wards and infection control measures (gloves, gowns, shoe covers, surgical masks, and eye protection) were employed (16). Airborne transmission could not be ruled out in this case.

Nevertheless, studies of other outbreaks argue strongly against a respiratory route of transmission. Most Ebola epidemics in Africa were ultimately controlled and ended without the use of specific airborne precautions. Airborne transmission of Marburg virus was not observed in the 1967 outbreak in Germany and Yugoslavia following the importation of infected African green monkeys (17). In 1975, only 1 in 35 health care workers exposed to Marburg disease without any barrier precautions became ill (18). In 1979, an outbreak of Ebola in Sudan infected 34 people. Twenty-nine cases of infection were reported among subjects who made direct physical contact, while no cases among 103 persons exposed in confined spaces without physical contact were reported (19). In 1994, only 1 of 70 contacts of an Ebola-infected patient acquired the disease despite no airborne precautions (20). In 1996, 300 contacts of Ebola-infected patients did not contract disease. These contacts were involved in numerous procedures prior to the patient's diagnosis with only standard blood and bodily fluid precautions. Again, no airborne precautions were taken (21).

ARENAVIRIDAE: LASSA FEVER AND NEW WORLD ARENAVIRUSES

Lassa fever and the New World arenaviruses (Lymphocytic Choriomeningitis virus, Junin virus, Machupo virus, Sabia virus, and Guanarito virus) are considered to have bioterrorism potential and are classified as Category A, or high priority, agents by the NIAID (2) and Category A (Biosafety Level 4) viruses by the CDC (3,4).

Rodents represent the natural reservoir for arenaviruses. Most Lassa virus infections can be traced to contact with the rodent, *Mastomys natilensis* (22). Argentine hemorrhagic fever, caused by Junin virus, is carried by the field mouse *Calomys colossus*. They can be transmitted to humans via inhalation of aerosolized particles from rodent urine/feces, direct contact with open wounds and mucous membranes, and ingestion of food contaminated with rodent excrement (23,24).

The primary route of person-to-person transmission is through direct contact with infectious blood or bodily fluids. There have been no documented cases of respiratory transmission of VHF arenaviruses; however, the possibility cannot be ruled out.

In 1970, a nosocomial outbreak of Lassa fever occurred in Nigeria. A single patient with pulmonary involvement caused 16 secondary cases of infection in subjects who shared the same hospital ward. Airborne transmission was believed to be the most likely cause of infection, but no definitive evidence of respiratory transmission was found, and the exact mechanism of disease transmission in this outbreak remains unknown (25). In 1971, a student became infected with Bolivian hemorrhagic fever watching a nursing instructor demonstrate the changing of bed linens of an infected patient. The student did not touch the bed linens nor any object in the room and kept a distance of approximately 6 feet from the patient. Approximately 80 other health care workers working with the patient, without respiratory precautions, did not become infected. Definitive evidence of person-to-person airborne transmission is lacking, but no alternative explanation to respiratory transmission was found for the single case of infection involving the student (26).

Findings that suggest a respiratory route of transmission is unlikely include the case of a single infected patient traveling from Sierra Leone to the United States. No secondary cases developed among 522 contacts (27). Another case involving a single infected patient traveling from Nigeria to St. Thomas (U.S. Virgin Islands) saw no secondary infections in 159 people who had direct contact with the patient (28).

Incubation periods vary between 5 and 17 days. There have been no documented cases of arenavirus transmission by infected persons during the incubation period (23,29). Disease transmission occurs primarily during the active phase of infection, but there have been reports of disease transmission from convalescing patients to spouses. Infectivity has been documented at 7 to 22 days after onset of illness (30) and Lassa fever virus has been detected in semen samples up to 3 months after acute infection (31). Mortality for Lassa fever ranges from 15% to 20%, while New World arenaviruses range from 15% to 30% (25,27,29).

BUNYAVIRIDAE: RIFT VALLEY FEVER, CRIMEAN CONGO HEMORRHAGIC FEVER, HANTAVIRUS

Rift Valley fever (RVF) and hantaviruses have been recognized as Category A, or high priority, agents by the NIAID, while Crimean Congo Hemorrhagic Fever (CCHF) has been classified as Category C by the same agency (2). The CDC places a lower priority on these agents with RVF and CCHF fitting the general definition of Category B agents and hantavirus listed among emerging pathogens in Category C (3,4,32).

The bunyaviruses are transmitted by both rodent and arthropod vectors. RVF is carried by mosquito vector,

CCHF is transmitted by a tick vector, and the hantaviruses have rodent vectors. All of these can be transmitted by bites, direct contact with infected animal tissues, or aerosolization of virus from infected animal carcasses.

RVF disease frequently resembles human influenza with fevers, fatigue, loss of appetite, and associated constitutional symptoms lasting for 2 to 5 days. In epidemic areas, human infection rates can be as high as 35% (33). Severe cases can cause significant morbidity from liver necrosis, hemorrhagic phenomena, retinitis with visual impairment, and meningoencephalitis (34,35), but fatality rates tend to stay relatively low <1% (36,37). There are no reported cases of person-to-person transmission of RVF (38). A group of World Health Organization (WHO) consultants have estimated that if 50 kg of RVF virus were released from an aircraft on a population of 500,000 persons, 400 would die and 35,000 would be incapacitated (39). Susceptible livestock could also become infected resulting in the potential establishment of disease in the environment (1).

CCHF fatality rates can be quite high with rates of 13% to 50% being reported in the literature (40). Humans may acquire the infection through tick bite, contact with blood or tissues from infected livestock, and infections of medical personnel treating or performing surgery on CCHF patients (41). There are reports that Iraq studied CCHF virus as a potential biological weapon and concluded that it was unsuitable as a biological weapon because it required vectors for dispersal (42). More recent reports, however, suggest that advances in viral replication technology may allow CCHF to be a viable aerosolized bioweapon (43).

Two diseases have been associated with the hantavirus genus: hantavirus with pulmonary syndrome (HPS) and hemorrhagic fever with renal syndrome (HFRS). Some strains of hantavirus have been cited as having fatality rates as high as 50% (44). The high fatality rate associated with HPS has given it some notoriety among laypersons, but it has little potential for development into a utilizable biological agent (45). With rapidly increasing knowledge about hantaviruses, many of the initial fears regarding their potential use as bioweapons have been put to rest. The CDC classifies it as a Category C virus, giving it low priority as a risk to national security. The reason it has fallen lower in the scope of potential VHF bioweapons is multifactorial:

1. Hantaviruses are hard to produce. They are extremely difficult to isolate (even in the most sophisticated laboratories) (46), dangerous for personnel involved in isolation, human viremia is low and short-lived (making capture even more difficult) (47,48), and adaptation of virus to growth in cell culture results in mutations and proliferation of strains that have reduced infectivity (49).

2. Hantaviruses are not easily transmitted. Infected rodents present only a limited period of viremia, after which they develop neutralizing antibodies. This means that blood from these rodents will not transmit disease and only a few excretory organs and their excreta could be considered as a source for terrorists seeking mass production of virus. This represents a difficult method of capture. Hantavirus-infected rodents also appear to be healthy, making it difficult to identify target specimens to obtain samples from. Human infection after a rodent bite is also highly exceptional (50).

3. Hantavirus infections can frequently be treated and prevented. Ribavirin has been shown to be active against hantavirus when given early enough and in sufficiently high intravenous doses. A field trial in China demonstrated that this treatment can be lifesaving (51). The same treatment was used in the management of HPS in the United States, but survival curves between treated subjects and nontreated subjects did not show an appreciable difference (52). Inactivated vaccines have been used for over a decade in South and North Korea (53). The protection rate among 1.2 million people was reported to be between 88% and 100% (54). Promising new vaccines are also being studied with potential for greater immunity to a broader range of hantavirus (55,56).

FLAVIVIRIDAE: YELLOW FEVER, DENGUE FEVER, OMSK HEMORRHAGIC FEVER, AND KYASANUR FOREST DISEASE

Dengue fever is a Class A pathogen according to NIAID categories, while Kyasanur Forest disease receives a rating of Class B, and yellow fever is Class C using the same rating system (2). The CDC considers these viruses Biosafety Level 4 (BSL 4) agents and would be Category B or C agents according to category definitions (3,4).

Humans acquire yellow fever and dengue fever from the bite of infected mosquitoes (57). Kyasanur Forest disease and Omsk hemorrhagic fever are transmitted by tick bites (58,59).

There have been no documented cases of person-to-person transmission or nosocomial spread of flaviviruses. As with RVF, there is a theoretical risk of flaviviruses becoming established in an environment following infection of susceptible arthropod vectors (1).

SIGNS AND SYMPTOMS

There are a variety of potential clinical manifestations following infection, but the dominant clinical feature of VHF syndrome is acute fever with changes in vascular permeability (hypotension, petechiae, unexplained hemorrhage, conjunctival infection, flushing, edema) (60). Other common presenting complaints include malaise, prostration, myalgias, rash, headache, nausea, arhtralgias, abdominal pain, and nonbloody diarrhea. Severe VHF typically evolves to shock and diffuse hemorrhage and is often accompanied by neurological, hematopoietic, or pulmonary sequelae.

TYPICAL PRESENTATION OF VHF

Previously healthy person who becomes acutely ill with high fever and the following signs and symptoms:

- Hemorrhagic manifestations (sometimes limited to conjunctival infection and nose bleeds)
- Maculopapular rash in the absence of other dermatologic lesions
- Rapidly progressing illness leading to intractable shock
- Absence of cough or rhinorrhea
- Death within one week

It is significant to note that in the absence of a known bioterrorist attack, the likelihood of acquiring VHF is extremely low unless patients, within three weeks before onset of fever, meet one of the following criteria (adapted from CDC) (61):

1. Traveled in the specific local area of a country where VHF has recently occurred

2. Had direct contact with blood, other bodily fluids, secretions, or excretions of a person or animal with VHF.

3. Worked in a laboratory or animal facility that handles hemorrhagic fever viruses.

4. The cause of fever in persons who have traveled to VHF endemic areas is more likely to be a different infectious disease (e.g., malaria or typhoid fever) than VHF; evaluation and treatment of these other potentially serious infections should not be delayed.

If there is a high suspicion for VHF, some clinical characteristics may help to distinguish between agents (although none are pathognomonic). Filoviruses, Rift Valley fever, and flaviviruses tend to have a more abrupt onset of symptoms, while arenaviruses have a more insidious onset. The filoviruses and CCHF produce large maculopapular rashes and may often be accompanied by profound hemorrhagic sequelae including disseminated intravascular coagulation (DIC) (Fig. 9-1). In contrast, hemorrhagic manifestations are much less pronounced in Lassa fever, yellow fever, and RVF. Jaundice is quite common in yellow fever, and retinitis can be a distinguishing finding in RVF.

Definitive diagnosis requires specific virologic diagnosis. The inoculation of cultured cells with serum, cerebrospinal fluid (CSF), or other body fluids or tissue extracts is the classical method to isolate and detect VHF viruses. Tests used to detect virus in acutely ill patients include antigen-capture enzyme-linked immunosorbent assay (ELISA), electron microscopy, reverse-transcription polymerase chain reaction (RT-PCR), modified conventional PCR (including nested, seminested, and Southern blotting), and real-time reverse-transcription PCR (62). Real-time reverse-transcription PCR has recently been shown to be a sensitive and rapid diagnostic test with the added capability of being able to screen for multiple pathogens simultaneously (63). These assays are currently only available at CDC or the U.S. Army Medical Research Institute of Infectious Diseases (USAMRIID) (63).

Several new tests are being developed to allow quick detection of virus-specific antibodies. The high virus concentration of Ebola and Lassa fever patients often facilitates antigen detection (less sensitive than PCR but quicker) (64). Another fairly simple test for Ebola virus can be performed by immunoperoxidase staining of formalin-fixed skin biopsies in infected individuals (65). This method has the advantage of being simple, specific, and safe (fixed material does not have to be handled in a BSL-4 laboratory). These tests could be of paramount importance in the future of bioterrorism preparedness and response. Early and timely detection of a VHF case will make it much easier to recognize additional victims and will also allow public health officials to dispatch appropriate information and precaution requirements. As new patients become diagnosed, they can be linked to common places and areas of potential exposure leading to identification of the index case/sentinel source.

If medical personnel suspect a diagnosis of VHF, they

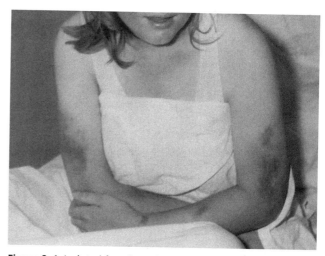

Figure 9–1. Isolated female patient diagnosed with Crimean-Congo hemorrhagic fever (CCHF). [Courtesy of Dr. B.E. Henderson, Center for Disease Control—Public Health Image Library (PHIL ID#2317).]

should immediately report the case to their local public health system, which will arrange for confirmatory testing to be performed. No material should be shipped to the CDC or USAMRIID laboratories without prior consultation. The following web sites offer more detailed instructions on packaging biological agents suspected of being BSL-4 agents:

http://www.bt.cdc.gov/labissues/PackagingInfo.pdf
www.cdc.gov/od/ohs/biosfty/bmbl4/bmbl4s1.htm.

MEDICAL MANAGEMENT

Supportive care is the mainstay of treatment for VHF. Special attention should be directed at maintaining fluid and electrolyte balance, circulatory volume, and blood pressure. In some cases, intravenous fluids may not be adequate to reverse hypotension and may contribute to pulmonary edema (61). If hypotension does not improve with fluid challenge, strong consideration should be given to early vasopressor support (1). Anticoagulants, nonsteroidal anti-inflammatory drugs, aspirin, and intramuscular injection are contraindicated. Transportation of patients by air is contraindicated due to effects of changes in ambient pressure on lung-water balance.

DECONTAMINATION

If the attack is ongoing or recently detected, it is imperative for patients directly exposed to the agent to take a full body shower with soap before entering the hospital. Weaponization of VHF in a liquid suspension may also prolong the life of the virus by several hours to several days depending on the transport medium so thorough decontamination of garments and bags is required.

If an undetected bioweapon is released, at least a week will elapse before significant numbers of patients become ill. After this period of time, it is highly unlikely that a VHF agent will remain in the environment so there is not likely to be a need for surface decontamination.

Decontamination is a significant concern for all virus-containing body fluids (emesis, diarrhea, blood, saliva) from sick patients. Filoviruses have the capability of surviving at room temperature in liquid or dried material for a number of days (depending on initial virus concentration) (66). Steam sterilization (thermal inactivation) is the most effective method of inactivating VHF agents (63). For the decontamination of objects and surfaces that cannot be sterilized by steam, the CDC recommends treatment with 1:100 dilution of household bleach or any standard hospital disinfectant registered with the U.S. Environmental Protection Agency (EPA) including quaternary ammonium compounds and phenol products.

Differential diagnosis should consider an extensive list of infectious diseases (influenza, septic shock, toxic shock syndrome, meningococcemia, Rocky Mountain spotted fever, leptospirosis, psittacosis, malaria, trypanosomiasis, plague, rubella, measles, hemorrhagic smallpox), and several noninfectious processes including idiopathic thrombocytopenic purpura, hemolytic uremic syndrome, and collagen vascular disease.

New technologies are being developed to more effectively inactivate VHFs. One of the more promising methods is inactivation with surfactant nanoemulsion (67). Nanoemulsions are a new form of disinfectant composed of detergents and vegetable oil suspended in water. These disinfectants have the ability to inactivate purified Ebola virus within 20 minutes. The advantage of nanoemulsions is that they are noncorrosive, simple to use (the majority of inactivation tools currently require additional protective measures from the disinfectant itself), very effective, and mild enough to be used in prevention of transmission through foodstuffs and skin/mucosa contact. Future studies on nanoemulsions are planned.

DRUG THERAPY

There are no antiviral drugs approved by the U.S. Food and Drug Administration (FDA) for the treatment of VHFs. Ribavirin has been used with varying amounts of success in cases of Lassa fever, New World hemorrhagic fever, RVF, and CCHF. Ribavirin is a nonimmunosuppressive nucleoside analog with broad antiviral properties. Treatment is most effective if begun within 7 days of onset. Current recommendations are to treat initially with ribavirin 30 mg/kg intravenously, followed by 15 mg/kg every 6 hours for 4 days, then 7.5 mg/kg every 8 hours for an additional 6 days (68). Ribavirin is not approved by the FDA for this indication and should be administered under an investigational new drug protocol. The primary adverse effect of ribavirin is a dose-related, reversible, hemolytic anemia. Some cardiac and pulmonary side effects have been reported with combination treatments of ribavirin-interferon therapy for hepatitis C (69). No other FDA-approved antiviral compounds are currently available for treatment of VHF.

VACCINES

There is a paucity of effective vaccines for VHF. The only licensed vaccine is a live attenuated vaccine for yellow fever. This has been shown to be highly effective in protecting travelers to endemic areas (70), but it has not been effective in postexposure prophylaxis. The short incubation period of yellow fever (3 to 6 days) does not provide adequate time for infected patients to develop neutralizing antibodies following vaccination.

Considerable research is being done in the development of future VHF vaccines. Promising results have been obtained in studies of laboratory animals. An experimental "accelerated vaccine" has been successful in providing immunity to non-human primates within 28 days (71). This is considered a significant development as previous Ebola vaccines required six months and multiple boosters to confer immunity on macaque monkeys (used in an attempt to prevent outbreaks in Africa). The speed of the new vaccine permits a strategy called ring vaccination, which aims to contain an outbreak by inoculating all possible contacts of the first detected cases. Ring vaccination is considered a viable option for dealing with other bioterrorist attacks (smallpox). A portion of the Ebola virus genome is "stitched" to a modified adenovirus, the virus responsible for the common cold, in order to develop the new vaccine. This generates an aggressive immune response from the host and teaches the immune system to recognize the protein encoded by the inserted gene. Should this vaccine prove effective in humans, it could form the template for developing emergency vaccines against numerous other diseases including viral bioweapons (72).

TRIAGE CONSIDERATIONS

Patients should be triaged according to their stage of disease and projected survivability based on the suspected agent. Patients with the best chance of surviving are those discovered in the early stages of disease.

Unfortunately, individuals with frank hemorrhage and evidence of end-organ damage are likely to progress to shock and death despite best medical care. These patients should be offered supportive care. It is also significant to note that patients in the latter stages of illness (characterized by vomiting, diarrhea, and hemorrhage) pose the greatest threat of transmission. These patients should be removed from public spaces such as an emergency department waiting room and quarantined if possible.

PERSONAL PROTECTION

Caution should be exercised in evaluating and treating patients with suspected VHF. The most common mechanism of human-to-human transmission and nosocomial infection is direct contact with blood, secretions, body fluids, and infected tissue. Particularly significant to hospital personnel is the finding that self-inoculation frequently occurs when virus-containing material on contaminated hands of caregivers makes contact with their own eyes and mouths (65). This mode of transmission was duplicated in laboratory experiments where monkeys were lethally infected by instilling drops of virus-containing fluid into their eyes and mouths (8).

Close attention to universal precautions should be used at all times. A consensus statement by 29 medical specialists (1) recommends "VHF-specific precautions" including: strict adherence to hand hygiene, double gloves, impermeable gowns, N-95 masks or powered air-purifying respirators, negative isolation room with 6 to 12 air changes per hour, leg and shoe coverings, face shields, goggles for eye protection, restricted access of nonessential staff and visitors to patient's room, and environmental disinfection with an EPA-registered hospital disinfectant or 1:100 dilution of household bleach. We also recommend hazard labeling of specimens submitted to the lab, limiting members of the patient care team to selected trained individuals, and special attention directed toward eliminating parenteral expo-

sures when possible (endoscopy, respirators, arterial catheters, phlebotomy, and laboratory analysis increase opportunities for dissemination of infectious blood and body fluids).

In past outbreaks, the greatest risk of transmission from sick to healthy people occurred during the opening phase when patients were being cared for by family members without appropriate precautions. Family members should receive appropriate instruction and education on precautions and risks.

SUMMARY Key Features of Viral Hemorrhagic Fevers

Family: Filoviridae
Genus: Filovirus
Virus (Disease): Ebola virus (Ebola hemorrhagic fever)
                Marburg virus (Marburg hemorrhagic fever)

- Vector in nature = Unknown
- Geographic distribution = Africa
- Person-to-person transmission = Yes (Direct contact)
- Incubation period = 2 to 21 days
- Mortality = 50% to 90%
- Treatment = Supportive

Family: Arenaviridae
Genus: Arenavirus
Virus (Disease): Lassa virus (Lassa fever)
                Junin virus (Argentine hemorrhagic fever)
                Machupo virus (Bolivian hemorrhagic fever)
                Sabia virus (Brazilian hemorrhagic fever)
                Guanarito virus (Venezuelan hemorrhagic fever)

- Vector in nature = Rodent
- Geographic distribution = West Africa (Lassa), South America (Junin, Machupo, Sabia, Guanarito)
- Person-to-person transmission = Yes
- Incubation period = 5 to 16 days
- Mortality = 15% to 20%
- Treatment = Ribavirin, supportive

Family: Bunyaviridae
Genus: Nairovirus, Phlebovirus, Hantavirus
Virus (Disease): Nairovirus (Crimean-Congo hemorrhagic fever)
                Phlebovirus (Rift Valley fever)
                Hantavirus (Hantavirus hemorrhagic fever)

- Vector in nature = Tick (CCHF)
                Mosquito (RVF)
                Rodent (HV)
- Geographic distribution = Africa, central Asia, eastern Europe, Middle East (CCHF)
                Africa, Saudi Arabia, Yemen (RVF)
                Asia, Balkans, Europe, Eurasia (HV)
- Person-to-person transmission = No
- Incubation period = 2 to 6 days
- Mortality = 3% to 50% (CCHF)
                <1% (RVF)
                50% (Hantavirus)
- Treatment = Supportive

SUMMARY Key Features of Viral Hemorrhagic Fevers *(continued)*

Family: Flaviviridae

Genus: Flavivirus

Virus: Dengue virus (dengue fever, dengue hemorrhagic fever, hemorrhagic fever with renal syndrome)

Yellow fever virus (yellow fever)

Omsk hemorrhagic fever virus (Omsk hemorrhagic fever)

Kyasanur Forest disease virus (Kyasanur Forest disease)

- Vector in nature = Tick (dengue fever and yellow fever)

Mosquito (Omsk and Kyasanur)

- Geographic distribution = Asia, Africa, Pacific, Americas (dengue fever)

Africa, tropical Americas (yellow fever)

Central Asia (Omsk hemorrhagic fever)

India (Kyasanur Forest disease)

- Incubation period = 3 to 5 days (dengue fever, but unknown for dengue hemorrhagic fever)

3 to 6 days (yellow fever)

2 to 9 days (Omsk and Kyasanur hemorrhagic fever)

Unknown for dengue hemorrhagic fever

- Mortality = 5% to 20% (dengue hemorrhagic fever)

3% to 6% (yellow fever)

0.5% to 10% (Omsk hemorrhagic fever)

3% to 10% (Kyasanur Forest disease)

- Treatment = Supportive

RESOURCES

1. In the event of an actual or threatened bioterrorist incident, immediately contact your state and local public health office (a list of these can be found at http://www.statepublichealth.org/index.php and the CDC web site: http://www.bt.cdc.gov/emcontact/index.asp).

2. For detailed packaging instructions on shipping BSL-4 agents, visit
http://www.bt.cdc.gov/labissues/PackagingInfo.pdf.
http://www.cdc.gov/od/ohs/biosfty/bmbl4/bmbl4s1.htm.

3. Borio L, Inglesby T, Peters CJ, et al. Consensus statement—hemorrhagic fever viruses as biological weapons: medical and public health management. JAMA. 2002;287(18):2391-405.

4. Drosten C, Kummerer BM, Schmitz H, Gunther S. Molecular diagnostics of viral hemorrhagic fevers. Antiviral Res. 2003;57:61-87.

QUESTIONS AND ANSWERS

1. The viral hemorrhagic fevers are a diverse group of enveloped RNA viruses. What type of virus are Ebola and Marburg examples of?
    A. Filovirus
    B. Flavivirus
    C. Arenavirus
    D. Bunyavirus
    E. Togavirus

2. Appropriate treatment for VHF patients include all of the following EXCEPT:
    A. Supportive measures
    B. Drug therapy when indicated
    C. Anticoagulation
    D. Early consideration of pressors when hypotension becomes an issue
    E. Hemodynamic monitoring

3. Laboratory methods for diagnosing VHF include
    A. Real-time reverse transcription PCR
    B. Electron microscopy
    C. Enzyme-linked immunosorbent assay (ELISA)
    D. Cell culture with anyline dye staining
    E. Immunoperoxidease staining of formalin-fixed skin biopsies

4. VHF precautions should include
    A. Double gloves
    B. N-95 masks
    C. Restricted access of nonessential staff and visitors to patient's room
    D. None of the above
    E. All of the above

ANSWERS

1: *A.* *Filovirus*
2: *C.* *Anticoagulation*

3: *D. Cell culture with anyline dye staining*
4: *E. All of the above*

REFERENCES

1. Borio L, Inglesby T, Peters CJ, et al. Hemorrhagic fever viruses as biological weapons: medical and public health management. JAMA. 2002;287(18);2391-405.
2. http://www.niaid.nih.gov/dmid/biodefense/bandc_priority.htm.
3. http://www.bt.cdc.gov/agent/agentlist-category.asp#a.
4. http://www.cdc.gov/ncidod/dvrd/spb/mnpages/disinfo.htm.
5. Leirs H, Mills JN, Krebs JW, et al. Search for the Ebola virus reservoir in Kikwit, Democratic Republic of the Congo: reflections on a vertebrate collection. J Infect Dis. 1999;179 (Suppl 1):S155-63.
6. Schou S, Hansen AK. Marburg and Ebola virus infections in laboratory nonhuman primates. Comp Med. 2000;50:2108-23.
7. Jaax NK, Davis KJ, Geisbert TJ, et al. Lethal experimental infection of rhesus monkeys with Ebola-Zaire (Mayinga) virus by the oral and conjunctival route of exposure. Arch Pathol Lab Med. 1996;120:140-55.
8. World Health Organization International Study Team. Ebola hemorrhagic fever in Zaire, 1976. Bull World Health Organ. 1978;56:271-93.
9. Emond RT, Evans B, Bowen ET, Lloyd G. A case of Ebola virus infection. Br Med J. 1977;2:541-4.
10. Dowell SF, Mukunu R, Ksiazek TG, et al. Transmission of Ebola hemorrhagic fever: a study of risk factors in family members, Kikwit, Democratic Republic of the Congo, 1995. J Infect Dis. 1999;179 (Suppl 1):S87-91.
11. Khan AS, Tshioko FK, Heymann DK, et al. The re-emergence of Ebola hemorrhagic fever, Democratic Republic of the Congo, 1995. J Infect Dis. 1999;179 (Suppl 1):S76-86.
12. Butler CJ, Kilmarx PH, Jernigan DB, et al. Perspectives in fatal epidemics. Infect Dis Clin North Am. 1996;10:917-37.
13. Jaax N, Jahrling P, Geisbert T, et al. Transmission of Ebola virus (Zaire strain) to uninfected control monkeys in a biocontainment laboratory. Lancet. 1995;346:1669-71.
14. Guimard Y, Bwaka MA, Colebunders R, et al. Organization of patient care during the Ebola hemorrhagic fever epidemic in Kikwit, Democratic Republic of the Congo, 1995. J Infect Dis. 1999;179 (Suppl 1):S268-73.
15. Centers for Disease Control and World Health Organization. Infection control for the hemorrhagic fevers in the African health care setting. Atlanta, GA: Centers for Disease Control and Prevention. Available at http://www.cdc.gov/ncidod/dvrd/spb/mnpages/vhfmanual.htm.
16. Center for Disease Control, Uganda Ministry of Health. Outbreak of Ebola hemorrhagic fever, Uganda, August 2000–January 2001. MMWR. 2001;50:73-7.
17. Slenczka WG. The Marburg virus outbreak of 1967 and subsequent episodes. Curr Top Microbiol Immunol. 1999;235:49-75.
18. Gear JS, Cassel GA, Gear AJ, et al. Outbreak of Marburg virus disease in Johannesburg. Br Med J. 1975;4:489-93.
19. Baron RC, McCormick JB, Zubeir OA. Ebola virus disease in southern Sudan. Bull World Health Organ. 1983;61:997-1003.
20. Fomenty P, Hatz C, Le Guenno B, et al. Human infection due to Ebola virus, subtype Cote D'Ivoire. J Infect Dis. 1999;179 (Suppl 1):S48-53.
21. Richards GA, Murphy S, Jobson RM, et al. Unexpected Ebola virus in a tertiary setting. Crit Care Med. 2000:28:240-4.
22. Jharling PB. Medical aspects of chemical and biological warfare. Chapter 29: viral hemorrhagic fevers. Walter Reed Army Medical Center. On U.S. Army Medical NBC Online Information Server. Available at: http://www.nbc-med.org/SiteContent/HomePage/WhatsNew/MedAspects/Ch-29electrv699.pdf.
23. Johnson KM, Mackenzie RB, Webb PA, et al. Chronic infection of rodents by Machupo virus. Science. 1965;150:1618-9.
24. Johnson KM, Kuns ML, Mackenzie RB, et al. Isolation of Machupo virus from wild rodent Calomys callosus. Am J Trop Med Hyg. 1966;15:103-6.
25. Carey DE, Kemp GE, White HA, et al. Lassa fever: epidemiological aspects of the 1970 epidemic, Jos, Nigeria. Trans R Soc Trop Med Hyg. 1972;66:402-8.
26. Peters CJ, Kuehne RW, Mercado RR, et al. Hemorrhagic fever in Conchabamba, Bolivia 1971. Am J Epidemiol. 1974;99: 424-33.
27. Zweighaft RM, Fraser DW, Hattwick MA, et al. Lassa fever: response to an imported case. N Engl J Med. 1977;297:803-7.
28. Cooper CB, Gransden WR, Webster M, et al. A case of Lassa fever: experience at St. Thomas's Hospital. Br Med J. 1982;285:1003-5.
29. Kilgore PE, Ksiazek TG, Rollin PE, et al. Treatment of Bolivian hemorrhagic fever with intravenous ribavarin. Clin Infect Dis. 1997;24:718-22.
30. Briggiler AM, Enria DA, Feuillade MR, et al. Contagio interhumano e infeccion clinical con virus Junin en matrimanos residents en el area endemica de fiebre hemorrhagic Argentina. Medicina (B Aires). 1987;47:565.
31. World Health Organization. Fact Sheet 179:Lassa fever. April 2000. Available at http://www.who.int/mediacentre/factsheets/fs179/en.
32. Sidwell RW, Smee DF. Viruses of the Bunya- and ogaviridae families: potential as bioterrorism agents and means of control. Antiviral Res. 2003;57:101-11.
33. Meegan JM, Watten R, Laughlin L, et al. Clinical experience with Rift Valley fever in human beings during the 1977 Egyptian epizootic. Conf Epidemiol Biostat. 1981;3:114-23.
34. Siam AL, Meegan JM, Gharbawi KF, et al. Rift Valley fever ocular manifestations: observations during the 1977 epidemic in Egypt. Br J Ophthalmol. 1980;64;366-74.
35. Meegan JM, Shope R. Emerging concepts on Rift Valley fever. Perspect Virol. 1981;11;267-87.
36. Gear JH. Clinical aspects of African viral hemorrhagic fevers. Rev Infect Dis. 1989;11 (Suppl. 4):S777-82.
37. Strausbaugh LJ, Laughlin LW, Meegan JM, et al. Clinical studies on Rift Valley fever, I: acute febrile and hemorrhagic-like diseases. J Egypt Public Health Assoc. 1978;53:181-2.
38. Jouan A, Coulibaly I, Adam F, et al. Analytical study of a Rift Valley fever epidemic. Res Virol. 1989;140:75-86.
39. Christopher GW, Cieslak TJ, Pavlin JA, et al. Biological warfare: a historical perspective. JAMA. 1997;278:412-7.
40. Swanepoel R, Gill DE, Shephard AJ, et al. The clinical pathology of Crimean/Congo hemorrhagic fever. Rev Infect Dis. 1989;11(Suppl.4): S794-800.
41. Nichol S. Bunyaviruses. In: Knipe D. et al., eds. Field virology. Philadelphia: Lippincott Williams & Wilkins.
42. Zilinskas RA. Iraq's biological weapons: the past as future? JAMA. 1997;278:418-24.
43. Bronze MS, Huycke MM, Machado LJ, et al. Viral agents as biological weapons and agents of bioterrorism. Am J Med Sci. 2002;323:316-25.
44. Duchin JS, Koster FT, Peters CJ, et al. Hantavirus pulmonary syndrome: a clinical description of 17 patients with a newly recognized disease. The Hantavirus study group. N Engl J Med. 1994;330;1949–55.
45. Clement JP. Hantavirus. Antiviral Res. 2003;57:121-7.
46. Monroe MC, Morzunov SP, Johnson AM, et al. Genetic diversity and distribution of Peromyscus-borne hantaviruses in North America. Emerg Infect Dis. 1999;5:75-86.
47. Galeno H, Mora J, Villagra E, et al. First human isolate of hantavirus (Andes virus) in the Americas. Emerg Infect Dis. 2002;8:657-61.
48. Peters CJ, Khan AS. Hantavirus pulmonary syndrome: the new American hemorrhagic fever. Clin Infect Dis. 2002;34:1224-31.
49. Lundqvist A, Cheng Y, Sjolander KB, et al. Cell culture adap-

tation of Puumula hantavirus changes the infectivity for its natural reservoir, Clethrionomys glareolus, and leads to accumulation of mutants with altered genomic RNA S segment. J Virol. 1997;71:9515-23.

50. Dournon E, Moriniere B, Matheson S, et al. HFRS after a wild rodent bite in the Haute-Savoie and risk of exposure to Hantaan-like virus in a Paris laboratory. Lancet. 1984;1:676—7.

51. Huggins JW, Hsiang CM, Cosgriff TM, et al. Prospective, double-blind, concurrent, placebo-controlled clinical trial of intravenous ribavirin therapy of hemorrhagic fever with renal syndrome. J Infect Dis. 1991;164:1119-27.

52. Chapman LE, Mertz GJ, Peters CJ, et al. Intravenous ribavirin for hantavirus pulmonary syndrome: safety and tolerance during 1 year of open label experience. Ribavirin study group. Antiviral Ther. 1999;4(4):211-9.

53. Kim RJ, Ru C, Kim GM. The special prevention of HFRS in P.D.R. of Korea. Chin Clin Exp Virol. 1991;4:487-92.

54. Lee HW, Ahn C, Song J, et al. Field trial of an inactivated vaccine against hemorrhagic fever with renal syndrome in humans. Arch Virol. 1990(Suppl. 1):35-47.

55. Choi Y, Ahn CJ, Seong KM, et al. Inactivated Hantaan virus vaccine derived from suspension culture of Vero cells. Vaccine. 2003;21(17-18):1867-73.

56. Hjelle B. Vaccines against hantaviruses. Expert Rev Vaccines. 2002;1(3):373-84. Review.

57. Monath TP. Yellow fever: Victor, Victoria? Conqueror, conquest? Epidemics and research in the last forty years and prospects for the future. Am J Trop Med Hyg. 1991;45(1):1-43.

58. Pavri K. Clinical, clinicopathologic, and hematologic features of Kyasanur Forest disease. Rev Infect Dis. 1989;11(May-Jun):S830-9.

59. Chumakov MP. Studies of virus hemorrhagic fevers. J Hyg Epidemiol Microbiol Immunol. 1959;7:125-35.

60. Peters CJ, Johnson ED, McKee KT. Filoviruses and management of viral hemorrhagic fever. In: Belshe RB, ed. Textbook of human virology. 2nd ed. St. Louis: Mosby-Year Book; 1991.

61. CDC. Notice to readers update: management of patients with suspected viral hemorrhagic fever—United States. MMWR. 1995; 44(25): 475-9.

62. Bray M. Defense against filoviruses used as biological weapons. Antiviral Res. 2003;57:53-60.

63. Drosten C, Gottig S, Schilling S, et al. Rapid detection and quantitation of RNA of Ebola and Marburg viruses, Lassa virus, Crimean-Congo hemorrhagic fever virus, Rift Valley fever virus, dengue virus and yellow fever virus by real-time reverse-transcription PCR. J Clin Microbiol. 2002;40:2323-30.

64. Bausch DG, Rollin PE, Demby AH, et al. Diagnosis and clinical virology of Lassa fever as evaluated by enzyme-linked immunosorbent assay, indirect fluorescent-antibody test, and virus isolation. J Clin Microbiol. 2000;38:2670-7.

65. Zaki SR, Shieh WJ, Greer PW, et al. A novel immunohistochemical assay for the detection of Ebola virus in skin: implications for diagnosis, spread, and surveillance of Ebola hemorrhagic fever. Commission de Lutte contre les Epidemies a Kikwit. J Infect Dis. 1999;179(Suppl. 1): S36-47.

66. Belanov EF, Muntyanov EP, Kryuck VD, et al. Survival of Marburg virus on contaminated surfaces and in aerosol. Voprosy Virusologii. 1996;41:32-4.

67. Chepurnov AA, Bakulina LF, Dadaeva AA, et al. Inactivation of Ebola virus with a surfactant nanoemulsion. Acta Tropica. 2003; 87:315-20.

68. CDC. Management of patients with suspected viral hemorrhagic fever. MMWR. 1988;37(Suppl. 3):1-16.

69. Rebetol product information. Available at http://www.hepatitisinnovations.com/pro/rebetol/rebetol_pi.html.

70. Monath TP. Yellow fever: an update. Lancet Infect Dis. 2001;1:11-20.

71. Sullivan NJ, Gelsbert TW, Gelsbert JB, et al. Accelerated vaccination for Ebola virus hemorrhagic fever in non-human primates. Nature. 2003; 424:681-4.

72. Clarke T, Knight K. Fast vaccine offers hope in battle with Ebola. Nature. 2003; 424:602.

10

Lesser Known Biological Agents and Potential Threats

Teriggi J. Ciccone and Seric S. Cusick

TULAREMIA

Tularemia is a bacterial zoonosis caused by *Francisella tularensis*, a facultative intracellular aerobic gram-negative coccobacilli. Several other names have been used to describe this disease, including rabbit fever, deerfly fever, market men's disease, or Francis disease. First described in rodents during the early 20th century in Tulare County, California, tularemia results in multiple clinical manifestations in infected humans (1). Clinical disease is caused by two isolates, known as Biovars Jellison Type A and B. This organism is found throughout most of the world with predominance in the Northern Hemisphere. Tularemia is endemic in the United States, northern Europe, Scandinavia, and the former Soviet Union. Cases have been reported in all of the continental United States, predominantly in southern and western states. From 1990 to 2000, 1,368 cases of tularemia were reported in the United States, with more than half of the cases occurring in Missouri, Arkansas, South Dakota, and Oklahoma (2).

THEORETICAL AND SCIENTIFIC BACKGROUND

Human tularemia infection occurs after exposure to the causative agent via insect bite or contact with contaminated substances. Arthropod vectors include ticks, deerflies, and mosquitoes. The natural reservoir for *F. tularensis* includes rabbits, rats, mice, squirrels, beavers, and deer. Infection can be introduced cutaneously or through mucous membranes after insect or animal bite, handling infected animal carcasses, or exposure to contaminated water. Respiratory exposure to tularemia occurs via inhalation of contaminated soil, dust, or other particles. Disease can also occur after ingestion of contaminated animal products or water. Human-

to-human transmission of tularemia has not been reported. Tularemia has been recognized as a possible bioweapon since the 1940s. The United States produced and maintained offensive tularemia during the 1950s and 1960s (3,4). A startling World Health Organization report from 1970 predicted that 50 kg of tularemia disseminated within a population of 5 million persons would result in 250,000 injuries and 19,000 deaths (5,6).

Tularemia is classified as a category A agent by the Centers for Disease Control and Prevention (CDC) (7) and represents a threat for several reasons. The Jellison Type A isolate is highly virulent, causing disease in humans with exposure to fewer than 10 bacteria when inhaled (8–10). This agent could be aerosolized and potentially spread over a large area causing pulmonary tularemia. Additionally, tularemia is a highly morbid disease, imposing a significant burden of disease on the victims, and untreated tularemia carries a mortality of upward of 33% (11). In addition to being highly virulent and morbid, *F. tularensis* can survive for prolonged periods of time in freezing conditions, making its storage and potential shipment relatively simple. Infected frozen rabbit meat has been shown to remain infective for greater than 3 years (12).

SIGNS AND SYMPTOMS

Tularemia causes multiple disease syndromes in infected humans depending on the site and amount of inoculum. Incubation periods after exposure generally range between 3 and 6 days. Initial symptoms are nonspecific and can mimic flulike or upper respiratory infections. Abrupt onset of fever with chills, myalgias, cough, fatigue, and sore throat are the earliest symptoms. Pulse-temperature disassociation has been noted in a large number of patients (11). Beyond this initial period, more readily identifiable syndromes develop.

Ulceroglandular tularemia is the most frequent naturally occurring form of the disease. Lesions on the skin or mucous membranes accompanied by regional lymphadenopathy characterize this form (13). Infection occurs after inoculation of skin or mucous membranes. A tender, erythematous papule develops a few days after inoculation. The lesion soon begins to ulcerate within a few days with the onset of systemic symptoms, with a granulomatous base and indurated, raised borders. Lesions range in size between 0.5 and 10 cm. As the disease process progresses, an eschar may form over the ulcer. Ulcers and lymphadenopathy may persist for months after onset if left untreated, with lymph nodes draining out onto the skin (13,14). Glandular tularemia is a syndrome in which regional lymphadenopathy occurs without a frank ulcer. Oculoglandular tularemia results from inoculation of the eye. Purulent, painful conjunctivitis, chemosis, and lymphadenitis are predominant features.

Tularemic pneumonia caused by inhalation of infectious particles produces a different symptom complex and occurs in approximately half of all cases of tularemia. This syndrome would be the one most likely occurring during bioterrorist attacks via airborne dispersion of infective particles. Patients become ill 3 to 5 days after exposure. Early constitutional symptoms are often noted before more specific pulmonary manifestations. After 3 to 6 days, sore throat, cough, dyspnea, pleuritic chest pain, and hemoptysis develop. In a majority of cases, patchy bilateral infiltrates or lobar consolidation with or without pleural effusions may make this disease indistinguishable from other pneumonias. More advanced cases of tularemic pneumonia cause pleuropneumonitis accompanied with hilar lymphadenopathy; however, these radiographic signs may be nonspecific or absent. Left untreated, tularemic pneumonia can lead to worsening respiratory failure and acute respiratory distress syndrome requiring assisted ventilation (12–14).

Oropharyngeal tularemia occurs after ingestion of contaminated water, plant, or animal products. This syndrome is characterized by pharyngitis, stomatitis, and prominent cervical lymphadenopathy, mimicking acute streptococcal pharyngitis (15,16). Ulcerations may form on the oropharyngeal mucosa. Abdominal pain, nausea, vomiting, and diarrhea may also occur.

Typhoidal tularemia occurs when systemic illness presents without a clear localizing source of inoculation. Tularemic sepsis is the most severe form of disease. The patient may present febrile, obtunded, and hypotensive and ultimately may develop multiorgan failure including disseminated intravascular coagulation, acute renal failure, and meningitis (14,15). Left untreated, this syndrome may result in a fatality rate up to 60% (8,12,13).

MEDICAL MANAGEMENT

The diagnosis of tularemia is challenging for a number of reasons. It is a relatively rare naturally occurring disease and thus not initially suspected by physicians. No specific rapid diagnostic test is readily available in most settings (8,13). From a laboratory perspective, the extremely high virulence of tularemia limits the number of laboratories that can safely work with this bacterium. Additionally, routine Gram stains and cultures from various sources are unreliable. Serological testing using latex agglutination or enzyme-linked im-

munosorbent assays are available; however, the utility of these studies in an acute outbreak is questionable because the serum antibodies required for serological testing do not develop for days to weeks after infection (13). More rapid diagnostic tests include direct fluorescence antibody and immunohistochemical studies. The use of these modalities is limited by the lack of appropriate equipment and personnel in many hospital laboratories. Most often these studies require samples to be sent to a reference laboratory, adding further delay to the diagnosis.

Given the nonspecific presentations of tularemia and the lack of rapid diagnostic testing, the physician's clinical suspicion becomes critically important. Tularemia should be suspected in cases where a large number of patients within a specific geographical area develop symptoms of severe respiratory and systemic infections. A cluster of atypical pneumonia with hilar lymphadenopathy in otherwise healthy patients should raise suspicion for possible bioterrorist attack and prompt further actions. Hospital infectious disease authorities should be notified, and a report should be made to local and regional health departments. Clusters of tularemic pneumonia should also be reported to local law enforcement agencies and the Federal Bureau of Investigation.

Routine laboratory data is nonspecific but may reveal a mild leukocytosis with a lymphocytosis (11,13,15,17). Chest roentgenograms should be obtained on all patients with nonspecific pulmonary symptoms searching for pleuropneumonitis and hilar lymphadenopathy. Cultures from blood, sputum, conjunctival, and oropharyngeal secretions should be collected and sent to appropriate laboratories for culture on glucose cysteine blood agar or thioglycollate broth (8,13).

Aminoglycoside antibiotics, specifically streptomycin, are considered the drugs of choice for the treatment of tularemia (8,12,13,15). Streptomycin is dosed as 1g intramuscularly (IM) twice daily for adults, and 15 mg/kg IM twice daily for children. Where streptomycin is unavailable or contraindicated, gentamicin at 5 mg/kg intravenously (IV) daily can be used for adults; 2.5 mg/kg IV three times a day can be used in children. Treatment should continue for 10 days. Alternative choices include doxycycline, chloramphenicol, and ciprofloxacin.

A bioterrorist attack has the potential to cause massive outbreaks of tularemia. Under such circumstances, the use of IV antibiotics on a large scale may not be feasible. The Working Group on Civil Biodefense recommends the use of oral antibiotics in mass casualty events (8). Both doxycycline and ciprofloxacin are recommended for both adults and children. Doxycycline dosing is 100 mg orally twice daily for adults and 2.2 mg/kg orally twice daily for children under 45 kg. Ciprofloxacin dosing is 500 mg orally twice daily for adults and 15 mg/kg orally twice a day for children. Treatment should continue for 14 days.

Methods of postexposure prophylaxis have been recommended for large-scale tularemia attacks. A study in the 1960s found human volunteers treated with tetracycline for 24 hours prior to aerosolized tularemia exposure were protected from disease (18). In the event of a known tularemia attack before the mass outbreak of symptoms, postexposure prophylaxis with doxycycline or ciprofloxacin should be administered to potential victims. In the event of an attack that is not apparent until patients begin manifesting signs and symptoms of tularemia, asymptomatic patients within the attack area should begin a fever watch and begin postexposure prophylaxis if fever develops (8).

TRIAGE CONSIDERATIONS

Because there has never been a reported case of tularemia spread between humans, no specific isolation is required for patients in whom this diagnosis is suspected. In the event of a mass casualty event, priority should be given to those patients with more severe respiratory signs and symptoms such as hypoxia, tachypnea, and respiratory failure. These patients may require immediate advanced airway interventions. The larger remainder of ambulatory patients with symptoms of pneumonia should be triaged based on acuity and comorbid factors. Children and the elderly may develop disease in a more rapid and severe fashion.

PERSONAL PROTECTION

Universal precautions should be observed for patients with suspected tularemia. A 0.5% hypochlorite solution can be used to sanitize bedding and surfaces contacted by patients with tularemia (19). Although no human-to-human transmission has been reported, the high virulence of tularemia in culture requires extreme caution for laboratory workers. Highly trained personnel should perform cultures in a specially equipped reference laboratory. Laboratory workers should wear impervious face masks, gloves, and gowns under negative-pressure microbiological cabinets (12).

Vaccination against tularemia was initiated in the 1930s in the former Soviet Union in endemic areas (20). A live attenuated vaccine has been used in a limited setting among high-risk personnel such as laboratory technicians in the United States. Use of this vaccine is currently under review by the Food and Drug Administration. The Department of Defense maintains this vaccine as an investigational new drug at the U.S. Army Medical Research and Material Command at Fort Detrick, Maryland (13).

SUMMARY

- Tularemia is an effective bioweapon due to its virulence, high morbidity and mortality, and ease of storage, transport, and dispersion by aerosol.
- Although tularemia causes multiple clinical syndromes, a primarily respiratory disease would result from a bioterrorist attack via aerosolized particles.
- Aminoglycosides, specifically streptomycin, are the treatments of choice for tularemia. In mass casualty events, oral doxycycline and ciprofloxacin should be used.

Q FEVER

Q fever is a febrile illness originally described in 1935 as Query fever prior to the discovery of the infectious agent *Coxiella burnetii*. This obligate intracellular, gram-negative coccobacillus has a worldwide zoonotic reservoir. The organism is located within the acidified phagolysosomes of eukaryotic cells and may sporulate in the presence of unfavorable environmental conditions.

THEORETICAL AND SCIENTIFIC BACKGROUND

An illness initially discovered during an outbreak among abattoir workers in Australia, Q fever remains a disease found primarily among persons in contact with infected livestock. Its zoonotic reservoir is broad, infecting mammals, birds, and arthropods. Arthropod carriage is thought to be an important source for enzoonotic transmission but not human infection (19). Cattle, sheep, and goats are the most common sources of human infection. The bacteria are concentrated in the placenta of mammals and may be shed in milk, urine, and feces. Inhalation of a single aerosolized bacterium may be sufficient to cause human infection. This respiratory route is the primary mode of transmission. Due to high concentration of organisms in birth products, persons in contact with parturient animals are at particularly high risk for contracting the disease. *C. burnetii* has a marked ability to resist heat and desiccation, and locations at which parturition occur may contain infective particles for weeks. Although less common, infection may also occur through ingestion of raw milk products, requiring a significantly larger inoculum (21). Human-to-human transmission is regarded as rare but has been reported in cases of blood transfusion, transplacental congenital infection, upon autopsy of infected cadavers, and by a case report of an obstetrician becoming infected while performing a therapeutic abortion on an infected woman (21). Sexual transmission has been demonstrated in the murine model and was recently reported in the case of an occupationally exposed man potentially transmitting the bacterium to his wife (22). The organism's potential infectivity is furthered by the ability to travel long distances windborne or upon contaminated fomites. Downwind reach of *C. burnetii* in a hypothetical biological attack is estimated to be 20 km (4).

Once infected, most often via the aerosol route, the organism replicates during a 1- to 6-week incubation period (19,21,23). Late in this phase, a transient bacteremia ensues, providing the opportunity for hematogenous seeding of multiple organ systems. Infection with *C. burnetii* may be asymptomatic in over 50% of cases (19,21). Acute Q fever is typically a self-limited, febrile illness. However it may also present as atypical pneumonia, hepatitis, myocarditis, pericarditis, or encephalitis. Mortality rates of untreated acute Q fever are 1% to 2% with mortality rates in treated patients being less than 1% (21). A chronic form of Q fever may ensue and is most commonly characterized by endocarditis and/or chronic granulomatous hepatitis. Persons with underlying cardiac valvular abnormalities and various immunodeficiencies are most susceptible to developing chronic Q fever.

The prevalence of acute Q fever is difficult to assess and varies dramatically worldwide. It is unclear whether this reflects actual difference in the number of cases, discrepancy in the level of physician awareness, a lack of diagnostic capabilities, or a combination of these factors. Annual incidence in the United States is reported as 20, with an unknown incidence worldwide (19).

C. burnetii has long been recognized as a potential biological agent, as evident by testing that began in the 1950s at Fort Detrick by the U.S. War Reserve Service (4). This microbe was maintained in the U.S. biological arsenal prior to the destruction of such materials in the early 1970s. More recently, the Japanese cult responsible for the March 1995 sarin attack of a Tokyo subway was found to be experimenting with several biological agents, including *C. burnetii*. This agent's utility in bioterrorist attacks is enhanced by high infectivity, expansive windborne reach, and its ability to resist unfavorable conditions. However, it is limited as a biological agent due to its prolonged and varied incubation period, the relatively low morbidity and mortality, and the near absence of person-to-person transmission.

SIGNS AND SYMPTOMS

Acute Q fever most commonly presents as a nonspecific febrile illness characterized by an acute onset of headache, fatigue, myalgias, fever, and chills. Another common and often misdiagnosed presentation is atypical pneumonia, which can range from an incidental finding on chest radiograph to, rarely, acute respiratory distress. Clinically evident hepatitis occurs in up to one-third of patients with acute Q fever and may be accompanied by nausea and vomiting, but it is rarely associated with abdominal pain, jaundice, or marked hepatic dysfunction (19,24). Additionally, it has become increasingly recognized that Q fever may be associated with various exanthems, including pink macules and purpura. Physical examination is often unrevealing but may be notable for inspiratory crackles, hepatomegaly, or splenomegaly, in addition to fever and cutaneous findings. The combination of fever, pneumonia, and acute hepatitis should alert the physician to the possibility of acute Q fever.

MEDICAL MANAGEMENT

Often the presentation of acute Q fever resembles that of other pneumonias or viral syndromes. Initial diagnostic evaluations may yield nonspecific results. A normal white blood cell count is found in the majority of patients. However, increased transaminase levels and an elevated erythrocyte sedimentation rate are present in over half of those presenting with acute Q fever (21,23,24). Thrombocytopenia and increased serum creatinine are present in a small fraction of patients. Chest radiographs may be consistent with atypical pneumonia, with increased reticular markings, multiple opacities, atelectasis, or pleural effusion. *C. burnetii* remains difficult to culture, and diagnosis requires serological tests with subsequent comparison between acute and convalescent phase sera. The diagnostic examinations of choice are indirect immunofluorescence (IFA) and enzyme-linked immunosorbent assay (ELISA).

Diagnosis of Q fever resulting from a bioterrorist attack may prove challenging for physicians. The prolonged incubation time and diverse, often nonspecific, symptoms contribute to the potential difficulty in diagnosis. An increasing number of otherwise healthy persons with a similar constellation of symptoms may allow the physician to consider a common exposure to *C. burnetii*.

Acute Q fever is often a self-limited disease that resolves without the administration of antimicrobial agents. However, a 5- to 7-day course of tetracycline (500 mg orally every 6 hours) or doxycycline (100 mg orally every 12 hours) is recommended as first-line therapy in order to reduce the rate of complications and the duration of illness. Fluoroquinilones may serve as an alternative in the case of meningoencephalitic disease or tetracycline intolerance (19,21).

TRIAGE CONSIDERATIONS

For nearly all persons with Q fever, triage will proceed according to standard emergency department practice. Patients with the rarer severe manifestations of Q fever should be triaged according to the presenting clinical picture. Respiratory isolation is not recommended given the absence of evidence supporting human-to-human transmission via respiratory droplets.

PERSONAL PROTECTION

Health care workers are advised to use standard precautions when caring for patients potentially afflicted with Q fever. One group recommends contact plus droplet precautions during obstetrical procedures for infected pregnant women (25). Given documented transmission among laboratory personnel, BSL3 containment practices are required. Decontamination may be performed using 0.5% hypochlorite, 1% Lysol, 2% formaldehyde, or 5% hydrogen peroxide. Postexposure prophylaxis should consist of doxycycline for 5 days, beginning 8 to 12 days after exposure (19). For those at high risk for contracting the disease, a vaccine may be obtained from USAMRIID (Fort Detrick, MD) as an investigational new drug.

SUMMARY

- Q fever is most often an asymptomatic or self-limited febrile illness caused by infection with *Coxiella burnetii*.

- The triad of fever, atypical pneumonia, and acute hepatitis may help identify cases of acute Q fever presenting to the emergency department.

- The use of *C. burnetii* as a biological weapon is aided by its stability, infectivity, and windborne reach but limited by the low morbidity/mortality, infrequent person-to-person transmission, and a prolonged incubation period.

BRUCELLOSIS

Brucellosis, also known as undulant fever, malta fever, and mediterranean fever, is caused by an aerobic, facultative, intracellular, gram-negative coccobacillus. It is categorized as a category B agent by the CDC (7). The organism is found throughout the world, with predominance in agrarian areas around the Mediterranean Sea, Middle East, Indian subcontinent, and Latin America with poor food sanitation standards. The disease is rare in the United States and generally confined to veterinarians and those with occupational exposure to livestock. Between 1992 and 1999, 813 cases of brucellosis were reported in the United States, with more than half occurring in California and Texas (26). Natural reservoirs include domesticated animals such as cattle, goats, pigs, sheep, and dogs. Several species are found in these different animal hosts. *Brucella abortus* occurs in cattle, *B. melitensis* in sheep and goats, *B. suis* in swine, and *B. canis* in dogs. Brucellosis is notable for its protean clinical manifestations and nonspecific presentations (15,27).

THEORETICAL AND SCIENTIFIC BACKGROUND

Humans become infected with brucellosis through a number of mechanisms. Most commonly, natural infection occurs after ingestion of contaminated animal products, particularly unpasteurized milk and cheese. Skin or mucous membrane contact with contaminated animal products also causes disease. Infection may occur via the respiratory tract through inhalation of infected particles. As with other potential bioterrorist agents, Brucella species are highly virulent when inhaled, with only 10 to 100 organisms required to cause infection (28). Spread of brucellosis between humans is not believed to occur. *Brucella*

use as a bioweapon is aided by its ability to survive under hostile conditions outside of the host for prolonged periods of time. *Brucella* bacterial may survive up to 10 weeks in water and soil (29).

Brucellosis was one of the first biological agents weaponized by the United States in the 1940s (19,29). However, despite its relative high virulence, its use as a potential bioterror weapon is limited. Unlike many other bioweapons, infection with brucellosis does not carry a high mortality rate. Untreated disease only causes death in about 2% of victims, usually from endocarditis (12,29–31). Additionally, a prolonged incubation period lasting up to months makes brucellosis a less effective bioweapon than other inhaled bacteria such as anthrax, plague, and tularemia.

SIGNS AND SYMPTOMS

After infection, the bacterium survives intracellularly in host monocytes and leukocytes and spreads hematogenously to various organs, leading to the wide variety of both systemic and localized disease noted in brucellosis infections. Incubation periods can range from 5 days to months after exposure. Most often, patients have nonspecific systemic complaints such as fever, chills, sweats, headache, fatigue, and weakness. The fever pattern is classically intermittent and irregular over weeks to months in the untreated patient.

Localizing symptoms involved the gastrointestinal tract in up to 70% of patients (29). Patients often present with anorexia, nausea, vomiting, diarrhea, and abdominal pain. Spread to the liver may cause liver abscesses, hepatitis, and hepatomegaly. Pancreatitis, cholecystitis, and splenic abscesses may result from hematogenous spread. Arthralgias of the axial skeleton and large joints, particularly sacroiliitis, occur in 20% to 60% of cases and can lead to osteomyelitis (29). Acute orchitis and epididymitis may occur in the setting of systemic illness (32). Pulmonic manifestations are rare, even if the organism infects the host via the respiratory tract (21). When present, pulmonic manifestations include interstitial pneumonitis, hilar lymphadenopathy, pleural effusions, and empyema. Less commonly, central nervous system (CNS) manifestations ranging from depression and difficulty with concentration to meningitis, encephalitis, and brain abscesses occur (27). Endocarditis occurs in less than 2% of cases but is the primary cause of death from brucellosis. Chronic forms of disease may result in prolonged complaints of fatigue, anorexia, and depression, mimicking chronic fatigue syndrome (15). Findings on routine laboratory data may reveal anemia with thrombocytopenia. The serum white blood cell count may be low or normal, with lymphocytic pleocytosis occasionally found. Mildly abnormal liver function tests may also be seen with hepatic involvement (29,30). Cerebrospinal fluid (CSF) analysis in cases of CNS involvement may reveal lymphocytic pleocytosis and an elevated protein level. CSF Gram stain and culture are often negative.

MEDICAL MANAGEMENT

The nonspecific protean presentations of brucellosis make it a difficult diagnosis. When suspected, blood or other potentially infected tissues should be sent for culture. Bone marrow culture has been found to have higher yield than blood cultures (27). *Brucella* species are exceeding slow to grow in culture, and the culture must be maintained for 4 to 6 weeks. In cases of a potential bioterrorist attack, a more rapid diagnostic test is required. Serum agglutination tests exist and can be performed more rapidly than cultures. Although most patients with active infection will have positive serological test results with titers greater than 1:160, diagnosis using these methods can result in false negative results (27,30).

In the setting of a possible bioterrorist attack, physicians noting a large number of otherwise healthy individuals with vague multisystem complaints and a lack of historic exposure to animal products or livestock need to consider brucellosis as a possible etiology. Because of the slow incubation period of brucellosis, these trends may only be noted over a matter of weeks to months.

Treatment of brucellosis requires multiple agents for a prolonged period of time to avoid relapse (27,29,30). In a majority of cases, doxycycline 100 mg twice daily plus rifampin 600 to 900 mg per day orally is the recommended treatment regimen. In more severe cases, rifampin should be substituted with streptomycin 1 g IM per day for the first 3 weeks (33). In children, trimethoprim-sulfamethoxazole has shown promise when combined with rifampin, although relapse rates are higher when compared with patients treated with doxycycline (34). CNS involvement may require a third-generation cephalosporin such as ceftriaxone (19,25). Corticosteroids have been recommended for cases of neurobrucellosis (19,27).

Postexposure prophylaxis for inadvertently inoculated persons consists of a combination of doxycycline and rifampin for 3 weeks. This regimen could theoretically be used in high-risk patients after a biological attack. There is no vaccine available for brucellosis.

TRIAGE CONSIDERATIONS

Because transmission of brucellosis between humans is not thought to occur, no specific isolation precautions are required in suspected cases. Because of the relatively indolent course of brucellosis and its low mortality, a true mass casualty scenario with a large number of critically ill patients arriving for medical treatment at the same time would be unlikely, even after a bioterrorist attack.

PERSONAL PROTECTION

Health care workers should practice universal precautions when caring for patients with brucellosis. Material and surfaces contacted by infected patients can be adequately disinfected with a 0.5% hypochlorite solution (19). Due to this agent's high virulence when inhaled, laboratory personnel should be trained in isolation measures and work with culture samples under negative-pressure precautions.

SUMMARY

- Brucellosis represents a moderate threat in a potential bioterrorist attack because of its high virulence when inhaled. However, a prolonged incubation period and low mortality make it a lesser threat than other inhaled bacteria.
- Brucellosis is known for its protean, multisystem manifestations and indolent course, making it an especially challenging diagnosis.
- Treatment of brucellosis requires prolonged treatment, ideally with doxycycline and rifampin.

FOOD AND WATERBORNE PATHOGENS

This group of agents includes those that cause acute diarrheal illness after ingestion of a contaminated food or water source. Several bacteria have been implicated in acts of biowarfare and/or mass epidemics, including *Vibrio cholerae*, *Shigella dysenteriae*, *Salmonella* species, and *Escherichia coli* O157:H7. Viral pathogens—such as rotavirus and Norwalk virus—are also frequent causes of outbreaks of gastroenteritis.

THEORETICAL AND SCIENTIFIC BACKGROUND

Vibrio cholerae is transmitted via the fecal-oral route, through contaminated water or vegetables, or by ingestion of undercooked marine shellfish serving as reservoirs. The organism may survive for 5 to 10 days on foodstuffs (35). It is a cause of epidemic diarrhea throughout much of the developing world. Large numbers of the organism must be ingested to cause disease because of its susceptibility to stomach acid. Toxins produced by the bacteria result in massive watery diarrhea due to chloride and water secretion. Electrolyte imbalance and dehydration are the primary cause of morbidity and mortality, with fatality rates as high as 50% in untreated cases yet limited to less than 1% if treated (36).

Shigella dysenteriae causes an inflammatory, bloody diarrhea that may be spread person to person via the fecal-oral route or less commonly by food- and waterborne outbreaks. An inoculum of as few as 100 organisms may result in disease. Following a 1- to 4-day incubation period, a self-limited 5- to 7-day illness ensues. Patients may shed the organism in fecal matter for weeks after symptoms subside. Mortality is rare in otherwise healthy individuals, but documented complications include hemolytic-uremic syndrome and toxic megacolon.

Salmonella species include those responsible for typhoid fever and those associated with enterocolitis. *S. typhi* and *paratyphi* cause systemic febrile illnesses that require person-to-person transmission. The mortality rate of treated typhoid fever is extremely low, but a chronic carrier state with fecal excretion of the bacteria may occur. The nontyphoidal species are commonly associated with food-borne outbreaks due to contamination with human or animal waste. The incubation period is 6 to 48 hours, and a self-limited diarrheal illness of 3 to 7 days follows. Severe disease may be observed in infants and the elderly, with mortality rates in the United States less than 1%.

Infection with *Escherichia coli* O157:H7 results in a toxin-mediated hemorrhagic colitis. It may be transmitted person to person, but the major source of infection is contaminated ground beef. The bacteria are relatively stable in the environment and may contaminate water supplies and other food sources. The illness is characterized by bloody stools and resolves within 1 week. A potential complication of this infection is hemolytic-uremic syndrome, which is associated with a 3% to 5% mortality rate.

Rotavirus is a common cause of gastroenteritis in children worldwide. It is transmitted primarily via the fecal-oral route. However, the virus exhibits marked stability in the environment and may be contracted by ingestion of contaminated food or water. Infection results in a nonbloody diarrhea after a 2-day incubation period. The virus replicates in the mucosa of the small intestine, impairing transport mechanisms. The illness is of concern only in young children who are susceptible to dehydration and electrolyte imbalances. Adults experience mild disease likely secondary to partial immunity.

Norwalk virus is named for an outbreak of gastroenteritis at a school in Norwalk, Ohio, in 1968. The virus is highly contagious, with as few as 10 viral particles sufficient to cause disease (37). Additionally, it is resistant to environmental factors. The primary mode of infection is through the fecal-oral route, but fomites and waterborne carriage are also implicated in transmission. Incubation period is typically 1 to 2 days and an acute, self-limited illness lasting 1 to 3 days follows.

Food- and waterborne illnesses have been previously identified and employed as biological agents. Japan utilized *Shigella* species, *Vibrio cholerae*, and *Salmonella* species (among others) in biowarfare experimentation on prisoners and in attacks on Chinese cities during the years 1932 to 1945 (4). More recently, intentional contamination of food supplies with *Salmonella* species and *Shigella dysenteriae* led to outbreaks involving 751 and 45 cases of gastroenteritis, respectively (38,39). The utility of these agents is aided by their stability and relative ease of dissemination via contamination of the food and water supply. They are fortunately limited in their efficacy as biological agents due to the relative low morbidity and mortality associated with the resultant illnesses.

SIGNS AND SYMPTOMS

Clinical presentation of the illnesses discussed is often that of an acute gastroenteritis that follows a benign, self-limited course. Patients may report abrupt onset of crampy abdominal pain or discomfort. A historical factor of diagnostic value is the character of the stools produced during the illness. Cholera is associated with "rice-water" stools of large volumes and in a minority of cases may be associated with overwhelming fluid loss. *Shigella* infections may begin with watery diarrhea, but classic findings of dysentery follow, with bloody-mucoid stools. The nontyphoidal *Salmonella* infections are varied and may or may not be associated with bloody diarrhea. Enterohemorrhagic *E. coli* strains cause bloody diarrhea without mucosal invasion. Microscopic examination of stool samples is negative for neutrophils, unlike other organisms causing bloody diarrhea. Rotavirus and Norwalk virus infections are both characterized by nausea, vomiting, and watery, nonbloody diarrhea. Signs and symptoms of dehydration should be identified during history and physical examination.

MEDICAL MANAGEMENT

Clinical diagnosis may be suggested by historical and epidemiological factors. Methylene blue staining of stool specimens distinguishes invasive from noninvasive forms of infectious diarrhea. Stool cultures allow diagnosis of bacterial agents responsible for such illnesses. In patients at risk for dehydration and electrolyte abnormalities, a basic chemistry panel should be obtained.

Physicians should be alerted to the possibility of an outbreak of a food- or waterborne illness based on the volume of similar complaints and any potential common exposures. Treatment must first address any hemodynamic instability or electrolyte abnormalities associated with volume loss. Antimicrobial therapy guided by in vitro susceptibility is indicated in severe cholera, nontyphoid salmonella infections requiring hospitalization, *Shigella* infections, and in immunocompromised patients, limiting duration of symptoms and time of excretion of organisms. Treatment should also occur in the immunocompromised. Antibiotics are not indicated in mild disease or in cases of *E. coli* O157:H7. Increased toxin release from the enterohemorrhagic *E. coli* may heighten the risk of developing hemolytic-uremic syndrome (40).

TRIAGE CONSIDERATIONS

Triage of patients presenting with symptoms suspicious for the illnesses just mentioned should proceed as per usual emergency department practices. Patients at risk for severe manifestations (infants, elderly, or immunocompromised) and those with signs or symptoms of profound dehydration should be managed appropriately. Isolation procedures are not necessary in this setting.

PERSONAL PROTECTION

Standard precautions should be utilized when caring for patients with presumed food- or waterborne illnesses. Contaminated surfaces should be treated with an EPA-registered hospital detergent-disinfectant. The vaccines in existence for typhoid fever have demonstrated poor efficacy and are no longer recommended by the CDC. Vaccines for cholera are not currently available in the United States but are in use in other countries. A live-virus vaccine developed for rotavirus is no longer recommended because of concerns over a potential relationship with intussusception in infants receiving the vaccine (41).

VIRAL ENCEPHALITIDES

Several viral agents with primary central nervous system (CNS) effects have the potential for use as bioweapons. This group of agents includes the alphaviruses, Venezuelan, eastern, and western equine encephalitides (VEE, EEE, and WEE, respectively), and West Nile virus, a flavivirus. The alphaviruses are enveloped RNA viruses. They were originally discovered as a veterinary illness from horses in the 1930s. EEE is the most common naturally encountered alphavirus causing CNS infection in the United States. Between 1983 and 2000, 182 cases were reported to the Centers for Disease Control. A majority of cases are found in Florida, Georgia, Massachusetts, and New Jersey, predominantly in coastal and swampy areas. Between 0 and 200 cases of WEE occur each year in the United States, generally in the western and Great Plain states. VEE occurs predominantly in Central and South America; however, cases have occurred in the Gulf states and southwestern United States. West Nile virus was first reported in Uganda in 1937. Since 1999, the number of West Nile cases in the United States has increased dramatically (42). In 2002, there were over 4,000 reported cases (43).

THEORETICAL AND SCIENTIFIC BACKGROUND

Natural transmission of these viruses to humans occurs via a bite by an infected mosquito vector. Human-to-human spread is not believed to occur. Seasonal variations in the incidence of viral encephalitis result from changes in the natural mosquito population. Peak incidence occurs in the summer months, corresponding to both an increase in the number of mosquitoes and more frequent outdoor activities by humans. After a bite from an infected mosquito, viral particles from the gut of the insect are inoculated into the skin and enter the lymphatic system. Initially, the virus replicates in lymphoid tissue. After replication, viral particles are released into the circulation, resulting in high levels of viremia and ultimately entry into the CNS (44).

EEE, WEE, and VEE are classified as category B agents by the Centers for Disease Control. These agents represent potential bioweapons because they are highly infectious when aerosolized (19). The first documented human cases of VEE occurred in laboratory workers in the 1940s (44). Additionally, these agents can be produced in large amounts and stored with relative ease. Morbidity and mortality rates vary. EEE carries a mortality rate of 30% to 75%, with children and the elderly being the most susceptible (19,45,46). EEE is also highly morbid, with permanent neurological sequelae occurring in 30% to

70% of cases. Fatality rates for WEE are approximately 10% (45). Although rarely fatal, VEE is a potential bioweapon because nearly all human cases become symptomatic (19,47). The case-fatality rate for West Nile virus ranges from 4% to 18% (48).

SIGNS AND SYMPTOMS

Incubation periods for the viral encephalitides range from 3 to 14 days. Most often a systemic febrile illness occurs with fever, chills, headache, myalgias, nausea, and vomiting. Upper respiratory symptoms including sore throat, cough, and pleuritic chest pain occur with WEE infections. Patients are often leukopenic during this phase of the illness. Elevated aspartate transaminase and lactate dehydrogenase levels are occasionally found with VEE infections. Progression of disease to CNS involvement results in altered levels of consciousness, nuchal rigidity, ataxia, focal motor and cranial nerve deficits, seizures, and frank coma (19,44,45). Cerebrospinal fluid (CSF) analysis typically reveals lymphocytic pleocytosis with elevated protein levels. Hyponatremia is sometimes noted in patients with neurological symptoms. Patients with VEE infections rarely develop neurological signs and symptoms, whereas EEE infections result in the most severe neurological abnormalities.

Most patients infected with West Nile virus are asymptomatic. Generally, a mild febrile illness occurs and resolves within 7 days. In addition to constitutional symptoms, lymphadenopathy and erythematous morbilliform rash may occur. Progression to severe neurological signs and symptoms occurs in less than 1% of infected patients (48).

MEDICAL MANAGEMENT

In the setting of a possible bioterrorist attack, the diagnosis of viral encephalitis should be considered when a large number of patients present over a relatively short period of time with febrile illnesses that progress to involve the CNS. Physicians should consider the local prevalence of the various viral encephalitides as well as seasonal and climactic variations in the mosquito population. Serum electrolytes and complete blood count should be obtained. Any patients with both fever and neurological signs and symptoms should undergo both a CNS imaging and lumbar puncture with CSF analysis for cell count, glucose, and protein levels. Both computer tomography (CT) and magnetic resonance imaging (MRI) have been used to demonstrate that a large number of neurologically impaired EEE patients have focal lesions in the basal ganglia, thalamus, and brain stem, with MRI considered the superior test (46). Serological assays or viral isolation are required to make a specific diagnosis. Both VEE and EEE can be isolated from serum during the early febrile phase of the illness; however, complement-fixing serological assays to detect IgM antibodies may be required during the encephalopathic phase due to low viremic loads (19,44).

Serological testing can also be performed on CSF samples. West Nile virus can also be diagnosed with serological assays for IgM in serum and CSF (48).

Treatment of viral encephalitis is generally supportive. Systemically ill patients may require antipyretics and intravenous hydration. Actively seizing patients should receive benzodiazepines and monitored care. Mechanical ventilation may be required for acutely encephalopathic patients. Ribavirin may have in vitro activity against these viruses; however, they are generally not used clinically (44,49).

TRIAGE CONSIDERATIONS

No specific isolation is required for viral encephalitis because no human-to human spread occurs. However, patients presenting febrile with neurological deficits may require negative-pressure isolation for the possibility of bacterial meningitis. Patients should be triaged according to the acuity of their systemic and neurological symptomatology.

PERSONAL PROTECTION

Mosquito control in endemic areas remains the most useful means of preventing zoonotic viral encephalitis. Practitioners caring for patients with viral encephalitis should maintain universal precautions. Laboratory workers should use negative-pressure cabinets and wear high-efficiency particle respirators (19). A live attenuated vaccine is available for VEE, used primarily for at-risk laboratory personnel. Inactivated vaccines are available in limited settings for EEE and WEE.

SUMMARY

- Viral encephalitides are potential bioweapons by means of inhalation of aerosolized particles.
- Viral encephalitides present initially as non-specific febrile illnesses that may progress to profound CNS signs and symptoms.
- No specific, effective treatment for zoonotic viral encephalitis exists.

SEVERE ACUTE RESPIRATORY SYNDROME (SARS)

The severe acute respiratory syndrome (SARS) is an acute, infectious, respiratory illness first reported in November 2002 in southern China. Subsequently, a novel coronavirus (SARS-CoV) responsible for this clinical syndrome was identified and further characterized in early 2003 (50–53).

THEORETICAL AND SCIENTIFIC BACKGROUND

In the Guangdong Province of China in late 2002, outbreaks of an atypical pneumonia were reported. The illness frequently progressed to respiratory failure and affected both casual contacts and exposed health care practitioners. An infected physician then traveled to Hong Kong where he resided in a hotel with international guests prior to his hospitalization. By March 2003 outbreaks of the illness termed SARS by the CDC had developed in Hong Kong, Singapore, Vietnam, and Toronto, each of which could be linked epidemiologically to this index case (54). These further outbreaks were described in the literature (55–58) and marked the beginning of a worldwide epidemic. As of September 2003, the World Health Organization (WHO) had identified 8,098 probable cases with a fatality rate of 9.6% and 29 reported probable cases in the United States (59).

By April 2003 several groups had identified the novel coronavirus, SARS-CoV, as the etiologic agent (50–53). The coronaviruses are a group of RNA viruses previously known to cause mild forms of respiratory and enteric diseases. The extent of the natural reservoir for this newly identified virus remains to be elucidated. However, similar strains have been identified in several animal species, including the masked palm civet, raccoon dog, and Chinese ferret badger, sold at markets in Guangdong (54).

The virus is transmitted primarily via respiratory droplets, although evidence indicates the virus may be shed in feces and urine as well (50). The observed incubation period ranges from 2 to 16 days, during which time the patient is not actively contagious. The stability of the virus outside the body has been preliminarily determined by the WHO to be 2 to 4 days in urine and feces. A majority of patients may continue to shed the virus up to 3 weeks after onset of symptoms (60).

Known development of SARS-CoV as a biological agent for warfare or bioterrorism has not been reported. The highly contagious nature of the virus, with significant person-to-person transmission, and the potential for mass morbidity and mortality are concerning features that lend to its use as a biological weapon. The stability of SARS-CoV in the environment is unclear and may limit its utility in such applications.

SIGNS AND SYMPTOMS

The initial manifestations of SARS are fever, myalgias, dry cough, headache, and dizziness. Less frequent symptoms may include coryza, sore throat, nausea, vomiting, and diarrhea. Common findings on physical examination include fever >38°C, hypoxia, inspiratory crackles, and dullness to percussion. For an unknown percentage of those infected, the clinical course may be asymptomatic or limited to a mild respiratory illness. However, within a week of symptom onset many patients will develop increasing dyspnea and clinical signs of a worsening pneumonia, with 25% of adult patients requiring intensive care.

MEDICAL MANAGEMENT

The clinical presentation of SARS often resembles that of an atypical pneumonia. Chest radiographs may reveal non-specific abnormalities including focal or patchy air space consolidations. CT of the chest demonstrates peripheral, subpleural, ground-glass opacities with air bronchograms. Initial laboratory evaluation may reveal leukopenia (34%), lymphopenia (70%), thrombocytopenia (45%), prolonged activated partial thromboplastin time (42%), elevated D-dimers (45%), and elevated lactate dehydrogenase (71%) (56). Early diagnostic evaluations required acute and convalescent sera for ELISA detection of antibody to SARS-CoV. The development of reverse transcription polymerase chain reaction testing has allowed for detection of viral RNA in clinical samples (61). These laboratory tests are available through the CDC Laboratory Response Network. A suspected or probable case may be identified in the setting of moderate to severe respiratory illness in the absence of an identifiable cause when combined with supporting epidemiological factors. These include contact with known or suspected SARS patients within 10 days or travel to regions listed under CDC travel alerts or advisories.

Several factors may alert the physician to the possibility of a SARS epidemic. A pattern of atypical pneumonia in large numbers of otherwise healthy individuals may be present. Given the highly infectious nature of SARS-CoV, afflicted health care practitioners and other clear epidemiological links may be identified.

The treatment of SARS is largely limited to supportive care. However, during the epidemic in Hong Kong, a combination of ribavirin and corticosteroids was used with reported favorable outcomes (58,62). This regimen has yet to be evaluated in controlled studies. In vitro studies have demonstrated the potential utility of human interferons in the treatment of infections with SARS-CoV (63).

TRIAGE CONSIDERATIONS

In the emergency department, suspected or probable cases of SARS should be placed in negative-pressure isolation. The disease is reportable to local and state health departments, which may assist in the identification of an outbreak and the quarantine of those exposed to suspected cases. Further triage of such patients should progress in concert with standard emergency medicine practices, providing supplemental oxygen and respiratory support as clinically indicated.

PERSONAL PROTECTION

The use of respiratory droplet and contact precautions is recommended for the prevention of nosocomial transmission of SARS (63,64). The CDC recommends the use of EPA-registered hospital detergent-disinfectant for cleaning potentially contaminated spaces. For laboratory investigations, BSL-2 or -3 practices are recommended to prevent infection of personnel. At the time of printing, no postexposure prophylaxis or vaccine exists.

SUMMARY

- The severe acute respiratory syndrome (SARS) is a febrile respiratory illness that may progress to acute respiratory failure in up to a fourth of those infected.
- The novel coronavirus that causes SARS is highly infective via respiratory droplets and has an incubation period of 2 to 16 days.

QUESTIONS AND ANSWERS

1. **Tularemia is a potent bioweapon due to all of the following factors EXCEPT:**
   A. Untreated cases carry a relatively high mortality rate
   B. Death in untreated cases can occur over a matter of hours after exposure
   C. Tularemia can be effectively spread via aerosolized particles
   D. A minimal number of infectious particles are required to cause disease
   E. Tularemia is a hardy bacterium that can survive for prolonged periods of time in hostile environments

2. **In patients presenting with acute febrile illnesses and focal neurological symptoms, the following diagnoses should be highly considered:**
   A. Eastern equine encephalitis
   B. Severe acute respiratory syndrome
   C. Q fever
   D. Brucellosis
   E. Venezuelan equine encephalitis

3. **Signs and symptoms of Q fever include all of the following EXCEPT:**
   A. Fever
   B. Pneumonia
   C. Diarrhea
   D. Hepatitis
   E. Rash

4. **Optimal treatment for brucellosis consists of:**
   A. Rifampin and ciprofloxacin
   B. Doxycycline and rifampin
   C. Ciprofloxacin
   D. Ampicillin
   E. Chloramphenicol

ANSWERS

1: **B.** *Death in untreated cases can occur over a matter of hours after exposure*
2: **A.** *Eastern equine encephalitis*
3: **C.** *Diarrhea*
4: **D.** *Ampicillin*

REFERENCES

1. Francis E. Tularemia. JAMA 1925; 84:1243-50.
2. Centers for Disease Control and Prevention. Tularemia: United States, 1990-2000. MMWR Mortal Wkly Rep 2002;51:182-4.
3. Evans ME, Gregory DW, Schaffner W, et al. Tularemia: A 30-year experience with 88 cases. Medicine 1985;64:251-69.
4. Christopher GW, Cielak TJ, Pavlin JA, et al. Biological warfare: a historical perspective. JAMA 1997;278:412-7.
5. Franz DR, Jahrling PB, Friedlander AM, et al. Clinical recognition and management of patients exposed to biological warfare agents. JAMA 1997;278:399-411.
6. Health aspects of chemical and biological weapons. Geneva, Switzerland: World Health Organization; 1970; 105-7.
7. Khan AS, Sage MJ. Biological and chemical terrorism: strategic planning, preparedness, and response. MMWR 2000;49:1-14.
8. Dennis DT, Inglesby TV, Henderson DA, et al. Tularemia as a biological weapon: medical and public health management. JAMA 2001;285:2763-73.
9. Salislaw S, Eigelsbach HT, Wilson HE, et al. Tularemia vaccine study I: intracutaneous challenge. Arch Intern Med 1961;107:121-33.
10. Salislaw S, Eigelsbach HT, Wilson HE, et al. Tularemia vaccine study II: respiratory challenge. Arch Intern Med 1961;107:134-46.
11. Kodama BF, Fitzpatrick JE, Gentry RH. Tularemia. Cutis 1994;54:279-80.
12. Chin J, Ashner MS eds. Control of communicable disease manual. 17th ed. Washington, DC: American Public Health Association; 2000.
13. Evans ME, Friedlander AM. Tularemia. In: Sidell FR, Takafuji ET, Franz DR eds. Textbook of military medicine: medical aspects of chemical and biological warfare. Washington, DC: Office of the Surgeon General, Department of the Army, United States of America, 1997; 503-12.
14. Burnett JW. Tularemia. Cutis 1994;54:77-8.
15. Quezner RW, Simpson GL. Acute undifferentiated multisystem infections. In: Brillman JC, Quenzer RW eds. Infectious disease in emergency medicine. 2nd ed. Philadelphia: Lippincott-Raven, 1998; 890-2.
16. Committee on R&D Needs for Improving Civilian Medical Response to Chemical and Biological Terrorism Incidents. Chemical and biological terrorism: research and development to improve civilian medical response. Washington, DC: National Academy Press, 1999.
17. Gelfand MS, Mehra N, Simmons BP. Tularemia and atypical lymphocytosis. J Tenn Med Assoc 1989;8:417-8.
18. Sawyer WD, Dangerfield HG, Hogge AL, et al. Antibiotic prophylaxis and therapy of airborne tularemia. Bacteriol Rev 1966;30:542-8.
19. Greenfield RA, Drevets DA, Machado LJ, et al. Bacterial pathogens as biological weapons and agents of bioterrorism. Am J Med Sci 2002;323:299-315.
20. Tigertt WD. Soviet viable francella tularensis vaccines: a review of selected articles. Bacteriol Rev 1962;26:354-73.
21. Maurin M, Raoult D. Q fever. Clin Microbiol Rev 1999;12(4):518-46.
22. Milazzo A, Hall R, Storm PA. Sexually transmitted Q fever. Clin Infect Dis 2001;33(3):399-402.
23. Raoult D, Marrie T. Q fever. Clin Infect Dis 1995;20:489-96.
24. Sampere M, Font B, Font J. Q fever in adults: review of 66 clinical cases. Eur J Clin Microbiol Infect Dis 2003;22:108-10.
25. Weber DJ, Rutala WA. Risks and prevention of nosocomial transmission of rare zoonotic diseases. Clin Infect Dis 2001;32:44.
26. Chang MH, Glynn MK, Groseclose SL. Endemic, notifiable bioterrorism-related diseases, United States, 1992-1999. Emerg Infect Dis 2003;9:323-30.
27. Young EJ. Brucella species. In: Mandell GL, Bennett JE, Dolin R eds. Principles and practice of infectious diseases. 5th ed., vol. 2. Philadelphia: Churchill Livingstone, 2000; 2386-93.
28. Bellamy RJ, Freedman AR. Bioterrorism. QJM 2001;94:227-34.
29. Franz DR, Jahrling PB, Friedlander AM, et al. Clinical recognition and management of patients exposed to biological warfare agents. JAMA 1997;278:399-411.
30. Young EJ. An overview of human brucellosis. Clin Infect Dis 1995;21:283-90.
31. Al-Harthi SS. The morbidity and mortality pattern of brucella endocarditis. Int J Cardiol 1989;25:321-4.
32. Khan MS, Humayoon MS, Al Manee MS. Epididymo-orchitis and brucellosis. Br J Urol 1989;63:87-9.
33. Ariza J, Gudiol F, Pallares R, et al. Treatment of human brucellosis with doxycycline plus rifampin or doxycycline plus streptomycin. Ann Intern Med 1992;117:25-30.
34. Lubani MM, Dudin KI, Sharda DC, et al. A multicenter therapeutic study of 1100 children with brucellosis. Pediatr Infect Dis J 1989;8:75-8.
35. World Health Organization. Cholera. http://www.who.int/inf-fs/en/fact107.html (accessed 9/2003).
36. Centers of Disease Control and Prevention. Cholera Technical Information. http://www.cdc.gov/ncidod/dbmd/diseaseinfo/cholera_t.htm (accessed 9/2003).
37. Centers for Disease Control and Prevention. Norovirus infection (Norwalk and Norwalk-like virus infection; cause of gastroenteritis). http://www.cdc.gov/ncidod/dvrd/revb/gastro/norovirus-factsheet.htm (accessed 9/2003).
38. Torok TJ, Tauxe RV, Wise RP, et al. A large community outbreak of salmonellosis caused by intentional contamination of restaurant salad bars. JAMA 1997;278:389-95.
39. Kovalic SA, Kimura A, Simons SL, et al. An outbreak of Shigella dysenteriae type 2 among laboratory workers due to intentional food contamination. JAMA 1997;278:396-8.
40. Wong CS, Jelacic S, Habeeb RL, et al. The risk of the hemolytic-uremic syndrome after antibiotic treatment of Escherichia coli O157:H7 infections. N Engl J Med 2000;342:1930-6.
41. Murphy TV, Gargiullo PM, Massoudi MS, et al. Intussusception among infants given an oral rotavirus vaccine. N Engl J Med 2001;344:564-72.
42. Petersen LR, Marfin AA. West Nile virus: a primer for the clinician. Ann Intern Med 2002;137:173-9.
43. Centers for Disease Control and Prevention. Provisional surveillance summary of the West Nile virus epidemic—United States, January-November 2002. MMWR Morb Mortal Wkly Rep 2002;51:1129-33.
44. Markoff L. Alphaviruses. In: Mandell GL, Bennett JE, Dolin R eds. Principles and practice of infectious diseases. 5th ed, vol. 2. Philadelphia: Churchill Livingstone, 2000; 1703-8.
45. Whitley RJ, Gnann JW. Viral encephalitis: familiar infections and emerging pathogens. Lancet 2002;359:507-14.
46. Deresiewicz RL, Thaler SJ, Hsu L, et al. Clinical and neuroradiographic manifestations of eastern equine encephalitis. N Engl J Med 1997;336:1867-74.
47. Weaver SC, Salas R, Rico-Hesse R, et al. Re-emergence of epidemic Venezuelan equine encephalomyelitis in South America. Lancet 2002;348:436-40.
48. Petersen LR, Marfin AA, Gubler DJ. West Nile virus. JAMA 2003;290:524-8.
49. Huggins JW, Robins RK, Canonico PG. Synergistic antiviral effects of ribavirin and the C-nucleoside analogs tiazofurin and selenazofurin against togaviruses, bunyaviruses, and arenaviruses. Antimicrob Agents Chemother 1984;26:476-80.
50. Drosten C, Gunther S, Preiser W, et al. Identification of a novel coronavirus in patients with severe acute respiratory syndrome. N Engl J Med 2003;348:1967-76.
51. Ksiazek TG, Erdman D, Goldsmith CS, et al. A novel coronavirus associated with severe acute respiratory syndrome. N Engl J Med 2003;348:1953-66.

52. Kuiken T, Fouchier RAM, Schutten M, et al. Newly discovered coronavirus as the primary cause of severe acute respiratory syndrome. Lancet 2003;362:263-70.
53. Peiris JS, Lai ST, Poon LLM, et al. Coronavirus as a possible cause of severe acute respiratory syndrome. Lancet 2003;361:1319-25.
54. Enserink M. SARS in China. Science 2003;301:294-6.
55. Hsu LY, Lee CC, Green JA, et al. Severe acute respiratory syndrome (SARS) in Singapore: clinical features of index patient and initial contacts. http://www.cdc.gov/ncidod/EID/vol9no6/03-0264.htm (accessed 9/2003).
56. Lee N, Hui D, Wu A, et al. A major outbreak of severe acute respiratory syndrome in Hong Kong. N Engl J Med 2003;348:1986-94.
57. Poutanen SM, Low DE, Henry B, et al. Identification of severe acute respiratory syndrome in Canada. N Engl J Med 2003;348:1995-2005.
58. Tsang KW, Ho PL, Ooi GC, et al. A cluster of cases of severe acute respiratory syndrome in Hong Kong. N Engl J Med 2003;348:1977-85.
59. World Health Organization. Summary of probable SARS cases with onset of illness from 1 November 2002 to 31 July 2003. http://www.who.int/csr/sars/country/table2003_09_23/en/ (accessed 9/2003).
60. Peiris JS, Chu CM, Cheng VC, et al. Clinical progression and viral load in a community outbreak of coronavirus associated SARS pneumonia; a prospective study. Lancet 2003;361:1767-72.
61. Centers for Disease Control and Prevention. RT-PCR testing at the Laboratory Response Network. http://www.cdc.gov/ncidod/sars/lab/rtpcr/index.htm (accessed 9/2003).
62. Wong GWK, Hui DSC. Severe acute respiratory syndrome (SARS): epidemiology, diagnosis and management. Thorax 2003;58:558-60.
63. Cinati J, Morgenstern B, Bauer G, et al. Treatment of SARS with human interferons. Lancet 2003;362:293-4.
64. Seto WH, Tsang D, Yung RWH, et al. Effectiveness of precautions against droplets and contact in prevention of nosocomial transmission of severe acute respiratory syndrome (SARS). Lancet 2003;361:1519-20.

11

Botulinum: The Most Toxic Substance Known

Robert Abar Timmons and Anthony Carbone

NAME AND DESCRIPTION OF AGENTS

Botulinum toxin is a potent protein neurotoxin that causes the paralytic condition known as botulism. This toxin has the distinction of being the most potent substance by weight known to science (1,2), requiring only 0.001 µg/kg body weight to kill 50% of animals in laboratory studies (3). Botulinum toxin type A is 15,000 and 100,000 times more toxic by weight than VX and sarin nerve gases, two of the well-known organophosphate nerve agents, respectively (3). It further has the singular distinction of being both a substance approved for medical treatment and a feared agent of biological terrorism. Currently, botulinum toxin is approved by the U.S. Food and Drug Administration (FDA) for use in treating neuromuscular disorders such as blepharospasm, strabismus, and torticollis. It also has several off-label uses, such as treatment of wrinkles, migraine headaches, chronic low back pain, stroke, traumatic brain injury, achalasia, and various dystonias (4). It should be noted that the licensed preparation is sufficiently dilute, containing only about 0.3% and 0.005% of the estimated human lethal inhalational and oral doses, respectively, that it is impractical for use as a bioterror weapon (4).

Botulinum toxin is elaborated by *Clostridium botulinum*, a spore-forming, gram-positive, anaerobic bacterium that is found throughout the world in soil and marine environments (5). Botulism is a neuroparalytic illness that results from the action of botulinum toxin. It typically begins with cranial nerve involvement and progresses caudally to involve the extremities (5). Because of botulinum toxin's extreme potency and lethality, ease of production and transport, and need for prolonged resource-intensive care of victims, it was one of the first agents to be considered for use in modern times as a biological weapon in warfare (6). Though the United States has renounced any further research in developing botulinum toxin as a biological weapon, concern remains that other countries or terrorist groups may still attempt to employ it (6). Currently it is one of six potential biological warfare agents listed by the Centers for Disease Control and Prevention (CDC) as a Category A agent, designating it as a high-priority biological agent of concern (7).

A German scientist, Justinius Kerner, first discovered botulism in 1793. Kerner traced the disease to spoiled sausage, a result of the crude means of sausage preservation at the time, and he named the substance "wurstgift" or sausage poison. This led to the origin of the term "botulism," as the Latin root word for sausage is *botulus*. *C. botulinum* was first described by Emile van Ermengem in 1897 after isolating the microbe while investigating a foodborne outbreak in Ellezelles, Belgium (8,9). Foodborne botulism remains the most common form of disease in adults. However, plant rather than animal products are the more common vehicles for poisoning, typically as a result of unregulated "home canning" or other improper food handling (8).

In humans, botulinum toxin inhibits the release of acetylcholine, leading to a characteristic flaccid paralysis (10). Four distinct forms of botulism can occur, depending on the mode of acquisition of the toxin. Cases may be classified as (a) foodborne botulism, resulting from ingestion of food contaminated with *C. botulinum* and containing preformed toxin (10); (b) wound botulism, caused by toxin produced in a wound contaminated by *C. botulinum* (10); (c) infant botulism, which is due to the endogenous production of toxin in the intestine of infants following ingestion of germinating spores of *C. botulinum* (10); or (d) inhalational botulism, a man-made form that results from inhaling aerosolized botulinum toxin (4). Intestinal botulism, a variation of infant botulism, can also occur in children or adults and is represented by those cases in which no food vehicle can be identified, there is no evidence of wound botulism, and there exists the possibility of intestinal colonization in a person older than 1 year of age (10).

Inhalational botulism has been demonstrated experimentally in primates (11), has been attempted by bioterrorists in recent times (12,13), and has been the intended outcome of at least one country's specially designed missiles and artillery shells (4,14,15). However, there has only been one report of three individuals suffering from accidental inhalational botulism, having occurred in three veterinary personnel in West Germany in 1962. All three individuals had detectable Type A botulinum toxin in their serum following exposure to reaerosolized botulinum toxin while disposing of lab animals whose fur was coated with aerosolized type A botulinum toxin (16).

THEORETICAL AND SCIENTIFIC BACKGROUND

C. botulinum is a species of four genetically distinct groups that have in common the production of antigenically distinct neurotoxin with a similar pharmacologic action but that otherwise would not be designated as a single species (4,17,18). *C. botulinum* organisms are straight to slightly curved, gram-positive (in young cultures), motile, anaerobic rods, 0.5 to 2.0 μm in width, and 1.6 to 22.0 μm in length, with oval, subterminal spores (8,19). There are seven distinct toxin types of *C. botulinum* described (A, B, C_1, D, E, F, and G), distinguished by the antigenic characteristics of the neurotoxins they produce (10). An eighth toxin type, C_2, is not a neurotoxin but actually a cytotoxin of unknown clinical significance (5). Toxin types A, B, E, and in rare cases F cause human botulism (8). Types C_1 and D cause disease in mammals and birds (5,10). Type G, now called *C. argentinense*, has been associated with sudden death, but not with neuroparalytic illness, in a few patients in Switzerland (5). Additionally, the rare clostridial strains of *C. baratii* and *C. butyricum* also have the capacity to elaborate botulinum toxin (4,5,20–22) (Figs. 11-1 and 11-2).

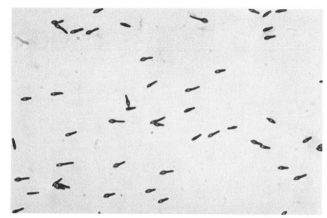

Figure 11–1. A photomicrograph of *Clostridium botulinum* type A viewed using a Gram stain technique. CDC/Dr. George Lombard (1978). The bacterium *C. botulinum* produces a nerve toxin, which causes the rare, but serious paralytic illness botulism. There are seven types of botulism toxin designated by the letters A through G; only types A, B, E, and F cause illness in humans. [Photomicrograph: Courtesy of Dr. George Lombard, Centers for Disease Control and Prevention– Public Health Image Library 1978 (PHIL ID#2131).]

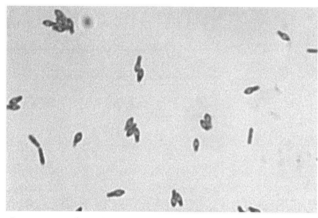

Figure 11–2. *Clostridium botulinum* spores stained with Malachite Green Stain. CDC/Courtesy of Larry Stauffer, Oregon State Public Health Laboratory (2002). The endospores of *C. botulinum* when stained using the Malachite Green staining method will appear as green spheres, while the bacilli themselves will turn purple in color. [Photomicrograph: Courtesy of Larry Stauffer, Oregon State Public Health Laboratory (2002). Centers for Disease Control and Prevention—Public Health Image Library 1978 (PHIL ID#1932).]

Each of the seven active neurotoxins has similarity in structure and mechanism of action, producing a polypeptide of 150 kDa, which is activated by proteases subsequent to bacterial lysis (8). Active botulinum neurotoxin is a simple dichain polypeptide consisting of a 100 kDa heavy chain (H), which is the fragment involved in neurospecific binding and translocation into the nerve cell, and a 50 kDa light chain (L), responsible for intracellular catalytic activity (5,8). The heavy and light chains are joined by a single disulfide bond (4,23). The heavy chain is composed of an amino-terminal 50 kDa domain (H_N) and a carboxy-terminal 50 kDa domain (H_C) (8). The light chain is a zinc-containing endopeptidase that blocks acetylcholine-containing vesicles from fusing with the terminal membrane of the motor neuron (4,24).

Neuronal cell intoxication involves four steps: (a) binding of the carboxy-terminal end of the heavy chain (H_C) to polysialoganglioside receptors on the neuronal membrane, (b) endocytotic internalization of active toxin into endosome-like compartments, (c) membrane translocation facilitated by the amino-terminal half of the heavy chain (H_N), and (d) enzymatic cleavage of SNARE proteins by the light chain (L), which prevents complete assembly of the synaptic fusion complex and thus blocks release of the neurotransmitter acetylcholine from synaptic terminals of the motor neurons in muscle (5,8). The muscle is unable to contract in the absence of acetylcholine release (8,25).

The light chain (L) of each neurotoxin type is a zinc-containing endopeptidase that is capable of cleaving a toxin-specific location of at least one of three proteins (4,8). Botulinum toxin types A, C, and E cleave the protein SNAP-25 (= synaptosomal-associated protein of 25 kd); types B, D, F and G cleave the protein synaptobrevin; and type C cleaves the protein syntaxin (4). These three proteins are members of a group of proteins known as SNARE proteins, or soluble NSF-attachment protein receptor (4,8). SNARE proteins are essential to the docking and fusion of synaptic vesicles with the presynaptic membrane (25).

As mentioned previously, botulinum toxins are the most toxic substances by weight known to science. The precise human lethal dose of botulinum toxin is not known but can be estimated from primate studies. The LD_{50}^H, or lethal dose to 50% of the human population exposed, for botulinum toxin has been estimated to be about 1 ng/kg (1,6). By extrapolation, the lethal amounts of crystalline type A toxin for a 70-kg human would be approximately 0.09 to 0.15 µg intravenously or intramuscularly, 0.70 to 0.90 µg inhalationally, and 70 µg orally (4,11, 26–28). All of the botulinum toxins are slightly less toxic by experimental models when exposure is by the pulmonary route, as estimates for the LD_{50} via inhalation is approximately 3 ng/kg based on experimental models (6,29). The oral route of exposure to botulinum toxin appears to be 2 degrees of magnitude less toxic than the intravenous or intramuscular routes.

The most likely scenario for terrorist or biological warfare use of botulinum toxin is an intentional aerosol release, or possibly an attempt to contaminate a food or water source (3). There has never been a reported case of waterborne botulism (4,8,30,31). Speculation has arisen that botulinum toxin may be used to contaminate a municipal water supply, but this scenario is not likely (4,32). One reason is that botulinum toxin is rapidly inactivated by standard potable water treatments such as chlorination and aeration (4,33). A second reason is that because of the slow turnover time of large capacity reservoirs, a comparable large inoculum of botulinum toxin would be required, and this would be technically infeasible to produce and deliver (4,34). However, botulinum toxin may remain viable in untreated water or beverages for several days; therefore, these items should be investigated in the absence of other identifiable sources of a botulinum index case or outbreak (4,33,35).

The three primary forms of naturally occurring botulism are foodborne, wound infection, and infant or adult intestinal botulism. The U.S. incidence of botulism is typically fewer than 200 cases of all forms annually (8). Foodborne botulism is a rare entity, as there are on average approximately 9 to 10 outbreaks and a median of 24 total cases of this disease per year in the United States (8). From 1950 through 1996, there were 444 outbreaks and 1,087 cases of foodborne botulism recorded in the United States (8). Both the average number of outbreaks per year and the average number of cases per outbreak has remained stable throughout the last century (8). The single largest outbreak of foodborne botulism in the United States in the last century occurred in Michigan in 1977, in which there were 59 cases as a result of eating home-preserved jalapeño peppers at a restaurant (4,36) (Figs. 11-3 and 11-4).

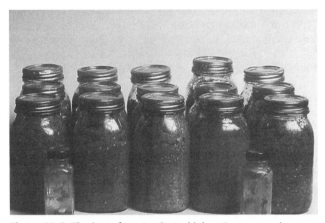

Figure 11–3. The jars of contaminated jalapeño peppers involved in an outbreak of botulism in Pontiac, Michigan, April 1977. CDC/Dr. Chas. Hatheway. The bacterium *C. botulinum* produces a nerve toxin, which causes the rare, but serious paralytic illness botulism. [Photograph: Courtesy of Dr. Chas. Hatheway, Centers for Disease Control and Prevention—Public Health Image Library, April, 1977 (PHIL ID#3355).]

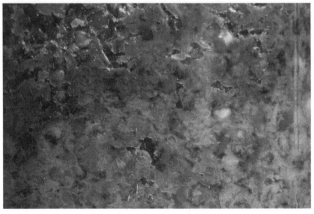

Figure 11–4. This is a close-up of contaminated jalapeño peppers involved in an outbreak of botulism in Pontiac, Michigan, April 1977. CDC/Dr. Chas. Hatheway. [Photograph: Courtesy of Dr. Chas. Hatheway, Centers for Disease Control and Prevention—Public Health Image Library (PHIL ID#3884).]

Of the 135 foodborne outbreaks in the United States from 1980 to 1996, toxin type A accounted for 54.1%, toxin type B for 14.8%, toxin type E for 26.7%, and toxin type F for 1.5% of these outbreaks, with 3.0% of the outbreak causes undetermined (4,8). Toxin types C and D cause botulism in wildlife and domestic animals, though it is thought that humans are susceptible based on primate studies (4,37–39). Toxin type G is produced by a bacterial species in South American soil and has never caused recognizable foodborne botulism (4,40).

Nearly all states have reported at least one outbreak of foodborne botulism since 1950; however, over half (53.8%) of all outbreaks reported have occurred in just five western states (California, Alaska, Washington, Colorado, and Oregon) (8). The geographic distribution of foodborne botulism cases by toxin type is closely correlated with the distribution of organism types found in the environment. Type A toxin is predominant west of the Mississippi River, and has accounted for 85% of foodborne outbreaks in this area (4,8). Type B toxin is distributed generally but more common in the eastern United States, where it has accounted for 60% of foodborne outbreaks east of the Mississippi River (4,8). Toxin type E predominates in the Pacific Northwest, Alaska, and the Great Lakes area, and foodborne outbreaks of type E toxin are commonly associated with fish products, especially native Inuit and Eskimo foods (4,5,8).

Any outbreak of botulism is a public health emergency and should include the possibility of bioterrorism (3,8,10). Certain features would be suggestive of a bioterrorist act or intentional release of botulinum toxin, such as a large number of patients presenting with acute flaccid paralysis and bulbar palsies, or patients presenting with an unusual toxin type not commonly associated with human botulism (4). Patients should be asked whether they know of any other persons with similar symptoms. A careful travel history is vital in this age of rapid and easily accessible airline travel. A dietary history is also valuable. Absence of a common dietary exposure among temporally clustered victims of botulism would suggest the possibility of inhalational botulism (4).

SIGNS AND SYMPTOMS

The onset of botulism can be quite striking, and very frightening to victims of poisoning. Whether botulinum toxin is ingested, produced in the intestine or an infected wound, or possibly inhaled, it enters the vascular system and is transported to peripheral cholinergic nerve terminals, including neuromuscular junctions, postganglionic parasympathetic nerve endings, and peripheral ganglia (5). Here it binds irreversibly to the nerve terminal. After binding, the toxin is internalized and enzymatically blocks acetylcholine release. Though all forms of botulism exhibit nearly identical signs and symptoms, foodborne botulism's neurologic signs may be preceded by abdominal cramps, nausea, vomiting, or diarrhea (4,41). However, these gastrointestinal symptoms are believed to be caused by other bacterial metabolites present in the food (4,17). Thus they may not occur if purified botulinum toxin is intentionally created and disseminated in food or aerosols (4).

The classic presentation or triad of botulism is that of a patient who is afebrile, develops a symmetric, descending flaccid paralysis that begins in the bulbar musculature, and

with a clear sensorium (4). Cranial nerve palsies almost always mark the onset of symptoms and are a key factor in distinguishing someone with symptomatic botulism (5). The central nervous system is not involved. While the extent or rate of onset of paralysis may vary among individual patients, the disease manifestations are similar regardless of toxin type (4,8,41–44). Severity of symptoms may range from mild symptoms that are barely noticeable on examination to paralysis so severe that patients appear comatose and require months of mechanical ventilatory support (4). Recovery ensues only after regeneration of motor axon twigs that reenervate paralyzed muscle fibers, a process that takes weeks to months in adults (4,45,46).

Frequently patients with botulism will present with vision problems, especially double or blurry vision, as well as difficulty speaking or swallowing (4). The prominent neurologic findings in all forms of botulism include diplopia, ptosis, blurred vision, dilated or poorly reactive pupils, dysarthria, dysphonia, and dysphagia (4,6,9,41,47). The oropharynx may appear dry and injected due to peripheral parasympathetic cholinergic blockade (4). Sensory changes are conspicuously absent, except for occasional patients with circumoral or peripheral paresthesias that typically result due to hyperventilation as a victim becomes distressed by the onset of paralysis (4). The prominent bulbar palsies are sometimes summarized as the 4 Ds: diplopia, dysphagia, dysarthria, and dysphonia (4).

Eventually the paralysis will extend beyond bulbar musculature, and generalized weakness and hypotonia will develop. There will be a loss of head control, and dysphagia and loss of a protective gag reflex may require intubation and mechanical ventilation. Untreated patients will suffer death from airway obstruction due to paralysis of pharyngeal and upper airway muscles and inadequate tidal volume due to diaphragmatic and accessory muscle paralysis (4).

Though botulism does not cause fever, secondary infections, such as aspiration pneumonia or genetically engineered strains of biological weapons that also contain botulinum toxin, may be present to cloud the diagnostic picture. The toxin does not penetrate brain parenchyma, so patients are not confused or obtunded, unless there is a secondary process interfering. However, patients may appear lethargic and have communication problems that can be mistaken for confusion or mental difficulties (4) (Figs. 11-5 and 11-6).

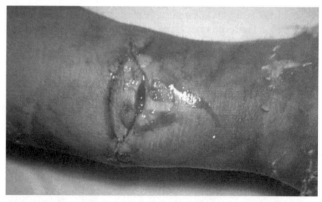

Figure 11–5. A 14-year-old-boy fractured his right ulna and radius and subsequently developed wound botulism. CDC PHIL, date unknown. [Photograph: Courtesy of Centers for Disease Control and Prevention—Public Health Image Library, date unknown. (PHIL ID#1936).]

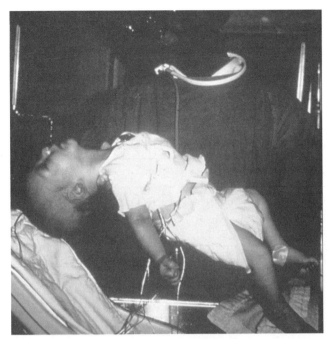

Figure 11–6. A young child with botulism, which is evident as a marked loss of muscle tone, especially in the region of the head and neck. CDC PHIL, date unknown. [Photograph: Courtesy of Centers for Disease Control and Prevention—Public Health Image Library, date unknown. (PHIL ID#1935).].

MEDICAL MANAGEMENT

Any case of suspected botulism should be considered a potential public health emergency due to the possibility that others are likely to be ill or exposed to toxin from a deliberate release or residual contaminated food (4,8–10). Clinicians caring for a patient with suspected botulism should immediately notify their local public health department and hospital infection control official to coordinate the shipment of therapeutic antitoxin, laboratory diagnostic testing, and epidemiological investigation (4,8). Botulism suspected solely on clinical grounds is a legally required reportable event to public health authorities in most U.S. jurisdictions, and tenacious execution of this task is essential (4).

The diagnosis of botulism relies on the astute clinician to recognize characteristic signs and symptoms of isolated cases or outbreaks and to suspect the disease in the context of a reasonable history (consumption of home-canned food or unreliable food source). Failure to suspect botulism and include it in the differential has led to misdiagnosis, including an illustrative outbreak in Canada where 28 people over a 6-week time period became ill before the diagnosis was made in a patient (2000 miles from the source!) and the cases were retroactively traced (4,48).

Botulism should be suspected in any adult who is afebrile, mentally intact, with cranial nerve dysfunction and symmetric descending flaccid paralysis without sensory findings, or in any infant with poor feeding, diminished sucking and crying ability, neck and peripheral muscle weakness, and/or ventilatory distress (5,8). Botulism is often misdiagnosed as Guillain-Barré or Miller-Fisher syn-

drome, myasthenia gravis, or a central nervous system disorder (4) (Table 11-1).

Unless there are secondary or underlying conditions, routine laboratory tests such as serum electrolytes, renal and liver function, complete blood counts, urinalysis, and electrocardiograms are not helpful in diagnosing botulism, but they may help differentiate other conditions that may appear similar (8). A normal cerebrospinal fluid (CSF) analysis may help distinguish botulism from Guillain-Barré syndrome, though the CSF may appear normal early in Guillain-Barré and can sometimes show slightly elevated CSF protein in botulism (8).

Currently only the CDC and approximately 20 state public health agencies are capable of performing laboratory diagnostic testing for botulism, and they should be consulted prospectively about specimen collection and processing (4,8). Samples to be collected include serum, stool, gastric aspirate, and, if available, vomitus and the suspected food source (4,8). All samples should be collected prior to giving antitoxin and then refrigerated (4,8,10). A medication list of the patient should accompany the samples because medications that are toxic to mice can be dialyzed from samples before testing (4).

Demonstration of toxin in serum and other specimens by mouse bioassay is the standard diagnostic test for botulism (4,26). The mouse bioassay can detect as little as 0.03 ng of botulinum toxin and can yield results in as little as 1 to 4 days, whereas culture of fecal and gastric specimens can take anywhere from 5 to 21 days (4,26). Samples should be collected as early as possible for two reasons. The first is that the likelihood of obtaining positive test results decreases with time (8). The second reason is that treatment with antitoxin needs to be initiated early in the course of neurologic dysfunction to be effective (8,49), and antitoxin will nullify the test results of the mouse bioassay. If inhalational botulism is suspected, the most likely means of laboratory diagnosis is through enzyme-linked immunosorbent assay (ELISA) identification of botulinum toxin from nasal mucosa swabs taken within 24 hours of exposure (6).

The mainstays of treatment for botulism are early administration of equine antitoxin and supportive care (8). Timely administration of passive neutralizing antibody may prevent progression of neurologic decline or shorten the duration of ventilatory failure (4). However it will not reverse existing paralysis, as it only neutralizes toxin unbound to nerve endings (4,8,42,49,50). Treatment with antitoxin should not be delayed for microbiological testing (4). Furthermore, aggressive respiratory monitoring and thorough intensive care must be maintained throughout any period of paralytic illness (8).

Botulinum antitoxin contains neutralizing antibodies against the three most common causes of human botulism, toxin types A, B, and E. This licensed trivalent formulation is available from the CDC via state and local public health departments. Currently the dose of licensed antitoxin is one 10-ml vial, diluted 1:10 in 0.9% saline solution, given by slow intravenous infusion (4,8). This provides serum levels of type A, B, and E antibodies capable of neutralizing serum toxin concentrations far in excess of those reported for foodborne botulism patients, so only one dose is required (4,8). For patients who may be intentionally exposed to unnaturally large amounts of botulinum toxin, such as from a biological weapon, the adequacy of neutralization can be con-

TABLE 11-1 Possible Mistaken Conditions for Botulism and Potential Distinguishing Features

CONDITIONS	POTENTIAL DISTINGUISHING FEATURES
Guillain-Barré syndrome* and variants (e.g., Miller-Fisher, which has a descending paralysis)	History of antecedent infection; paresthesias; ascending paralysis; early areflexia; CSF protein increase; EMG findings
Myasthenia gravis*	Recurrent paralysis; EMG findings; sustained response to anticholinesterase therapy
Stroke*	Asymmetric paralysis; abnormal CNS image
Other intoxication (e.g., alcohol, CO, nerve gas, organophosphates)	History of intake or exposure; excessive drug levels in body fluids
Lambert-Eaton syndrome	Increased strength with sustained contraction; evidence of lung carcinoma
Tick paralysis	Paresthesias; ascending paralysis; attached tick
Poliomyelitis	Antecedent febrile illness; asymmetric paralysis; CSF pleocytosis
CNS infections, especially of brainstem	Mental status changes; CSF and EEG abnormalities
CNS tumor	Paralysis often asymmetric; abnormal CNS image
Streptococcal pharyngitis	Absence of bulbar palsies; positive rapid antigen test or throat culture
Psychiatric illness*	Normal EMG in conversion paralysis
Viral syndrome*	Absence of bulbar palsies and flaccid paralysis
Inflammatory myopathy*	Elevated creatinine kinase levels
Diabetic complications*	Sensory neuropathy; few cranial nerve palsies
Hyperemesis gravidarum*	Absence of bulbar palsies or acute flaccid paralysis
Hypothyroidism*	Abnormal thyroid function test results
Laryngeal tumor*	Absence of flaccid paralysis; dysphonia without bulbar palsies
Overexertion*	Absence of bulbar palsies or acute flaccid paralysis

Adapted from Arnon SS, Schecter R, Inglesby TV, et al. Consensus statement—botulinum toxin as a biological weapon: medical and public health management. Table 3. *JAMA*. 2001 Feb 28:285(8);1059-70.

CSF indicates cerebrospinal fluid; EMG, electromyogram; CNS, central nervous system; EEG, electroencephalogram.

*Misdiagnosis made in large outbreak of botulism in Canada (4,48).

firmed by retesting serum for toxin after treatment (4). In the event that another toxin type was intentionally disseminated, the U.S. Army maintains an investigational heptavalent (ABCDEFG) antitoxin, though the time required for toxin typing prior to administration of this antitoxin decreases its utility in an outbreak (4,51).

The safety of botulinum antitoxin is uncertain. Approximately 9% of patients treated with equine antitoxin have experienced some sort of hypersensitivity reaction (4,8,52), though the recommended dose was previously larger than current rec-

ommendations. Skin testing should be performed prior to administration of antitoxin. Patients responding to challenge with a substantial wheal and flare reaction may be desensitized over 3 to 4 hours before additional antitoxin is given (4,8). Clinicians should review the package insert and instructions with public health officials prior to using antitoxin.

Infant botulism requires supportive care, and use of antitoxin is of questionable benefit in light of the risk of inducing lifelong hypersensitivity to equine antigens (8). A human-derived botulism immune globulin is currently under investigation in California (4,8,42,53,54). As for other special populations with botulism, based on limited information, children, pregnant women, and immunocompromised persons with botulism should be treated by standard therapy (4). Both children (4,55,56) and pregnant women (4,57,58) have received equine antitoxin without apparent short-term adverse effects, though the risks to fetuses of exposure to equine antitoxin are unknown (4).

Antibiotics have no known use for treatment of botulism, but they may be required for treatment of secondary infections, or treatment of wound botulism based on wound culture results (4,5,8). Aminoglycoside antibiotics and clindamycin are contraindicated because of their ability to exacerbate neuromuscular blockade (4,59,60). Activated charcoal may be given for detoxification prior to availability of antitoxin, but there is no data on its usefulness (4,61). Emetics and gastric lavage can be used if the time since ingestion is brief (5). In the absence of ileus, cathartics and enemas may also be used to purge the gut of toxin (5).

A pentavalent (ABCDE) botulinum toxoid vaccine has been in use by the CDC for lab workers and by the military for protection of troops (3,4,62). A recombinant vaccine is also in development (4,63). The toxoid is not useful for post-exposure prophylaxis, as it induces immunity over several months (4). Furthermore, mass immunization is not feasible and possibly undesirable, due to scarcity of the toxoid, rarity of disease, and loss of potential therapeutic benefit of medicinal botulinum toxin (3,4).

TRIAGE CONSIDERATIONS

In the event of a large-scale exposure to botulinum toxin, one must consider certain aspects of triage that may need to be employed. Patients who are victims of botulinum toxin poisoning may progress to respiratory failure within hours to days of the first onset of symptoms. These patients would require ventilatory support. However, neuromuscular recovery would ensue only after regrowth of new axon terminals, a process that takes 2 to 3 months or longer. Thus any large-scale exposure of populations to botulinum toxin would easily overwhelm an institution's, or even an entire metropolitan area's, available mechanical ventilation resources. For this reason, supplementary support measures should be coordinated with appropriate agencies, institutions, and neighboring facilities in advance of such an occurrence (10,47,64).

PERSONAL PROTECTION

Since botulism is an intoxication rather than an infection, it is not transmissible from person to person. Also, botulinum toxin does not penetrate intact skin. Thus medical personnel caring for patients with suspected botulism should use standard precautions. Furthermore, patients with suspected botulinism do not need to be isolated. However, those with flaccid paralysis in whom there is a suspicion of meningitis do require droplet precautions until this is ruled out (4,9,10,65).

SUMMARY

The seven serotypes of botulinum toxin produced by *Clostridium botulinum* are the most toxic substances known (6). They cause the disease known as botulism, a rare but potentially fatal illness, usually from the ingestion of preformed toxin in improperly preserved foods. A single gram of crystalline toxin could kill more than one million people, though technical factors concerning dissemination would make such a scenario difficult (4). Though botulism is not an infectious disease, and is not spread person to person, even one suspected case constitutes a medical and public health emergency to provide necessary treatment and intervention to prevent additional cases.

Due to their extreme potency and lethality, wide availability, ease of production, and need for prolonged intensive care among affected persons, botulinum toxins have been evaluated by several countries as a potential biological weapon (6). Terrorists have already attempted use of botulinum toxin as a bioweapon, when the Aum Shinrikyo cult in Japan made three attempts at aerosol dispersion between 1990 and 1995; luckily each one was unsuccessful (4,12,13). Nevertheless, botulinum toxin remains on the list of Category A agents of bioterrorism with the CDC (7).

Botulinum toxin works by irreversibly blocking the action of the neurotransmitter acetylcholine at the neuromuscular junction, causing a characteristic flaccid, descending paralysis, along with cranial nerve palsies. Diagnosis is made clinically, with treatment required prior to laboratory confirmation at a limited number of federal and state laboratories. Treatment consists of intensive supportive care, including prolonged mechanical ventilation in some patients, and administration of antitoxin maintained by the CDC.

RESOURCES

In the event of an actual or threatened bioterrorist incident, immediately contact your state and local public health office (a list of these can be found at http://www.statepublichealth.org/index.php and the CDC web sites: www.bt.cdc.gov/protocols.asp, www.bt.cdc.gov/emcontact/ index.asp).

1. Websites Relevant to Bioterrorism Response and Readiness Pertaining to Botulinum Toxin
   http://www.apic.org
2. CDC Bioterrorism Web Pages
   http://www.bt.cdc.gov/
   http://www.bt.cdc.gov/agent/botulism/index.asp

3. Agency for Toxic Substances and Disease Registry—USA, Global Information System
http://www.atsdr.cdc.gov/gis/conference98/gisindex.html

4. Medical NBC Information Online Server
http://www.nbc-med.org/ie40/Default.html

5. Center for Civilian Biodefense Strategies Johns Hopkins University Web Pages
http://www.hopkins-biodefense.org/
http://www.hopkins-biodefense.org/pages/agents/tocbotox.html

6. Association of Public Health Laboratories
http://www.aphl.org/

7. Association of State & Territorial Health Officials
http://www.astho.org/

8. U.S. Army Medical Research Institute of Infectious Diseases (USAMRIID)
http://www.usamriid.army.mil/education/bluebook.html

9. NOVA: PBS series on Bioterrorism
http://www.pbs.org/wgbh/nova/bioterror/

10. National Institute of Allergy and Infectious Diseases (NIAID): Bioterrorism
http://www.niaid.nih.gov/publications/bioterrorism.htm

11. Federation of American Scientists: Working Group on Biologic and Toxin Weapons
http://www.fas.org/bwc/index.html

12. Center for Infectious Disease Research and Policy, University of Minnesota
http://www.cidrap.umn.edu/cidrap/

13. Center for Non-proliferation Studies—Monterey Institute of International Studies
http://cns.miis.edu/

14. U.S. Food & Drug Administration
http://www.fda.gov/oc/opacom/hottopics/bioterrorism.html

15. Health Agency Locator
http://www.statepublichealth.org/index.php

16. National Association of County & City Health Officials (NACCHO). Bioterrorism & Emergency Response Program
http://www.naccho.org/project90.cfm

17. National Library of Medicine: Biological Warfare
http://www.sis.nlm.nih.gov/Tox/biologicalwarfare.htm

18. USAMRIID. Phone: (301) 619-2833.
Email: USAMRIIDweb@amedd.army.mil

19. CDC: CDC's 24-hour telephone number for state health departments to report suspected botulism cases, obtain clinical consultation on botulism cases, and request botulinum antitoxin release has changed. State health departments should call 770-488-7100. The call will be taken by the CDC Emergency Operations Center, which will page the Foodborne and Diarrheal Diseases Branch medical officer on call. All other aspects of the botulism emergency response system will remain unchanged. Medical care providers who suspect a diagnosis of botulism in a patient should immediately call their state health department's emergency 24-hour tele-

phone number. The state health department will contact CDC to arrange for a clinical consultation by telephone and, if indicated, release of botulinum antitoxin.

20. U.S. Public Health Service. Phone: 1 (800) 872-6367

21. National Response Center. Phone: 1 (800) 424-8802

22. Domestic Preparedness Information. Phone: 1 (800) 368-6498

23. Arnon SS, Schecter R, Inglesby TV, et al. Consensus statement—botulinum toxin as a biological weapon: medical and public health management. JAMA. 2001 Feb 28:285(8);1059-70.

QUESTIONS AND ANSWERS

1. Which of the following statements is/are true regarding the epidemiology of botulism?
A. Foodborne botulism is the most common form of botulism.
B. The incubation period is dose-dependent and, in a biological attack, could be less than typically observed in foodborne illness.
C. Inhalational botulism occurs naturally in cannery employees.
D. Mortality in treated patients is 30%.

2. Which of the following is a true statement regarding the clinical presentation of botulism?
A. Botulism presents as an initial nonspecific febrile illness.
B. Paralysis begins in the bulbar musculature.
C. Paresthesias are secondary to sensory nerve damage.
D. Respiratory failure is not likely to occur.

3. Which of the following is a true statement about botulinum antitoxin?
A. It is effective against all seven types of botulism.
B. It reverses paralysis upon administration.
C. It must be obtained from CDC through the local and/or state health department.
D. It is recommended for prophylaxis of close contacts of cases.
E. All of the above.

4. Which of the following is a true statement about the diagnosis of botulism?
A. It is confirmed by blood culture.
B. It must be confirmed in a public health laboratory.
C. It is supported by pathognomonic findings on EMG.
D. All of the above.
E. None of the above.

ANSWERS

1: B. *Naturally occurring forms of botulism include infant, wound, and foodborne botulism. Infant botulism is the most common form. Inhalational botulism does not occur naturally and would most likely result secondary to the deliberate release of a botulism aerosol. The incubation period of foodborne botulism is 12 to 72 hours and is dose-dependent. Aerosol exposure is likely to* *result in a shorter incubation period. Death occurs in 60% of untreated cases, but <5% of treated.*

2: B. *Botulism patients present with the acute onset of an afebrile, symmetric descending flaccid paralysis. Paralysis begins in the bulbar musculature, with cranial palsies. Respiratory failure can occur in as little as 24 hours. Sensory changes are not present, with the exception of paresthesias secondary to anxiety with subsequent hyperventilation.*

3: C. *Trivalent botulinum antitoxin is effective against toxin types A, B, and E and is available from CDC. An investigational heptavalent toxin is held by the U.S. Army, but it is not currently available for use in the general population. Antitoxin prevents binding of toxin to the acetylcholine receptor, subsequent to its administration, but it does not reverse the effects of already-bound toxin. Botulism is not transmitted from person to person: therefore, prophylaxis is not necessary for contacts of cases.*

4: B. *Laboratory confirmation of botulism is by mouse bioassay, available at CDC and certain public health laboratories. EMG findings are nonspecific but may be useful in ruling out other potential causes of paralysis.*

REFERENCES

1. Gill MD. Bacterial toxins: a table of lethal amounts. Microbiol Rev. 1982;46(1):86-94.
2. National Institute of Occupational Safety and Health. Registry of toxic effects of chemical substances (R-TECS). Cincinnati: National Institute for Occupational Safety and Health; 1996.
3. Kortepeter M, Christopher G, Cieslak T, et al. USAMRIID's medical management of biological casualties handbook. 4th ed. Fort Detrick, MD: Operational Medicine Department, USAMRIID; 2001. pp. 70-5.
4. Arnon SS, Schecter R, Inglesby TV, et al. (Working group on civilian biodefense). Botulinum toxin as a biological weapon; medical and public health management. JAMA. 2001;285:1059-71.
5. Abrutyn E. Botulism. In: Harrison's principles of internal medicine. 15th ed. New York: McGraw-Hill; 2001. pp. 920-1.
6. Franz DR, Middlebrook JL. Botulinum toxins. In: Sidell FR, Takafuji ET, Franz DR, eds. Medical aspects of chemical and biological warfare. Washington, DC; Office of the Surgeon General, United States Army; 1997. pp. 643-54. (Textbook of military medicine; part I, vol. 3).
7. Centers for Disease Control and Prevention [online]. September 8, 2003; Available from URL:http://www.bt.cdc.gov/agent/agentlist-category.asp#catdef.
8. Centers for Disease Control and Prevention. Botulism in the United States, 1899-1996. Handbook for epidemiologists, clinicians, and laboratory workers. Atlanta: Centers for Disease Control and Prevention; 1998.
9. Shapiro RL, Hatheway C, Swerdlow DL. Botulism in the United States: A clinical and epidemiological review. Ann Intern Med. 1998;129:221-8.
10. APIC Bioterrorism Task Force (English JF, Cundiff MY, Malone JD, Pfeiffer JA). CDC Hospital Infections Program Bioterrorism Working Group (Bell M, Steele L, Miller JM). Bioterrorism readiness plan: a template for healthcare facilities. April 1999.
11. Franz DR, Pitt LM, Clayton MA, et al. Efficacy of prophylactic and therapeutic administration of antitoxin for inhalational botulism. In: Das-Gupta BR, ed. Botulinum and tetanus neurotoxins: neurotransmission and biomedical aspects. New York: Plenum Press; 1993. pp. 473-6.
12. Tucker JB, ed. Toxic terror: assessing the terrorist use of chemical and biological weapons. Cambridge, MA: MIT Press; 2000.
13. WuDunn S, Miller J, Broad WJ. How Japan germ terror alerted world. New York Times. 1998 May 26: A1, A10.
14. United Nations Security Council. Tenth report of the executive chairman of the special commission established by the secretary-general pursuant to paragraph 9(b)(l) of Security Council resolution 687 (1991), and paragraph 3 of resolution 699 (1991) on the activities of the special commission. New York: United Nations Security Council, 1995. pp. S/1995/1038.
15. Zlinskas RA. Iraq's biological weapons: the past as future? JAMA. 1997;278:418-24.
16. Holzer VE. Botulism from inhalation [in German]. Med Klin. 1962;57:1735-8.
17. Smith LDS. Botulism: the organism, its toxins, the disease. Springfield, IL: Charles C Thomas Publisher; 1977.
18. Hatheway CL, Johnson EA. Clostridium: the spore-bearing anaerobes. In: Collier L, Balows A, Sussman M, eds. Topley & Wilson's microbiology and microbial infections. 9th ed. New York: Oxford University Press; 1998. pp. 731-82.
19. Cato EP, George WL, Finegold SM. Genus Clostridium. In: Sneath PHA, Mair NS, Sharpe ME, et al., eds. Bergey's manual of systematic bacteriology. vol. 2. Baltimore: Williams & Wilkins; 1986. pp. 1141-1200.
20. Hall JD, McCroskey LM, et al. Isolation of an organism resembling Clostridium baratii which produces type F botulinal toxin from an infant with botulism. J Clin Microbiol. 1985;21: 654-5.
21. Aureli P, Fenicia L, Pasolini B, et al. Two cases of type E infant botulism caused by neurotoxigenic Clostridium butyricum in Italy. J Infect Dis. 1986;154:207-11.
22. Arnon SS. Botulism as an intestinal toxemia. In: Blaser MJ, Smith PD, Ravdin JI, et al., eds. Infections of the gastrointestinal tract. New York: Raven Press; 1995. pp. 257-71.
23. Lacy DB, Tepp W, Cohen AC, et al. Crystal structure of botulinum neurotoxin type A and implications for toxicity. Nat Struct Biol. 1998;5:898-902.
24. Montecucco C, ed. Clostridial neurotoxins: the molecular pathogenesis of tetanus and botulism. Curr Top Microbiol Immunol. 1995;195:1-278.
25. Schiavo G, Montecucco C. The structure and mode of botulinum and tetanus toxins. In: Rood J, McClane BA, Songer JG, Titball RW, eds. The clostridia. Molecular biology and pathogenesis. San Diego: Academic Press; 1997. pp. 295-322.
26. Schantz EJ, Johnson EA. Properties and use of botulinum toxin and other microbial neurotoxins in medicine. Microbiol Rev. 1992;56:80-99.
27. Herrero BA, Ecklung AE, Streett CS, et al. Experimental botulism in monkeys: a clinical pathological study. Exp Mol Pathol. 1967;6:84-95.
28. Scott AB, Suzuki D. Systemic toxicity of botulinum toxin by intramuscular injection in the monkey. Mov Disord. 1988;3: 333-5.
29. McNally RE, Morrison MB, Berndt JE, et al. Effectiveness of medical defense interventions against predicted battlefield levels of botulinum toxin A. vol 1. Joppa, MD: Science Applications International Corporation; 1994. p. 3.
30. Gangarosa EJ, Donadio JA, Armstrong RW, et al. Botulism in the United States, 1899–1969. Am J Epidemiol. 1971;93:93-101.
31. Hauschild AH. Epidemiology of human foodborne botulism. In: Hauschild AH, Dodds KL, eds. Clostridium botulinum: ecology and control in foods. New York: Marcel Dekker; 1993. pp. 69-104.
32. Wannemacher RW Jr, Dinterman RE, Thompson WL, et al. Treatment for removal of biotoxins from drinking water. Frederick, MD: US Army Biomedical Research and Development Command; Sep 1993. Technical Report 9120.
33. Siegel LS. Destruction of botulinum toxin in food and water. In: Hauschild AH, Dodds KL, eds. Clostridium botulinum: ecology and control in foods. New York: Marcel Dekker; 1993. pp. 323-41.

34. Burrows WD, Renner SE. Biological warfare agents as threats to potable water. Environ Health Perspect. 1999;107:975-84.

35. Kazdobina IS. Stability of botulin toxins in solutions and beverages [in Russian with English abstract]. Gig Sanit. 1995 Jan–Feb:9-12.

36. Terranova W, Breman JG, Locey RP, Speck S. Botulism type B: epidemiological aspects of an extensive outbreak. Am J Epidemiol. 1978;109:150-6.

37. Gunnison JB, Meyer KF. Susceptibility of monkeys, goats and small animals to oral administration of botulinum toxin types B, C and D. J Infect Dis. 1930;46:335-40.

38. Dolman CE, Murakami L. *Clostridium botulinum* type F with recent observations on other types. J Infect Dis. 1961;109:107-28.

39. Smart JL, Roberts TA, McCullagh KG, et al. An outbreak of C botulism in captive monkeys. Vet Rec. 1980;107:445-6.

40. Giménez DF, Ciccarelli AS. Another type of Clostridium botulinum. Zentralbl Bakteriol [Orig]. 1970;215:221-4.

41. Hughes JM, Blumenthal JR, Merson MH, et al. Clinical features of types A and B food-borne botulism. Ann Intern Med. 1981;95:442-5.

42. Arnon SS. Infant botulism. In: Feigen R, Cherry J, eds. Textbook of pediatric infectious diseases. 4th ed. Philadelphia: WB Saunders; 1998. pp. 1570-7.

43. Wilson R, Morris JG, Snyder JD, et al. Clinical characteristics of infant botulism in the United States: a study of the non-California cases. Pediatr Infect Dis. 1982;1:148-50.

44. Merson MH, Dowell VR. Epidemiologic, clinical, and laboratory aspects of wound botulism. N Engl. J Med. 1973;289:1005-10.

45. Duchen LW. Motor nerve growth induced by botulinum toxin as a regenerative phenomenon. Proc R Soc Med. 1972;65:196-7.

46. Mann JM, Martin S, Hoffman R, Marrazzo S. Patient recovery from type A botulism: morbidity assessment following a large outbreak. Am J Public Health. 1981;71:266-9.

47. Franz DR, Jahrling PB, Friedlander AM, et al. Clinical recognition and management of patients exposed to biological warfare agents. JAMA. 1997;278:399-411.

48. St. Louis ME, Peck SH, Bowering D, et al. Botulism from chopped garlic: delayed recognition of a major outbreak. Ann Intern Med. 1988;108:363-8.

49. Tackett CO, Shandera WX, Mann JM, et al. Equine antitoxin use and other factors that predict outcome in type A foodborne botulism. Am J Med. 1984;76:794-8.

50. Sugiyama H. Clostridium botulinum neurotoxin. Microbiol Rev. 1980;44:419-48.

51. Hibbs RG, Weber JT, Corwin A, et al. Experience with the use of an investigational F(ab´)2 heptavalent botulism immune globulin of equine origin during an outbreak of type E botulism in Egypt. Clin Infect Dis. 1996;23:337-40.

52. Black RE, Bunn RA. Hypersensitivity reactions associated with botulinal antitoxin. Am J Med. 1980;69:567-70.

53. Center for Disease Control. Botulism type F—California. MMWR. 1966;15:359.

54. Arnon SS. Clinical trial of human botulism immune globulin. In: DasGupta BR, ed. Botulinum and tetanus neurotoxins: neurotransmission and biomedical aspects. New York: Plenum Press; 1993. pp. 477-82.

55. Weber JT, Goodpasture HC, Alexander H, et al. Wound botulism in a patient with a tooth abscess: case report and literature review. Clin Infect Dis. 1993;16:635-9.

56. Keller MA, Miller VH, Berkowitz CD, Yoshimori RN. Wound botulism in pediatrics. Am J Dis Child. 1982;136:320-2.

57. Robin L, Herman D, Redett R. Botulism in a pregnant woman. N Engl J Med. 1996;335:823-4.

58. St. Clair EH, DiLiberti JH, O'Brien ML. Observations of an infant born to a mother with botulism. J Pediatr. 1975;87:658.

59. Santos JI, Swensen P, Glasgow LA. Potentiation of Clostridium botulinum toxin by aminoglycoside antibiotics: clinical and laboratory observations. Pediatrics. 1981;68:50-4.

60. Schulze J, Toepfer M, Schroff KC, et al. Clindamycin and nicotinic neuromuscular transmission. Lancet. 1999;354:1792-3.

61. Olson KR, ed. Poisoning and drug overdose. 3rd ed. Stamford, CT: Appleton & Lange; 1999.

62. Siegel LS. Human Immune response to botulinum pentavalent (ABCDE) toxoid determined by a neutralization test and by an enzyme-linked immunosorbent assay. J Clin Microbiol. 1988; 26:2351-6.

63. Byrne MP, Smith LA. Development of vaccines for prevention of botulism. Biochimie. 2000;82:955-66.

64. American Public Health Association. Control of communicable disease in man. Washington, DC: American Public Health Association; 1995.

65. Centers for Disease Control and Prevention, the Hospital Infection Control Practices Advisory Committee (HICPAC). Recommendations for isolation precautions in hospitals. Am J Infect Cont. 1996;24:24-52.

12

Toxins
Section A: Staphylococcal Enterotoxin Type B

Sophia Dyer and Stephen Traub

STAPHYLOCOCCAL ENTEROTOXIN B

Staphylococcal enterotoxin B (SEB) is one of many enterotoxins produced by the *Staphylococcus* organism. *Staphylococcus* species and other bacterial organisms produce many enterotoxins that are responsible for a myriad of effects in the animal or human serving as host for the organism. Due to their clinical effects and mode of action, these are sometimes referred to as superantigens or pyrogenic toxins. In total, seven enterotoxins have been identified. The type B serotype is the agent that has been most extensively studied as a biological weapon. The U.S. military considered SEB as a weapon in the 1960s (1,2).

THEORETICAL AND SCIENTIFIC BACKGROUND

SEB is frequently classified as an "incapacitating agent" because it does not in general produce mortality. Its military usefulness is based on the belief that this agent would be effective to halt troop movements; within the civilian population, it would produce a large number of ill persons over a short period of time. This wave of patients could overwhelm the medical care system, and the enterotoxin could also be mistaken for more lethal biological agents, promoting fear and terror.

Enterotoxins in general are exotoxin products of bacteria, that is, secreted toxins. "Entero" means these toxins are predominantly identified as causing illness to the gastrointestinal system. Some clinicians may not be familiar with the term "SEB"; however, most are well acquainted with the toxin-caused staphylococcal food poisoning syndrome: abdominal pain, nausea, vomiting, and diarrhea with onset within a few hours of ingestion of the offending food product. With staphylococcal food poisoning, enterotoxins are responsible for the clinical syndrome. Naturally occurring strains of staphylococcus aureus produce enterotoxins when allowed to grow in milk products, meats, and bakery products. Staphylococcal enterotoxins are protein complexes, many with similar amino acid sequences (1). Other enterotoxins are identified as having distinct protein compositions from staphylococcus aureus. These are classed as A through G, but type B can be taken as an example of the entire class.

Another enterotoxin to produce disease is the toxic shock syndrome toxin (TSST-1). This toxin shares some structural relations to SEB as well as other staphylococcal toxins. Streptococcal species produce several toxins as well.

The concept of SEB classification as incapacitating agents is reflected in the differences between the effective dose versus the lethal dose of this toxin. Effective dose is also considered the incapacitating dose. This is represented by the concepts of effective/incapacitating dose for 50% of an exposed population (ED50) and lethal dose for 50% of an exposed population. The reported incapacitating dose for 50% of a population exposed to SEB is 0.0004 micrograms/kg with inhalation exposure, as compared to the lethal dose (LD50), which is an exponentially larger dose of 0.02 micrograms/kg (2). These doses are less than lethal doses for many chemical exposures.

SEB, like many similar toxins in its family, causes its effects by its tendency to activate the immune system nonspecifically. The chemical interaction responsible for this stimulation occurs on multiple levels; SEB affects both T-cell antigen receptors and MHC (major histocompatibility complex) class II components of the immune system. The MHC class II molecules are found on the cell surfaces of what is frequently termed "antigen presenting cell" macrophages, dendritic cells, and B-cells. The subsequent stimulation of CD-4 helper T-cells results in the release of cytokines and further activation of the immune system. Proliferation of these stimulated T-cells is believed to be at the heart of the effect of SEB (4). The end result of this immune system activation is release of cytokines. Cytokines released include interferon gamma, interleukin-6, and tumor necrosis factor (3). The effect of this "cytokine storm" is to produce the inflammation and hence clinical syndrome of SEB poisoning. Gastrointestinal disease from SEB may also result from the release of other substances such as histamine and leukotrienes.

In addition to SEB's ability to generate release of cytokines and activate an immune system response that results in a clinical syndrome, it possesses other characteristics that make it plausible for use as a biological weapon. One of these characteristics is the toxin's stability with respect to temperature, solubility in water, and stability in air. SEB could be delivered by an aerosol mechanism or solubilized in water, representing an ingestion hazard from contaminated foodstuffs or potable water. (Note: Chlorination of water should eliminate the toxin.)

In addition to recognition of the clinical signs of SEB exposure, detection of SEB is possible in environmental and biological samples. Available technologies include ELISA and TRF (time-resolved fluorometry). Note that other biological weapons of concern detected by TRF techniques include *Francisella tularensis* and *Clostridium botulinum* toxin A/B (5). Reverse passive latex agglutination (RPLA) tests can identify SEB in food. Polymerase chain reactions can be used to identify the staphylococcal aureus genome. Retrospective diagnosis can be attempted with the use of serological tests for SEB in victims.

SIGNS AND SYMPTOMS

Signs and symptoms of illness differ by the route of exposure to this superantigen. Because SEB is one of the frequently suspected etiologies of naturally acquired food-borne illness, it could be difficult to differentiate between exposure to SEB as acquired from a culinary misadventure or illness as the result of an intentional contamination of food products. One leading point might be the type of food ingested because naturally occurring staphylococcal enterotoxin food poisoning typically is seen in dairy products, pastry (especially cream-filled pastry), custard, ham, and potato salad. The clinician should be cognizant of the potential for victims exposed to inhalational SEB to have combined symptoms of inhalational exposure and signs and symptoms of ingestion of SEB, if during the inhalational exposure the victim swallowed the toxin in addition to inhaling.

Ingested SEB food-borne illness is typically self-limited. Incubation period can be as short as 1 hour after ingestion of the food substance, with a general range of 1 to 6 hours after exposure for the onset of symptoms. Predominating symptoms are nausea and vomiting with abdominal cramping (9). Fever and diarrhea are not seen in all patients. Many patients begin to recover after 24 hours. Other food-borne toxins that present with nausea and vomiting as predominant symptoms are *Bacillus cereus* and Norwalk-like virus. *Bacillus cereus* is typically associated with starch-rich foods such as rice and recognized as the etiology of a vomiting illness associated with fried rice dishes. Norwalk-like virus (norovirus) is a common source of food-borne illness (10). Norwalk-like virus can be contracted via food products and has been associated with shellfish. It can also be contracted via contact with contaminated surfaces, then through hand-to-mouth activity that transmits the virus. The presenting symptoms are similar to SEB ingestion. Norwalk-like virus (norovirus) has an incubation time of 24 to 48 hours. Vomiting and diarrhea are typically both present. With SEB, diarrhea is less prevalent and generally nonbloody. Other symptoms found with all of these exposures may include fever, generalized myalgias, and fatigue (11). Several outbreaks of norovirus on cruise ships have been documented and may give a sense of how a localized bioterrorism outbreak may present. In one report, vomiting and diarrhea were present in the majority of the patients stricken (12).

Most patients recover without significant morbidity and mortality from SEB food-borne illness. The clinician should consider testing of food product or vomitus for the SEB toxin to confirm the etiology of the illness. Ingestion exposures would not be expected to present the constellation of respiratory symptoms described later. However, ingestion of SEB after inhalation exposure can demonstrate both symptoms of inhalation exposure and ingestion in the same victim.

One of the best documentations of exposure to the inhalational form of the SEB agent is chronicled in the text *Medical Aspects of Chemical and Biological Warfare* published by the Surgeon General of the U.S. Army. In this report the exposure event was a laboratory accident affecting nine laboratory workers (14). It appears that all patients exposed became symptomatic, but biological or environmental sampling is not described in the authors' report of the exposure. Two additional workers were in the vicinity but believed not to have been exposed. Nonproductive cough was found in all patients. Onset averaged at approximately 10 hours after exposure. Other respiratory findings included inspiratory and expiratory rales, orthopnea, and varying degrees of dyspnea. Exertional dyspnea persisted for 10 days in one patient. Chest pain accompanied with respiratory symptoms in many patients presented around the same time of onset of the nonproductive cough. Chest radiograph findings included pulmonary edema, interstitial edema, peribronchial cuffing, atelectasis, and even "normal" chest radiograph interpretation. Fever was found in all patients. Duration of fever was up to 5 days. Shaking chills and onset of fever was estimated at 8 to 20 hours after suspected time of exposure. Myalgias were also seen in this case series. Headache was also a common presenting sign, even as early as 4 hours after exposure. Similar to myalgias, average time to onset of headache symptoms was 13 hours. Symptom control of headache was achieved with oral medications. Interestingly, nausea, anorexia, and vomiting were demonstrated in this series of patients. Some of the vomiting was posttussive in nature. No diarrhea was seen. In terms of length of illness, the results are of concern when considering the potential impact to the health care structure. Cough may persist for up to 4 weeks, and return to work may take up to 2 weeks. Adult respiratory distress syndrome (ARDS) could develop in some patients, severely taxing the critical care system (13). Differential diagnosis should include common community-acquired pneumonias, influenza, and mycoplasma respiratory illnesses. Most of these illnesses would not be expected to either occur in a small number of patients (i.e., most community-acquired pneumonia and mycoplasma) or to have an epidemiological pattern more consistent with a natural movement of an infectious disease through a population, as would be the case with influenza.

MEDICAL MANAGEMENT

Most of the treatment options for either gastrointestinal presentation of SEB or the inhalation form of the illness focus on supportive care. Fever and myalgias can be treated with antipyretics. Some patients with gastrointestinal symptoms may require support with intravenous fluids. Antiemetics could also be utilized to control vomiting and encourage self-hydration. Cough suppressants can provide symptomatic relief. Of most concern would be the progression of respiratory compromise to require supplemental oxygen and potentially in some cases the need for endotracheal intubation and mechanical ventilation. Antibiotics are not believed helpful, except in the event of secondary infection in the patient with respiratory compromise. Other work has explored the possibility of blocking the effects of superantigens from both staphylococcal aureus and streptococcus species. Peptide antagonists have been found to decrease mortality by inhibiting the immunological cascade before activation in a mouse model (6). Of concern, many staphylococcus species produce some variant form of toxin, not necessarily SEB, requiring specific tailoring of a peptide antagonist. A vaccination candidate has been developed against SEB with the production of a recombinant SEB strain using *E. coli* as an intermediate step. The product reduced lethality by elicitation of an immune response able to respond to a challenge with SEB (7). A future possibility is the use of antibodies against SEB. Passive transfer of immunoglobulins produced in chickens offered protection against a lethal challenge of SEB in rhesus monkeys even if administered after exposure (8). As of this writing, no human vaccination is currently available.

TRIAGE CONSIDERATIONS

In the case of exposure to gastrointestinal SEB, most patients are expected to have a self-limiting course of illness. Antiemetic therapy may allow for early discharge to home, and not all patients require intravenous fluid rehydration. Consider clinical signs and symptoms of dehydration as decision points for the utilization of medical resources with intravenous fluids. Small children and the elderly may not tolerate dehydration well and should be triaged accordingly. For an inhalation exposure, it would be prudent to focus attention on those with underlying respiratory illness, immunocompromise, and the extremes of age. Other groups of concern would be those with abnormal oxygen saturation, hypotension not quickly reversed with fluid resuscitation, and abnormal chest radiograph (especially findings consistent with pulmonary edema or ARDS).

PERSONAL PROTECTION

SEB is not spread person to person. Universal precautions should be in place with patient contact activities.

SUMMARY

SEB can affect the victim via ingestion or inhalation. Ingestion of toxin results in symptoms generally within 6 hours: nausea, vomiting, on occasion fever, and diarrhea. Most illness is self-limiting.

Inhalation of toxin results in fever, nonproductive cough, myalgias, and chest pain and can result in pulmonary edema or ARDS. Cough may be a prolonged symptom. There is no person-to-person spread.

RESOURCES

PUBLICATIONS

1. Ulrich RG, Sidell S, Taylor TJ, et al. Staphylococcal enterotoxin B and related pyrogenic toxins. In: Textbook of military medicine. Part I. Warfare, weaponry and the casualty. Vol. 3. 1997;621-31.

2. Briggs S, Brinsfield KH eds. Advanced disaster medical response manual for providers. Harvard Medical International Trauma and Disaster, 2003.

3. Medical management of biological casualties handbook. Frederick, MD: U.S. Army Medical Research Institute of Infections Diseases, Fort Detrick.

WEB SITES

1. Center for Disease Control: www.cdc.gov.

2. U.S. Department of Agriculture, food-borne illnesses: www.usda.gov.

QUESTIONS AND ANSWERS

1. **SEB can develop in improperly refrigerated foodstuffs. Which of the following is not commonly associated with SEB?**
   A. Pastry
   B. Milk products
   C. Starchy foods
   D. Potato salad
   E. Cream fillings

2. **Different presentations are possible for SEB. Which of the following would not typically be associated with SEB infection?**
   A. Nausea, vomiting
   B. Nonproductive cough, fever
   C. Myalgia, headache
   D. Bloody diarrhea
   E. Normal chest radiograph

3. Which of the following statements are false regarding SEB?

A. May occur not associated with a terrorist event
B. Is a common cause of food-borne illness
C. Inhalation exposure frequently presents with respiratory symptoms rather than gastrointestinal
D. A human vaccine is currently available
E. Cough symptoms may last for more than 1 week

4. The differential diagnosis for inhalational exposure to SEB could include which of the following?

A. Botulism toxin
B. Nerve agent exposure
C. Influenza
D. Shigella
E. Anthrax

ANSWERS

1: C. *Starchy foods*
2: D. *Bloody diarrhea*
3: D. *A human vaccine is currently available*
4: C. *Influenza*

SECTION A REFERENCES

1. Ulrich RG, Bavari S, Olsen M. Bacterial superantigens in human disease: Structure, function and diversity. Trends Microbiol 1995;3:463-8.
2. Hursh S, McNally R, Fanzone J, et al. Staphylococcal enterotoxin B battlefield challenge: modeling with medical and nonmedical countermeasures. Joppa, MD: Science Applications International Corp; 1995. Technical Report MBDRP-95-2.
3. Stiles BG, Bavari S, Krakauer T, et al. Toxicity of staphylococcal enterotoxins potentiated by lipopolysaccharide: major histocompatability complex class II (MHC class II) molecule dependency and cytokine release. Infect Immun 1993;61:5333-8.
4. Kappler J, Kotzin B, Herron L. Vbeta-specific stimulation of human T-cells by staphylococcal toxins. Science 1989;244:813-7.
5. Peruski AH, Johnson LH, Peruski LF. Rapid and sensitive detection of biological warfare agents using time-resolved fluorescence assays. J Immunol Methods 2002;263:35-41.
6. Kaempher R, Arad G, Levy R, et al. Defense against biological warfare with superantigen toxins. IMAJ 2002;4:520-3.
7. Coffman JD, Zhu J, Roach JM, et al. Production and purification of a recombinant Staphylococcal enterotoxin B vaccine candidate expressed in Escherichia coli. Protein Expr Purif 2002;24(2):302-12.
8. LeClaire RD, Hunt RE, Bavari S. Protection against bacterial superantigen staphylococcal enterotoxin B by passive vaccination. Infect Immun 2002;70:2278-81.
9. Balaban N, Rasooly A. Staphylococcal enterotoxins. Int J Food Microbiol 2000;61:1-10.
10. Mead PS, Slutsker L, Dietz V, et al. Food-related illness and death in the United States. Emerg Infect Dis 1999;5:607-25.
11. Dolin R, Treanor JJ, Madore HP. Novel agents of viral enteritis in humans. J Infect Dis 1987;155:365-76.
12. Anon. Outbreaks of gastroenteritis associated with noroviruses on cruise ships—United States, 2002. Mor Mortal Wkly Rep 2002;51:1112-5.
13. Franz DR, Jahrline PB, Friedlander AM, et al. Clinical recognition and management of patients exposed to biological warfare agents. JAMA 1997;278:399-417.
14. Ulrich RG, Sidell S, Taylor TJ, et al. Staphylococcal enterotoxin B and related pyrogenic toxins. In: Zajtchuk R, Bellamy RF eds. Textbook of military medicine. Part I. Medical aspects of chemical and biological warfare. Washington, DC: Office of the Surgeon General, Department of the Army, 1997.

Section B: Trichothecene Mycotoxins

Sophia Dyer

TRICHOTHECENE MYCOTOXIN, T-2 MYCOTOXIN, "YELLOW RAIN"

THEORETICAL AND SCIENTIFIC BACKGROUND

Mycotoxins have provided many benefits for society: penicillin-based antibiotics; cyclosporine A (an important immunosuppressant for transplant patients); even cholesterol-lowering drugs (such as lovastatin) are based on mycotoxins. Even outside the realm of biological weapons, however, mycotoxins are the source of significant human suffering. Aflatoxin contamination of food is a major source of illness in the form of a potential etiology of hepatocellular carcinoma. Another mycotoxin still in use today medically, but also with severe potential toxic effects, is ergotamine. A contamination of rye with ergotamines is believed by some to be the cause of behavioral changes that led to the Salem witch trials in 1692.

Trichothecenes compose a group of mycotoxins. These mycotoxins are derived from many different fungi: fusarium, myrothecium, stachybotrys, trichoderma, and cephalosporium. Fusarium is the source of weaponized trichothecene T-2 mycotoxin. Although other mycotoxins may also possess the potential for human toxicity, the focus here is on what is known about T-2 mycotoxin as a biological weapon, due to known experience weaponizing this toxin. Another member of the trichothecene mycotoxin family is vomitoxin, with the physiological effects directly related to the toxin's name. Between 1997 and 1998, an estimated 1,700 children in the United States became ill with nausea, abdominal cramps, and of course vomiting after suspected vomitoxin contamination of burritos at a level of less than 1 part per billion in the contaminated food (1). Reports of trichothecene-induced illness from contaminated food date back to 1913 Siberia (2). T-2 mycotoxins have relevance to more modern history. Many are familiar with the "yellow rain" attacks in Southeast Asia in the 1970s, but also in Afghanistan in the late 1970s and reportedly in the Iraqi research weapons machine (3,4). Some believe T-2 mycotoxins were used in Iraqi warheads released in Desert Storm. T-2 mycotoxin has several properties that increase its utility as a biological weapon: It is resistant to UV light degradation, has high heat stability, and although not soluble in water, it

is soluble in solvents such as ethanol, methanol, propylene glycol, and dimethyl sulfoxide (DMSO) (5). An unconfirmed report from the Iran-Iraq war suggested that T-2 mycotoxin was mixed with mustard (a blister agent) (6). Similar to ricin, T-2 mycotoxin can represent not only an inhalation hazard but ingestion in foodstuffs.

T-2 mycotoxins are generally nonvolatile stable compounds. Although stable in high heat, 3% to 5% sodium hypochlorite solution will inactivate the toxins, thus making this the decontamination solution for surfaces and equipment (7). The T-2 mycotoxins' mechanism of action is complex. Several possible sites of cellular damage exist. Most of the focus on T-2 mycotoxin damage is its effects on protein synthesis. T-2 mycotoxin binds to 60S ribosome, affecting peptidyltransferase and peptide bond formation (8), protein elongation, and protein synthesis termination (9). The inhibition of protein syntheses caused by T-2 mycotoxin starts as soon as 5 minutes after exposure in a cell study (10). Trichothecene mycotoxins can cross cell membranes, and their lipophilicity allows for absorption through skin, gastrointestinal, and respiratory systems.

Other research points to the ability of these toxins to cause cellular apoptosis as demonstrated in an animal model with thymus, spleen, liver, and Kupffer cells affected (11). Apoptosis in intestinal crypt cells has been seen (12) with DNA fragmentation potentially initiating apoptotic changes (13). In addition to cellular damage, direct interference with the proper functioning of brain monoamines is possible as demonstrated in the cerebral changes in T-2 mycotoxin–exposed rats (14).

A victim can be exposed to T-2 mycotoxin by several different routes: aerosol, droplets, or dust. Lethality appears to be a factor of route of exposure. The lethal concentration of 50% of an exposed population (LCt50) is given a range of 200 to 5,800 mg min/m^3 (15–17). For skin injury, T-2 mycotoxin is actually more potent than the vesicant mustard with an LD50 of 2 to 12 mg/kg^3. These mycotoxins do not appear to bioaccumulate (18). Metabolism involves utilization of glucuronide conjugation, oxidation, hydrolysis, deepoxidation (19), and enterohepatic recirculation (20).

SIGNS AND SYMPTOMS

Acute inhalation exposure could be expected to involve the entire respiratory system. Inhalation of the toxin will lend itself to potentially swallowing the toxin, thus gastrointestinal symptoms may appear as a component of the respiratory exposure. Respiratory symptoms reported include rhinorrhea, epistaxis, nasal pain and itching, sore throat, aphonia, change in vocal quality, cough, dyspnea, and chest pain (21). Ocular exposure can be assumed to have occurred in most situations that include respiratory exposure to the toxin. Ocular irritation, tearing, blurred vision, and corneal injury could be expected and may last up to 7 days (22,23). Other related symptoms can include anorexia, lethargy, nausea, hypotension, and shock related to gastrointestinal symptoms of diarrhea that can proceed to bloody diarrhea and hematemesis. Symptoms have developed within minutes to hours of exposure. Acute ingestion of the toxin from contaminated food or water supply would be expected to yield these gastrointestinal and systemic presenting symptoms also.

Acute dermal exposures begins to become symptomatic within a few hours after dermal contact. Redness, cutaneous irritation followed by desquamation, as well as the possibility of vesicles increasing to bullae, may result, with symptoms slow to resolve over weeks. Maximal damage is likely seen by 48 hours (21). Differential diagnosis should include exposure to vesicants (such as mustard and Lewisite). Note that, as with mustard agents, T-2 mycotoxin effects do have similarities to radiation exposure and could thus be called a radiomimetic toxin.

Detection can be accomplished in environmental and agricultural samples using GLC (gas-liquid chromatography), TLC (thin-layer chromatography), and HPLC (high-performance liquid chromatography). In biological samples, urine can be analyzed using TLC as well as gas chromatography and mass spectrometry. In the exposed patient, an initial elevation of neutrophil counts followed by falling neutrophil counts, elevation of prothrombin, and partial prothrombin time may be seen. Electrolyte abnormalities may result from gastrointestinal fluid/electrolyte losses as well as anemia if significant hemorrhage occurs or is due to bone marrow injury. Radioimmune assays and enzyme-linked immunoassays for exposure assessment are other technologies that may be available (24).

MEDICAL MANAGEMENT

Exposed skin should be washed with soap and water to prevent further absorption and secondary contamination with the toxin. In an animal study, washing even up to 6 hours after exposure prevented dermal lesions (25). Consideration should be given to the use of activated charcoal in the event of direct oral exposure to T-2 mycotoxin or for inhalation exposure that can lead to secondary ingestion of particles residing on the oral mucosa. Activated charcoal and superactivated charcoal has been found to be useful in reducing mortality in avian and mouse models (26–27). Eye irrigation for ocular exposures may reduce the burden of the toxin. Skin care should comprise decontamination and supportive care with soothing lotions such as calamine. Respiratory care is supportive (humidified supplemental oxygen if indicated, bronchodilators if needed, and cough suppressants). Intravenous hydration may be needed for gastrointestinal losses and hypotension if present. In animal research, selenium pretreatment (acting as a free radical scavenger) reduced toxicity of T-2 mycotoxin (28). Other antioxidants that have been considered include vitamin C and vitamin E in cell-line studies (29).

TRIAGE CONSIDERATIONS

Patients with respiratory symptoms of dyspnea, respiratory distress, and/or pulmonary edema should be carefully observed for the need for potential airway support. Throat irritation and cough are early indicators that respiratory exposure has occurred; those patients should be observed for worsening respiratory symptoms. Patients with gastrointestinal exposures should be considered at risk for dehydration, vomiting, hematemesis, watery or bloody diarrhea, and shock. Neutropenia and/or thrombocytopenia should be screened for because of the radiomimetic effects of this agent.

SUMMARY

- T-2 mycotoxin dermatological exposure: burning, skin inflammation, necrosis, vesicles to bullae.
- T-2 mycotoxin respiratory exposure: cough, throat irritation, chest pain, dyspnea, pulmonary edema to ARDS.

QUESTIONS AND ANSWERS

1. **T-2 mycotoxin dermal exposure can appear similar to which of the following exposures?**
   A. Mustard
   B. Anthrax
   C. Smallpox
   D. Nerve agent
   E. Staphylococcus enterotoxin B

2. **Complications of T-2 mycotoxin can include which of the following?**
   A. ARDS
   B. Shock
   C. Hematemesis
   D. Corneal irritation
   E. All of the above

3. **T-2 mycotoxin causes damage to which of the following cellular components or functions?**
   A. Lipid manufacturing
   B. Protein elongation
   C. Golgi apparatus
   D. Mitochondrial function
   E. Reproductive cell damage only

ANSWERS

1: *A. Mustard*
2: *E. All of the above*
3: *B. Protein elongation*

RESOURCES

1. Tucker JB. Mycotoxins and Gulf War illness: a possible link. The National Gulf War Resource Center, Inc. (www.ngwrc.org/research/exposure/tucker.htm). An interesting alternative account of Gulf War illness.

2. Haig AM. Chemical warfare in Southeast Asia and Afghanistan. Washington, DC: U.S. Government Printing Office; Report to the Congress.

3. Bibliography of all T-2 symptoms with references: Deborah Cazden, 2001: http://www.mycotoxicosis.com/tricothecene.html.

4. Medical management of biological casualties handbook. Frederick, MD: U.S. Army Medical Research Institute of Infectious Diseases, Fort Detrick.

SECTION B REFERENCES

1. Centers for Disease Control and Prevention. Outbreaks of gastrointestinal illness of unknown etiology associated with eating burritos—United States, October 1998, MMWR 1999; 152:210-3.

2. Joffe AZ. Foodborne diseases. In: Rechcegle M ed. Handbook of foodborne disease of biological origin. Boca Raton, FL: CRC Press; 1983;351-495.

3. Rosen RT, Rosen JD. Presence of four Fusarium mycotoxins and synthetic materials in "yellow rain": evidence for the use of chemical weapons in Laos. Biomed Mass Spectrom 1982;9:443-50.

4. The United Nations Blue Book Series. Vol. 9. The United Nations and the Iraq-Kuwait conflict, 1990-1996. New York: United Nations, Department of Public Information, 1996;784.

5. Cole RJ, Cox RH. The trichothecenes. In: Cole RJ, Cox RH eds. Handbook of toxic fungal metabolites. New York: Academic Press, 1981;152-263.

6. Embers LR, Sorenson WG, Lewis DM. Charges of toxic arms use by Iraq escalate. Chem Engineer News 1984;62:16-18.

7. Wannemacher RW, Bunner DL, Dinterman RE. Inactivation of low molecular weight agents of biological origin. In: Proceedings for the Symposium on Agents of Biological Origins. Aberdeen Proving Ground, MD: U.S. Army Chemical Research Development and Engineering Center, 1989.

8. Cundliffe E, Davies JE. Inhibition of initiation, elongation, and termination of eukaryotic protein synthesis by trichothecene fungal toxins. Antimicrob Agents Chemother 1977; 11:491-9.

9. Murthy MR, Radouco-Thomas S, Bharucha AD, et al. Effects of trichothecenes (T-2 mycotoxin) on protein synthesis in vitro by brain polysomes and messenger RNA. Prog Neuropsychopharmacol Biol Psychiatry 1985;9:251-8.

10. Thompson WL, Wannemacher RW. Detection and quantitation of T-2 mycotoxin with a simplified protein synthesis inhibition assay. Appl Environ Microbiol 1984;48:1176-80.

11. Ihara T, Sekijima M, Okumura H, et al. Apoptotic cellular damage in mice after T-2 toxin-induced acute toxicosis. Toxin 1997;5:141-5.

12. Li G, Shinozuka J, Uetsuka K, et al. T-2 toxin induced apoptosis in intestinal crypt epithelial cells of mice. Exp Toxicol Pathol 1997;49:447-50.

13. Islan A, Nagase M, Ota A, et al. Structure-function relationship of T-2 toxin and its metabolites in inducing thymic apoptosis in vivo in mice. Biosci Biotechnol Biochem 1998;62: 1492.

14. Wang J, Fitzpatrick DW, Wilson JR. Effects of the trichothecene mycotoxin T-2 toxin on neurotransmitters and metabolites in discrete areas of the rat brain. Food Chem Toxicol 1998;36:947-53.

15. Creasia DA, Thurman JD, Wannemacher RW, et al. Acute inhalation toxicity of T-2 mycotoxin in the rat and guinea pig. Fundam Appl Toxicol 1990;14:54-9.

16. Marrs TC, Edginton JA, Price PN, et al. Acute toxicity of T2 mycotoxin to the guinea-pig inhalation and subcutaneous routes. Br J Exp Path 1986;67:259-68.

17. Creasia DA, Thurman JD, Jones LJ. Acute inhalation toxicity of T-2 mycotoxin in mice. Fundam Appl Toxicol 1987;8:230-5.

18. Sudakin DL. Trichothecenes in the environment: relevance to human health. Toxicol Letters 2003;143:97-107.

19. Yagen B, Bialer M. Metabolism and pharmacokinetics of T-2 toxin and related trichothecenes. Drug Metab Rev 1993;25: 281-323.

20. Coddington KA, Swanson SP, Hassan AS, et al. Enterohepatic recirculation of T-2 toxin metabolites in the rat. Drug Metab Dispos 1989;17:600-5.

21. Wannemacher RW, Wiener ST. Trichothecene mycotoxins. In: Zajtchuk R, Bellamy RF eds. Textbook of military medicine. Part I. Medical aspects of chemical and biological warfare. Washington, DC: Office of the Surgeon General, Department of the Army, 1997.

22. Wannemacher RW, Bunner DL, Neufeld HA. Toxicity of trichothecenes and other related mycotoxins in laboratory animals. In: Smith JE, Henderson RS eds. Mycotoxins and animal foods. Boca Raton, FL: CRC Press, 1991;499-552.

23. Watson SA, Mirocha CJ, Hayes AW. Analysis for trichothecenes in samples from Southeast Asia associated with "yellow rain." Fundam Appl Toxicol 1984;4:700-17.

24. Fan TS, Zhang GS, Chu FS. An indirect enzyme-linked immunosorbent assay for T-2 toxin in biological fluids. J Food Prot 1984;47:964-7.

25. Wannemacher RW, Bunner DL, Pace JG, et al. Dermal toxicity of T-2 toxin in guinea pigs, rats and cynomolgus monkeys. In: Lacey J ed. Trichothecenes and other mycotoxins. Chichester, England: Wiley, 1985;423-32.

26. Edrighton TS, Kubena LF, Harvey RB, et al. Influence of a superactivated charcoal on the toxic effects of aflatoxin or T-2 toxin in growing broilers. Poult Sci 1997;76:1205-11.

27. Fricke RF, Jorge J. Assessment of efficacy of activated charcoal for treatment of acute T-2 toxin poisoning. J Toxicol Clin Toxicol 1990;28:421-31.

28. Yazdanpanah H, Roshanzamir F, Shafaghi B, et al. Assessment of possible protective roles of selenium, zinc, and cis-silben oxide against acute T-2 toxin poisoning: a preliminary report. Toxin 1997;5:133-5.

29. Shokri F, Heidari, Gharagozloo S, Ghazi-Khansari M. In vitro inhibitory effects of antioxidants on cytotoxicity of T-2 toxin. Toxicol 2000;146:171-6.

Section C: Ricin

Stephen Traub

RICIN

Ricin is a toxin found in castor beans, which are the seeds of the plant *Ricinus communis*. Ricin poisons mammalian ribosomes, that part of the cell responsible for protein synthesis. It is extraordinarily potent, with a lethal dose of 500 to 700 micrograms for the average human adult when inhaled or injected. The U.S. Centers for Disease Control (CDC) classifies ricin as a Class B biological terrorism threat (1,2), identifying it as an agent that can be disseminated with moderate ease and that would be expected to cause significant morbidity.

The processing of castor beans to castor oil, a commonly available consumer product, produces a residue that is rich in ricin. This residue is then heated to deactivate the toxin and used for agricultural purposes. It is conceivable that the residue could be diverted before heating, however, and purified for terrorist purposes.

Ricin is toxic by oral, injected, and inhaled routes. Should ricin ever be used as a weapon of mass destruction, it would most likely be disseminated by aerosolization.

THEORETICAL AND SCIENTIFIC BACKGROUND

MOLECULAR BASIS OF RICIN TOXICITY

Ricin toxin is composed of two protein chains, A and B, which are joined together by a chemical linkage of two sulfur atoms. The ricin A chain produces the biochemical changes that produce cellular toxicity, whereas the ricin B chain governs the entrance of ricin into susceptible cells.

Ricin binds through the B chain to cell surface carbohydrates. These cell surface carbohydrates are ubiquitous within the human body, and thus ricin can bind to and subsequently enter many different types of cells. The exact mechanism by which ricin enters the cell is not completely understood and may involve several different pathways (3).

Once ricin enters the cell, the chemical linkage between the A and B chain is broken. The free A chain then acts as an enzyme that chemically alters mammalian ribosomes (4), rendering them dysfunctional. Because the A chain is an enzyme, which promotes a destructive chemical reaction but is not consumed by it, each ricin A chain molecule is capable of inactivating over 1,000 ribosomes. This, in part, is responsible for ricin's potency because a single molecule can disrupt the protein-synthesis machinery of a cell.

Because ribosomes are crucial to normal protein synthesis, their deactivation by ricin disrupts normal cellular function. Cells incapable of producing the proteins crucial to their survival soon die, producing the cascade of symptoms seen in ricin poisoning.

TECHNICAL CONSIDERATIONS REGARDING RICIN AS A WEAPON OF MASS DESTRUCTION

Contamination of food or water supplies could produce epidemic oral ricin poisoning. This mode of attack would likely be less appealing to terrorists, however, because ricin is several orders of magnitude less toxic when administered by the oral route. Inhalation would likely be the route by which bioterrorists would deliver ricin because it can be stored as a powder, aerosolized without losing its biological activity, and is extremely potent when delivered in this fashion. Although injection can produce severe morbidity and mortality, obvious technical barriers make the use of ricin by this route as a weapon of mass destruction unlikely.

This does not mean it cannot be used by this route as an agent of terror or murder, however. Georgi Markov was an exiled Bulgarian dissident living in London during the height of the Cold War, who was broadcasting scathing anti-Soviet views on the BBC. He was almost assuredly assassinated by a ricin-containing pellet, delivered by means of a modified umbrella (5).

SIGNS AND SYMPTOMS

The signs and symptoms of ricin poisoning depend on the mode of exposure. Scenarios involving oral, injected, and inhaled poisoning are all possible.

Oral. The symptoms encountered in epidemic oral ricin toxicity would likely resemble cases of castor bean ingestion reported in the medical literature (6–9). As such, health care providers should expect to see abdominal pain, nausea, vomiting, and diarrhea occurring within several hours of ingestion; the vomiting and diarrhea may be bloody. This initial gastrointestinal phase may be followed by hypovolemia and circulatory collapse. Hepatotoxicity may occur several days later in moderate to severe cases.

Inhalation. Ricin might be aerosolized for use as a bioweapon. In humans, fulminant inhalational ricin toxicity has not been reported. Inhalational ricin toxicity has been studied in animals, however (10,11), and human inhalational ricin poisoning would likely resemble the symptoms seen in these experimental models. Health care providers should expect to see toxicity developing several hours after exposure. This dose-related toxicity may range from a simple cough in cases of trivial exposure to pulmonary edema and acute respiratory failure in more severe cases.

Injection. Because injection of ricin would involve person-by-person contact between terrorists and their victims, it is the least likely route to be involved in an attack. Health care providers should know the signs and symptoms of ricin injection, however, especially in light of the fact that this toxin has been used as an agent of terror in the past.

Several cases of human ricin poisoning by injection (5,12,13) suggest a clinical syndrome. Pain at the injection site is followed by local lymphadenopathy, after which nausea, vomiting, and gastrointestinal hemorrhage may ensue. Renal, hepatic, and respiratory failure may occur, and in two cases death occurred approximately 3 days after exposure to the toxin.

MEDICAL MANAGEMENT

Treatment of ricin toxicity is entirely supportive. No antidote is available. The initial assessment of the ricin-poisoned patient begins with an assessment of the patient's airway, breathing, and circulation. Patients who are moribund from the latter stages of oral or injectional ricin poisoning, as well as those with respiratory failure from inhalational ricin poisoning, should be intubated endotracheally. Supplemental oxygen should be administered to assure adequate tissue oxygenation; very high levels will likely be required in patients with lung damage from inhalational ricin toxicity. Hypovolemia is expected in virtually all cases of significant ricin poisoning and should be treated with aggressive infusion of crystalloid. Patients who remain hypotensive after appropriate fluid resuscitation require vasopressor therapy. Late complications, such as renal and/or hepatic failure, are managed with aggressive supportive care as well.

TRIAGE CONSIDERATIONS

The triage of ricin-poisoned patients must take into account two factors: the route of exposure and the severity of the patient's illness. Exposure route is important in that inhalational toxicity will produce symptoms more quickly than ingestion or injection. Pulmonary deterioration should be predicted, and patients should be triaged to an appropriate area or facility.

Severity of patient illness should govern other triage decisions, with the most ill-appearing patients addressed first. Because there is no antidote for ricin poisoning, there is no pressure to deliver these patients to a hospital quickly for preemptive treatment.

PERSONAL PROTECTION

Water precautions. Ricin is stable in water and resistant to traditional chlorine decontamination techniques. The reverse osmosis water purification unit used by the U.S. military effectively purifies drinking water. An easier approach to purification of potentially ricin-tainted potable water is boiling for 10 minutes, which inactivates the heat-labile toxin (14).

Respiratory precautions. Appropriate respiratory precautions will prevent inhalation of ricin in the event of an aerosolized attack. Standard U.S. military issue M17 or M40 masks are acceptable respiratory precautions (15), and civilians would likely rely on level C or better "hazmat" gear.

Vaccination. Vaccination with inactivated ricin toxoid attenuates ricin-induced lung injury in experimental animal models. Protection has been demonstrated whether the toxoid is delivered orally (16), subcutaneously (17), or directly into the lung (18). Although such work is encouraging, it should be noted that vaccination would have to occur days or weeks prior to exposure to have any benefit. Furthermore, this experimental work is at this time confined to animal models.

SUMMARY

Ricin is a potent, naturally occurring toxin that poisons mammalian cells by disrupting normal protein synthesis. It is toxic by the oral, inhaled, and injected routes. Symptoms vary depending on dose or route of exposure, but pulmonary toxicity from inhalational exposure and hypovolemia regardless of route of exposure are the most feared sequelae. Care is supportive because no antidote to ricin poisoning exists.

RESOURCES

Centers for Disease Control and Prevention: Ricin: http://www.bt.cdc.gov/agent/ricin/faq/index.asp.

QUESTIONS AND ANSWERS

1. **Ricin is an extremely potent toxin. Which of the following represents a potentially lethal dose of inhaled ricin?**
   A. 500 micrograms
   B. 5 grams
   C. 50 grams
   D. 500 grams

2. **Ricin may produce toxicity via several mechanisms of exposure. Which of the following is NOT a route of exposure that would be expected to cause toxicity?**
   A. Dermal

B. Oral
C. Injected
D. Inhaled

3. Which of following is NOT a clinical feature of ricin poisoning?

A. Acute lung injury
B. Vomiting and diarrhea
C. Hypotension from circulatory collapse
D. Paralysis

4. Which of the following statements about the treatment of ricin poisoning is FALSE?

A. The initial treatment of dehydration and/or hypotension is aggressive crystalloid infusion.
B. Hypotension unresponsive to crystalloid infusion may require vasopressor therapy.
C. Hypoxia should be treated with supplemental oxygen.
D. The ricin antidote, if delivered within 2 hours of exposure, will prevent the development of any clinical symptoms.

ANSWERS

1: *A. 500 micrograms. One half of one gram represents a lethal dose of inhaled ricin. Aerosolization of even a few hundred grams of ricin, therefore, could easily produce a mass casualty incident.*

2: *A. Dermal. The skin provides an effective barrier against ricin because the protein does not penetrate intact integument. Oral toxicity from ricin poisoning may occur, although higher doses of ricin would be needed to produce toxicity by this route. Injected or inhaled ricin is expected to cause serious morbidity or mortality in doses of less than 1 gram.*

3: *D. Paralysis. Answers a, b, and c are all symptoms that one might see after ricin poisoning. Paralysis is a common finding in poisoning by nerve agents and might be seen after poisoning by botulinum toxin, but it is not an expected finding in ricin poisoning.*

4: *D. The ricin antidote, if delivered within 2 hours of exposure, will prevent the development of any clinical symptoms. Answers A, B, and C all represent appropriate therapy for ricin poisoning. At the present time, there is no antidote for ricin poisoning; treatment is supportive.*

SECTION C REFERENCES

1. Centers for Disease Control and Prevention. Biological and chemical terrorism: strategic plan for preparedness and response. Recommendations of the CDC Strategic Planning Workgroup.
2. MMWR Recomm Rep 2000;49(RR-4):1-14.
3. Lord MJ, Jolliffe NA, Marsden CJ, et al. Ricin: mechanism of cytotoxicity. Toxicol Rev 2003;22(1):53-64.
4. Endo Y, Tsurugi K. The RNA N-glycosidase activity of ricin A-chain. The characteristics of the enzymatic activity of ricin A-chain with ribosomes and with rRNA. J Biol Chem 1988;263(18):8735-9.
5. Crompton R, Gall D. Georgi Markov—death in a pellet. Med Leg J 1980;48(2):51-62.
6. Aplin PJ, Eliseo T. Ingestion of castor oil plant seeds. Med J Aust 1997;167(5):260-1.
7. Challoner KR, McCarron MM. Castor bean intoxication. Ann Emerg Med 1990;19(10):1177-83.
8. Kopferschmitt J, Flesch F, Lugnier A, et al. Acute voluntary intoxication by ricin. Hum Toxicol 1983;2(2):239-42.
9. Wedin GP, Neal JS, Everson GW, et al. Castor bean poisoning. Am J Emerg Med 1986;4(3):259-61.
10. Griffiths GD, Rice P, Allenby AC, et al. Inhalation toxicology and histopathology of ricin and abrin toxins. Inhal Toxicol 1995;7;269-88.
11. Brown RF, White DE. Ultrastructure of rat lung following inhalation of ricin aerosol. Int J Exp Pathol 1997;78(4):267-76.
12. Fine DR, Shepherd HA, Griffiths GD, et al. Sub-lethal poisoning by self-injection with ricin. Med Sci Law 1992;32(1):70-2.
13. Targosz D, Winnik L, Szkolnicka B. Suicidal poisoning with castor bean (*Ricinus communis*) extract injected subcutaneously: Case report [abstract]. J Toxicol Clin Toxicol 2002;40:398.
14. Burrows WD, Renner SE. Biological warfare agents as threats to potable water. Environ Health Perspect 1999;107(12):975-84.
15. Wiener SL. Strategies for the prevention of a successful biological warfare aerosol attack. Mil Med 1996;161(5):251-6.
16. Kende M, Yan C, Hewetson J, et al. Oral immunization of mice with ricin toxoid vaccine encapsulated in polymeric microspheres against aerosol challenge. Vaccine 2002;20 (11-12):1681-91.
17. Griffiths GD, Lindsay CD, Allenby AC, et al. Protection against inhalation toxicity of ricin and abrin by immunisation. Hum Exp Toxicol 1995;14(2):155-64.
18. Griffiths GD, Bailey SC, Hambrook JL, et al. Liposomally-encapsulated ricin toxoid vaccine delivered intratracheally elicits a good immune response and protects against a lethal pulmonary dose of ricin toxin. Vaccine 1997;15(17-18):1933-9.

Nuclear Terrorism

13

Types of Radiation: Basic Theory Explained for the Nonphysicist

Greene Shepherd

THEORETICAL AND SCIENTIFIC BACKGROUND

What are radiation and radioactivity? What are the immediate and long-term threats to life and health that can result from exposure? How is it detected? What safety measures are needed? Where can I find expert help? These are questions that many health care professionals are uncomfortable answering. The next several chapters are devoted to addressing such questions for the clinician. The goal of the current chapter is to provide a clear and user-friendly description of radiological principles.

Radiation is simply the release of energy from atoms in the form of particles or waves. To understand how radiation is generated, a basic understanding about the structure of atoms is needed. Atoms are the basic building blocks of all matter (Fig. 13-1). The atom consists of a central nucleus, with shells of electrons orbiting around this nucleus. Electrons are very small relative to the size of the nucleus and are negatively charged. The nucleus carries a positive charge and is made up of protons and neutrons. Each element has a defined number of protons. These protons, which are posi-

tively charged, have the tendency to repel each other. Neutrons also exist in the nucleus of atoms, except for hydrogen, which only has one proton. Neutrons are roughly the same size as protons, but they do not carry a charge. Think of neutrons as spacers that keep the positively charged protons from repelling each other. In most atoms there is an average ratio of 1.2 neutrons for every 1 proton. When such a balance exists, the nucleus of the atom is very stable and emits little energy except under very extreme conditions. When there is an imbalance of this ratio of protons to neutrons, an element is radioactive. Often the imbalance is due to an excess of neutrons. An element with an unbalanced nucleus is referred to as an isotope or radionuclide. Different isotopes of the same element are identified based on the difference between the atomic weights. For example the atomic weight of iodine is normally 125.9 g/mol while the most common radioactive isotope weighs 131 g/mol. The extra weight in this case comes from excess neutrons. In order for the nucleus of the atom to return to a stable or balanced condition it will release energy. This release of energy is referred to as radioactive decay or simple decay (Fig. 13-2). This process will continue until enough energy has been released for the nucleus to stabilize.

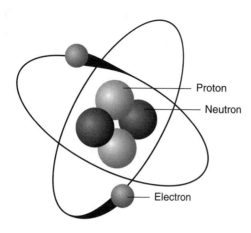

Figure 13–1. The basic structure of an atom.

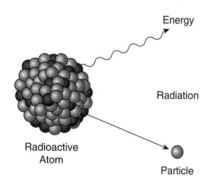

Figure 13–2. Emission of energy from a radioactive atom in the form of a wave (**top**) and a particle (**bottom**). (From the Nuclear Regulatory Commission: http://www.nrc.gov/reading-rm/basic-ref/glossary/radioactivity.html.)

The energy is released in two forms that can be described as particles and waves. The first form of radiation is tiny fast-moving particles that have both energy and mass (weight). The other form of radiation is pure energy with no weight. This kind of radiation is vibrating or pulsating waves of electrical and magnetic energy. It is also referred to as electromagnetic waves or electromagnetic radiation. Another way of describing radiation is in terms of how it interacts with matter; it can be classified as ionizing or nonionizing. Ionization is the process of removing electrons from atoms, leaving two electrically charged particles (ions) behind. Ionizing radiation comes in the form of atomic particles and waves that deliver a large amount of energy. Nonionizing radiation does not have sufficient energy to remove electrons from atoms (1,2).

An unstable nucleus can become stable by changing a neutron into a proton with the ejection of a negative bit of matter (a beta particle or electron). Conversely, a proton can change into a neutron with the ejection of a positively charged bit of matter (a positron or positively charged electron). The nucleus of large unstable atoms can reach stability by ejecting larger particles that consist of two protons and two neutrons (an alpha particle). Since the number of protons can change as an atom reaches stability, the resultant element can be different than the original one.

Because energy is released at predictable rates, we are able to calculate the half-life ($t_{1/2}$) of the radioactive element. This is simply the amount of time it takes for the amount of a radioactive isotope to decrease by 50% as it loses energy to become a stable element. These half-lives can be very short (technetium 99m, $t_{1/2}$ = 6 hours) or very long (Uranium 235, $t_{1/2}$ = 7.1 _ 10^8 years). It is important to remember that even a tiny amount of a substance (say a milligram) will contain millions of individual atoms. When thinking about radioactive decay, we are really dealing with the conversion of individual atoms. When we talk about half-life, we are talking about how many atoms are decaying over a period of time. For example if we started with 100 atoms of a radioactive element, the half-life would indicate how long it would take for 50 of the atoms to decay to a stable configuration. Half-lives will not be the same for different isotopes. Table 13-1 contains a list of common isotopes with half-lives and types of radiation emitted. When all the excess energy and mass is given off, the resultant element finally becomes stable. For all practical purposes, any amount of radioactive material will be completely depleted after 10 half-lives.

The most common types of ionizing radiation are alpha particles, beta particles, protons, gamma rays, and x-rays. Alpha particles usually have high energies (4 million to 8 million electron volts, or MeV), and they consist of two protons and two neutrons. They travel a few centimeters in air and up to 60 micrometers into tissue. The high energy and short path result in a dense track of ionization along the tissues with which the particles interact. Alpha particles will not penetrate the stratum corneum of the skin, and thus they are not an external hazard. However, if alpha-emitting elements are taken into the body by inhalation or ingestion or from open wounds, serious problems such as cancer may develop. Alpha emitters are primarily uranium isotopes and are generally found in nuclear chemistry laboratories and isotope production facilities. They can also be found in hospitals that offer nuclear medical services. They are not likely to be used as a weapon unless combined with a conventional explosive device (Chapter 17). The path length of a proton is somewhat longer than that of an alpha particle of equivalent energy. Beta particles interact much less readily with matter than do alpha particles and will travel up to a few centimeters into tissue or many meters through air. Exposure to external sources of beta particles is potentially hazardous, but internal exposure is more hazardous. Examples of beta-particle emitters are the isotopes carbon-14, gold-198, iodine-131, radium-226, cobalt-60, selenium-75, and chromium-51. Protons with energies of a few million electron volts can be produced by high-energy accelerators and are quite effective in producing tissue ionization. They are similar to alpha particles but have a longer path length and are more likely to produce hazardous effects. Gamma rays are electromagnetic energy emitted from the nucleus. They have a range of many meters in air and many centimeters in tissue and, like beta particles, constitute a biologic hazard both internally and externally. Examples of gamma emitters are cobalt-60, cesium-137, iridium-192, and radium-226. X-rays, like gamma rays, are high-energy electromagnetic energy with short wavelengths. X-rays and gamma rays are sometimes referred to as photons. These waves or rays are very penetrating and can ionize atoms deep within the body. X-rays generally have longer wavelengths and lower frequencies relative to gamma rays; consequently, they have lower energies. The biologic effects of x-rays and gamma rays are better known than any of the other forms of ionizing radiation.

| TABLE 13-1 | Isotopes Listed Alphabetically* |

ISOTOPE	PHYSICAL HALF-LIFE	EFFECTIVE HALF-LIFE	RADIATION TYPE
Americium-241	458 yr	139 yr	a, e-, g
Americium-243	7950 yr	194 yr	a, g
Antimony-122	67 h	—	b-, b+, g
Antimony-124	60 d	—	b-, g
Antimony-125	2.7 yr	—	b-, e-, g
Argon-37	35 d	—	g
Arsenic-74	18 d	17 d	b-, b+, g
Arsenic-76	26.5 h	—	b-, g
Arsenic-77	39 h	24 h	b-, g
Barium-131	12 d	—	g, e-
Barium-133	7.2 yr	—	g, e+
Barium-137m	2.55 min	—	g, e-
Barium-140	13 d	11 d	b-, e-, g
Beryllium-7	53 d	—	g
Bismuth-207	30 yr	—	e-, g
Bismuth-210	5.01 d	—	a, b-, g
Bromine-82	35.34 h	—	b-, g
Cadmium-109	453 d	140 d	e-, g
Cadmium-115	53.5 h	—	b-, g
Cadmium-115	43 d	—	b-, g
Calcium-45	165 d	162 d	b-
Calcium-47	4.5 d	4.5 d	b-, g
Californium-243	2.6 yr	2.2 yr	g, a, N
Carbon-11	20.3 min	—	b+, g
Carbon-14	5730 yr	12 d	b-
Cerium-141	33 d	30 d	b-, e-, g
Cerium-144	284 d	280 d	b-, e-, g
Cesium-131	9.70 d	—	g
Cesium-134	2.05 yr	—	b-, g
Cesium-137	30.0 yr	70 d	b-, e-, g
Chlorine-36	3.1 _ 105 yr	—	b-, g
Chromium-51	27.8 d	27 d	e-, g
Cobalt-57	270 d	9 d	e-, g
Cobalt-58	71.3 d	8 d	b+, g
Cobalt-60	5.26 yr	10 d	b-, g
Copper-64	12.8 h	—	b-, e-, b+, g
Curium-242	163 d	155 d	a, N, g
Curium-243	32 yr	27.5 d	a, g
Curium-244	17.6 yr	16.7 yr	a, N, g
Dysprosium-159	144 d	—	e-, g
Erbium-169	9.4 d	—	b-, e-, g
Europium-152	13 yr	3 yr	b-, b+, e-, g
Europium-154	16 yr	3 yr	b-, e-, g
Europium-155	2 yr	1.3 yr	b-, e-, g
Fluorine-18	2 h	2 h	b, g
Gadolinium-153	242 d	—	e-, g
Gallium-67	78.1 h	—	g
Gallium-68	68.3 min	—	b+, g
Gallium-72	14.1 h	12 h	b, g
Germanium-71	11.4 d	—	g
Gold-195	183 d	—	e-, g
Gold-198	2.7 d	2.6 d	b-, e-, g
Gold-199	75.6 h	—	b-, e-, g
Hafnium-181	42.5 d	—	b-, e-, g

| TABLE 13-1 | Isotopes Listed Alphabetically* (continued) | | |

ISOTOPE	PHYSICAL HALF-LIFE	EFFECTIVE HALF-LIFE	RADIATION TYPE
Holmium-166	26.9 h	—	b-, e-, g
Hydrogen-3	12 yr	12 d	b-
Indium-111	2.8 d	—	g
Indium-113m	100 min	—	e-, g
Indium-114	72 sec	—	b-, b+, g
Indium-114m	49 d	27 d	e-, g (DR)
Iodine-123	13 h	—	g
Iodine-125	60 d	42	e-, g
Iodine-129	1.7 _ 107 yr	—	b-, e-, g
Iodine-130	12.4 h	—	b-, g
Iodine-131	8.05 d	8 d	b-, e-, g
Iridium-192	74 d	—	b-, e-, g
Iridium-194	17.4 h	—	b, c, g
Iron-52	8.3 h	—	b-, g
Iron-55	2.6 yr	1 yr	g
Iron-59	45 d	42d	b-, g
Krypton-81m	13.0 sec	—	g
Krypton-85	10.76 yr	—	b-, g
Lanthanum-140	40.22 h	—	b-, g
Lead-210	2 yr	1.3 yr	a, b-, e-, g
Lutetium-177	6.7 d	—	b-, e-, g
Magnesium-28	21 h	—	b-, e-, g
Manganese-54	303 d	—	e-, g
Mercury-197	2.7 d	2.3 d	e-, g
Mercury-197m	24 h	—	e-, g
Mercury-203	4 d	11 d	b-, e-, g
Molybdenum-99	67 h	1.5 d	b-, g
Neodymium-147	11.1 d	—	b-, e-, g
Neptunium-237	2 _ 106 yr	200 yr	a, g (DR)
Neptunium-239	2.3 d	2.3 d	b, g
Nickel-63	92 yr	—	b-
Niobium-95	35 d	—	b+, g
Osmium-191	15 d	—	b-, e-, g
Oxygen-15	124 sec	—	b+, g
Palladium-103	17 d	—	g
Palladium-109	13.47 h	—	b-, e-, g
Phosphorus-32	14 d	14 d	b-
Plutonium-238	88 yr	63 yr	g, a
Plutonium-239	2.4 _ 104 yr	197 yr	g, a
Polonium-210	138 d	46 d	a, g
Potassium-42	12 h	12 h	b-, g
Praseodymium-142	19.2 h	—	b-, g
Praseodymium-143	13.6 d	—	b-
Praseodymium-144	17.3 min	—	b-, g
Promethium-147	2.6 yr	1.6 yr	b-
Promethium-149	2.2 d	2.2 d	b-, g
Protactinium-233	27.0 d	—	b-, e-, g
Protactinium-234	6.75 h	—	b-, e-, g
Radium-224	3.6 d	3.6 d	g, a (DR)
Radium-226	160 yr	44 yr	a, e-, g (DR)
Rhenium-186	90 h	—	b-, e-, g
Rhodium-106	30 sec	—	b-, g
Rubidium-82	1.3 min	—	b+, g
Rubidium-86	19.0 d	13.2 d	b-, g

| TABLE 13-1 | Isotopes Listed Alphabetically* *(continued)* |

ISOTOPE	PHYSICAL HALF-LIFE	EFFECTIVE HALF-LIFE	RADIATION TYPE
Ruthenium-97	2.9 d	—	e-, g
Ruthenium-103	39.6 d	—	b-, g
Ruthenium-106	367 d	2.5 d	b- (DR)
Samarium-151	87 yr	—	b-, e-, g
Samarium-153	47 h	—	b-, e-, g
Scandium-46	84 d	40 d	b-, g
Selenium-75	120.4 d	—	e-, g
Selenium-77m	17.5 sec	—	g
Silver-110	24.4 sec	—	b-, g
Silver-110m	253 d	5 d	b-, e-, g
Silver-111	7.5 d	—	b-, g
Sodium-22	2.60 yr	11 d	b+, g
Sodium-24	15 h	14 h	b-, g
Strontium-85	64 d	64 d	e-, g
Strontium-87m	2.83 hr	—	e-, g
Strontium-89	52 d	—	b-, g
Strontium-90	28 yr	15 yr	b- (DR)
Sulfur-35	88 d	44 d	b-
Tantalum-182	115 d	—	b-, e-, g
Technetium-99	2.12 _ 105 yr	20 d	b-
Technetium-99m	6.0 h	—	e-, g
Tellurium-132	78 h	—	b-, e-, g
Terbium-160	72.1 d	—	b-, e-, g
Thallium-201	73 h	—	g (DR)
Thallium-204	3.8 yr	—	b-, g
Thorium-230	8 _ 104 yr	200 yr	a, g

* a, alpha; b, beta; e, electron; g, gamma; DR, daughter radiation; N, neutron.

Adapted from Ellhorn, M.J. ed. Ellenhorn's medical toxicology: diagnosis and treatment of human poisoning. 2nd ed. Baltimore: Williams & Wilkins; 1997.

Nonionizing radiation is quite common and consists of low-energy electromagnetic waves. This includes the visible spectrum, infrared, and ultraviolet light. Low-energy electromagnetic energy such as radio waves and microwaves are also nonionizing forms of radiation. Nonionizing radiation lacks the energy to dislodge orbital electrons or destroy the physical integrity of an impacted atom. Generally speaking, nonionizing radiation is not able to cause mass casualties. Although largely improbable, nonionizing electromagnetic devices such as lasers or electromagnetic pulses could theoretically be used by terrorists to damage structures or interrupt the function of electronic devices.

RADIATION UNITS

Like most drugs or chemicals, there is a relationship between radiation dose and its effect on the body. To quantify the varying effects of radiation exposure, one must be able to understand the dose of radiation. Most drug dosing can be thought of as an amount (grams, etc.) per unit of body weight (kilograms or pounds). Radiation dosing can be thought of as an amount of energy absorbed by the body.

The dosing can be acute, a one time exposure, or chronic, a cumulative dose over time. Table 13-2 contains definitions of the units and terms that are used to describe radiation and its dosing. Currently, two systems of units describing radiation are widely used. In the United States the older terms "rads," "rems," and "curies" are frequently used, while newer units consisting of "gray," "sievert," and "becquerel" are used internationally. Table 13-3 shows the relationship between the different systems of units. The international system is becoming more popular because it produces numbers that are more practical to use when describing effects of commonly encountered doses. For the purpose of this section, the older and more familiar terms will be used followed by the newer units in parentheses where appropriate.

The basic unit for measuring radiation is the rad (or the international Gy). The rad is defined as the deposition of 0.01 joule of energy per kilogram of tissue. Think of rad (Gy) as a one time dose, like an x-ray. To quantify the amount of damage that is suspected from a radiation exposure, rads (or an equivalent number of Gy) are converted into rems, which at one time stood for Roentgen Equivalent Man. The rem (or the similar international unit sievert, or Sv) is adjusted to reflect the type of radiation absorbed and the likelihood of damage (Table 13-2). Think of rem (Sv) as

TABLE 13-2 Radiation Measurements and Definitions (S1 Units in Descriptions)

CHARACTERISTIC	UNITS	DESCRIPTION
Energy	Electron volt (eV) or Joule (J)	eV = Kinetic energy of an electron as it moves through a potential difference of 1 volt. J = the kinetic energy of an object with a mass of 2 kilograms moving with a velocity of one meter per second.
Half-life	Time	The time required for the radioactivity of an isotope to decrease by 50%.
Rate of radioactive decay	Curie (Ci) or Becquerel (Bq)	Radioactivity emitted per unit of time 1 Ci = 3.7 _ 10^{10} disintegrations per second. 3.7 _ 10^{-10} Ci = 1Bq = 1 disintegration per second.
Air exposure	Roentgen (R)	Used to quantify ionization caused by x-rays or gamma radiation in air. One roentgen of exposure will produce about 2 billion ion pairs per cubic centimeter of air.
Absorbed dose	Rad or Gray (Gy)	The amount of ionizing radiation that the body absorbs. One rad results in the absorption of 0.01 Joule (1 Gy = 1 Joule) of ionizing radiation per gram of medium.
Biologic effectiveness	Rem or Sievert (Sv)	Dose of any form of ionizing radiation that produces the same biological effect as 1 roentgen; 1 rem = 1 rad × Penetrating Factor (PF), where the value of PF depends on the type of radiation as follows:
		x-radiation = 1.0 gamma radiation = 1.0 beta = 1.0 alpha = 20 neutrons = 5 to 20, depending on their energy

Agency for Toxic Substances and Disease Registry. Toxicological profile for ionizing radiation. Atlanta: U.S. Department of Health and Human Services, Public Health Service; 1993.

TABLE 13-3 Conversions Between New and Old Units Used for Describing Radiation

QUANTITY	OLD UNIT	SYMBOL	NEW UNIT	SYMBOL	RELATIONSHIP
Activity	curie	Ci	becquerel	Bq	1 Ci = 3.7 _ 1010 Bq
Absorbed dose	rad	rad	gray	Gy	1 rad = 0.01 Gy
Dose equivalent	rem	rem	sievert	Sv	1 rem = 0.01 Sv

the cumulative dose. In most cases of one time "flash" exposure, the rad (Gy) and rem (Sv) will be equivalent. For example, a standard x-ray machine was used to deliver 100 rads of radiation. If you get exposed every day for 10 days your cumulative dose (100 rads per day) would be 1000 rem (Tables 13-1 to 13-3).

Radiation is measured by a variety of instruments (Chapter 14). The instrument used depends on the type of radiation being emitted. Personnel who have a potential for radiation exposure will need to work with badges or other devices to measure their exposure levels. This will allow planning for how to rotate staff and to know who might require treatment.

RADIATION DOSES IN PERSPECTIVE

Radioactivity has existed for millions of years in the crust of the earth, in building materials, in the food we eat, in the air we breathe, and in virtually everything that surrounds us. Radiation from these materials, as well as cosmic radiation from the sun and universe, makes up the natural background radiation to which we are constantly exposed.

Most individuals are exposed to about 360 millirems (3.6 mSv) per year from natural and man-made sources.

Smoking 1.5 packs of cigarettes a day for 1 year produces an accumulative radiation dose of 16 rem (0.16 Sv) to the bifurcation of the bronchus. If an individual is exposed to more than 100 rads (1 Gy) at one time, predictable signs and symptoms will develop within a few hours, days, or weeks depending on the dose. Fifty percent of individuals exposed to a single dose of 450 rads (4.5 Gy) of penetrating radiation will die without medical intervention, within 60 days.

The dose of radiation a person receives and the likelihood of adverse effects from radiation exposure depend on four factors: source of radiation, distance from the source, duration of exposure, and shielding. Identifying the radiation *source* is important because the magnitude and type of radiation being released can be determined from it. As previously discussed, penetrating forms of ionizing radiation are the most concerning. It is also important to appreciate how much radioactive source material is present. The dose of radiation decreases dramatically as the *distance* away from the source of radiation is increased. Avoiding direct physical contact with the source is important in limiting exposure. If a person is forced to work in close proximity to a radiation source, he or she should be allowed to use tools that allow the person to work at a distance from the source. Even simple tools such as poles, rakes, or shovels can dramatically reduce the dose. A general rule of thumb is that by doubling the distance from the radiation an individual will get four times less radiation. If the distance between the individual and the source is halved, exposure will increase by a factor of four. This phenomenon is described by a mathematical model known as the inverse square law (Fig. 13-3). The further the person is away from the source, the lower the radiation dose will be. *Duration* of exposure is another important factor in estimating the total dose absorbed. The shorter the time within in a radiation field, the less the radiation exposure. Limiting time in close proximity to the radiation source will dramatically decrease the total dose absorbed. *Shielding* refers to anything that can be placed between the individual and the radiation source to block its effects. Radiation can also be blocked or reduced by various materials. In general, dense materials are better shields than materials with low density. However, there are some exceptions. Alpha radiation can be stopped by a sheet of paper. Alpha particles travel approximately 1 to 2 inches in air and cannot penetrate unbroken skin. Beta particles travel up to 10 feet in air and can penetrate a few millimeters of tissue. They can be stopped by light layers of clothing, aluminum foil, or an average book. Gamma rays are only reduced by dense materials such as steel, concrete, earth, or lead. Gamma rays can travel several hundred feet in air and penetrate the human body. Neutrons can travel several hundred feet in air and are very damaging to cells. They can be slowed or stopped by hydrogenous materials (wax, water, or plastics). Do *not* shield neutron-producing sources with lead or dense materials. The neutrons will collide with the atoms in these materials and emit gamma rays in the process. Using wax, water, or plastic as a covering for more dense shielding will minimize secondary radiation from neutrons. This approach offers the safest shielding when dealing with an unidentified source

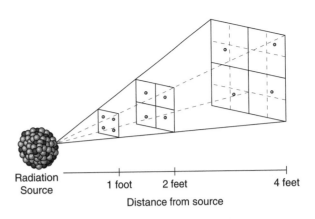

Figure 13–3. The inverse square law demonstrates how the radiation dose decreases as you move away from the source of the radiation. Notice how the spacing between the particles increases as they move away from the source.

of radiation. When dealing with radiation, the factors of distance, duration, and shielding can be manipulated to decrease health risks.

TYPE OF RADIATION EXPOSURE

Three types of radiation exposure can occur: external irradiation, contamination, or incorporation. *External* irradiation occurs when all or part of the body is exposed to penetrating radiation from an external source. During exposure, this radiation can be absorbed by the body or can pass completely through it. A similar thing occurs during an ordinary chest x-ray. This type of exposure can occur all at once, like a single x-ray, or on a chronic basis, as with a person who works with radium every day. Following external exposure, an individual is not radioactive and can be treated like any other patient. *Contamination* means that radioactive materials in the form of gases, liquids, and/or solids are on/in a person's body are said to be contaminated. An external surface of the body, such as the skin, can become contaminated, and if radioactive materials get inside the body (through the lungs, gastrointestinal tract, or wounds), the contaminant can become deposited internally. Contaminated individuals are at significant risk due to close proximity to the radiation and the potential for a long duration of exposure unless they are decontaminated. *Incorporation* refers to the uptake of radioactive materials by body cells, tissues, and target organs such as bone, liver, thyroid, or kidney. In general, radioactive materials are distributed throughout the body based upon their chemical properties. Incorporation cannot occur unless internal contamination has occurred. Individuals who are contaminated can pose a risk to other people. These three types of events (i.e., external irradiation, contamination, and incorporation) can happen in combination and can be complicated by physical injury or illness.

Radioactive iodine is probably the most common and significant of isotopes that can be incorporated into the body. The thyroid is the only organ in the body that uses iodine. Blocking available sites for iodine in the thyroid with nonradioactive iodine prevents incorporation. When the thyroid is properly blocked, radioactive iodine has nowhere else to go and will be eliminated in the urine without noticeable effect, no matter how much an individual is exposed to. Unfortunately, the nonradioactive iodine has to get there before the radioactive iodine, so potassium iodide must be administered within 4 hours of the exposure to be effective. After 12 hours, there is no protective effect. Elimination of internal contamination with other isotopes such as uranium and tritium may be hastened through urinary alkalinization and forced fluids to reduce the potential for injury.

MEDICAL MANAGEMENT

The most immediate source of expertise on patients who are exposed or contaminated by radioactive substances will likely be a medical physicist, nuclear pharmacist, or radiation safety officer. Most governments require that any health facility that administers radiation to patients (as diagnostic studies or therapy) have a person with significant training and experience assessing and treating the effects of radiation on people. Such individuals will also be very familiar with how to activate the assistance of governmental resources if needed. Due to their wide distribution and specialized knowledge, such individuals are invaluable local resources when planning, doing training exercises, or responding to actual threats.

SUMMARY

Radiation is energy released from unstable atoms. It can be released as particles or as waves. If the radiation has enough energy, it can produce dangerous ionizing interactions with living tissue. The dose absorbed depends on the source of the radiation, the distance from it, shielding, and the duration of exposure. Knowledge of these factors can help to minimize exposures.

COMMON FORMS OF IONIZING RADIATION

- Alpha particles—Intermediate energy and low penetration
- Beta particles—Low energy and intermediate penetration
- Gamma rays or x-rays—High energy and high penetration

PRINCIPLES FOR MINIMIZING EXPOSURE

- Stay as far away from the source as practical.
- Use appropriate shielding.
- Limit exposure time.

QUESTIONS AND ANSWERS

1. Which of the following is NOT a common type of ionizing radiation?
   A. Beta particles
   B. Electrons
   C. Gamma rays
   D. Protons
   E. X-rays

2. Which of the following is NOT TRUE regarding alpha particles?
   A. Alpha particles usually have low energies.
   B. Alpha particles consist of two protons and two neutrons.
   C. Alpha particles will not penetrate the stratum corneum of the skin.
   D. Alpha particles travel a few centimeters in air and up to 60 micrometers into tissue.
   E. Alpha particle emitters are primarily uranium isotopes and are generally found in nuclear chemistry laboratories and isotope production facilities.

3. Which of the following statements is FALSE?
   A. If an individual is exposed to more than 100 rads at one time, predictable signs and symptoms will develop within a few hours, days, or weeks depending on the dose.
   B. All individuals exposed to a single dose of 450 rads of penetrating radiation will die within 60 days if they receive no medical intervention.
   C. Most individuals are exposed to about 360 millirems per year from natural and man-made sources.
   D. Alpha radiation can be stopped by a sheet of paper.
   E. Gamma rays are only reduced by dense materials such as steel, concrete, earth, or lead.

4. Which of the following is NOT CORRECT?
   A. A rem is the dosage of any ionizing radiation that will cause biologic injury to human tissue equal to the injury caused by 1 roentgen of x-ray or gamma-ray dosage.
   B. A rad is a unit that measures the absorbed dose of ionizing radiation.
   C. A roentgen is a unit of measure quantifying ionization produced by x-radiation or alpha-ray radiation.
   D. A curie is a measure of a substance's radioactivity.
   E. Radioactive half-life is the time required for the radioactivity of an isotope to decrease by 50%.

ANSWERS

1: *B. Electrons.*
2: *A. Alpha particles usually have low energies.*
3: *B. All individuals exposed to a single dose of 450 rads of penetrating radiation will die within 60 days if they receive no medical intervention.*
4: *C. A roentgen is a unit of measure quantifying ionization produced by x-radiation or alpha-ray radiation.*

REFERENCES

1. Agency for Toxic Substances and Disease Registry. Toxicological profile for ionizing radiation. Atlanta: U.S. Department of Health and Human Services, Public Health Service; 1993.
2. Agency for Toxic Substances and Disease Registry. Toxicological profile for ionizing radiation. Atlanta: U.S. Department of Health and Human Services, Public Health Service; 1999.

14

Detection of Nuclear Radiation

Keith Edsall and Daniel C. Keyes

INTRODUCTION

Ionizing radiation is not detectable by any natural means. Specific devices are necessary to detect alpha, beta, gamma, x-rays, and neutrons. Medical staff must learn to use simple portable instruments and interpret the findings, and they must also be aware of the associated pitfalls when using these instruments. Understanding the technical aspects of the working of the instrument is not essential, but those interested can obtain the information from any nuclear physics textbook. Note that this chapter uses the units of rads and rems, currently used in the United States. See Chapter 13 for a discussion of newer international units of measurement used in discussing radiation.

RADIATION DETECTION INSTRUMENTS

Instruments used to detect radiation can be divided into three major categories: portable instruments, laboratory instruments, and personnel and area dosimeters (Table 14-1).

TABLE 14-1 Instrument Requirements Based on the Type of Radiation Incident

TYPE OF INCIDENT	INSTRUMENT REQUIRED	COMMENTS
Sealed beta gamma source	Geiger Müller (GM) instrument; ionizing chamber instrument; dose-rate/meter	GM instrument is used for low dose rates and counts. An ionizing chamber instrument is used to measure high dose rates.
Unsealed beta gamma sources	Instruments as above, together with air samplers	Instruments as above. Also an air sampler may be used to determine the concentration of radioactive material in the air in the working environment.
Known neutron source	Neutron meter	These instruments can measure high doses of neutrons.
Alpha sources	Instrument using an alpha probe; air sampler	Use of this instrument requires special training. The probe must be held very close without touching the skin. These probes are easy to contaminate.
Contained criticality	Ionizing chamber; dose rate meter; neutron meter	Requires a high dose rate meter and also a neutron meter.
Uncontained criticality	All those required for "contained criticality" along with an air sampler	Initial radiation will consist of high dose gamma and neutrons. However, all types of radiation will be produced by the fission products formed, which are radioactive
Unknown radioactivity	All of the above	Assuming the worst, all such instruments may be required. It is easy to scale down in an incident; it is very difficult to scale up.

Note: Regular training in instrument use is essential not only in aiding the treatment of the patient but also protection of the medical staff.

PORTABLE INSTRUMENTS

The portable instruments that hospital and prehospital personnel use are capable of detecting contamination on the patient and also the dose rate coming off the patient as a result of external or internal contamination. Many medical decisions can be made from the information gained.

The Geiger-Müller "Counter"

The most common type of portable instrument used is the Geiger Müller, known familiarly as the "Geiger counter." It is constructed using either an end window probe to detect beta and gamma radiation or a pancake probe to detect alpha, beta, and gamma radiation (Fig. 14-1).

Chapter 13 describes the penetrating characteristics of the different types of radiation and how to provide protection. Alpha radiation can be completely shielded by a simple piece of paper; beta particle shielding can be achieved by using a light material such as aluminum. Gamma radiation can only be attenuated by using heavy materials such as lead, depleted uranium, or blocks of concrete; and finally, neutrons are shielded by materials with a high hydrogen content such as polystyrene or wax.

The Geiger counter detects beta and gamma irradiations using the end window device. With the window facing the contamination, two types of radiation can be detected, beta and gamma. By turning the end window 90 degrees, the casing of the end window probe, which is made of metal, only permits gamma radiation through, shielding out beta radiation. Therefore the types of radiation can be differentiated.

The Pancake Probe

The typical pancake probe, more sensitive than the end window, is capable of detecting alpha, beta, and gamma radiations. However, it is inefficient when it comes to detecting alpha radiation. Special probes are used with a thin Mylar

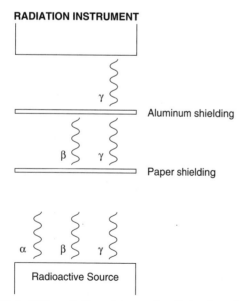

RADIATION INSTRUMENT

Figure 14–1. Differentiation of types of radiation by using shielding.

film cover containing zinc sulphide. Scintillation is used to measure alpha radiation, requiring a scintillation material known as a phosphor. When a phosphor material is exposed to ionizing radiation, it causes excess energy due to electron excitation and produces a flash of light. These flashes of light are directed onto a photo multiplier tube that changes them into electrical pulses, and by means of electronic circuits is able to record readings on an instrument scale.

The scintillation counter's advantages over a Geiger-Müller instrument are that it has greater range for measuring dose rate, is capable of measuring higher count rates, and demonstrates improved accuracy when measuring dose rates. Removing the protective cover from the pancake probe, one can detect the three types of radiation, which can be differentiated by using simple shielding.

Placing a piece of paper between the radiation source and the probe of the instrument shields out alpha, allowing only the beta and gamma radiation to reach the probe of the instrument. Placing a thin piece of aluminum between the radiation source shields out beta radiation and also alpha radiation, allowing only gamma to reach the probe. The pancake probe casing is generally made out of aluminum. By turning the head 180 degrees, the beta radiation is shielded out. Therefore users have a good idea of what types of radiation they are dealing with and what radiation is the main contributor.

The Geiger-Müller instrument can be used to measure counts per minute or dose rate in mR/Hr. 1 mR/Hr corresponds to approximately 2,000 to 3,000 counts per minute. A word of caution: These instruments only detect low levels of gamma, and they can saturate with high-count levels giving a zero reading. Typical range for a Geiger-Müller counter is up to 80,000 counts per minute and up to 20 m/R per hour. Note that these instruments are calibrated against a known gamma source. For higher levels of gamma, a different type of instrument is required (e.g., an ionizing chamber, which can read levels up to 500R/Hr), and assistance should be obtained from a nuclear health physicist.

The Geiger-Müller instrument only distinguishes types of radiation, but it does not indicate what specific isotope or isotopes are causing the radiation. Identification of isotopes can only be achieved by using specialized laboratory techniques such as a mass spectrometer. Thus contaminated clothing, wound dressings, and other related samples should be sent as soon as possible to the designated nuclear laboratory for identification of radioactive isotope/isotopes.

Generally speaking, these types of instruments have a low sensitivity, in the range of 10%. Therefore only part of the irradiation/contamination present is being measured.

BACKGROUND RADIATION AND INTERPRETATION OF DETECTION DEVICES

We live in a "radiation environment." The annual background radiation and human-made radiation in the United States is estimated as 360 m/rem. The contributions are 87% natural occurring, approximately 11.5% medical, 0.5% weapon fallout, 0.5% air travel and luminous dials, and 0.5 % occupational exposure.

We are continuously exposed to natural occurring sources including cosmic radiation, terrestrial gamma rays, internal radiation, and decaying products such as radon. We also have internal radiation: We are all "radioactive" with carbon 14 (C14) and potassium 40 in our bodies in very small amounts. C14 is produced by cosmic radiation interacting with nitrogen in the upper atmosphere changing N14 to C14. The C14 diffuses down into the lower atmosphere where it is absorbed by live tissue, and radioactive potassium 40 is found in the soil.

We are also exposed to human-made radiation, especially from medical sources including x-rays, nuclear medicine procedures, and radiotherapy procedures. Nuclear weapon tests also contribute to background exposure, but this is declining since the cessation of atmospheric testing in the mid-1960s. Other trivial contributions come from the nuclear industry.

It is important to know the level of background radiation in your area. Background radiation varies from area to area and from day to day. If you live in a mountainous region, the background radiation is much higher than in a "sedimentary," or low-altitude region. Measure the background radiation in your area regularly so that in a radiation incident you will be able to calculate the increase above this background level. There have been cases in which it was erroneously assumed some individuals were contaminated, when in fact it was background radiation being measured. In areas of low natural radiation, the background count might be approximately 20 to 30 counts per minute. In areas with greater natural background levels, the count would be much higher. Therefore it is essential you measure the background for that particular day, especially before patients arrive at your hospital. You are looking for any increase in the instrument count level above background.

Many common errors occur with radiation instruments, and adequate training for medical staff in the use of the instruments accompanied by regular practice sessions is essential. Experience dictates that most serious incidents occur at inconvenient hours when the staffing levels are at a minimum. Therefore all key staff must know how to use these instruments.

Common errors that occur using radiation detection instruments include the following: (a) not checking batteries regularly; (b) leaving the batteries in the instrument, which corrodes the connecting terminals; (c) using the wrong scale on the instrument, resulting in misinterpretation of the readings; (d) not calibrating the instrument regularly; and (e) covering the alpha probe head with a surgical glove to prevent the probe becoming contaminated. Putting a surgical glove over the probe is fine to measure beta or gamma radiation, but it is contraindicated when measuring alpha radiation. If alpha radiation cannot penetrate through a piece of paper, it certainly will not penetrate a surgical glove. During exercises, people have made the simple error of putting a surgical glove over the probe to protect the alpha probe. This resulted theoretically in the medical facility becoming completely contaminated when they were under the impression they were free from contamination.

Monitor slowly, moving the probe at a rate of about an inch a second. Make sure you monitor the whole body, especially paying close attention to the back and head including the hair. The use of the probe varies depending on which type of radiation you are measuring. Hold the probe about 1 centimeter away from the skin to pick up beta and gamma radiations. If measuring alpha, hold the alpha probe closer to the skin, that is, only a few millimeters, otherwise you will miss alpha radiation. Note that when detecting alpha radiation, it is very easy to contaminate the probe so make sure spare alpha instruments are available and you have an adequately trained staff member to perform the detection process. It requires considerable practice to use an alpha probe competently.

Develop a procedure to monitor the body so you do not miss any part of the body. If you find contamination on the person's clothing, stop monitoring, remove the clothing, and then remonitor from the beginning. Handle the instruments with care because they are delicate and sensitive. Always transport the instruments in their carrying case.

NEUTRON METER

Neutron meters are straightforward but do require instruction and practice to be effective. Neutrons, as the name implies, are neutral and do not produce ionization directly. They are detected via indirect methods. One common method is to use an instrument that contains helium gas. When the helium gas is bombarded with neutrons, the neutron is absorbed into the nucleus and a proton is ejected, changing helium into tritium. This proton causes ionization in the instrument, thereby indirectly demonstrating the presence of neutrons.

CRITICALITY INCIDENT

Under normal conditions, reactors are kept below a "critical mass." If this minimum threshold amount of nuclear material is reached, it can cause a propagating nuclear reaction that goes out of control. It occurs when sufficient fissile material is present (fissile materials are those containing atoms with nuclei capable of splitting). One such material is uranium-235 (U-235), which in the correct geometrical arrangement can start a chain reaction. When a U-235 atom is bombarded with a thermal neutron, it causes the uranium atom to split. This creates two fragments, each of which are new elements that may or may not be radioactive, plus energy, plus on average three new free neutrons. The three new neutrons go on to split another three atoms of U-235, producing nine new neutrons, and so on, to cause a chain-reaction "cascade" and uncontrolled fission. This is referred to as a *criticality incident.*

An example was the Tokai Mura criticality accident on September 30, 1999. After too much enriched U-235 was dissolved in nitric acid, the critical threshold was reached. The quantity of uranium used and the geometrical shape was such as to cause "criticality," resulting in pulsed high levels of neutron and gamma emissions. The reaction produced large amounts of energy in the form of heat, which changed the geometrical configuration and the mass became noncritical. However, on cooling, the geometric configuration returned to the ideal and the solution became critical, resulting in intermittent criticality. Therefore with respect to fissile material it is essential that a critical mass is not inadvertently assembled, which could cause a serious radiation accident.

In a criticality incident, a person may be exposed to a flux of neutrons. As a result of the neutron exposure, the patient may actually emit radiation in the form of "secondary gamma." This is one of the few times when the victim can actually become a radiation source. Radiation emission by the patient can be detected by placing a beta gamma detector on the abdomen of the patient and having the patient bend over the probe.

PERSONNEL DOSIMETERS

Several types of dosimeters can be used by the medical staff. However, patients will not have been wearing one of these devices when they were exposed. Therefore calculating the dose of the patient will be a very difficult task for the nuclear health physicist. Arrangements must be made to provide these devices for the staff prior to initiating work in an at-risk environment. The dosimeters must be worn on the anterior thorax. Note that the dose recorded is the dose to the dosimeter and does not necessarily represent an accurate whole-body dose to the individual, especially in a nonuniform radiation field. Some dosimeters may not have a very high maximum measurement. If an individual wearing such a badge experiences a very high exposure, it may be impossible to determine the actual dose received. Typically, hospital staff members receive very low doses. Higher, more dangerous doses would only be expected at the incident site, and then only when entering the cordoned-off area (Table 14-2).

The types of dosimeter recommended for medical staff include the thermo luminescent dosimeter, a quartz fiber dosimeter, and an instantaneous electronic readout dosimeter. In the case of a criticality accident, a neutron dosimeter is also required. Air sampling systems can also play a role. There are other types of dosimeters, but these are the essential ones required for hospital staff.

THERMOLUMINESCENT DOSIMETER (TLD)

Two main types of thermoluminescent dosimeters (TLD) are in common use: the one positioned on the anterior chest and the finger-tip dosimeter. These dosimeters use the property of certain crystals with impurities added into the crystal. In simple terms, these crystals can trap radiation energy within their structure. Typically, lithium fluoride is used and impurities such as copper within the crystal serve as electron traps between the valence and conduction band within the crystal. When radiation enters the TLD, electrons are caught in these electron traps. To release trapped electrons to their stable state, heat is applied to the crystal (200° to 300°C) resulting in the emission of light, which can be detected by using a photo multiplier tube and thereby enabling the dose to be calculated.

This type of device has many advantages. The dose response is linear, up to 10 grays (1,000 rads). It can be measured rapidly within a few minutes, but typically the dosimetry laboratory is not in close proximity to the hospital. Quite often these laboratories are in distant cities, making "real-time" use impractical. The crystal material used in the dosimeter reacts just like human tissue (known as "tissue equivalent"), and so it provides an accurate estimate of tissue dose. This type of dosimeter can also be modified into a finger-tip device, giving an indication of the dose received to the fingers of emergency staff or surgical staff carrying out surgical procedures.

QUARTZ FIBER DOSIMETER

The quartz fiber dosimeter can measure beta, gamma, and x-rays. Its range can be up to 200mR per hour, and there are various designs depending on the radiation ranges being detected. The dosimeter is pen shaped and worn just inside the neck margin of the surgical gown. It is an ionization chamber of the capacitor type. These devices require charging, and an ionizing current is allowed to disperse the charge. The quartz fiber is supported by a wire. When these compo-

---

TABLE 14-2 Characteristics for Use of Personal Dosimeters

TYPE OF INCIDENT	DOSIMETER	COMMENTS
Sealed source: alpha, beta, gamma radiation	Thermo-luminescent dosimeter (TLD); quartz fiber dosimeter (QFD)	TLD legal requirement: to be worn under a surgical gown on the anterior chest. QFD is worn inside the neck of the surgical gown. These are very sensitive. Do not knock or drop them. They will give a falsely high reading.
Unsealed radioactive source: alpha, beta, gamma	TLD, QFD, and also a personal air sampler	A personal air sampler should be as close to the nose and mouth as possible and positioned on the superior anterior chest.
Criticality accident	TLD, QFD, neutron dosimeter (e.g., criticality lockout)	In this situation high doses are to be expected. Expert advice is required.

Adapted from Wald N. Ionizing radiation. ATSDR. 1993 Oct.

nents are both charged to positive polarity, they cause a deflection of the quartz fiber. When ionizing radiation enters the ion chamber, a "leakage current" flow discharges the device and causes the quartz fiber to move toward the positive support wire.

NEUTRON PERSONNEL DOSIMETERS

The neutron personnel dosimeter uses a type of plastic called CR39, the same plastic often used in the manufacture of lenses of glasses. In simple terms, neutrons cause tracks in the plastic and these are used to estimate the dose of radiation exposure (1).

CRITICALITY LOCKETS

Criticality lockets are used when fissile material is handled in the environment of nuclear reactors and in reactor fuel ponds. These devices measure very high neutron doses. Neutrons are measured indirectly via bombardment of certain materials that release beta particles. These beta particles can be counted and the neutron dose calculated. Later neutron dosimeters use a type of plastic called CR39, the same plastic often used in the manufacture of lenses of glasses. As just described, the neutrons cause tracks in the plastic that are used to estimate the dose of radiation caused by neutrons.

ELECTRONIC READOUT INSTRUMENTS

These compact instruments give an instantaneous readout of the dose. They can be worn by the response team or placed in strategic positions inside the work environment. They have an audible alarm that can be set to activate upon reaching a specific dose.

AIR SAMPLERS

The personal air sampler is worn on the chest as close to the nose and mouth as possible and usually positioned on the neck collar. Another type, the static sampler, is placed in strategic positions in the hospital emergency department or at the incident site. Some of the static air monitors are provided with an audible alarm that can be set to a certain level of contamination by the health physicist. These devices are used to monitor the contamination levels of radioactivity in the working environment and measure the radioactive particles suspended in the air. This is achieved by drawing a known quantity of air through a filter paper. A health physicist then counts the filter paper under correct conditions. The airborne activity is calculated from the count rate on the filter paper.

THE IMPORTANT ROLE OF THE HEALTH PHYSICIST

The health physicist complements the role of the doctor and must exercise his or her role on a regular basis. Leaving it to the time of the nuclear incident will be too late. Also, the health physicist must be experienced with trauma. It would not be the first time an individual has fainted at the sight of blood. R. E. Toohey wrote an excellent review of the role of the health physicist (2).

SUMMARY

The medical staff in the emergency department, which includes doctors, nurses, and ancillary staff, require proper training in the use of radiation instruments. Provision of or access to these instruments, as well as personnel dosimeters, is essential. Regular training with these instruments is key to maintain staff competence in their use (Figs. 14-2–14.5).

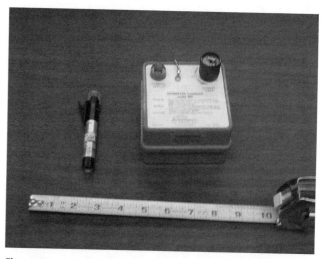

Figure 14–2. Quartz fiber pen dosimeter with its charger.

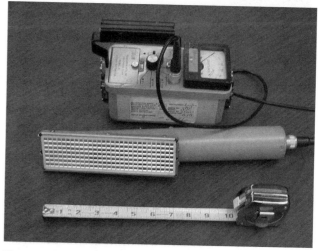

Figure 14–3. Radiation instrument with alpha probe.

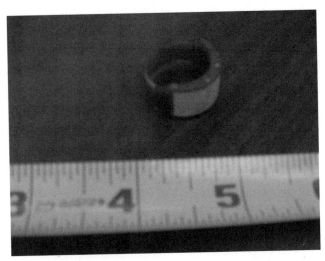

Figure 14–4. Finger dosimeter.

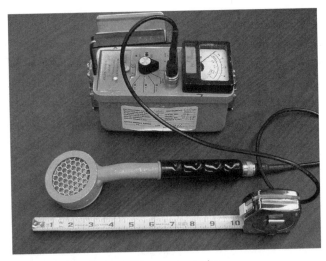

Figure 14–5. Radiation with pancake probe.

QUESTIONS AND ANSWERS

1. **With what radiation must most care be taken when trying to detect it with the appropriate instrument?**
   A. beta
   B. gamma
   C. neutrons
   D. alpha

2. **Common error(s) that occur while using radiation detection instruments include:**
   A. Finding the batteries are dead when the instrument is needed
   B. Leaving the batteries in the instrument, which corrodes the connecting terminals
   C. Using the wrong scale on the instrument, which results in misinterpretation of the readings

   D. Covering the alpha probe head with a surgical glove to prevent the probe becoming contaminated
   E. All of the above

3. **Regarding air samplers:**
   A. Personal ones are usually positioned on the thigh.
   B. A static sampler is typically placed in strategic positions in the hospital emergency department or at an incident site.
   C. Some static air monitors are provided with flashing lights and a silent alarm that can be set to certain levels of contamination by health physicists.
   D. They cannot be used to monitor contamination levels of radioactivity in the working environment
   E. They may be used to measure water contamination as well as air.

4. **Which of the following is FALSE?**
   A. Neutrons can produce ionization directly.
   B. Under normal conditions, reactors are kept below a "critical mass." If this minimum threshold amount of nuclear material is reached, it can cause a propagating nuclear reaction that goes out of control.
   C. The annual background radiation and human-made radiation for the year in the United States is estimated to be 360 m/rem. Major contributions are 87% natural occurring and approximately 11.5% medical.
   D. Specific devices are available to detect alpha, beta, gamma, x-rays, and neutrons.
   E. Beta particle shielding can be achieved by using a light material such as aluminium.

ANSWERS

1: D. *alpha*
2: E. *All of the above*
3: B. *A static sampler is typically placed in strategic positions in the hospital emergency department or at an incident site.*
4: A. *Neutrons can produce ionization directly.*

REFERENCES

1. Matiullar, KJ, Durrani SA. A flat dose-equivalent dosimeter for fast neutrons using a CR-39 polymeric track detector with front radiators. Radiation Protection Dosimetry 1986;17:149-52.
2. Toohey RE. The role of the health physicist in dose assessment: the medical bases of radiation accident preparedness. Fourth International REAC/TS Conference, Parthenon Publishing Group, Orlando, FL, March 2001.

SUGGESTED READINGS

1. Martin A, Harbinson SA. An introduction to radiation protection. London: Chapman and Hall, 1972.
2. NRCP Report 45. Natural background in the USA, 1975.
3. NRCP Report 57. Instrumentation and monitoring methods for radiation protection, 1978.

15

Personal Protection and Decontamination for Radiation Emergencies

Keith Edsall and Daniel C. Keyes

PERSONAL PROTECTION

Personal protection for incidents involving radioactive materials should be integrated into an all-hazards approach to disaster planning. Important features to include in such planning are (a) predetermination of hospital and emergency department layout and staffing for triage, decontamination, and management of victims; (b) proper training and availability of equipment for use of personal protection; (c) knowledge of where expert advice can be obtained over the telephone and the time interval it would take for experts to arrive on request; and (d) awareness of specialized centers in the area where patients can be transferred if needed and preexisting written understandings with these institutions. Finally, regular exercises will be needed to reinforce learning and to correct deficiencies in the overall process.

Personal protection is based specifically on proper consideration of the type of radiation involved, whether alpha, beta, gamma or neutron, and the ever-important features of *time*, *distance*, *shielding,* and *quantity* (Chapter 13). One must also know what the basic radiation detection instruments are and understand how to interpret the readings of these instruments (Chapter 14). Individual staff members need to know about the types of personal dosimeter to use and where to place them on oneself. In this chapter, we discuss which type of protection must be worn in the hospital environment, as well as accepted practices and procedures for the decontamination of patients.

Radiation can either be caused by *particles*, including beta or alpha particles or neutrons, or *electromagnetic waves*, including gamma rays and x-rays. Particular radiation can be blocked completely by proper shielding; however, electromagnetic radiation can only be decreased (attenuated). It is not completely stopped by shielding. However, if the proper amount of shielding is used, the amount of radiation that penetrates will be so low as to be of no biological signifi-

cance. By carrying out set procedures correctly, it is possible to limit the dose to the medical staff and also prevent both external and internal contamination from occurring.

PROTECTION AGAINST ALPHA RADIATION

Alpha particles, which produce dense ionization, can only travel 1 or 2 centimeters in air and only up to about 70 micrometers into tissue. The penetrating power of alpha particles is very poor and can be stopped completely by a piece of paper. Since the outer layers of skin are dead and generally thicker than 70 micrometers, alpha particles externally would not generally cause biological damage. On the other hand, alpha particles that enter into the body present a more serious situation because the alpha particles are now adjacent to live tissue and could cause serious biological damage within that 70-micrometer track length. Inhalation and ingestion of alpha particles are therefore the primary concern with respect to personal protection. If a patient has been exposed to alpha radiation but is not contaminated, there is no need for personal protection whatsoever. However, if the patient has been contaminated with alpha-containing material, then removal of clothing and washing should be sufficient to protect the medical personnel from risk. In addition, application of a face mask and standard "universal precautions" (which will be described later in this chapter) should be sufficient for this purpose.

PROTECTION AGAINST BETA RADIATION

Beta particles have a range of energies, and their penetrating power depends on the initial energy of the particle concerned. There tends to be a range or *spectrum* of energies for beta particles. Beta particles typically travel 1 to 3 meters in air and just a few millimeters into tissue. Beta particles of higher energies can penetrate deeper into tissue. With internal intake of beta particles, the depth of penetration into live tissue would be the same. These particles can cause severe beta burns of the skin as was seen in the Chernobyl accident. They may also cause severe internal damage if they enter the body via inhalation, ingestion, or wounds. To shield against beta particles, a light material such as aluminum is all that is required. In fact, it is preferable to use materials such as aluminum to prevent *Bremsstrahlung radiation.* Bremsstrahlung radiation occurs when beta particles come under the influence of a positive nucleus. As a result of such close proximity and bending around the nucleus, they slow down. As this occurs, it gives off heat and x-ray electromagnetic radiation. This is more likely to occur if a heavy material is used, such as tungsten. This is the principle of an x-ray machine.

PROTECTION AGAINST GAMMA RADIATION

Gamma rays, as with ordinary x-rays, penetrate right through the body. The gamma radiation interacts with the biological tissues and causes damage. Therefore this type of radiation can produce the *acute radiation syndrome* (Chapter 16). Shielding required for this type of radiation requires lead, concrete, or depleted uranium. Shielding attenuates this type of radiation but does not completely shield against it; however, the amount of gamma rays that penetrates the shield is so small that it is of no biological significance. An important point to mention here is that if a patient who has been irradiated by gamma rays only, this patient is not radioactive and is of no danger to the medical staff. The opposite may actually be true: the medical staff, with the bacteria they normally carry, can endanger an immunocompromised patient. The reason in mentioning this point is that there have been a few cases around the world where patients have been refused admission into the hospital because of concerns that they might contaminate the hospital. In these cases, there is no contamination, and there is no residual irradiation on the patient. There is therefore no danger the hospital or hospital staff. Consider a routine chest radiograph. After patients have a chest x-ray, they do not walk out of the x-ray department radioactive. The same principle applies to gamma exposures.

NEUTRONS

Criticality accidents involving neutron exposures may actually cause the patient to become radioactive. The sodium in our body has an affinity to capture neutrons, and in so doing it changes from the normal Na-23 to radioactive Na-24, which has a half-life of 15 hours. This can be detected simply by placing an instrument on the abdomen of the patient and having the patient bend over the instrument. The axillae may also be used for this purpose. The instrument will then detect any secondary gamma radiation. Neutrons are highly penetrating and are shielded by material of high hydrogen content such as wax or polystyrene.

TIME

Time is an important factor with respect to exposure; ideally the time spent in a radiation environment should be as short as possible. Experts, either at the scene of the incident or at the hospital emergency department, set specific limits of dose for responders in an emergency. The fact that such threshold levels are set does not mean that the responders really receive this dose of radiation. Ideally, one should rotate staff so that the dose is "shared," keeping individual doses to a minimum. There is a much greater risk of exposure to high doses at the incident scene than in the hospital emergency department. In the hospital environment, the dose received by hospital staff is generally low. Nevertheless, the practice of rotating staff is important in both settings.

DISTANCE

Distance is an important factor to take into consideration when dealing with radiation. A useful rule of thumb is to remember the inverse square law: by doubling the distance the dose is reduced to a quarter. In practical terms, the radiation dose will be markedly reduced if one works a few extra feet from the radiation source. If one considers being one foot away from a radioactive source and the dose recorded from the instrument reads 80 cGy (centi-Gray) by doubling the distance to 2 feet the instrument would read 20 cGy, a quarter of the original dose. By doubling the distance again to 4 feet, the dose would again be reduced by a quarter to 5 cGy. Therefore, by increasing the distance to 4 feet, the dose has reduced from 80 cGy to 5 cGy, for a total reduction in dose of 75 cGy.

SURGERY AND OTHER WORK VERY CLOSE TO RADIOACTIVE SOURCES

When working very close to a contaminated patient, the converse of the inverse square law applies. If performing surgery or otherwise working in close proximity to the patients, the doses increase by the same "inverse square" principle. By halving the distance the dose would go up fourfold. As one approaches the source, the dose rapidly rises. On actual direct contact with the source, the dose could be very significant. It is important to remember to *never pick up a source with your fingers,* no matter how small it is. When working directly on wounds, it is preferable to use 6-inch swab forceps not your fingers. The dose resulting from direct contact of the wound with your fingers could be significant compared to the dose 6 inches away using forceps.

QUANTITY

The quantity of radiation can be modified rapidly in a contaminated radiation incident simply by removing the clothing. This is particularly important if a large number of contaminated casualties arrive at your facility. Taking off the clothing reduces the contamination of the patient by approximately 85% to 90%. Each individual's clothing should be double-bagged using polyethylene bags, which are labeled with the patient's name, date of birth, and time the clothing was removed. This clothing must not be kept in the emergency department but instead should be placed outside the hospital in a designated area as determined by the health physicist. In this way, a build-up of radioactive material in the emergency department can be avoided, and the staff will not be exposed to unnecessary irradiation. It is also important to remove all radioactive waste from the emergency department as soon as possible.

The preceding discussion endeavors to illustrate how the important principles of time, distance, shielding, and quantity of radiation are the key concepts to remember in protecting hospital personnel.

TRIAGE CONSIDERATIONS

It may be anticipated that many otherwise healthy but concerned individuals will arrive at the hospital, demanding treatment and reassurance. As such, it is recommended that an area be designated to provide personnel for monitoring and counseling. (See also Chapter 41.)

Individuals, who believe that they have been contaminated or irradiated but who have been shown not to be, tend to suffer from stress, in some cases severe. In the experience of the author, the counseling team should consist of a health physicist, a physician conversant with radiation, a psychiatrist, and a radiation safety officer with instrumentation. Patients benefit from seeing the instruments used. By using these devices, the counseling team can clearly demonstrate that the patients have no contamination on them. This counseling center should be positioned away from the emergency center but within a short distance of it. If the hospitals and emergency services are forewarned that a nuclear terrorist event has taken place before the public are aware, then receiving centers can be set up before victims arrive. One option is to use a nearby public venue such as a sports arena. Triage can be set up there and only patients requiring hospital treatment need to be transferred to the hospital.

MEDICAL MANAGEMENT

PREPARING THE HOSPITAL AND STAFF TO RECEIVE CONTAMINATED PATIENTS WITH TRAUMA

Emergency departments are often accustomed to receiving occasional chemical casualties, and usually a small area of an emergency department is designated for decontamination and care of these patients. Such a small area will most likely not be adequate in a terrorist event. Most of the area in the emergency department will be required for this type of event, remembering that it is easy to scale down but very difficult to scale up in an emergency. It is essential for the emergency disaster plan to include the possibility of radiation incidents. In a terrorist event, the number of people arriving at the emergency department may range anywhere from just a few people to a crowd involving thousands of people. With most serious disasters around the world, only the most seriously injured people have stayed at the accident site for initial triage. The vast majority of patients either found the hospital on their own or used public transportation. This was seen in the 1995 Japanese terrorist attack with sarin nerve agent. In that incident, approximately 500 people were taken to the hospital by the general public before the first ambulance arrived. Therefore, it is important that the hospital's emergency plans be designed to cater to large numbers of people who require triage and decontamination.

As with chemical incidents, patients should be properly disrobed and decontaminated prior to passing into the emergency department. Triage is required to differentiate the type of patient you are dealing with. If the patient is contaminated without any trauma, then facilities must be put in place to enable removal of clothing. This includes washing facilities for decontamination of hair and showering, biological sampling, and the provision of replacement clothing. Ideally, the only patients who should then be seen in the emergency department are those who have been traumatized, have been irradiated to significant levels, or have any likelihood of heavy contamination externally or internally. Ultimately they will be given treatment depending on the radioactive isotope identified. Many patients may be followed up as an outpatient.

PREPARATION OF THE EMERGENCY DEPARTMENT

Ideally, the emergency department should be divided into two major areas: (a) a "dirty area" (contaminated) and (b) a "clean area" (kept free of contamination). A third area may be used in case of overload (Fig. 15-1). The ventilation system to the emergency department should be completely isolated from the rest of the hospital, and even shut down if necessary. This prevents the transmission of radioactive contamination to other parts of the hospital. All unnecessary equipment should be removed from the designated dirty area of the emergency department. Anything that cannot be removed should be covered with drapes. The floor should be covered with an impervious material and "taped down." A typical practice is to use common "butcher's paper" and tape it down. Demarcate the dirty area from the clean area by using colored floor tape. Butcher's paper is a good choice for a number of uses. It is very strong and inexpensive. If there are any splashes decontaminating a patient, the paper absorbs the liquid and is easily identifiable. Once the splashing is identified, one should mark around it with a marker pen and cover with a spare piece of the paper. Then one writes on the patch the word "contamination." Once all the patients have been dealt with, the specialist team will concentrate on the splashed areas first, by decontaminating the area. When this has been completed, the rest of the paper on the floor is removed and bagged. Final monitoring of the area is carried out, and the emergency department can then be used again for its normal functions.

X-ray facilities are an important consideration because it is relatively easy to contaminate this department. For this reason, it may be advisable to use only portable x-ray machines. The machines should be positioned on the edge of the clean area. The x-ray head and arm of the machine can be covered with a polythene bag so that the arm can

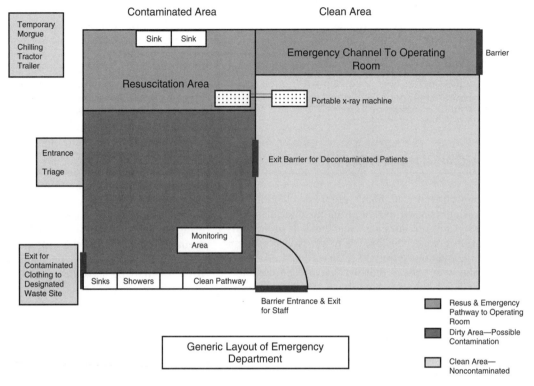

Figure 15–1. Generic layout diagram of a hospital emergency department.

be maneuvered into the dirty area without contaminating the x-ray machine. X-ray film cassettes should be placed in a polyurethane bag before being transferred into the dirty area.

Part of your resuscitation facility should be within the dirty area to deal with emergency traumatized patients. You must deal with the trauma first before considering the irradiation or contamination problem. If an endotracheal tube is being inserted into a patient, a good practice is to put a surgical hat over the patient's hair. Following this practice will prevent the clothing of the resuscitator from becoming contaminated when inserting the tube, checking placement, or auscultating the chest with a stethoscope.

The dirty area should contain wash basins and a shower, if possible, with a designated pathway to the clean area for movement of patients. An operating theater should be designated for severely injured patients. If possible, this should be situated close to the emergency department. A patient requiring a life-saving surgical procedure then may be taken directly to the operating theater. There may be concern about contaminating an operating room. However, these theaters are designed to be decontaminated as a result of viral and bacterial agents so they can also be decontaminated as a result of radioactive contamination. Patients who are being transferred to the operating room may be covered with a clean drape. To prevent contamination of the hospital by the wheels of the gurney, one may roll the wheels of the gurney onto duck tape, at the demarcation of the dirty and clean area barrier. This will trap any potential contamination on the gurney wheels. There should be provision for a designated pathway for emergencies through the clean area if necessary to access the operating room.

PERSONAL PROTECTION

PROTECTIVE CLOTHING REQUIRED BY HOSPITAL STAFF

Hospital staff working in the "dirty" area should wear surgical greens and gown, as well as work with "universal" (body secretion) precautions. Surgical hood, mask and face shield, and shoe covers or surgical boots are also included in this uniform. Two pairs of surgical gloves are generally recommended, with the inner pair being a different color than the outer. The second color of the outer surgical gloves allows for changing as one moves from patient to patient. On some occasions people have taken off the outer gloves and forgotten to put a new set on. The practice of using two colors allows the staff to be reminded when they take off the outer gloves. If the inner gloves become contaminated, they can be removed under controlled conditions and under the watchful eye of the health physicist. They may then be replaced with two new sets of gloves. The inner set of surgical gloves should be taped to the sleeves of the surgical gown; the outer set of gloves is not taped. Also the opening on the back of the surgical gown should be taped, just as the surgical trousers should be taped to the surgical boots. It is also advisable to wear a lightweight waterproof plastic apron over the other garments.

DOSIMETERS

Dosimeters should be provided for each member of staff entering the dirty area. The characteristics of these devices are described in Chapter 14 and include a quartz fiber dosimeter (QFD) worn just inside the neck of the surgical gown for easy access. The health physicist will monitor the dose received by the members of staff in the dirty area periodically. These devices give an instantaneous readout. Dosimeters should be handled very carefully, as these devices are sensitive to knocks or being dropped. Another personal measuring device that, by law, must be worn is a thermoluminescent dosimeter. This is worn on the anterior chest underneath the surgical gown. The thermoluminescent dosimeter cannot be read immediately and must be sent to a registered dosimetry laboratory to be read. It is important that you know in advance where this laboratory is situated. Arrangements should be made with this laboratory in the event of an emergency. There should also be provision for supply of these dosimeters in the event of a nuclear incident; however, the hospital should already have a limited stock of dosimeters and should provide for the rapid acquisition of additional supplies if needed.

Instantaneous readout dosimeters are electronic devices that can be worn by the individual or placed in a strategic position both in the dirty and clean areas so that everyone can see what dose is accumulating in that particular area. Individuals need to wear personal dosimeters because our body senses cannot detect irradiation. They also serve to reassure the individual staff members because the actual dose received will generally be very low.

In a radiation incident, staff should be committed into the designated dirty area only as they are needed. This situation is different from the normal trauma disaster where staff members are already at their designated positions. The hospital will not know initially how many patients it will be receiving; it could be one or two, or it could be hundreds. The staff assigned to the dirty area will need to undress in a specific order, handing over their dosimeters, and to be fully monitored from head to toe to rule out contamination. When done correctly, this procedure should take between 5 and 10 minutes for each individual. Thus if 30 people are in the dirty area, it will take a few hours to monitor the last staff members out of the dirty area if there is only one exit monitoring team. Rotate staff as much as possible to share the dose. Also staff members should be informed not to eat, drink, or smoke in or near the treatment or decontamination sites. Also it is a good idea to remind staff to use the rest room before entering the dirty area, as they could be there for a long period of time. If possible, a counseling team should be assigned specifically to the emergency staff. The emergency staff will not have deep knowledge of radiation. Following the incident, all staff members will need to be monitored fully, their doses assessed, and reassurance provided by an expert. There often will be a need for psychological support both during and after the incident.

All hospital emergency staff should be able to use radiation instruments in an emergency and differentiate among alpha, beta, and gamma radiation. Unfortunately, quite often these events happen during "off hours," with a minimum staff level. Not knowing how to use these instruments correctly can lead to major problems. Only by regular practice with these radiation instruments will the staff become competent. Common failures with instrumentation are covered in Chapter 14.

REMOVING CLOTHING FROM THE PATIENT

There is a slight difference between the patient arriving by ambulance and the patient arriving at the door of the emergency department. The patient arriving by ambulance may already be wrapped in blankets. Before transferring the patient onto a hospital gurney, place two sheets on the gurney and then transfer the patient. The contamination is contained on the inner surface of the blankets that the patient is wrapped in, and on the outer surface of the patient's clothing. One should roll the blankets from the outside in, thus trapping the contamination, which is on the inside of the blanket. While being conscious of the potential for contamination on the outside of the patient's clothing, carefully cut the clothing away from the face down both arms and legs. Do not put the clothing under tension when cutting because this tends to release contamination into the air in the region of the faces of the emergency staff carrying out the procedure. Once the clothing is cut, roll the clothing from the inside out to trap the contamination inside the clothing. There will be two rolls on either side of the patient, including the clothing along with the blankets. One side of the top sheet is carefully folded, placed by the side of the patient, and then rolled up. The same procedure is carried out on the other side. The patient can then be rolled over onto the second clean sheet. The top sheet, which now contains the contaminated clothing and blankets, is folded at both ends to prevent venting of the radioactive material when rolling up the contaminated clothing. This clothing is then carefully placed in a polyethylene bag and sealed. Footwear is removed by encasing each shoe in a polyethylene bag and then pulling the shoe off. The contaminated shoe is then contained in the polythene bag.

The contents of the bag are then placed in another polyethylene bag and labeled with the patient's name, date of birth, and the time the clothes and shoes were removed. The contaminated clothing is immediately removed from the emergency department to the designated contamination collection site outside the hospital. At a later stage, the contaminated clothing will be assessed by health physicists to determine the amount of contamination each individual was subjected to and to aid in determining what contribution to the total dose the patient received.

Patients who walk into the hospital should wear a mask prior to and during the removal of contaminated clothing to prevent inhalation of airborne particles. A staff member should aid the patient in carrying out this procedure. Once the clothing has been removed from these patients, the patients should be surveyed with the radiation instruments, and any necessary biological samples should be then taken from the patient. Typically these samples include nasal swabs, nose "blows," throat swabs, all urine, feces, and a blood sample.

Great care must be taken with decontamination because significant amounts of fluid are required. It is very easy to contaminate oneself by not following the correct procedures. In general, the priority is to decontaminate wounds first and then to decontaminate the remaining skin. To care for a wound, place a cover over the area, and surround the wound with waterproof drapes. These drapes must be taped down. The drapes should be arranged to provide a run-off for the irrigation fluid into a collecting container, such as a polyethylene bag placed into a garbage can. The initial count reading of the radiation instrument is recorded. The wound is then irrigated with sterile saline using a 50 cc syringe several times, ensuring that all the washings are collected into the polyethylene bag. The drapes around the wound are removed and placed in the same bag as the washings. The wound is then dried and monitored again. It is important that the drapes be removed prior to conducting these repeat measurements because these drapes can cause false readings on the measuring device. After irrigation, the radiation count of the wound should be reduced. This procedure may be repeated several times until the wound is completely free of contamination. Ideally, the wound will be irrigated until the radiation count has become equal to the background radiation. However in some instances complete decontamination of the wound cannot be achieved. Such cases require referral for surgical debridement of the wound.

If there is localized contamination of the skin adjacent to the wound, then the same procedure is carried out with respect to draping the area. However, one should apply soapy swabs, working from the outside edge of the contaminated skin to the center. This procedure is usually repeated several times. A detailed procedure is described in Chapter 16.

All the washing fluid and material removed from the wound are collected and saved for future analysis by the health physicist to determine the dose received to the tissues of the wound in order to determine if there will be any long-term effects as a result of radiation exposure from the radioactive contamination. Sometimes large quantities of sterile normal saline are used to decontaminate a wound. It is critical that these procedures be carried out meticulously so that the medical staff do not become contaminated.

SHOWERING

In the current atmosphere of terrorism preparedness, many hospitals are becoming prepared to perform showers on large numbers of people. (See also Chapter 29.) In the terrorist situation, the hospital could be faced with hundreds of people requiring radioactive decontamination. If the hospital receives warning about an incident before the general public becomes aware, then one option might be to use a sports stadium or other large venue that has both showers and toilet facilities. The hospital will undoubtedly be inundated with large numbers of individuals who suddenly arrive, creating a difficult problem. Of course, it is not possible to produce showers immediately without advanced preparation. If such an irrigation system is not immediately available, it may be necessary to transfer the patients to another site that has these facilities.

Typically showers may be set up in a large covered parking area with plumbing. Both hot and cold water terminals are required. Garden hoses and showerheads could be attached to these terminals. One method of decontamination involves the use of showers at two levels: high and low. The lower level shower head is used to decontaminate only the hair on the head, while the higher shower is used to decontaminate the whole body. The hair of the head should be decontaminated first. This is achieved by

bending the patient over the improvised container, while making sure to avoid runoff of contaminated water onto the rest of the body. If this is not done properly, runoff may contaminate hair in the chest, axilla, and pubic region. Once the hair has been decontaminated, then the patient is placed under the shower. In colder climates, temporary winter heating is used to prevent hypothermia. The contaminated water should also be collected. Proper screening should be provided to allow discreet lanes for males and females. After decontamination, clean clothing will be required for all patients. Protective clothing is required for hospital personnel who assist patients with decontamination. This typically consists of waterproof clothing and boots together with a mask and splash visor and a waterproof hood. Hospital staff must also wear the relevant dosimeters as discussed previously.

In conclusion, personal protection against irradiation and contamination involves the provision of protective clothing and dosimeters to members of the staff, as well as the ability to carry out decontamination procedures correctly. Staff members should also be trained in the proper use of radiation instruments and interpretation of the results. Ultimately, this requires regular training and exercises.

Staff members will initially be very apprehensive about treating irradiated or contaminated patients. With proper training and preparation of the hospital facilities, exposures will be kept to very low, safe levels. However, if the correct procedures are followed, the dose to the staff will be very minimal. International incidents involving exposure to radiation have illustrated this point. An example of this was seen in an incident in Goiania, Brazil, where a number of patients were heavily contaminated both externally and internally. Some of these patients also suffered from acute radiation syndrome and required treatment for several months. In spite of this, the average dose received by the medical support team was less than 1 rem (5 MSv) radiation because of the proper attention to the procedures described in this chapter.

SUMMARY

If faced with an irradiated or contaminated patient, medical staff will be very apprehensive about providing treatment because their medical training did not cover managing this type of patient. It is essential that medical staff be trained to deal with these patients and at the same time know how to protect themselves. After the medical staff has been trained, their fear of treating patients who have been irradiated or contaminated will disappear. Exercises on relevant procedures on a regular basis should be carried out to reinforce and maintain knowledge and skills. The training for doctors, nurses, paramedics, and health physicists can be obtained. One center that provides training on a regular basis is the Radiation Emergency Assistance Center/Training Site (REAC/TS). See the resources section for more information.

RESOURCES

1. Radiation Emergency Assistance Center/Training Site (REAC/TS) Web Address:
   http://www.orau.gov/reacts/default.htm

QUESTIONS AND ANSWERS

1. **Personal protection for incidents involving radioactive materials should be integrated into an all-hazards approach to disaster planning. Important features to include in such planning include all of the following, EXCEPT:**
   A. Predetermination of hospital and emergency department layout and staffing for triage, decontamination, and management of victims
   B. Distribution of alpha-detectors and potassium iodide pills to all medical personnel before radiation accidents
   C. Proper training and availability of equipment for use of personal protection
   D. Knowledge of where expert advice can be obtained over the telephone and the time interval it would take for experts to arrive on request
   E. Awareness of specialized centers in the area where patients can be transferred if needed, and preexisting written understandings with these institutions

2. **What is the source of radiation?**
   A. Alpha and beta particles
   B. Neutrons
   C. Electromagnetic waves including gamma and x-rays
   D. A + C
   E. A + B + C

3. **Which of the following statements about alpha particles is FALSE?**
   A. Alpha particles, which produce dense ionization, can only travel in air a centimeter or two and only up to about 70 micrometers into tissue.
   B. The penetrating power of alpha particles is very poor and can be stopped completely by a piece of paper.
   C. Since the outer layers of skin are dead and generally thicker than 70 micrometers, alpha particles externally generally do not cause biological damage.
   D. If an alpha particle enters the body, it may be adjacent to live tissue and can cause serious biological damage within that 70-micrometer track length.
   E. If a patient has been contaminated with alpha-containing material, potassium iodide will completely obliterate any adverse effects.

4. **Which of the following statements about gamma rays is FALSE?**
   A. A patient who has been irradiated by gamma radiation is likely radioactive and is generally dangerous to the medical staff.
   B. Gamma rays, as with ordinary x-rays, penetrate right through the body.
   C. Gamma radiation interacts with the biological tissues and causes damage; therefore, it can produce the acute radiation syndrome.
   D. Shielding required for this gamma radiation requires lead, concrete, or depleted uranium.
   E. Shielding attenuates gamma radiation, but does not completely shield against it; however, the amount of gamma radiation that penetrates the shield is so small that it is of no biological significance.

ANSWERS

1: B. *Distribution of alpha-detectors and potassium iodide pills to all medical personnel before radiation accidents.*

2: E. *Alpha and beta particles, neutrons, and electromagnetic waves including gamma rays and x-rays.*

3: E. *If a patient has been contaminated with alpha-containing material, potassium iodide will completely obliterate any adverse effects.*

4: A. *A patient who has been irradiated by gamma radiation is likely radioactive and is generally dangerous to the medical staff.*

SUGGESTED READINGS

1. 10-90 Gold NBC. Response plan procedures and support activities developed by the defense protective service for response to a nuclear, biological or chemical incident within DPS jurisdiction. June 1996.
2. Berger M, et al. Transport of radioactive materials, Q & A about incident response. REAC/TS Medical Sciences Division, Oak Ridge Associated Universities; 1992.
3. Dons RF, Cerveny JT. Triage and treatment of radiation injured mass casualties. In: Textbook of military medicine, part 1: warfare, weaponry and the casualty. (Medical consequences of nuclear warfare; vol. 2.) Washington DC: Office of the Surgeon General; 1989.
4. Hubner KF, Fry SA. The medical basis for Radiation Accident Preparedness II, Clinical experiences and follow up since 1979. In: Ricks RC, Fry SA, eds. REAC/TS Conference, 1998 Oct. New York: Elsevier.
5. Markovechick V. Radiation Injuries. In: Tintinalli E, et al. eds. A comprehensive study guide, 4th ed. New York: McGraw-Hill; 1996.
6. Mettler FA Jr, et al. Medical management of radiation. Boca Raton FL: CRC Press;1990.
7. Mettler FA Jr, Moseley RD. Medical effects of ionising radiation. New York: Grune & Stratton; 1985.
8. National Council on Radiation Protection and Measurements. Management of persons accidental contaminated with radionuclides, Bethesda, MD: NRCP Publications. Report No 65;1993.
9. Ricks RC. Prehospital management of radiation accidents. Oak Ridge, TN: Oak Ridge Associated Universities; 1984.
10. Jarret DG. Nuclear nightmares. Emergency Medical Services; 1996.
11. Ricks RC. Hospital emergency department management of radiation accidents. Oak Ridge, TN: Oak Ridge Associated Universities, Medical and Health Science Division; 1984.

16

Treatment of Radiation Exposure and Contamination

Keith Edsall and Daniel C. Keyes

Most physicians have little knowledge about treating radiation injuries because the subject is not included in the medical school curriculum. Radiation accidents are not common events; however, a number have occurred throughout the world in recent years. Several international terrorist events have demonstrated the threat of biological, chemical, and nuclear terrorism. Experts worldwide agree that the possibility of a nuclear terrorist threat exists. Since the devastating attack on the World Trade Center in New York, the sarin attack on the subway system in Japan, the train bombings of Madrid, Spain, in 2004, and various other terrorist bombings, concerns have now changed from "if" to "when" terrorists will attempt a nuclear attack of some sort.

This chapter discusses how to diagnose, investigate, and provide initial treatment with respect to irradiation and contamination of patients. Every specialty within the hospital will be involved in one way or another with the treatment of these patients. These include emergency physicians, hematologists, pathologists, microbiologists, toxicologists, general and plastic surgeons, dermatologists, nutritionists, and intensive care specialists, to name but a few. There will also be a requirement for nuclear, medical, and health physics specialists such as those from REAC/TS (Radiation Emergency Accident Center and Training Site) located in Oak Ridge, Tennessee, to be involved. REAC/TS is one of the World Health Organization–designated collaboration centers for support and advice in the event of a radiation accident. However, these specialists will take time to get to you, with delays estimated at 12 to 24 hours depending on your geographical location. Thus for the first few hours you will be on your own. But you should plan to have a direct communication link with an organization such as REAC/TS, which will be able to offer advice.

In the terrorist event you will not know what radioactive isotope/isotopes you are dealing with initially, and this will take time to identify. If a dispersal device using explosives has been used, your facility could receive hundreds of worried people. Some of these individuals will be traumatized, irradiated, and contaminated, some without trauma but exposed to radiation, and some who are possibly contami-

nated. It may be assumed that the majority of people who believe they have been irradiated or contaminated in actual fact are not. With most disasters people tend to go straight to the hospital and not wait for emergency services to arrive. This has been well documented after many major disasters that have occurred around the world. If instead sealed sources were strategically placed or an isotope was dispersed without the use of explosives, the patients would likely arrive at different hospitals or medical facilities over a period of time complaining of various ailments that initially would not be attributed to irradiation. Therefore vigilance is of prime importance, and radiation should be added to the differential diagnosis.

ACUTE RADIATION SYNDROME

Before discussing acute radiation syndrome (ARS), the concepts of both cell death and the LD_{50} must be understood. *Cell death* is defined as the stopping of cell division and not the killing of the cell outright. Significant doses of radiation can prevent cell division, whereas very high doses are required to kill the cell outright. Rapidly dividing cell populations within the body are very sensitive to radiation such as the hematopoietic cell lines of the bone marrow and the epithelial cells lining the small intestine.

Our body senses cannot detect radiation, so we must rely on instruments to measure any exposure. Experiments were carried out on animals in the late 1940s and early 1950s to determine the acute dose of whole body exposure required to kill 50% of the animals in a set period of time, usually 30 days, known as the $LD_{50/30}$. The dose required varied from animal species to species. In general, the smaller the animal, the higher the $LD_{50/30}$. For example, the goat requires only 3.5 Gy (350 rads), whereas the frog must receive the higher dose of 7 Gy (700 rads). Other factors influence the susceptibility to radiation, including age, sex, genetic considerations, health, and the nutritional status of the animals. With respect to humans, very limited information is available to be certain of the LD_{50}. With information from accident data and results from human studies on patients after the dropping of the atomic bombs on Hiroshima and Nagasaki, the LD_{50} for humans is believed to be in the region of 2.5 to 4.5 Gys (250 to 450 rads). ARS in humans takes longer to express itself compared to animal data and is closer to 60 days. Therefore in humans we talk about the $LD_{50/60}$, defined as the lethal dose required to kill 50% of the population within 60 days.

To produce classical ARS, certain parameters are required. Of particular importance is the presence of a high dose delivered very rapidly at a high dose rate. Also the radiation must be penetrating, and it is usually the result of whole body exposure. Note that the source of radiation is not important. It is immaterial what the radioactive source is, whether the source is from a reactor or from sealed or unsealed containers used in industry or medicine. If the dose is high enough, it will produce the same biological damage.

ARS follows a set course, which will express itself within hours to weeks depending on the level of dose received. The syndrome can be divided into four phases: (a) the prodromal phase, (b) the latent phase, (c) the illness phase, and (d) the phase of final outcome, either recovery or death. ARS can be expressed as injury to several major organ systems including the hematopoietic, gastrointestinal, pulmonary, and finally the cardiovascular and central nervous system (CVS/CNS) syndrome. The expression of damage to these organ systems depends on the dose received. The hematopoietic syndrome is seen within the dose range of 2 to 8 Gy (200 to 800 rads). The gastrointestinal syndrome is seen in the dose range of 8 to 30 Gy (800 to 3,000 rads). The CVS/CNS syndrome is in the range of 30 Gy (3,000 rads) and upward. Note that as the dose increases, the survival time decreases. If untreated, death from the hematopoietic syndrome will occur within 60 days. Death from the gastrointestinal syndrome will occur within 1 to 2 weeks, and CVS/CNS syndrome death is the most rapid, usually occurring within 48 hours (Table 16-1).

THE PRODROMAL PHASE

After exposure to radiation, several vague, nonspecific symptoms begin to occur, known as the *prodromal* phase. The time to onset of the prodromal phase of signs and symptoms can be from minutes to hours depending on the dose received. Anorexia, vomiting, and diarrhea are the main symptoms and signs. *The most important indicator of prognosis is the time of onset of vomiting following irradiation.* Vomiting within 2 to 4 hours is an indication of a high dose of radiation. Other signs and symptoms are the development of headache and a rise in core temperature. At doses below 1 Gy (100 rads) there are very few signs and symptoms, and

these patients can be sent home and followed up on an outpatient basis. At doses of 1 to 2 Gy (100 to 200 rads), vomiting will develop in a number of patients, and it is advisable to admit these patients for observation. At doses in the range of 2 to 4 Gy (200 to 400 rads), vomiting is noted in the majority of patients. This occurred within the first 2 to 8 hours. In doses of 4 to 8 Gy (400 to 800 rads), vomiting occurs in only 2 hours. At doses above 8 Gy, vomiting is severe, starting much earlier, within the first hour or so.

POTENTIALLY MISLEADING PRESENTATIONS

A word of caution is warranted from the experience of several radiation accidents around the world. The prodromal phase is sometimes misdiagnosed or not even seen. In several cases the patients were thought to have "food poisoning," and it was only after a fall in the white cell count (lymphocytes, granulocytes, and platelets) that medical personnel realized they were dealing with a radiation incident. Another lesson to be learned was from the Goiania accident in Brazil, where out of the 112,000 people monitored, approximately 8,000, who had no radiation exposure presented with either erythematous rashes or nausea or vomiting. Of course these people were concerned that they, too, might have been exposed (1).

THE LATENT PHASE

During the latent phase, the patient appears asymptomatic. This phase typically lasts from 2 to 4 weeks. However, if the dose received by the patient is very high, the latent phase can be shortened. Occasionally, the patient goes directly into the illness phase. During the latent phase, the patients are asymptomatic; however, it is during this period that rapidly dividing cell populations become depleted and patients begin to develop infections. These patients will usually require prophylactic antibiotics, antiviral agents, and antifungal agents.

THE ILLNESS PHASE

The illness phase is expressed by the damage to the specific organ system and depends on the level of whole body exposure dose received by the patient. Great strides have been made toward treatment of the hematological system, but unfortunately this is not the case for the "full-blown" gastroin-

TABLE 16-1 Characteristics Features of Clinical Syndromes Resulting from Radiation Exposure

SYNDROME	KEY CHARACTERISTICS	DOSE RANGE	USUAL TIME TO DEATH
CVS/CNS	Cardiovascular and brain failure	30 Gy (3,000 rads)	48 hours
Gastrointestinal	Small intestine failure	18 to 30 Gy (800 to 3,000 rads)	1 to 2 weeks
Hematopoetic	Bone marrow failure	2 to 8 Gy (200 to 800 rads)	60 days

testinal syndrome or the CVS/CNS syndrome. For the latter two, at present no treatment is available that can confidently bring about a full recovery.

DEFINITIVE OUTCOME: THE PHASE OF RECOVERY OR DEATH

Recovery of these patients can take weeks to months and follow-up will be required for the rest of their lives.

ASSESSING AN IRRADIATED CASUALTY

When assessing a casualty from a terrorist event, a number of distinct scenarios are possible. The patient could have injuries resulting from the use of explosives. The patient may have received whole body or partial body irradiation, and the patient may be *externally* or *internally* contaminated. Various combinations of these may occur together in a single patient. The time interval between when patients received the dose to when they develop signs and symptoms could range from a few days up to 3 weeks.

Remember that the irradiated patient is not a "medical emergency." No immediate intervention will make a difference to the survival of the patient. When caring for a traumatized irradiated patient, your first priority is to stabilize the patient for the trauma, not radiation. After the patient has been stabilized, proceed to focus on the problems of irradiation and contamination. Note that radiological contamination differs from *chemical* decontamination, where early decontamination is the rule. This is because with radiation exposures, the causative agent can be detected immediately with instrumentation. Also, staff members are wearing protective clothing with dosimeters. It is therefore possible to monitor them and have them rotate into or out of the environment if needed. Hence, with respect to radiation, it is often said, "You will be thanked for a live contaminated patient; however, you will not be thanked for a clean corpse."

IMPORTANT CLUES FROM THE PATIENT'S HISTORY

Several important variables may be obtained from simply talking to the awake and oriented patient. For example, did the patient develop nausea, vomiting, and diarrhea recently? What time did the symptoms start, how long did they last, and was it diagnosed as food poisoning? Did the patient receive any treatment for the vomiting? Other important information may be obtained by directed questions. Were any other people involved? Was the patient aware of where he or she was on that particular day? If the patient noticed skin redness, when and where did it occur? Did it disappear, has it reoccurred, and are there any areas of dry peeling or blistering of the skin?

The past medical history of the patient is also important. Ask if there is any history of renal disease, for example, because most interventional drugs used for removal of internal radioactive contamination are excreted through the kidneys. Has the pa-

tient had any nuclear medicine procedures with radioactive isotopes? If so, when were these performed? There has been the odd case where it was believed the patient was contaminated with radiation, only to learn later the patient had a recent nuclear medicine procedure. Inquire about the family medical history, and then carry out a full medical examination. If anything suggests radiation injury, photograph the involved site (2).

BIOLOGICAL SAMPLING: LABORATORY TESTS FOR PATIENTS WITH ACUTE RADIATION EXPOSURES

BLOOD

1. Obtain a complete blood count and white cell differential. Repeat every 4 to 6 hours, especially monitoring the lymphocyte count. By plotting the lymphocyte curve and comparing it to the *Andrews lymphocyte curves,* you can predict the prognosis and clinical course of the patient (3,4) (Fig. 16-1).

2. Obtain a full hospital biochemical laboratory screening as baseline information.

3. If you believe you are dealing with a criticality incident with the possibility of exposure to *neutrons*, send blood sample for identification of radioactive sodium. Natural body sodium 23 (Na_{23}) has the affinity of absorbing neutrons, changing it into *radioactive* Na_{24}, which is a beta and gamma emitter. Na_{24} has a half-life of approximately 15 hours.

4. Take a blood sample for cytogenetic analysis, and send it to a designated laboratory capable of doing chromosome analysis. They will be looking for "dicentric malformations" in the chromosomes. The dose to the patient (up to

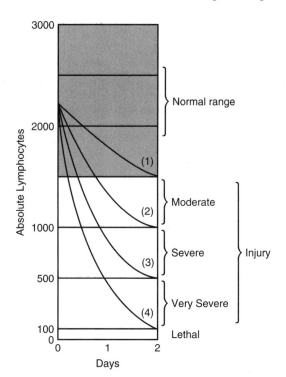

Figure 16–1. Andrews lymphocyte—prognosis nomogram.

10 Gy) can be determined. The lower limit of detection is in the region of 150 to 200 mGy (15 to 20 rads). Lymphocytes are required for this analysis. The lymphocytes are made to divide, fixed in metaphase, and the dicentric lesions are counted. The results of this laboratory test will not be available for a few days. Bender first proposed the use of dicentrics as a biological marker of radiation injury (5). However, some limitations exist with the interpretation of these results (6).

5. Take a blood sample for full human leukocyte antigen (HLA) typing. Also ABO blood typing and Rh blood grouping should be performed in case the patient requires blood transfusions or stem cell transplantation later.

6. For patients with potential or confirmed *internal contamination,* several samples are required. Save urine and fecal samples. Fecal samples are very important with respect to intake of insoluble radioactive isotopes located in the lungs or gastrointestinal tract. Fecal samples are often very difficult to obtain, especially in those individuals who are treated as outpatients. Stress the importance of these samples to the patients. Biological models used by the health physicist can determine the body burden of the relevant organ by the radioactive isotope involved using these samples.

7. Take a nasal swab specimen from each nostril, recording the time the swabs were taken and also the time the patient was removed from the radiation environment. Approximately 5% of the total radioactive material is held in the nares in the 1.5 hours after exposure. After this time, there tends to be clearance from the nose. Hence if you obtain a low reading from the nasal swabs more than 1.5 hours following exposure, this reading could represent a falsely low reading. The patient may have inhaled a significant amount of radioactivity (7). Be sure to record the time the swab samples were taken following exposure.

8. Other nonbiological samples to be taken are from the clothing and wound dressings of the patient. These should be sent to a nuclear laboratory to identify the isotopes you are dealing with, if you are dealing with a contamination. However, with the instrumentation used in your clinical setting, only the *types* of radiation produced are detected, not the actual isotopes. You may also take samples from metal objects such as jewelry and even the patient's medication. In the early 1980s, a radiation accident occurred in Norway. In this case, the health physics specialists at the time were able to calculate the dose to the patient by measuring the dose received to his angina medication (nitroglycerine tablets). This was achieved by using a technique known as *electron spin resonance dosimetry* (8).

ASSESSING THE PATIENT

The key blood test to monitor is the white cell differential count, which should be obtained every 4 to 6 hours for the first 24 to 48 hours. You may then display your results graphically and determine the prognosis of the patient.

An indication of the dose the patient has received can be estimated from the time of onset of vomiting initially, as already mentioned. The major problem is the time the patient presents to you after irradiation. Immediately following the ra-

diation exposure, there will be a rise in granulocytes, which is considered the trauma steroid response ("demargination"), followed shortly by a fall in the lymphocyte count. The lymphocyte cell line is very sensitive to irradiation. As described earlier, the Andrews lymphocyte curves can give an indication of the severity of the effect of irradiation on the hematopoietic system (9).

The Andrews nomogram gives a useful indication of the prognosis with respect to the patient. At very high dose ranges, the lymphocyte pool can be completely depleted within a 24- to 48-hour period. Therefore if the patient arrives for medical assessment more than 48 hours after the exposure and has received a significant high dose of irradiation, the patient will have no lymphocytes for the dicentric chromosomal analysis mentioned earlier (Fig. 16-2).

When one follows the general trend of the fate of the granulocytes, the nadir (lowest point) usually occurs at around 20 to 30 days after the exposure, with recovery taking place at around 30 to 40 days, depending on the dose of radiation received. At very high doses, one can expect no recovery at all. In the dose range of 2 to 4 Gy (200 to 400 rads), one might see an "abortive attempt" of granulocyte recovery. This may mislead the clinician into thinking the patient is recovering. The platelets are also very sensitive to irradiation, and their nadir tends to be slightly later than the granulocytes. The consequences of failure of these three cell lines will finally lead to severe infection and hemorrhage if not properly treated.

SPECIFIC TREATMENT FOR RADIATION INJURY

Treatment of radiation exposure depends largely on the organ systems involved and the extent of exposure. Among those who survive trauma and the initial phase of radiation sickness, the hematopoietic system is the most important focus of treatment in these patients.

Treatment of the hematopoietic syndrome is quite a sophisticated undertaking, often involving the use of cytokines, peripheral blood stem cells, platelet growth factors, platelet transfusions, cord blood stem cells, and bone marrow transplants. These approaches have sometimes been successful in supporting the patient during the hematopoietic crisis. Treatment in a number of cases was given in the nadir phase of the syndrome because the radiation accident was not identified until the latter part of the latent phase. The consensus now is to give cytokine treatment as soon as possible if the dose received was high enough to severely affect the stem cell lines.

CYTOKINES IN THE TREATMENT OF THE HEMATOPOIETIC SYNDROME

A specific class of drugs used to stimulate the bone marrow stem cells is the *cytokines.* These include granulocyte colony stimulating factor (G-CSF filgrastim) and granulocyte macrophage colony stimulating factor (GM-CSF sargramostim). The current drug of choice is G-CMF because it has fewer side effects. However, it tends to delay the recovery of platelets, and platelet transfusions are generally required.

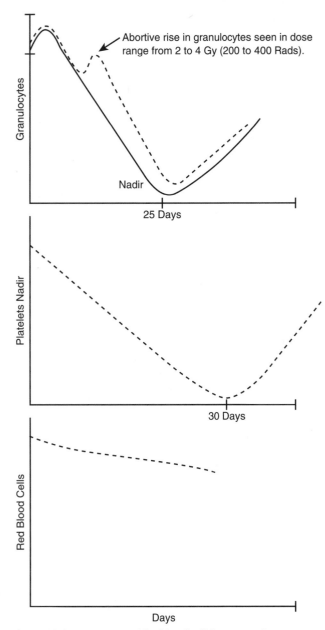

Figure 16–2. Damage to white blood cell lines over time.

When using G-CSF, platelet recovery ensues only after administration is stopped. In various accidents around the world, both G-CSF and GM-CSF have been used. GM-CSF was used in Goiania (3) where the patients were in the nadir phase. This resulted in recovery of some patients, but for those who did not survive it was believed no stem cells were left for the cytokines to act on. In the case of the Soreq accident in Israel, the patient was given GM-CSF within the first 24 hours and also received a bone marrow transplant 4 days following the accident (10). This was the first patient to receive the cytokine within the first 24 hours. Unfortunately, the patient succumbed to pneumonia and multiorgan failure and died approximately a month later.

Peripheral blood progenitor cells (PBPC) have also been used to treat the hematopoietic syndrome. Approximately 10% of peripheral blood is made up of these progenitor cells. These may be obtained by apherisis and expanded by cytokines in vitro and then transferred back into the patient (11).

One newer technique involves the use of hematopoietic *cord* blood cells (stem cells). These are obtained from the um-

bilical cord of the placenta at the time a baby is delivered. The cord blood is screened at the time of collection to rule out infectious diseases and then HLA typed. It is stored in liquid nitrogen. Umbilical cord blood has been used to treat a number of genetic and malignant diseases in children; a single collection would be sufficient to treat a child. So far cord blood transplants have been associated with reduced graft versus host disease (GVHD). In fact, in some cases full HLA typing was not achieved where cord blood stem cells were used. Very little is known about treating the adult in the accident situation. Umbilical cord blood transplant was used to treat one of the patients in the Tokaimura accident in Japan.

An excellent discussion about the management of hematological cell transplantation has been published (12,13). It has shown experimentally that cord blood cells can be obtained from delivery wards; matched for HLA, ABO, and Rh; and stored at normal blood storing temperatures of 4°C. Using this technique, cells were viable for another 10 to 21 days using gas permeable bags perfused with oxygen (14). This resulted in a reduction in the T-cell lymphocytes at a later stage. Hence it may be useful to consider this approach during radiation emergencies.

The major problem of HLA mismatch is it can cause GVHD. In this condition, the implanted blood progenitor cells react against the patient in whom they were implanted. Cord blood cells may have fewer problems with GVHD. It is known, for example, that some children treated for cancer with cord blood stem cells without full HLA typing did very well. The numbers of cord blood stem cells required for an adult in an emergency are not known; however, it is known that there are more stem cells per milliliter of cord blood compared to bone marrow. The concept of using cord blood in an emergency in the future is that these cells will be harvested at the time of each individual's birth. They are then stored in case they are needed at some future time. There is no invasive painful harvesting procedure as there is in bone marrow harvesting. Usually patients who require transplant receive their transplants within 3 to 5 days (15).

Platelet growth factors, thrombopoietin (TPO), and megakaryocyte growth and development factor (MGDF) are other modalities currently under investigation for the stimulation of platelet production to prevent hemorrhage (15). Before the introduction of these growth factors, the only treatment available was platelet transfusion. TPO administered immediately postirradiation is recommended by most specialists; however, it has not always been successful, and further research is required to define its role fully in treating victims of radiation illness.

TREATMENT OF THE GASTROINTESTINAL SYNDROME AND CVS/CNS SYNDROME

There is currently no treatment for full recovery for either of these syndromes. If a high level of radiation exposure occurred, the gastrointestinal syndrome will ensue and patients will suffer from vomiting and diarrhea. Sometimes the diarrhea will be bloody and explosive. Injury from irradiation is mostly confined to the lining of the small intestine, especially the villi and crypts. This results in shrinkage, ulceration, bleeding and sloughing of the internal lining, and loss of function. The inner lining loses its integrity, resulting in loss of electrolytes and important fluid loss. Also there is invasion by bacteria or bacterial toxins through this defective barrier. This usually leads to infection, septicemia, and death.

Vomiting can be treated with odansetron, a 5-HT3 receptor antagonist (16). The commonly recommended practice is to "sterilize" the intestines by using prophylactic antibiotics. Treatment of these syndromes is being investigated, but currently there are not many satisfactory alternatives.

LOCAL INJURIES

Local injuries, including trauma and radiation skin injuries, are very important. If the patient is suffering with the acute radiation syndrome *and* trauma, there is only a 24- to 48-hour window of opportunity available to operate. After this time, patients typically develop the hematological syndrome and become immunocompromised. Patients who receive surgery during this time are prone to develop serious infections, often leading to death. If this window of opportunity is missed, surgery must be delayed until recovery of the bone marrow has taken place. Note that for patients with both trauma and irradiation, the dangers are far greater than with irradiation alone.

Skin injuries can reveal a probable dose that the patient has received to the particular part of the body. The clinical expression of skin injuries can be divided into epilation, erythema, dry desquamation, wet desquamation, and finally necrosis. These are deterministic effects, in that there is a threshold dose for each one of these.

Epilation is the loss of body hair. The dose required to produce this is 3 Gy (300 rads). It usually takes 2 to 3 weeks to fully develop, and it is important to examine the whole body, especially arms and legs and chest. If a lesion is present, it is useful to take photographs.

Erythema is manifested at various times depending on the dose. If a part of the body is exposed to 3 Gy, the erythema takes 3 weeks to occur. At a dose of 6 Gy, the erythema will occur in only 24 to 48 hours. It then tends to disappear and reoccurs a few days later. Therefore the patient must be checked on a regular basis in the initial phase and serial photographs should be taken of the injury. Erythema that occurs minutes after exposure may be due to the chemical nature of the radioactive isotope and does not necessarily have any prognostic significance.

Dry desquamation is a dryness or peeling of the skin similar to that seen with sunburn without blisters. The dose required to produce this effect is 10 Gy (1,000 rads), and the time to expression is 2 to 4 weeks. *Moist desquamation* can present with small blisters, and as the dose increases these can coalesce into large blisters. The dose range for this lesion is from 15 to 25 Gy, and the expression of these injuries occurs after about 2 to 8 weeks depending on dose. Finally *necrosis* of the skin results with doses above 50 Gy (5,000 rads), occurring from days to weeks. By examining these types of injury one is able to achieve a rough assessment of the dose the patient has received to that particular part of the body.

CONTAMINATION

Contamination can be divided into external and internal, and both of these can occur at the same time. The radioactive material can either be in a gas, liquid, or solid form and can therefore contaminate a victim in several ways.

External contamination is most often the result of radioactive material being released into the atmosphere ("fallout"). The fallout settles on individuals or populations within a limited region. Since 90% of one's body is covered with clothing, simply by removing the clothing carefully one can eliminate 85% to 90% of the contamination. The remaining exposed parts include the head (hair, face, neck) and hands, providing there has been no damage to the clothing. Simply shampooing the hair a few times will result in effective decontamination of the hair. If the patient is ambulatory, the hair can be washed in the barber position over a sink. If you are faced with the situation where radioactive material can still be detected after several washings, cut off the hair with scissors. Never use a razor to shave the head because this can produce small cuts and provide a pathway for internal contamination. However, it is very uncommon for hair removal to be necessary. Ideally one should collect the contaminated water by disconnecting the waste pipe of the sink and allowing the water to drain into a container. This simple technique may not be practical if a large number of people must be decontaminated. The face, eyes, ears, and nostrils also require irrigation and decontamination.

For *skin decontamination*, simple washing with soap and water is usually all that is necessary. The technique involves washing from the outside toward the center, and it may have to be repeated many times. The goal is to detect a decrease in the instrument count after every wash. Acceptable decontamination can be defined as a decrease in radiation instrument count to no more than twice the background level. If this simple procedure is unsuccessful, use light abrasive techniques such as the use of cosmetic puff pads or a mild abrasive paste such as ground corn with washing powder. Diluted bleach has also been used, but it is not suitable for use on the face. If the skin becomes red, stop the procedure.

Another method used is known as the "sweat technique." Place a gauze pad over the contaminated area. Cover the site with polythene that is taped down and left in position for 4 to 6 hours. Remove the dressing and wash the area again. Note that these sweat dressings are not to be left on overnight. The final method is using a gauze dressing or a cotton glove and changing the dressings daily. The basis of this procedure is that 13% of epithelial skin is shed daily.

It is sometimes possible to make the isotope more soluble and thereby simplify its removal. In the Goiania, Brazil, incident, acetic acid solution was successfully used to decontaminate Cesium 137 from the skin (17). In the past it was considered acceptable to use potassium permanganate as a stripping agent for the outer layers of skin, but this is no longer utilized because of the strong oxidizing character of this agent.

INTERNAL CONTAMINATION

The three major routes by which internal contamination can occur are inhalation, ingestion, and through a wound. In unusual cases, absorption of the radioactive isotope can also occur through the intact skin, as with radioactive isotope tritium. The water form of this isotope can be absorbed through the intact skin.

When the information becomes available, it is helpful to be aware of the characteristics of each isotope involved in the radiation incident. Knowing what isotope you are dealing with gives an indication of what the target organ is likely to be. Examples include radioactive iron, which principally affects the bone marrow and the liver. Radioactive iodine 131 targets the thyroid gland. Heavy metals such as plutonium exert their effect principally on bone and liver.

The physical form of the isotope is also important whether it is in gaseous, liquid, or solid form. In the case of tritium, the radioactive isotope can either be in gaseous or liquid phase. The target organ in this case depends on the solubility of the isotope. Tritium in the gaseous form is insoluble, and the target organ is only the lungs. Tritiated water is soluble and the whole body would be irradiated.

Another important factor is the half-life of the isotope. Depending on the isotope, this can range from seconds to thousands of years. The definition of the *physical* half-life is the time it takes the radioactive isotope to decay to half its value. Ten half-lives are considered to be the time for the isotope to decay completely. The *biological* half-life is the time for half of the isotope to be excreted from the body. The combination of the physical and biological half-lives is called the *effective* half-life and can be derived by using the following formula:

$$\text{Effective half-life} = \frac{\text{biological half-life} \times \text{physical half-life}}{\text{biological half-life} + \text{physical half-life}}$$

If the isotope of concern is insoluble, the injury is limited to the organ of entry. Examples of target organs affected in this way include the lungs (inhalation), gastrointestinal tract (ingestion), or direct absorption across wounds. The most common site of injury for these insoluble isotopes is the lungs, resulting from inhalation of contaminated air. Taking nasal swabs within the 1.5 hours will give an indication of the lung burden the patient has received. Approximately 5% of the intake is contained within the anterior nares during this time period. The particle size of an inhaled isotope is also important to determine. However, this information will not be available until some time after the event. Particles between 1 and 10 microns tend to get trapped in the terminal bronchioles, which are not lined with ciliated epithelium. Larger particles are transported up the bronchial tree with the aid of the ciliated epithelium, which acts as an escalator. When these particles reach the back of the trachea, they are either expelled by coughing or swallowed, thereby contaminating the gastrointestinal tract. Collect all fecal samples. This measurement of contamination in fecal samples allows the nuclear health physicist to calculate the lung burden. When patients have received a very large intake of radioactive material into their lungs, especially isotopes with very long half-lives, medication is required to aid excretion of these isotopes. If this fails, broncheoalveolar lavage may be considered. The procedure consists of washing out the lungs with isotonic saline under a general anesthetic. The washing procedure is repeated several times, and an estimated 25% to 50% of the intake can be removed by this method (18).

CONTAMINATED WOUNDS

Wounds contaminated with radioactive material resulting from trauma must be treated after stabilization of the patient and before decontamination of the skin. Copious irrigation of the wound with normal saline is required. Surround the wound with waterproof drapes and save all washings for analysis at a later stage. The wound may require several irrigations. After each irrigation, monitor the wound with a radiation instrument. If the count from the instrument is still decreasing, continue irrigating. The goal is to arrive at less than twice the background levels of radiation. If after several washings of the wound decontamination has not been achieved, refer the patient for surgical debridement. Surgical debridement of wounds requires consideration of function and cosmetic result. Surgical management of the irradiated, traumatized patient has been described in the medical literature (19).

TREATMENT OF INTERNAL CONTAMINATION

Several drugs can be used to aid excretion of radioactive isotopes, but some of these have limiting side effects and are only used in an emergency. A detailed account of drugs used for various isotopes can be found in the NCRP Report No. 65 (20). A few examples follow.

Cesium 137 (Cs_{137}) was the major isotope of concern in the Goiania, Brazil, accident, and it was also one of the major isotopes released in the Chernobyl accident. Cesium is a beta gamma emitter with a physical half-life of 36 years and an effective half-life of approximately 40 days. Its chemical properties are similar to those of potassium. Prussian blue (ferric ferrocyanate) has been used for treating exposure to this isotope. The first time this drug was reported was in Goiania (21). Because Cs is in the same group as potassium in the periodic table, it was assumed Cs would act similarly to potassium and be excreted with the aid of diuretics. However, this was not the case. As a result, Prussian blue was introduced, and it was found that Cs_{137} was excreted at a ratio of 4:1 via the fecal pathway, compared to urine. It was thought that Prussian blue works via a mechanism of enterohepatic circulation. This drug was given orally to patients, who received doses from 3 to 20 grams a day. However, some patients could not tolerate these high doses of the drug due to the side effect of gastritis. These effects improved upon reduction of dose. There were some cases of long-term gastritis, with improvement after 18 to 24 months. Gastroscopy and gastric biopsies were carried out over this period of time and showed no pathological lesions.

Tritium, the third isotope of hydrogen, comes in two main forms: tritiated gas, which is insoluble, and tritiated water, which is soluble. It has a physical half-life of 12.6 years and an effective half-life of 12 days, giving off low beta radiations.

Virtually all of tritiated *gas* is exhaled directly to the atmosphere. Therefore in this situation it is especially important to evacuate the building and open all windows, thereby allowing the tritiated gas to escape. In the case of tritiated water, the tritium is in the soluble form and ends up in the water pool of the body. The treatment of choice here is copious fluid, 4 to 5 liters a day, to exchange the pool of body water. Enhancing fluid intake in this manner reduces the effective half-life of tritium from 12 days to about 4 days.

Many other important isotopes are not discussed here, such as iodine-131, cobalt-60, strontium-90, plutonium-239, and uranium-235. Many of these have specific forms of supplementary treatment (20).

LOGISTICS INVOLVED IN TREATING RADIATION INCIDENTS

In an incident involving radioactivity, you might be dealing with a few exposed individuals from a limited exposure or thousands of patients. In the latter case, large numbers of individuals require testing to rule out radiation injury or contamination, even though perhaps only a small number will have suffered actual exposures. Many individuals in these situations are frightened about the consequences of exposure regardless of whether they are actually injured or not. It is best to plan for the availability of counseling for people who are concerned about a possible exposure. Ideally, support centers should be set up away from the accident site or hospital. A typical team would be staffed with a team that includes a physician knowledgeable about radiation health, a health physicist, a psychiatrist and/or a psychologist, and a radiation safety officer with instrumentation.

Finally, medical staff must be fully trained to deal with irradiated contaminated casualties and regular exercises carried out to maintain the individual and team skills.

PSYCHOLOGICAL CONSIDERATIONS

The patient will be understandably worried about the consequences of irradiation. Most people relate to Hiroshima and Nagasaki. It is important to explain to the patient what radiation is and how it affects an individual. These patients must be supported through their stress and be advised and supported by a team as just described.

DEALING WITH FATALITIES AND PASTORAL SUPPORT

Not many people give thought to the proper disposition of bodies in radiation incidents until it is upon them. It is important to plan for temporary mortuary facilities. Generally, you do not want to use the hospital mortuary because it puts the Pathology Department out of action. The ideal temporary mortuary facility to use is a mobile chilling unit such as those used to transport food. Note that the goal of such a chilling unit is not to freeze the remains because this will destroy some of the forensic evidence.

Another important factor is religious considerations. In cases where contamination with radioactive materials exists, the bodies may not be cremated unless they are first decontaminated. Religious practices for dealing with the death of a family member vary. Arrangements should exist to provide special dispensation for the religion of concern, thereby reducing as much stress as possible to the relatives.

SUMMARY

The treatment of irradiated contaminated patient depends on the dose the patient has received, whether it is whole body or partial body exposure or a combination of both, and to this can be added the problem of internal or external contamination.

Signs and symptoms are very limited initially, but one can determine the probable outcome. At very high doses it can be determined whether the individual is developing the classic radiation syndromes. As stated, for the full-blown gastrointestinal syndrome and the CVS/CNS syndrome, there is at present no treatment to aid in patient recovery. However, with respect to the hematopoietic syndrome, significant advances have been made.

When dealing with these patients, every specialty within the hospital will be involved. Also radiation specialists will be involved; however, these people will not be available immediately, but advice initially can be obtained by telephone until the radiation specialists arrive to support the relevant hospital staff concerned.

The Radiation Emergency Assistance Center/Training Site (REAC/TS) is a good resource for radiation expertise. This organization, which is part of the U.S. Department of Energy response network, makes available medical experts, radiobiologists, and health physics experts. It has responded to several major radiation accidents and also provides training for doctors, nurses, and health physicists in the treatment and managing of irradiated/contaminated casualties, treatment capabilities, and consultant assistance on a 24-hour basis.

RESOURCE

Radiation Emergency Assistance Center/Training Site (REAC/TS). Web site: http://www.orau.gov/reacts/default.htm.

QUESTIONS AND ANSWERS

1. **Acute radiation syndrome (ARS) follows a set course, which will express itself within hours to weeks depending on the level of dose received. ARS can be divided into each of the following phases, EXCEPT:**
   A. The prodromal phase
   B. The precipitant phase
   C. The latent phase
   D. The illness phase
   E. The phase of final outcome, either recovery or death

2. **Laboratory tests that should be initiated for patients with acute radiation exposures include each of the following, EXCEPT:**

A. T3 resin uptake
B. Complete blood count
C. Blood sample for cytogenetic analysis
D. Human leukocyte antigen (HLA) typing
E. Full hospital biochemical laboratory screening

3. Approaches that have sometimes been successful in supporting the patient during a radiation-induced hematopoietic crisis include:

A. Cytokines
B. Platelet transfusions
C. Bone marrow transplants
D. A + B
E. A + B + C

4. Routes by which internal radiation contamination can occur include all of the following, EXCEPT:

A. Inhalation
B. Ingestion
C. Through a wound
D. Occasional absorption of radioactive isotope through intact skin
E. Bony absorption through carious teeth

ANSWERS

1: *B.* *The precipitant phase*
2: *A.* *T3 resin uptake*
3: *E.* *A + B + C*
4: *E.* *Bony absorption through carious teeth*

REFERENCES

1. International Atomic Energy Agency, The Radiological accident in Goiania, IAEA, Vienna, 1988.
2. International Atomic Energy Agency. How to recognize and initially respond to an accidental radiation injury. Rev. ed. Vienna: IAEA-TECDOC-953, IAEA, 2000.
3. Andrews GA, Auxier JA, Lushbaugh CC. The importance of dosimetry to the medical management of persons accidentally exposed to high levels of radiation. In: Personnel dosimetry for radiation accidents. Vienna International Atomic Emergency Agency 1965;3-16.
4. Andrews GA. Medical management of accidental total body irradiation. In: Hubner KF, Fry SA eds. The medical basis for radiation accident preparedness. North Holland: Elsevier 1980;297-301.
5. Bender, MA. Chromosome aberrations in irradiated human subjects. Ann NY Acad Sci 1964;114:249-51.
6. Littlefield LG, Lushbaugh CC. Cytogenetic dosimetry for radiation accidents: the good, the bad, and the ugly. In: Ricks RC, Fry, SA eds. The medical basis for radiation accident preparedness. North Holland: Elsevier, 1990.
7. Hyde KR, Jech, JJ. Assessing the probable severity of plutonium inhalation cases. Health Physics 1969;17:433-47.
8. Sagstuen E, Theisen H., et al. Dosimetry by ESR spectroscopy following a radiation accident. Health Phys 1983;45 (5): 961-8.
9. Bennder M. Chromosome aberrations in irradiated human subjects. Ann NY Acad Sci 1964; 114:249.
10. Andrews, GA. Radiation accidents and their management. Radiat Res Suppl 1967;7:390-7.
11. Bensinger WI, Clift R, Martin P, et al. Allogeneic peripheral blood stem cell transplantations in patients with advanced haematological malignancies: a retrospective comparison with bone marrow transplant. Blood 1996;88:2794-800.
12. Confer DL, Stroncek DF. Bone marrow and peripheral stem cell donors. In: Thomas ED, Blume KG, Foreman SJ eds. Haemopoietic cell transplantation. Boston: Blackwell Scientific, 1999;421-30.
13. Ende N, Lu S, Ende M, et al. Potential effectiveness of stored cord blood (non frozen) for emergency use. J Emerg Med 1996;14(6):673-7.
14. Ende N, Lu S, Mack R, et al. The feasibility of using blood bank-stored (4c) cord blood, unmatched for H.L.A. for marrow transplantation. Am J Clin Pathol 1999;111:773-81.
15. Schiffer CA, Anderson K. Platelet transfusion therapy. In: Asco 2000 syllabus. Alexandria, VA: American Society of Clinical Oncology, 2000;290-8.
16. Priestman TJ. Clinical studies with odansetron in the control of radiation induced emesis. Eur J Cancer Clin Oncol 1989;25(Suppl 1):S29-S33.
17. Rosenthal JJ, de Almeida CE, et al. The radiological accident in Goiania: the initial remedial actions. Health Phys 1991; 60(1):7-15.
18. Muggenburg BA, Mauderly JL, et al. Prevention of radiation pneumonitis from inhaled cerium-144 by lung lavage in beagle dogs. Am Rev Respir Dis 1975;111(6):795-802.
19. Hirsch EF, Bowers GJ. Irradiated trauma victims: the impact of ionizing radiation on surgical considerations following a nuclear mishap. World J Surg 1992;16(5):918-23.
20. Management of persons accidentally contaminated with radionuclides. NCRP Report no. 65.
21. Melo DR, Lipsztein JL, et al. 137Cs internal contamination involving a Brazilian accident, and the efficacy of Prussian Blue treatment. Health Phys 1994;66(3):245-52.

17

Radiation Dispersal Devices, Dirty Bombs, and Nonconventional Radiation Exposure

Madison Patrick, Keith Edsal, and Daniel C. Keyes

The author T. S. Elliot once said, "Give me a handful of dust, and I will show you true fear." He was referring to radioactive contamination.

The nuclear threat is an invisible threat and the biological effects that occur depend on the dose received and the dose rate. To produce *acute radiation syndrome* (Chapter 16), the radiation must be penetrating, and the whole body must be exposed to the radiation. The expression of these biological effects may be delayed for hours, days, or even years. Risk to the individual depends on the route of exposure and the type of radiation produced. Two important methods of exposure are discussed in this chapter: the "dirty bomb" and a hidden radiation source.

A radiation dispersal device (RDD) is essentially the combination of a conventional explosive and radioactive material. In an RDD, the explosion spreads the radioactive material, but there is no nuclear detonation. This might be similar to an actual nuclear bomb that fails to cause a nuclear detonation, but scatters radioactive material when the conventional explosives in the weapon explode. Individuals who are near the device might be injured or killed by the explosion, and the radioactive material would be scattered causing additional injuries, contamination of the survivors, emergency personnel, and area. A recent article in *Time* magazine reports that Osama Bin Laden has threatened to use the so-called dirty bomb and notes that U.S. officials even raise the possibility of Al Qaeda trying to acquire nuclear weapons, allegedly from Pakistan (1). It is thought that Al Qaeda has attracted sympathetic individuals from among Pakistan's nuclear scientists. The *Time* article states, "In the past eight years, 175 cases have been recorded worldwide of nuclear materials (not bombs) being smuggled out of former Soviet territories and other countries." In addition, the threat of this actually happening in the United States has risen since a U.S. citizen was arrested for allegedly working with Al Qaeda to detonate an RDD within the United States. Weapons-grade nuclear material could also come from the loss of the small nuclear bombs during the breakup of the Soviet Union (2).

There have been several recorded incidences of theft of weapons-grade materials including plutonium and enriched uranium-235. In 1993 at the shipyard in Murmansk, parts of nuclear fuel assemblies were stolen. In October 1993, police in Istanbul seized 2.5 kilograms of uranium-238. In Prague, 2.7 kilograms of highly enriched uranium-235 was seized. In the early 1990s, several incidences in Germany with respect to smuggling both real and fake nuclear material occurred, and at that time the frequency of such cases appeared to be increasing (3,4).

INJURIES DUE TO BLAST EFFECTS

Injuries may be differentiated between those caused by a conventional blast and those resulting from radiation exposure. One of the authors had a personal experience that demonstrated some of the concerns of a potential radioactive dispersion associated with an explosive event.

Basic characteristics of blast injuries will be introduced here, but they are present in greater detail in Chapter 20.

Blast effects will depend on the amount of explosive used in the device. The blast injuries depend on the magnitude of the explosive charge and how close the victims are to the blast. There are several explosive properties to be considered. *Primary blast injuries* are those that occur when the blast wave travels through the body causing damage to the organs and tissues that have air and fluid interfaces, in contact with each other, such as in the lungs. When the blast wave goes through the body, the fluid is noncompressible and it is thrown or pulled into the less dense tissue. In such cases, when the blast wave goes through the chest, blood is forced into the air cells of the lungs causing additional hemorrhage. As the blast wave goes through the lung, more blood is "pulled" into the lung tissue and more hemorrhage results. Tearing of the lung tissue also results in air and blood vessels being in contact, and potential air embolism can result. The patient can clinically have difficulty breathing, tachycardia, hypoxia, chest pain, altered mental status, and anxiety. The patient may have a syncopal episode (loss of consciousness) as well as anxiety. These patients are at risk for air embolism (air in the blood vessels) or a pneumothorax (free air in the pleural cavity). All these injuries can be serious and/or life threatening. *Secondary blast injuries* are those injuries caused by flying debris from the blast. Depending on the size of the blast, glass and shrapnel can penetrate the body causing major wounds and fractures. The result is that the trauma is applied directly to the body and traumatized tissue. Suicide bombings frequently include shrapnel, and these materials can contribute greatly to injury and death. *Tertiary blast injuries* result from the victim being thrown by the blast force against stationary objects. It is thought that the majority of injuries from the Oklahoma City terrorist event were due to secondary and tertiary blast injuries (5,6). In addition to long bone fractures and some complete amputations, skull fractures were common, and 17 children had open brain trauma. Miscellaneous blast effects, such as burn, inhalation of gases, and other types of trauma, may also occur. Falling structures may induce crush injuries, which are discussed in Chapter 21. These patients will need appropriate trauma and burn care.

INJURIES DUE TO RADIOLOGICAL EFFECTS

Radiological effects from an explosive device will be dependent on the amount and type of the radioactive source(s) used. The radioactive exposure will depend on the type of radioactive source, how large it was, how close the victims were to it, and how long the victims were exposed to it.

SOURCES OF RADIATION USE IN RADIATION DISPERSAL DEVICES

Numerous sources of radioactive material are in normal use today. In the medical field, radioactive isotopes are used in the treatment of cancer modalities and include cesium-37, cobalt-60, and iridium-192. Nuclear medicine departments use certain radioactive tracer elements for investigations. In industry, radioactive isotopes are used for testing the integrity of welds in oil pipes and for detecting metal stress fractures in aircraft. Large activity radioactive sources are used in the sterilization of medical products such as syringes and intravenous drip bags. They are also used in food preparation to reduce the bacterial count of food, therefore increasing the food shelf life. They have been used to irradiate seeds. Enriched uranium-235, used as fuel rods for reactors, is also applied as a high activity source for research. It is interesting to note that the majority of serious radiation accidents that have occurred around the world have been due to accidents with industrial sources or medical therapy sources used in the treatment of cancer. The accountability of radioactive sources in the Western countries is good due to strict regulations. Departments that use these materials

are required to register them as radioactive sources, and inventories together with regular spot check inspections are mandatory. In the case of a radiation accident occurring, the source and the activity of the source will be known. Unfortunately, these crucial last two factors will not be known in a terrorist event.

There are millions of packages containing radioactive materials shipped annually. Since there has not been a transportation accident resulting in a radiation exposure death since the start of radioactive materials transportation over 40 years ago, it has become standard practice to ship radioactive materials. Radiation sources from shipped packages could potentially be used as a terrorist weapon in an RDD.

RADIATION THREAT SCENARIOS

To fully understand the impact of RDDs, we must put them into perspective with other methods of distributing radiation. *A simple radiological device* is defined as a method of spreading radioactive material *without* the use of an explosive device. An example of this type of device could be the placement of a device where unsuspecting people could be exposed to the radiation. Surreptitious exposure of hidden isotopes without a blast

A terrorist could place a high activity source in a highly populated location where the movement of people is relatively stationary, such as at queues or a conference venue. These sources could be placed under seats or around bars or even under buffet tables; as a result, people could receive a significant dose of radiation and develop nausea and vomiting a few hours later, blaming this on food poisoning. Generally the majority of people who develop nausea and vomiting tend to take care of themselves over the first 24 hours and not go to a doctor. If they did go to a doctor, the doctor would most often diagnose food poisoning and usually radiation would not be in the differential diagnosis. People could also develop skin lesions, such as erythema, desquamation, blisters, or even ulcers. This would generally be misdiagnosed as dermatitis, mycosis, allergies, chemical burns, or even pemphygus skin lesions. Initially, this would not be associated with ionizing radiation.

As discussed in previous chapters, this type of exposure has already occurred in Goiania, Brazil, in 1987, where thieves stole a radiotherapy source from an abandoned clinic, and broke it apart (7,8). They actually were able to get to the source of 1375 curies of radioactive cesium-137 and were heavily exposed to the radiation. They sold the machine to a scrap metal dealer. The scrap dealer, his family, friends, and others suffered from exposure, and four died. It took about two weeks to realize that this was radiation exposure. The exposure was discovered when the wife of the scrap dealer took some of the cesium source into town on a bus (exposing more people) to deliver it to a town official. The source was placed on the desk of the official where it was recognized as a high-level radiation source the following day. A major radiation accident was announced to the local population, and over 112,800 people had to be monitored, 249 were contaminated, 129 were both internally and externally contaminated, 49 were hospitalized, 28 had local radiation injury, and 4 died. There had to be extensive cleanup over several months with several homes demolished and containerized. This caused substantial fear in the local population with travel restricted in the area and an embargo of the produce of the area. A terrorist could cause such fear by hiding a similar radioactive source in a heavily populated or trafficked area, thus exposing many.

RADIATION DISPERSAL DEVICE

An RDD, or dirty bomb, is formed by combining an explosive agent (such as TNT) with radioactive material. These devices can cause conventional blast injuries as well as radiation injuries resulting from the dispersion of the radioactive material to the environment and surrounding population. This would be one of the easier radiation devices for a terrorist to use. It would not be difficult to obtain a radiation source or the explosives. Significant amounts of radioactive materials could be spread this way with additional conventional blast injuries.

An airplane used as a "suicide bomb" as in 9/11 could have radioactive material in it and could, on impact, spread radioactive material over a wide area. This would provide a great challenge to rescue efforts since the radioactive dust might contaminate the victims and the rescue workers as well as equipment. A similar issue was raised with the firefighters who initially did not have respiratory protection during the Twin Towers attack on September 11, 2001. The problem of inhaled contaminants and pulmonary toxicology would be compounded if they were breathing radioactive dust. Even with respiratory protection, they would still be contaminating their clothing.

If terrorists managed to obtain weapons-grade material such as enriched uranium-235 or plutonium-239, they could also use these materials in a conventional explosive device. This would cause major problems not in the short-term radiation sense, but as a result of contamination of the environment. Plutonium-239 and uranium-235, both nuclear weapons-grade materials, have very long physical half-lives and require thousands of years to decay completely. This would produce areas of contamination that would be considered as "no go" areas until decontamination was completed, which could take months to years to achieve.

Radiation monitoring devices were described previously in Chapter 14. In the event of an RDD explosion, these instruments would be used to measure radiation in a fixed location, self standing or attached to people. These instruments should be in fire departments and other emergency response agencies. It has been suggested that there should be radiation monitoring and detection devices strategically placed around a city to monitor any potential radioactive material from a blast where potential radioactive material could have been used, such as if radioactive material were spread by means of an RDD. With an alarm, notification would go to the appropriate law enforcement agency and the FBI, since this would be a potential "weapon of mass destruction." A series of local, state, and federal responses and other notifications would result, depending on the situation.

INITIAL EVALUATION AND TREATMENT FOR RDD DETONATION

Emergency treatment should take precedence over other care since resuscitation and life/limb saving care has the highest priority. If the patient is contaminated, decontamination should be a high priority also. Staff protection with appropriate personal protective equipment (PPE) and personal dosimeters will be necessary. *Radiological survey* (specialized history, physical examination, and radiation detection) of the patient is the initial starting point for care of a contaminated patient and is described more completely in Chapter 16. The patient should be interviewed to obtain the history of the exposure. Information should be gathered on the type and source of exposure if possible, as well as the distance from the source and the amount of time exposed. Other pertinent information includes determining if there were other victims and obtaining information necessary to assist in the criminal investigations.

Signs and symptoms assist in determining prognosis. Nausea, vomiting, and anorexia are important symptoms to note. If they occur earlier, this is an indication of a severe exposure (see Chapter 16). Severe exposure may result in transient loss of consciousness. There may also be trauma with the exposure, so trauma life support may be initiated as appropriate. If surgery or orthopedic care is needed, it should be done in the first 2 days before bone marrow depression occurs. Otherwise, there will be a wait of about 2 months while the blood cells return to normal.

LABORATORY TESTS

Patients who have been exposed to an RDD generally should receive a complete blood count (CBC) with differential. Platelet count and absolute lymphocyte count are also important prognostic indicators. Samples must be taken if internal contamination is suspected. These include swabs of nares, oropharynx, and wounds to check for internal contamination. Stool, emesis, sputum, and urine samples for baselines are important, and they should be repeated daily for 4 days to monitor excretion rate. A heparinized blood sample for chromosomal abnormalities in circulating lymphocytes is useful as well.

TREATMENT

Emergency treatment of the victim of an RDD is based first on the type of injury suffered by the patient. Life-threatening injuries should take precedence. Treatment should begin in the "hot zone" to stabilize the patient along with decontamination. It will be important to have the radiation protection officer (RPO) or other appropriate radiologically trained person do an expeditious survey of the patient in case gross contamination is present. These patients should be transferred to appropriate hospitals for definitive care. The receiving hospital should be informed of the patient's contamination status and survey readings so that they can prepare the response personnel with appropriate PPE as well as prepare the decontamination/treatment area for receipt of contaminated patients.

DECONTAMINATION

If the patient was only irradiated, then decontamination will not be necessary. If an RDD is suspected, decontamination will be necessary. It will be important to know which has occurred and to survey the patient to make certain. Decontamination of externally contaminated body surface includes the removal of the clothing, which will take care of the majority of the body. The exposed parts of the body, including the head and the extremities, should be carefully cleansed to prevent the spread of contaminants to any parts of the body that were not initially contaminated.

INTERNAL CONTAMINATION

The most likely form of internal contamination from an RDD is from inhalation of particles of debris contaminated with small amounts of radioactive material. Inhalation of radioactive material is difficult to remove since it may be insoluble and remain in the lung. This would cause ongoing radiation to the sensitive lung tissues. Lung lavage may be required (9).

DECONTAMINATION OF WOUNDS

Wound decontamination needs to be done by irrigation with sterile saline or water to remove any radioactive material. Decontamination may need to be repeated, and measurements should be taken of the wound after each irrigation (Chapter 16). It is helpful to know if it emits beta, gamma, and/or alpha radiation. The commonly used instruments measure beta and gamma radiation. Alpha radiation is much more difficult to detect, and it should be performed by a trained and experienced person. The contaminated wounds may be difficult to clean and may require repeated irrigations, debridement, and/or decorporating agent treatment and monitoring. As long as the contamination is being reduced, it should be continued. Surgical care may be needed to remove contaminated tissue. Survey of the cleansed areas must be done, especially for wounds, to make certain that they are clean.

DECONTAMINATION OF THE GASTROINTESTINAL TRACT

If the gastrointestinal (GI) tract was contaminated, or is highly suspected to be so, then gut decontamination will be

necessary, since uptake from the gut leads to incorporation into the body and internal organs. It is significantly more important to treat internal contamination since the radioactive material continues to irradiate tissues until it decays to a stable isotope or is biologically eliminated. Incorporation may take place if the isotope is absorbed and distributed in the body. The biochemical nature of the radionuclide determines whether it is disseminated throughout the body or goes to a specific organ, such as the thyroid. The term *critical organ* is used for the organ that receives the highest dose of radiation or is the site of the most significant biological damage.

IDENTIFICATION AND MEASUREMENT

The way to determine if there is internally deposited radionuclide is by radioanalysis of the substances excreted from the body such as sputum, urine, and fecal specimens. Radioactivity in the body may also be measured by a whole body counter, which primarily measures gamma emitters and some high-energy beta radiation. Such whole body counters are not usually practical in the emergency setting.

GENERAL TREATMENT

The different radioisotopes have differing methods for removal and are only briefly introduced here. The main goal of removal is to reduce absorption, or hasten elimination. Identification is possible using radiochemical identification of radionuclides but may take several days. If the substance was inhaled, bronchopulmonary lavage may be required. When the radioactive material crosses into the extracellular fluid, it is incorporated. There are several ways to *decorporate* including blocking agents, isotopic dilution, displacement, mobilization agents, and chelation (9). Incorporation is not usually a hazard to medical personnel because they are wearing protective clothing. *Blocking agents* reduce the uptake of the radioisotope at an organ or metabolic site by saturating the site with a stable form of the isotope, for example by using KI (potassium iodide) to saturate the thyroid with stable iodide (KI, oral 300 mg/day for 7 to 14 days). For children, a KI cough syrup is used. *Isotopic dilution* is a method of decreasing the concentration of the radioactive form of the isotope so it will be excreted (e.g., for tritiated water contamination). This is typically done by the oral intake of water (3 to 4 liters daily). *Chelation* therapy uses organic compounds that provide an ion exchange matrix; it is one method of *decorporation*. The radioactive isotope exchanges with an inorganic ion resulting in a nonionized ring complex that can be excreted (e.g., DTPA, 1 g/day for 5 days). *Mobilizing agents* may be used to induce body tissues to release radioisotopes by increasing the natural turnover process. These methods are designed to increase the rate of elimination. Mobilizing agents such as these are most effective when given early after the exposure. The efficacy of these interventions diminishes with time (9). *Alpha contamination* is a particularly important case, sometimes requiring decorporation. Since alpha contamination causes potentially significant damage when internalized, early *chelation* is sometimes useful (within 1 to 2 hours after exposure), with Ca-DTPA (calcium diethylenetriamine pentaacetic acid) or the zinc form being recommended. Other heavy metal contamination is also effectively chelated by using these forms. Ca-DTPA is preferred due to the metallic taste of the zinc form.

EXTERNALLY IRRADIATED PATIENTS—GENERAL CONCEPTS

MANAGEMENT OF THE CONTAMINATED PATIENT

The contaminated RDD victim may have a complex radiation exposure: external, internal, contamination, and injury. Priority of treatment includes the serious medical or surgical conditions first. Protection of the providers is next. Decontamination of the patient follows. Counseling of the patient concerning the significance of the radiation may be necessary. External contamination is usually on clothing and exposed skin—hands, face, and head.

MEDICAL MANAGEMENT

Personal protective equipment is an important consideration for health care providers. References that describe appropriate PPE are available (10), and general characteristics are discussed in Chapter 28. Protecting the airway, eyes, and mouth of each medical provider, with surgical-type scrub suits and double gloves, is the goal of PPE here. All workers will also need radiological monitoring devices worn on their PPE suits. Patient management should be conducted in the *radiation emergency area* (REA). Access by clinic staff and other patients should be restricted to the clinical staff caring for the patient to minimize the possibility of spreading contamination to other areas of the clinic.

SPECIAL CONSIDERATIONS FOR FIELD RESCUE FOR VICTIMS OF RDD

As soon as the patient is stabilized, decontamination should commence in the field. The decontamination process not only reduces the patient exposure by decreasing the total amount of surface contamination but also minimizes the opportunity for the contamination to be ingested or inhaled. Decontamination also removes the material from wound sites to assist in preventing incorporation. Field decontamination also reduces exposure to the staff, other patients, and the facility. Removal of the contaminated clothing will eliminate the majority of the contamination. During the decontamination, care must be taken to prevent the patient from being internally contaminated, through inhalation or ingestion or across contaminated wounds. Definitive, methodical decontamination should be performed at the hospital with the guidance of the RPO. Patients transported in advance of decontamination should be wrapped in blankets to minimize/eliminate the spread of the contamination.

WOUND DECONTAMINATION

Wounds may be difficult to clean if contaminated since the tissues, fluids, and the like can mask the alpha emitters such as plutonium, and alpha particles can be readily absorbed by body fluids. Tissue samples from wounds may have to be sent for laboratory analysis to be certain if they are clean. Special low-energy x-ray detectors operated by highly trained and experienced personnel may be necessary to examine wounds. It is clear that if there were many radioactively contaminated personnel from an explosion of a radioactive weapon such as an RDD with resultant contaminated wounds, there would be a need for many experienced radiation personnel to assist.

If the mouth is involved, it should be rinsed well with much water. Assistance may be necessary to accomplish this. Obtain swabs of orifices during the irrigation procedures. Save all irrigation fluids for analysis. Name, date, site, and time of sampling should be noted on the container. These samples can be evaluated for radiation. Based on the number of counts above the background radiation, they are then classified as low level (up to thousands of counts) or high level (many thousands of counts). Copious amounts of water should be used first, and soap is also needed, to remove heavy high-level surface contamination. Soft surgical sponges should be used to prevent damage to the skin. After the survey results, the highest level of contamination should be cleaned first. Use clean 4x4 gauze pads for each swab to avoid cross-contamination. The areas to be cleaned must be isolated with waterproof drapes to prevent contamination of other areas of the body. Lower-level intact skin should be next, and it should be cleaned appropriately similar to the skin in the high-level areas.

Eyes—Treatment of the eyes should be similar to standard treatment of a foreign body, with the additional issue of radioactivity. Removal of any foreign bodies and then irrigation with analysis for radioactivity is required. Irrigation of the eyes should be in the direction from the inner canthus to the outer canthus to limit the possibility of contaminating the lacrimal duct.

Thermal and Chemical Burns—These areas need cleansing like other burns with additional precautions of saving all rinsing fluids and surveying all materials used for cleaning the areas. Dressings need to be labeled and saved for analysis when removed.

Lacerations—Gentle irrigation with copious amounts of water or saline are needed. Special use of cleaning with hydrogen peroxide and surgical scrubs may be necessary. Save all wound drainage. Leave open if unable to determine if clean.

Puncture Wounds—It may be necessary to surgically remove some contaminated tissue, but caution should be exercised to prevent further damage.

TABLE 17-1 Guideline for Response to a Radiation Accident or a Dirty Bomb for a Hospital

1. Radiation accident hospital response notification
   a. Number of patients
   b. Type of injury/illness
   c. Is the patient contaminated?
   d. Staff/REA preparation
2. Patient arrival
   a. Medical report
   b. Radiological report
   c. Clean team transfer
3. Triage/evaluation/treatment
   a. Cut away clothing
   b. Isolate contaminated area
4. Dry decontamination
   a. Remove contaminated articles from patient/staff
5. Radiological assessment
   a. Survey/document
   b. Sample orifices and contaminated area/label
6. Wet decontamination
   a. Priorities
      i. Wound/orifices
      ii. Intact skin
   b. Methods
      i. Drape
      ii. Wash
      iii. Rinse
      iv. Dry
      v. Survey
7. Patient exit
   a. Clean pathway
   b. Clean team transfer
   c. Final survey at control line
8. Staff exit
   a. Remove anti-contamination clothing
   b. Survey at control line
9. REA cleanup

EMERGENCY MEDICAL SERVICE PERSONNEL

Prehospital personnel, who have provided care for the patient in the emergent situation, must remain in a controlled area until they can be properly surveyed and cleared from contamination. The same is true for any of their equipment that may have been used in the care of the patient and potentially contaminated. If contaminated, the equipment must be cleaned or discarded.

Treatment Area—The treatment area must be surveyed for any residual contamination after the "clean" patient has been finally transferred to ongoing care in the hospital. State, contractor, or Department of Energy personnel may assist in the survey, cleanup, and restoration of the room for use.

Radiation Emergency Area—The REA is where the radiation-contaminated patient is managed and grossly decontaminated. It is discussed and diagrammed in Chapter 15. The patient must be decontaminated before being transported to an outlying facility. To prevent contamination of the transport equipment, contaminated clothing and external exposed parts such as exposed skin and hair will at least need to undergo gross decontamination before the patient can be moved to definitive care (Table 17-1).

SUMMARY

- Radiation exposure can occur by several routes. These include placing a radioactive source near the public, exploding a conventional bomb contaminated with radioactive materials, or detonating an actual nuclear weapon. The first two are thought to be the most likely to be used by terrorists.
- RDDs are formed by combining an explosive agent (such as TNT) with radioactive material. These devices can cause conventional blast injuries as well as radiation injuries.
- Victims may suffer internal contamination by inhaling debris from an RDD blast.
- Emergency treatment of the victim of an RDD is based first on the type of injury suffered by the patient. Life-threatening injuries should take precedence. Treatment should begin in the hot zone to stabilize the patient along with decontamination.
- The immediate treatment of these victims involves caring for traumatic injury.
- Training and regular exercise of the correct procedures will instill confidence into the medical and emergency responders resulting in the elimination of the fear of the unknown.
- Principles of management of the victim of RDDs are discussed in greater depth in the other radiation chapters in this text.

RESOURCES

1. Radiation Emergency Assistance Center/Training Site (REAC/TS) at Oak Ridge, TN, with 24-hour response. Daytime phone: (865) 576-3131. After hours phone: (865) 576-1005.
2. Armed Forces Radiobiology Research Institute (AFRRI) with 24-hour response to include the Medical Radiobiology Assistance Team (MRAT). Phone: (301) 295-0316/0530.

Case Study

Depleted Uranium-Containing Explosions

One of the authors was in the Army on active military duty in Kuwait during "Operation Desert Storm" in 1991. He was the incoming commander of a forward medical unit when nearby a series of tank explosions occurred. In this incident, a tank filled with munitions caught on fire causing munitions to explode. This, in turn, caused a series of other tanks to explode. These explosions also resulted in the destruction of the field hospital, which the writer was in at the time—I thank the Almighty that I am alive. The explosions caused over a hundred injuries to personnel. Some of the munitions contained depleted uranium (DU). Although DU is only minimally radioactive and this was an accident, this type of incident could fall in the category of a "dirty bomb" had it been done by a terrorist. Some of the casualties could potentially have received internal fragments or even dust that was contaminated with DU. Here the major focus was to triage the more serious casualties to Kuwaiti hospitals. Conventional blast and fragments caused the majority of the injuries.

QUESTIONS AND ANSWERS

1. **Which of the following is LEAST likely to be used for radiation dispersal by terrorists?**
   A. A radiation source may be placed in a food line at a buffet or cafeteria, resulting in delayed diagnosis and treatment.
   B. Radioactive materials from medical sources may be placed within a conventional explosive device.
   C. There exists a remote possibility that terrorists could obtain an actual nuclear bomb.
   D. Nuclear weapons grade materials may be embedded in a conventional explosive device, making environmental decontamination difficult.
   E. An actual nuclear device could be detonated.

2. **The most probable injuries of a dirty bomb may include all the following EXCEPT:**
   A. Infection with the AIDS virus
   B. Contamination with weapons-grade radioactive materials like plutonium
   C. Secondary blast injuries, caused by flying debris from the blast
   D. Crush injury from falling structures
   E. Contamination of lungs or eyes, requiring special techniques of decontamination

3. **Priorities in the initial emergency care of RDD victims INCLUDE which of the following?**
   A. Ensuring ability-to-pay and insurance status on all victims prior to treatment
   B. Determining the exact isotope involved in the blast
   C. Treating life-threatening injuries first
   D. Transporting the victims to special radiation treatment centers and bypassing all other health facilities
   E. Contacting family members to determine living-will status as a part of initial triage

4. **News reports in the popular media raise the possibility of a nuclear terrorist attack from which of the following types of devices?**
   A. Radioactive materials from medical sources
   B. Weapons-grade nuclear materials
   C. Detonation of an actual nuclear device
   D. Bombs made with radioactive materials purchased from criminal sources
   E. All of the above

ANSWERS

1: *E. An actual nuclear device could be detonated.*

2: *A. Infection with the AIDS virus.*

3: *C. Treating life-threatening injuries first.*

4: *E. All of the above.*

REFERENCES

1. Karon T. The "dirty bomb" scenario. TIME.com. June 10, 2002. http://www.time.com/time/nation/article/0,8599,182637,00.html; Accessed April 22, 2004.
2. Public Broadcasting System (PBS). An interview with Alexei 1999. PBS online and WGBH/FRONTLINE. Complete interview available at http://www.PBS.org. Accessed on April 23, 2004.
3. Mathew S, Slater MD, Donald D, Trunkey MD. Terrorism in America. Arch Surg. 1997;132:1063.
4. Wossner WP. The real threat of nuclear smuggling. Sci Am. 1996:274;40-4.
5. Quintana DA, Parker JR, Jordan FB, et al. The spectrum of pediatric injuries after a bomb blast. J Pediatr Surg. 1997:32 (2):307-10; discussion 310-1. [Erratum appears in J Pediatr Surg. 1997 Jun;32(6):932].
6. Leibovici D, Gofrit ON, Stein M, et al. Blast injuries: bus versus open-air bombings—a comparative study of injuries in survivors of open-air versus confined-space explosions. J Trauma. 1996;41(6):1030-5.
7. International Atomic Energy Agency (IAEA). The radiological accident in Goiania. Vienna: IAEA; 1988.
8. International Atomic Energy Agency (IAEA). Dosimetric and medical aspects of the radiological accident in Goiania in 1987. Vienna: IAEA: 1998. TECDOC-1009.
9. National Council on Radiation Protection and Measurements (NCRP). Management of persons accidentally contaminated with radionuclides. 22 Sep 1997; pp. 155-8. NCRP report no. 65.
10. National Council on Radiation Protection and Measurements (NCRP). Management of terrorist events involving radioactive material. Bethesda, MD: NCRP Publications. Report no. 138; 24 Oct 2001.
11. Radiation Management Consultants, Inc. Hospital emergency preparedness and response. Philadelphia: U.S. Department of Energy, Carlsbad Area Office.

SUGGESTED READING

1. Messerschmidt O. Medical procedures in a nuclear disaster. In: Pathogenesis and therapy for nuclear-weapons injuries. Turner JE, Turner RG, trans. Hanle W, Pollermann M, eds. München: Verlag K. Thiemig; 1979.

18

Detonation of a Nuclear Device

Cham E. Dallas

INTRODUCTION

The increasing likelihood of the use of weapons of mass destruction (WMD) on large civilian populations has been described in international government alerts (1), U.S. congressional hearings (2) and research studies (3), and numerous scientific publications. The Islamic terrorist attacks on New York and Washington, D.C., have accentuated the reality of this threat. There is continued concern over the security of the enormous arsenal of nuclear, chemical, and biological agents left over in Russia as a result of the Cold War. It is known that Libya, Iran, Syria, Iraq, and North Korea have been actively recruiting the scientists who constructed this massive stockpile, and it is not certain where many of these experts are now (4). In just the case of biological weapons, at least 17 countries are believed to be in possession of or actively developing these agents (5). Although the terrorist use of nuclear weapons has a certainty of mass casualties, empirical analysis of the historical trends of terrorist events have shown that chemical and biological agents were employed far in excess of nuclear or radiological materials (6).

As the threat of the use of WMD on the civilian population increases, data suggest that hospitals and medical providers in general are significantly unprepared for a biological, chemical, radiological, or nuclear incident, with a nuclear weapon attack presenting the greatest degree of a lack of preparedness. Radiological attacks are defined as involving the release of radioactive materials into the proximity of people without a nuclear explosion and typically involve far fewer and less consequential casualties than nuclear detonations. Only in some regions of the former Soviet Union have there been significant casualties from the release of radionuclides into the environment without atomic detonation (7,8). Use of a nuclear weapon will involve a nuclear detonation, with the accompanying massive explosion, devastating fireball, extensive burns in patients, trauma victims, blindness, and short- and long-term radiation sickness. This chapter focuses on specific medical response procedures for treating patients resulting from the use of nuclear weapons, including the unique aspects of dealing with mass casualties.

Although the preparation of hospitals using the principles inherent in hazardous materials (hazmat) training has provided some degree of response capability, there are significant additional concepts for an overwhelming impact on public services. Medical as well as law enforcement personnel will need to understand the unique challenges in dealing with the intense public fear of radiation, which will significantly impact on the apprehension of perpetrators as well as maintaining public order (especially in nuclear attacks, with the attendant widespread destruction). Public health officials will learn of the potential radiological monitoring of patients and the environment, dealing with the likelihood of a large number of "worried well," transportation difficulties inherent in mass casualty management, and the sheer magnitude of nuclear attacks in general. Pharmacists must understand their critical role in the rapid dispersion of iodide tablets for the prevention of radiation-induced thyroid cancer, the pharmaceutical agents of most importance in nuclear attack medical response, and the agents for removal of internal radioactive contaminants from exposed patients.

THEORETICAL CONCERNS RELATED TO NUCLEAR BLAST

Radiation exposure involves various particles (i.e., beta, alpha, neutrons) or rays (gamma) generated from the unstable elements released into the environment (see Chapter 13). Gamma rays and some of the more intense beta particles (electrons emitted from radioactive materials) can be detected at a distance, and scanning the individuals and samples taken from them can generate relatively rapid indications of exposure. Unfortunately, alpha particles (a low-penetration particle consisting of two protons and two neutrons) cannot be detected with standard detection devices, so plutonium exposures, for example, are harder to detect. Because nuclear weapons generate a wide range of radiations and radioactive particles, the scanning of patients and the environment for gamma and beta detection is sufficient to determine an overview of the exposure potential for an individual patient.

TABLE 18-1 Patient Categories Based on USSR Chernobyl Classification

PARAMETER	1st DEGREE	2nd DEGREE	3rd DEGREE	4th DEGREE
Prodromal onset (hours)	>3	1-3	0.5-1	<0.5
Latent period (days)	>30	15-25	8-17	6-8
Lymphocytes/ul (3 to 6 days)	600-1,000	300-500	100-200	<100
Granulocytes/ul*	3,000-4,000	>1,000	<1,000	<500
Platelets/ul†	40,000-60,000	40,000	<40,000	<40,000
Total body dose (rads)††	100-200	200-400	420-630	600-1,600
Estimate of survival	Probable without treatment	Possible without treatment	Probable with treatment	Unlikely

Modified from F. Fong, Nuclear detonations: evaluation and response, which was based on Barabanova, Complete Union of Soviet Socialist Republics Classification of Chernobyl Victims

* Data from 1st and 4th degrees based on 7-9 days, 2nd for 15-20 days, and 3rd for 8-20 days.

† 1st degree based on 25-28 days, 2nd on 17-24 days, 3rd on 10-16 days, 4th on 8-10 days.

†† Values in grays are 1st degree: 1-2; 2nd degree: 2-4; 3rd degree: 4.2-6.3; 4th degree: 6-16.

Classification of both nuclear detonation and radiological contamination patients in the event of a nuclear detonation is significantly expedited by evaluation of hemodynamic parameters, as well as the time of prodromal onset, as discussed in Chapter 16 (10). The rapid decline in blood lymphocytes induced by significant radiation exposure is particularly useful. Data gathered for the large number of highly exposed cleanup workers (known as "liquidators") and others following the Chernobyl nuclear disaster provide an example of the classification of radiation patients as to outcome (Table 18-1). Lymphocyte counts were found to be highly correlated with the treatment categories, with very low numbers found in patients who did not survive and progressively higher counts found in groups that had probable survival with treatment, possible survival without treatment, and probable survival without treatment, respectively. Granulocytes had a similar utility and over a larger range of values (11). Platelets were useful in distinguishing between the lower exposed groups but had less utility in distinguishing between higher exposed groups (12). If hemodynamic parameters are not available or of questionable quality, the onset of the prodromal syndrome will still have considerable utility in patient classification. Indeed, prodromal onset may be better correlated with radiation dose than blood parameters. If both are available, they can be used to verify each other in patient category designation. The health provider will have to be careful in using vomiting as a parameter, however, because it is likely that many patients will present this symptom for psychological reasons (13). Generally, patients with very low or undetectable lymphocyte counts, prodromal onset of less than 30 minutes, and very severe (i.e., 60% of the body) burns are likely to be in the expectant category. Every case should be evaluated separately, however, on the judgment of the provider on site (Table 18-1).

One of the most feared long-term effects of radiation exposure is the subsequent induction of cancer (14,15). It has been found after tracking survivors of the Hiroshima and Nagasaki atomic bomb attacks that there is a series of long latent periods followed by a detectable incidence of radiation-induced cancers (Table 18-2). Because some of the nuclear weapons available today have far greater yields than the atomic bombs used on Hiroshima and Nagasaki, the degree of cancer incidence may be considerably greater. Even the latent periods may be shorter, as was seen following the Chernobyl nuclear accident with the much shorter incidence (presumably due to the much higher dose rates for radioiodine) for thyroid cancer (16,17) (Table 18-2).

TABLE 18-2 Radiation-induced Cancer Induction Following Atomic Bomb and Nuclear Reactor Airborne Releases

CANCER	HIROSHIMA/NAGASAKI	CHERNOBYL	LATENT PERIOD (YEARS)
Leukemia	(+)	(-)	6 +
Lymphoma	(+)	(-)	9 +
Thyroid cancer	(+)	(+)	5 + (Chernobyl); 15 + (H/N)
Stomach cancer	(+)	(-)	20 +
Lung cancer	(+)	(-)	20 +

UNSUBSTANTIATED FEAR OF RADIATION-INDUCED BIRTH DEFECTS

One of the most entrenched concepts in the general public concerning radiation is the fear of birth defects induced by radiation exposure. Certainly, it has been shown that intense x-ray exposure has produced birth defects in humans (17,18,20) and there have been a very limited number of defects reported in Hiroshima and Nagasaki atomic bomb survivors (21–23). Indeed, many of these survivors were avoided socially in relation to marriage selection because of a fear of birth defects in subsequent offspring. However, the actual incidence of teratogenicity resulting from radiation exposure has been highly overrated, based on numerous historical radiation exposures worldwide (24).

The most distinctive example of how this fear of birth defects impacts on a medical response to ionizing radiation was the Chernobyl experience (25,26). Over 100 times the amount of radioactivity generated by both the Hiroshima and Nagasaki atomic bomb detonations was released into the air after the Chernobyl nuclear accident (27). In the immediate aftermath of the accident, over 30,000 women terminated their pregnancies directly as a result of fear of the birth defects from their radiation exposure. These are women who would have had the babies otherwise, so their decision (supported by medical providers) was completely due to the accident. Subsequent analysis of the 60,000 other equally exposed women who did have their babies, however, revealed no statistically significant incidence of birth defects. Clearly, the information given to the women concerning relative risk of birth defects was false and misleading. In conjunction with the very low incidence of birth defects after the atomic bomb detonations in Japan, a fear of significant numbers of birth defects is not justified. In both the immediate aftermath and long-term medical response to nuclear weapon use and in radiological exposures, therefore, termination of pregnancy due to the anticipation of radiation-induced birth defects is not a scientifically justified course.

DETECTION AND MEDICAL SURVEY FOLLOWING NUCLEAR BLAST

Radiation detection was discussed in Chapter 14. Radiation exposure to humans can result from irradiation from a distance, contamination on the skin, hair, and clothing, and from internal contamination of radioactive materials from inhalation or ingestion (28). In a long-distance irradiation (gamma, beta, and neutron), internal injury can occur due to the penetrating power of the particular radiation. One intense source of this external irradiation occurs in the blast of radiation emitted from a nuclear weapon at the time of detonation, and decreases in intensity (not counting shielding) are evident with distance from ground zero. Evaluating an individual for possible contamination or radiation emission using detection de-

vices is referred to as a *radiation survey*. A radiation survey does not, except for some neutron-induced activity, detect a person's exposure to radiation. A radiation survey is useful for the radiation that occurs as a result of fallout or the contamination from radiological exposure. Therefore, the radiation survey helps identify those individuals who have been exposed and is invaluable in protecting those serving the victims (and preventing further exposure). It can only be expected, though, to give an approximation of the extent of exposure that actually occurred (29).

If the emergency unit does not possess a gamma-counting device, state and federal authorities must be contacted and a detection instrument procured *immediately*. Along with survey instrumentation, at least one trained person should accompany the device, and this training must be transmitted to as many personnel on site as quickly as possible upon arrival. Fortunately, basic radiation survey can be conveyed to a wide variety of personnel fairly quickly, although the overall process must be under the authority of the incident commander and the local physicians and other health care professionals. If patients have detectable radiological contamination, their clothes must be removed, and these individuals examined and treated as potential radiation victims.

In a radiological terrorism event, as well as in some accidental radiation exposures, the specific radionuclide used determines the specificity and efficacy of scanning and detection (30). If strontium-90 was the agent of concern, for example, the radiation monitoring would have to focus on beta detection. From the consideration of the penetration potential of various radiations, gamma and neutron radiation have the highest penetrating power (i.e., through walls), beta is less penetrating (i.e., most will not pass all the way through the body), and alpha particles will not even penetrate a piece of paper (29,31). However, penetrating power only determines the mode in which the various radiations can exert physiological injury. Gamma and beta radiation can be a health hazard from a distance due to their penetrating power. Although alpha particles would not be dangerous outside the body (i.e., on clothing), once they are inhaled or ingested into the body, they have a very high radiation energy with a significant potential of generating toxic injury in the tissues immediately next to them.

The initial radiation survey technique is provided in Table 18-3 and describes a generalized overview of the approach to be taken in surveying patient populations for radiation exposure and potential decontamination. Whenever possible, a health physics practitioner should be included in the radiation survey team. Because properly trained individuals are few in number, this may be hard to accomplish if there is a large-scale event. The extent of the survey would depend to some extent on the number of potential victims as well as the size of the medical response team. Whenever time and resources are sufficient, and especially when the patient population is lower, the survey should be conducted as thoroughly as possible. This radiation survey is not specific only to nuclear detonation but may be used in any radiation exposure (Table 18-3).

Monitoring of clothing is usually considered to be extraneous to the mission, and the clothing should be

TABLE 18-3	Basic Radiation Survey Technique for Patients

1. Conduct a background radiation check to determine contamination of the immediate environment.
2. Cover probe with a disposable glove to prevent contamination of the probe during the initial survey.
3. Remove patient's clothing (separate monitoring of clothing is labor intensive) and store it away.
4. Have the patient stand with extremities extended slightly to avoid confusion of radiation source.
5. Move probe 1 inch above the body at a rate of 1 inch/second or less.
6. Monitor the entire body, including soles of feet, armpits, groin, and hair.
7. Indicate the places in which contamination are found on a simple diagram chart.
8. If contamination with patient seems remote (cooperation), conduct survey without glove.
9. Remove the glove and replace with another before the next patient survey.
10. Repeat the background radiation check of the immediate environment periodically.

bagged for later disposal. It is important to protect the probe from contamination with a glove because in most emergency settings a replacement will not be available. Therefore, complete protection of the probe becomes a serious limiting factor. If the monitoring crew has sufficient confidence, and the patient is very cooperative, one might consider using the probe without the glove. This would increase the sensitivity of the probe for weak beta particles and perhaps some alpha contamination. However, the most important consideration is to protect the probe for subsequent use (which in mass casualty situations would mandate the use of a glove even with the availability of multiple probes). Checking the background of the examining area should be done at periodic intervals in order to remove the confounding interference with the patient measurements. For every patient, a record of his or her contamination (or lack thereof) should be made for future reference. A simple schematic of body surfaces (front: with top of feet shown; back: with bottom of feet shown; right face; and left face) would be used to indicate the presence (and absence) of contamination. The type of survey meter shown and its settings should also be indicated, along with the patient name, date, and time.

Further radiological surveys are usually beyond the capabilities of most emergency settings, but additional information gathered can be useful to subsequent treatment. Blood samples can be taken and lymphocyte counts made over time, which would be plotted out on an *Andrews nomogram* (Chapter 16). This profile would provide an indication of the likely impact on the blood elements of the affected individual after the initial crisis is over. Whole-body counting can be employed to determine the extent of internal radionuclide contamination in patients, after decontamination. These counters are relatively scarce but have considerable utility in delineating patient dosimetry for long-term health care planning. Additional scarce, but highly useful techniques can also be employed in long-term follow-up, such as lymphocyte cytogenetics, fixed in situ hybridization (FISH) techniques, "chromosome painting," and electron spin resonance. Chromosome analysis for dicentric malformations was described in Chapter 16. Expertise and equipment for these approaches can be identified by contacting the Armed Forces Radiobiology Research Institute (AFRRI) in Washington, D.C., or the Lawrence Livermore Laboratory in San Francisco.

NUCLEAR WEAPON DETONATION

With the demise of the Cold War, the possibility of devastating attacks with multiple nuclear weapons (known as mutual assured destruction, or MAD) has decreased dramatically. However, the new asymmetric threat for a nuclear weapon involves small terrorist groups or rogue states detonating a single nuclear weapon in a population center using covert delivery (e.g., a delivery van). The "nuclear club" of countries possessing nuclear weapons now includes North Korea, Pakistan, possibly Iran, and other nation-states who have been willing to export this technology freely. Although there has been a precipitous decline recently in the number of active nuclear warheads in the U.S. and Russian nuclear arsenals, it is unfortunate that none of the weapons-grade material removed from the deactivated warheads has been destroyed. Instead, the plutonium and uranium pits from these thousands of nuclear warheads have simply been stored away. Possible theft of small portions of the tons of this stored nuclear material, especially from the Russian arsenal, is a constant source of concern. Additional efforts by unstable and even aggressive nations (e.g., North Korea, Iran) to produce nuclear material for use in warheads also heightens the tension.

BLAST DYNAMICS

Upon detonation of a nuclear device in an urban area, a series of events would result in a spectrum of injuries requiring a massive medical response (32). The impact of a medium-sized nuclear detonation on an urban population, including the health care system, is depicted in Figure 18-1. Commensurate with conventional explosion blasts, there would be a pressure change decreasing in intensity with the distance from the blast (31). With nuclear detonations, of course, the degree of pressure change is larger and covers a greatly enhanced area relative to conventional blasts. A shock wave emanates from the blast with a pressure change that will result in the destruction of buildings (generally decreasing in intensity with distance from ground zero), eardrum damage in humans, and the intense movement of air containing radioactive materials and massive amounts of

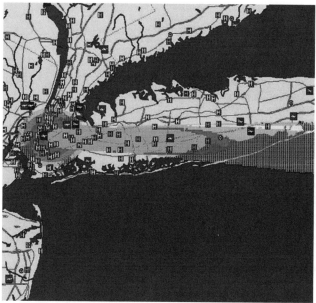

Figure 18–1. A 350 KT nuclear detonation in New York City is depicted, with the casualty plumes depicted over the ensuing 24 hours. The circle of casualties at ground zero on Manhattan represent deaths, trauma victims, and burn patients resulting from the blast, shock wave, and fireball. The comet-shaped plume extending eastward across most of Long Island represents the subsequent casualties from the short-term (first 24 hours) fallout from the blast. Together, one million casualties could be expected. The major hospitals are shown with the letter H, with airports delineated by an airplane. It is evident that a single medium-sized nuclear detonation will result in the inactivation of a majority of the health care centers in the metropolitan area, which would put an even greater (and overwhelming) stress on the remaining hospitals.

debris. The destruction of buildings and the movement of materials in the shock wave can be expected to generate very large numbers of trauma injuries, amounting to hundreds of thousands of trauma patients in a highly populated urban area.

RADIATION BURNS AND FLASH INJURIES

A daunting array of burn injuries will result in all directions from a nuclear blast as a result of the explosion fireball released. A nuclear fireball is at least four orders of magnitude (10,000 times) hotter than that produced by a conventional explosive, with the resulting dramatic increase in fires and thermal burns in the affected population. The fireball can be expected to result in a *large number of burn victims*, which will create one of the most perplexing logistical medical issues in a nuclear weapon response. The fireball will expand in a full circle around ground zero, creating burn victims in all directions in a continuous wave over many square miles of territory. With a large nuclear weapon in a major urban area, several hundred thousand serious burn victims could be presented to the medical response community. The intense flash of visible light at detonation can by itself cause the ignition of fires as well as external flash burns in hu-

mans. The most common result of this initial flash is flash blindness, which involves primarily a temporary loss of sight. A far more serious (but less common) injury is the retinal burn, which is permanent and can result in blindness (33). The instinctive reflex to cover the eyes in a flash will aid significantly in many cases in reducing these injuries. The distances at which burn and flash injuries will occur can be calculated based on the size of the nuclear detonation.

IMMEDIATE AND DELAYED RADIATION TOXICITY

Both immediate and delayed radiation exposures occur following nuclear detonations. Gamma irradiation occurs from the detonation as well as from fission products resulting from the blast (34). Neutrons emitted in the blast are believed to be considerably more hazardous than the gamma rays, and neutrons are unique in that they can make other materials (including living tissue) radioactive. Both gamma and neutron radiation can pass through average walls to induce radiation damage in people. Delayed radiation exposures can occur when people encounter materials that have been induced to become radioactive by neutron and gamma radiation. Exposures to delayed radioactivity can occur over very wide areas due to the airborne dispersion of fission products that condense and return to the ground as what is known commonly as fallout. Airborne detonations produce considerably less fallout than surface bursts. The dispersion of fallout is dictated primarily by the prevailing winds in the first days after the detonation, with winds at higher altitudes often traveling in very different directions than on the surface (35). In the early fallout in the first 24 hours (Fig. 18-1), most hazardous exposures are due to external radiation sources, and the fallout particles tend to be larger. Smaller particle sizes of the subsequent late fallout keep them aloft longer, but the levels of radioactivity are lower. Less penetrating beta particles and low-penetration (but high-energy) alpha particles are more of a hazard when taken into the body (36). Some higher energy beta radiation can also be an external hazard as well. Internal contamination of gamma or neutron emitting materials also results in considerable human health hazards. One variant with nuclear weapons is the use of a neutron bomb, which is reputed to employ only a small blast area. Instead, it would emit a large amount of deadly neutron irradiation that would kill people and animals but leave most buildings intact (there may be unpredictable health effects on the periphery of the attack area, outside of where people are actually killed). However, it is unlikely a terrorist group will acquire a neutron bomb.

RADIOLOGICAL EXPOSURES

It is valuable to consider release of smaller amounts of radiation into the environment to contrast these with the effect of a nuclear detonation. Radiological exposures can result from the deliberate or accidental release of radionuclides into the air, water, food supplies, or on surfaces that people contact (37). The resulting health hazards can be similar to those experienced following early and delayed fallout. Recently, there have been a number of alleged threats from Islamic terrorists considering the use of "dirty bombs," or conventional explosive devices that have radioactive materials encased around them. The intent would be for the explosion to distribute the radioactive materials over a certain area. Usually there will be few immediate health effects, unless the radiation source is especially intense. The danger for human exposure will be primarily from the ingestion or inhalation of radioactive particles. Commensurate with the time-honored radiation protection maxim of time, distance, and shielding, the best immediate action is to decrease the length of exposure, increase the distance of the victims from exposure, and put appropriate shielding in between the patient and the radiation exposure source. If a radiological source is located in the vicinity of a population, the primary danger is from a lack of detection. Once a hazard is identified, people can be removed relatively quickly and further exposure averted.

ORGANIZATION OF THE MEDICAL RESPONSE TO NUCLEAR DETONATION AND RADIOLOGICAL EVENTS: THE U.S. GOVERNMENT MODEL

All responses to major disasters, including nuclear and radiological attacks, are by nature initially local events. A common misconception of the public, and many medical providers, is that state and especially federal response assets will be on the scene of an attack within hours or even minutes of an attack. It is now widely estimated by these state/federal response groups that it will not be uncommon for 24 or even up to 72 hours to elapse before substantial specialized personnel and equipment begins to arrive at the scene of an attack with weapons of mass destruction. There is a further delay, of course, as these assets are deployed and set up in field applications and still more delay during intelligence gathering and decision making. This mandates that the appropriate entity should be contacted absolutely as soon as possible, so a further increase in this inherent latent period of response is avoided. Another source of delay will be the jurisdiction of local and especially state authorities in a crisis, in that federal institutions must be approached through appropriate channels (i.e., the state governor's office) before the federal mobilization can even begin. It is also incumbent on health care responders to notify authorities because *they are required to do so by law*, and penalties for noncompliance may be severe.

In most crises that could be envisioned as a result of radiological and nuclear attacks, the initial authority rests with the government of the state in which the attack occurs. The first responders on the scene of most attacks will be municipal and county officials, but these personnel will immediately report and respond to the authority of the state governor. The governor would then make the decision to call in federal assets (Table 18-1), which would likely occur in most cases soon after the attack.

The initial phase of an attack with weapons of mass destruction is known as the crisis management phase, and the lead federal agency is the Federal Bureau of Investigation (FBI). All aspects of the initial federal response would be under the authority of the FBI, which would include the collection of evidence, the pursuit and capture of perpetrators, management of medical resources, and coordination of local, state, and federal response entities. After the initial crisis management period has transpired, disasters are categorized as moving into the consequence management phase, where primary responsibility moves to the Federal Emergency Management Agency (FEMA). FEMA will coordinate the movement of the massive supplies and large numbers of support personnel needed in the response that would ensue over the weeks and months after a major tragedy. Whenever medical personnel are considering acquiring an array of resources for dealing with the crisis, FEMA should be contacted to determine the availability of resources as well as their overall authority in the response.

MASS CASUALTY ISSUES

One of the most daunting prospects for the emergency community response to a nuclear weapon attack is the very large numbers of real patients that are likely to be generated (38). These groups of patients will descend on the local hospitals and designated emergency response centers in large unorganized masses. Even more thousands will lie where they are or wander about until emergency responders can reach them, often within environments that are not conducive to transport. Unless they are separated and organized quickly into manageable treatment groups, at best many of these individuals will be lost unnecessarily, and at worst the entire medical system could be swept away in just the initial stages of the crisis. By contrast, in radiological events the actual number of real injured patients (particularly in short-term response) is likely to be quite small, and triage will not be a major issue.

Because of the large numbers of patients and worried well, and due to the special issues of decontamination, security of the medical response area following a nuclear weapon attack is an initial primary concern. As large numbers of these people arrive at emergency rooms or even hospital entrances, all subsequent health care will be disrupted, and it might cease altogether. The incident commander for the event will decide where to set up areas for receiving and processing patients, which will include not only hospitals but large public areas such as schools, government buildings, and even shopping malls. A major priority will be to have a security perimeter placed around these areas as quickly as possible. Initially, local police would be employed, of course, but the size of the areas to be covered would entail the incorporation of additional nonmedical personnel from the local municipal authorities, at least until state and federal resources arrive. It would be expected that the state national guard would take over most of the security functions once they are mobilized and arrive at the scene. However, it cannot be overemphasized how much the local authorities will be on their own in the first hours and even days into a crisis.

UNIQUE SECURITY ISSUES

A major tactical and legal issue will be the degree of force to be used to protect the health care perimeter. Because of the panic and loss of confidence in public institutions likely to ensue following the devastation of a nuclear attack, the loss of restraint in the patients and worried well on the perimeters of the health care system is likely to be striking (39). Once the perimeter is breached in even one area, the sequential breakdown of order within the perimeter might be precipitous (40). Another related concern will be the manner in which the security personnel will conduct their duties and prevent contamination of themselves and the facility while still serving the patient community. It should be remembered that radioactive contamination of patients, unlike highly toxic chemicals, is not going to have an immediate effect on the security people. If they become contaminated by contact with the public in protecting the perimeter, this can be detected by the radiation survey personnel and they can simply be decontaminated and return to protecting the perimeter. As with all radioactive contamination issues, *the major exposure to avoid is inhaling or ingesting radioactive particles*. Therefore, the security force would need to avoid eating or drinking on the perimeter, and they could consider wearing a face mask with an appropriate filter if a concern for inhalation of particles on the perimeter is verified by the radiation survey team. The degree of verified hazard would dictate the decision (to be made by the incident commander, not by the security personnel) of the degree of force to be used at the perimeter.

SEPARATION OF RADIATION INJURIES AND "WORRIED WELL"

Because of the extensive trauma injuries involved in nuclear weapons attacks, the precautions established for advanced trauma life support take precedence, of course, over all considerations of the involvement of radiation. Although severe consequences have been reported on occasion following exposure of first responders and medical personnel to biologically and chemically contaminated patients, there have been very few reports of medical personnel suffering ill effects from radiological contamination from patients. Upon consideration of the primacy of trauma support issues, establishing the truth and extent of radiation exposure is an essential initial process in patients potentially involved in a nuclear or radiological event (41).

Because of the widespread and intense fear of radiation in the public, it is likely that in many instances the "worried well," or the uncontaminated and uninjured population insistent upon treatment that the medical provider will directly encounter, will far outnumber the actual nuclear/radiological-injured patients (42,43). Therefore, the inundation of hospitals and other emergency provider sites with a mixture of real patients and worried well will require a rapid, accurate, and convincing protocol for delineating the two groups. In the case of a nuclear attack in a major urban area, it is conceivable the worried well would number in the hundreds of thousands or even in the millions. Radiological attacks would generate far fewer actual patients than nuclear weapon attacks, but the number of worried well could still be very high (44).

HEALTH HISTORY CONSIDERATIONS

In the event of a nuclear weapon detonation, it is highly likely that the health care system will be inundated with severely injured patients, patients who will exhibit injury at a later date (but are not immediately obvious), and very large numbers of worried well. The health history would be of critical benefit in delineating between these groups. In the absence of a radiation survey, of course, the entire subsequent treatment plan will depend on the history outcome and analysis. The interviewer will have to establish the immediate previous history of the individual as well as current symptoms. In the event of an overwhelming number of worried well, an initial interview using several salient questions would be able to separate out large numbers of these individuals who can be established as not being in danger. For instance, with a nuclear weapon dispersion of radionuclides in the air, knowledge of the direction of the fallout plume will give the interviewer the ability to determine quickly whether exposure was possible. Having a large map available would allow a quick reference for these worried well to be identified, perhaps even in large groups. It would also be very useful to have a large number of volunteers who are willing to spend time with the groups of worried well, in order to comfort them, prevent them from spreading their panic to others, and identify individuals within the group who may indeed have been exposed and require treatment or decontamination (45). These volunteers need not be medical personnel or municipal employees (fire, police) but average citizens with good verbal skills, a minimal level of training on procedure and outcomes (which could be done on site), and who will follow orders from legitimate authority.

Many, perhaps even most, patients being examined for potential radiation exposure will not be expected to exhibit significant symptoms at the time of presentation, even if they received significant radiation exposure. This is because of the characteristic delayed onset of symptoms following radiation exposure. As the delay of symptom onset decreases (symptoms appear more rapidly), it can be expected that the severity of symptoms will increase. There is therefore a real danger of missing the potential exposure severity with an examination of only the symptoms at hand. Follow-up examination over the next hours and days is essential to establishing the true nature and extent of exposure. Establishing the time that individuals were in a potential exposure area is important, as well as the potential for ingestion or inhalation of radioactive materials. Because of the intense public fear of radiation, it should be expected that considerable panic and even exaggeration of symptoms are likely in a typical population (46). However, all claims must be considered and balanced with the likelihood of being in tandem with an expected radiation exposure.

FEDERAL RESOURCES IN THE UNITED STATES: COMMUNICATION AND COORDINATION

Federal emergency response authorities are being coordinated under the new Department of Homeland Security, which will have a series of notification requirements established. There are separate responsibilities for the distinct federal agencies. The large number of agencies to be notified in a radiation-related crisis (Table 18-4) may seem daunting, but it is imperative that emergency and other health care responders understand the various federal responsibilities and lines of authority to be followed. Unfortunately, many people in a disaster will not understand these and can be expected to circumvent them and advise others to do so. In most cases, the FBI, FEMA, and the incident commander will inform people of the proper notification requirements in a particular crisis, but it is incumbent on response personnel to know who to notify in order to maximize response and maintain compliance with the law.

Whenever nuclear reactor materials are involved in the crisis, the Nuclear Regulatory Commission (NRC) would be contacted. This would involve the release (or potential release) of radioactive agents directly from an operating reactor or the dispersion of materials that originated from a nuclear reactor (i.e., stolen reactor waste, fuel rods). One of the more frequently ignored federal notification requirements is that of derangements with the transportation of nuclear materials. All transportation of nuclear and other radioactive materials is strictly regulated by the Department of Transportation (DOT), and any radiation hazard that results from the release of an agent during or following transport must be reported to the department.

There has been considerable concern voiced over the large-scale transportation of radioactive waste materials for permanent burial because they could be intercepted by terrorists desiring to use them in radiological terrorist attacks. One of the most time-sensitive aspects of responding to a nuclear weapon attack or nuclear reactor fire would be the distribution of iodide tablets to the affected population. If iodide tablets are taken within 12 hours (ideally within 4 hours) of exposure to radioactive iodine, the incidence of radiation-induced thyroid cancer (especially in children) can be prevented. The National Pharmaceutical Stockpile (NPS), run by the Centers for Disease Control (CDC), should be contacted immediately for this and other emergency medical needs (Table 18-4).

The actual weapons-grade nuclear materials are produced and owned by the Department of Energy (DOE), which must be notified if any portion of them becomes compromised in any way. Tracking and monitoring of these materials can also be provided by DOE in a crisis. The operational nuclear weapons in the U.S. arsenal are under the authority of the Department of Defense (DOD), so any problem (or hint of a problem) with a weapon would be reported to DOD. In most cases, the FBI or one of the other agencies would contact the DOD whenever such a problem was even suspected. Whenever foreign nationals or people in contact with them are found to be involved in any way with radioactive materials, the Central Intelligence Agency (CIA) should be contacted. Especially in the current environment with dedicated Islamic terrorists pursuing American targets, the CIA has the responsibility of vigorously pursuing potential leads to interdict these individuals before an event. Whenever radioactive materials are released into the environment, the Environmental Protection Agency (EPA) should be contacted so officials can make plans to decrease the spread of agents and remediate the existing hazard.

TABLE 18-4 Notification of Federal Agencies

NOTIFICATION OF FEDERAL AGENCIES	
Terrorist attacks and all criminal activity with radioactive agents	Federal Bureau of Investigation (FBI)
Nuclear reactor materials (accidents or intentional use)	Nuclear Regulatory Commission (NRC)
Transport of radioactive materials (hazards from legal or illegal transport)	Department of Transportation (DOT)
Distribution of medicines in a crisis (i.e., iodide tablets)	Centers for Disease Control (CDC)
Nuclear weapons materials (components, production materials)	Department of Energy (DOE)
Operational nuclear weapons	Department of Defense (DOD)
International citizens involved with radioactive materials and/or weapons	Central Intelligence Agency (CIA)
Environmental contamination	Environmental Protection Agency (EPA)
Mobilization of medical resources	Federal Emergency Management Agency (FEMA)
Coordination of federal and local response to all major attacks	Department of Homeland Security

TRIAGE AND TREATMENT OF NUCLEAR AND RADIATION EVENT PATIENTS

The conventional triage system of immediate, delayed, minimal, and expectant can be used in nuclear/radiological triage, with the additional modifiers of radiation dose (if known) and onset of symptoms that aid in classification. If the radiation dose is less than 150 rads, it can be expected that the onset of prodromal symptoms will be in less than 3 hours, and patients may present in all four categories. If doses increase beyond this range up to 450 rads, the onset of symptoms could decrease to as little as 1 hour, and all categories but immediate will simply become expectant patients. Once the dose exceeds 450 rads, nearly all patients can be expected to be in the expectant category (47–49). At these higher doses, all of these patients would likely present prodromal symptoms in less than an hour (Table 18-5).

Nuclear and radiological medical treatment is similar to other conventional trauma treatment approaches in that life-threatening complications like airway blockage and shock must be addressed before other issues, even radiological concerns. Thus conventional trauma treatment takes precedence over all other priorities (Table 18-5), and the ATLS protocols should be followed. The incident commander will make corporate decisions about the relative importance of decontamination, but it is likely that at least some initial radiation survey will be done at the perimeter before the patient arrives at the site of the medical provider (50). Again, it should be remembered that radioactive contamination does not hold the immediate health hazard that toxic chemical and contagious biological agents hold, and decontamination is generally much easier to conduct.

TREATMENT OF RADIATION/THERMAL BURN PATIENTS IN LARGE-SCALE EVENTS

The aspect of nuclear war casualties that might be the hardest to address appropriately in terms of patient outcome is *the overwhelming number of burn victims* that will result. It has been estimated that just one medium-sized nuclear weapon will fill every burn bed in the eastern United States. The speed with which burn victims need to be treated to avoid the high level of pain presented as well as to achieve survival is almost certain to preclude a successful transport of large numbers (i.e., hundreds of thousands) of these patients to stationary current facilities capable of treating them.

About one out of eight burn victims will die as a direct result of the event; slightly less than half will die of infection. Most of the remainder will be lost as a result of organ failure. The high degree of mortality due to infection dictates the use of antimicrobials. When feasible, the support of immune mechanisms of defense by the patient is also important. It is critical to eliminate reservoirs of infections on the patient as well as ensure that the transfer of infection to other sites and to other patients does not occur. Mafenide acetate cream can be used to treat the burns, which may be significant and cover large areas. Standard burn approaches such as debridement, surgical removal, and the use of skin grafts and covering with nylon fabrics can be employed depending on the patient load and resources. In the Chernobyl experience, nearly all victims with significant burns had received very high doses of radioactivity (mostly firemen in close proximity to the reactor fire) and died (51,52). With a nuclear device detonation, there is likely to be a more heterogeneous population, and some portion of the burn victims will have received a low enough dose of radioactivity to survive if their burns are treated in time.

The major problems in burn treatment for nuclear detonation victims is going to be transport, time from injury to treatment, and availability of trained personnel to enable treatment. With only a handful of facilities even in peacetime capable of handling severely burned patients, the prospect of treating large numbers (i.e., thousands) requires a rapid expansion of burn treatment capability in the vicinity of the disaster and rapid transport to those sites. The key problem is time because the burn victims will be in severe pain during the delay, and infection will be setting in during this interim period. As mentioned, arrival of state and federal assets will be delayed at best for hours, and perhaps days after the detonation, and it is these assets that will be critical for large-scale burn treatment. For this reason, many analysts have concluded that most severe and even moderately burned victims would perish before an adequate response can be mounted. This was the case for the severely burned firemen and other workers coping with the Chernobyl nuclear disaster. Therefore, it is essential that local authorities devise emergency response plans that mobilize burn treatment, and especially trained health care providers, rapidly on the immediate periphery of a nuclear detonation disaster area. Transport will also be very difficult in a devastated urban area. It is likely that most roads will have debris hindering or even preventing the rapid movement of patients that would be necessary. An organized helicopter transport system would be useful, but the large number of likely victims might overwhelm the capacity of this approach.

An important point to stress, however, is that *health care providers should not write off burn victims as a group, and they*

TABLE 18-5 Triage Priorities for Combined Nuclear Weapon Injuries

1. Presence of trauma dictates the immediate need for medical care.
2. Burn victims must be categorized as to extent of burns, survival prospect, and resources.
3. Time of onset from nuclear detonation to prodromal symptoms (vomiting could be psychogenic).
4. Decline in lymphocyte count (when possible, use more than one value to determine a trend).
5. As always, the immediate availability of personnel dictates triage priority outcome.

should not just transfer all resources to other patients. The best effort possible with existing personnel should be made, and the most promising prospects for treatment selected, so some of these victims survive. The incident commander and decision makers should be aware that burn treatment and radiation-induced skin burns will be labor intensive, but with proper selection of patients for treatment a higher percentage of these burn victims will be saved than might be expected (53,54). With careful management of the flow of nonburn patients and their providers, resources can be transferred where feasible to burn treatment, with the purpose of expanding capacity whenever possible. Those patients classified as expectant should be given pain relief, of course, as supplies are available. Every effort should be made to bring the immediate burn victims to the health care site, even if capacity seems to be saturated. With the constant flux in resources and the arrival of new assets over time expected as medical response unfolds, these patients might be squeezed in if they are present.

TREATMENT STRATEGIES TO ENHANCE ELIMINATION OF RADIONUCLIDE BODY BURDENS

Once people have been exposed to radionuclides due to nuclear weapon detonation or other radiological release, pharmaceutical approaches can be taken to lower the amount of radionuclides taken up by the patient (Table 18-6). The intention is to lower the relative risk to the patient by decreasing the subsequent body burden of the toxins that the patient will carry over a lifetime. Therefore, it is not necessary in all exposures that these decorporation interventions be initiated during the medical crisis response. However, once patients are in the care of the medical provider, enhanced elimination could be used when other response work requirements allow them. Note that some analysts question the utility of some enhanced elimination strategies because there is limited human data to verify the utility demonstrated in animal studies. Clearly, enhanced elimination approaches should be used only when high levels of radionuclide uptake can be substantiated.

Following a nuclear weapon detonation or with a nuclear reactor fire (like Chernobyl), very large amounts of radioactivity will be released into the air, including both particulate and gaseous radioactive *iodine*. These radioactive agents will be inhaled and ingested by large numbers of people in the radioactive plume, which may have long-term health consequences. Following the Chernobyl nuclear disaster, when over 100 million curies of radioactivity were released (100 times as much as the Hiroshima and Nagasaki atomic bomb detonations combined), thousands of people contracted radiation-induced thyroid cancer years later (55,56). The real tragedy of this occurrence was that it was almost totally preventable. The Soviet authorities did not issue potassium iodide tablets until 72 hours after the reactor fire issued radioactive iodine into the air (radioactive iodine is much more of a hazard for a nuclear reactor fire than for a nuclear detonation), by which time they were useless.

It is a very time-sensitive mandate that the successful response must have *iodide tablets* issued to radiation-exposed people within 4 hours after the initiation of exposure, and no later than 12 hours after exposure begins. The iodide tablets bind up all sites within the thyroid before the radioactive iodine

arrives at the target site, and because no other organ in the body utilizes iodine, all subsequently inhaled/ingested radioiodine will simply be eliminated. The most critical population to be reached are children because the majority of radiation-induced thyroid cancer cases have appeared in patients who were children or teenagers at the time of exposure. Therefore a major priority of the security personnel, those in patient registration, the decontamination squads, radiation survey teams, and health care responders in the first hours after the release of radioactivity suspected of radioiodine content is to distribute the iodide tablets. After more than 12 hours have elapsed, this priority is eliminated entirely. It should be noted that some individuals may enter the radioactive plume or become exposed to a radiological release later than others, so knowledge of when the plume has moved over the area the patient was in may justify issuing iodide tablets in time periods later than 12 hours following detonation or initiation of radiological agent release.

Plutonium and the transuranics (artificially made elements that are heavier than uranium, including plutonium, americium, neptunium, and curium) are known to be highly toxic in humans, with very long half-lives. The use of chelators to remove them could be justified depending on the relative degree of exposure. The agent *diethylenetriamine pentaacetic acid (DTPA)* has been shown to remove 90% of the soluble plutonium (even from bone, the major sink for plutonium in humans) from an exposed individual if given within 1 hour of exposure (57). Some of the more soluble transuranics can also be removed using DTPA, although not as efficiently. The calcium (Ca)-DTPA would be used if given early (i.e., 1 hour) after exposure for maximum efficacy. Subsequent doses after this initial Ca-DTPA dose or if the first dose is given hours after exposure would utilize *zinc-DTPA* (in order to lower the risk of zinc depletion). Cesium forms a sizable portion of the radioactive components formed by nuclear and radiological events, so it can be expected to be taken up by most people who are in the vicinity of these events. Because it is an efficient gamma emitter, scanning for multiple radionuclide exposures is often really based on the cesium exposure that has occurred. *Insoluble Prussian blue* has been shown to be effective in binding cesium in the intestinal tract and decreasing the cesium physiological half-life in the body (58). The Prussian blue itself is not absorbed, but it can cause gastrointestinal disturbances at doses exceeding 20 grams/day (Table 18-6).

A daily dose of 300 mg of potassium iodide is recommended for 7 to 14 days to prevent the uptake of radioiodine. As noted previously, the dose needs to be initiated within 12 hours following the initiation of the exposure of the individual (not necessarily since radiation release). The World Health Organization recommends lower daily doses, with 100 mg for adults, 50 mg for children (3 to 12 years), 25 mg for infants (1 month to 3 years), and 12.5 mg for neonates (birth to 1 month). Increased removal of tritium operates under the simple principle of increasing water intake to 4 liters/day, which has been shown to reduce the tritium physiological half-life by up to half. A reduction in absorption of over 80% in radiostrontium uptake has been shown following 100 ml of *aluminum phosphate* (59). Additional oral administration of *ammonium chloride* enhances this removal rate. A significant removal of uranium has been shown by the *alkalinization of urine* (increased to a pH of 7.5 to 8) with sodium bicarbonate (60). This also serves to protect the individual from uranium-induced renal toxicity. Supplemental augmentation with *potassium chloride* may also be used.

TABLE 18-6 Pharmaceutical Intervention Strategies

Calcium-DTPA	Early doses after exposure to more soluble transuranics[†], plutonium
Zinc-DTPA	Subsequent doses, late administration to transuranics,[†] plutonium
Insoluble Prussian blue	Cesium
Potassium iodide[*]	Radioactive iodine, Technetium
Radiostable water	Tritium
Aluminum phosphate, ammonium chloride	Radiostrontium
Sodium bicarbonate, potassium choride	Alkanization of urine (pH of 7.5 to 8) for removal of uranium

* Potassium iodide must be orally administered within 1 to 4 hours to be maximally effective; if more than 12 hours has elapsed since exposure, it will be of dubious value.

† The *transuranics* are artificially made elements that are heavier than uranium, including plutonium, americium, neptunium, and curium. They are all alpha emitters.

QUESTIONS AND ANSWERS

1. Which of the following is FALSE?
   A. The initial phase of an attack with weapons of mass destruction is known as the crisis management phase, and the lead federal agency is the Central Intelligence Agency (CIA).
   B. After the initial crisis management period has transpired, disasters are categorized as moving into the consequence management phase, in which primary responsibility moves to the Federal Emergency Management Agency (FEMA).
   C. Many patients being examined for potential radiation exposure will not be expected to exhibit significant symptoms at the time of presentation, even if they received significant radiation exposure.
   D. The National Pharmaceutical Stockpile (NPS) is run by the Centers for Disease Control (CDC) and should be contacted immediately after a nuclear attack to distribute pills that may prevent the ultimate development of thyroid cancer.
   E. Actual weapons-grade nuclear materials are produced and owned by the Department of Energy (DOE), which must be notified if any portion of them becomes compromised in any way.

2. Which of the following has been shown to remove 90% of soluble plutonium (even from bone, the major sink for plutonium in humans) from an exposed individual if given within 1 hour of exposure?
   A. Diethylenetriamine pentaacetic acid (DTPA)
   B. Potassium iodide
   C. Aluminum phosphate
   D. Diethyldithiocarbamate
   E. Calcium EDTA

3. Which of the following is FALSE?
   A. The actual incidence of teratogenicity resulting from radiation exposure has been highly overrated, based on numerous historical radiation exposures worldwide.

   B. Regarding the penetration potential of various radiations: gamma and neutron radiation have the highest penetrating power (i.e., through walls), beta is less penetrating (i.e., most will not pass all of the way through the body), and alpha particles will not even penetrate a piece of paper.
   C. With a large nuclear weapon in a major urban area, several hundred thousand serious burn victims could be presented to the medical response community. The intense flash of visible light at detonation can by itself cause the ignition of fires as well as external flash burns in humans.
   D. Delayed radiation exposures can occur when people encounter materials that have been induced to become radioactive by neutron and gamma radiation.
   E. It is expected that state and especially federal response assets will be on the scene of a nuclear attack within hours or even minutes of an attack.

4. If _____ tablets are taken within 12 hours (ideally within 4 hours) of exposure to radioactive iodine, the incidence of radiation-induced thyroid cancer (especially in children) can be prevented.
   A. Strontium chloride
   B. Potassium iodide
   C. Calcium carbonate
   D. Levoxyl (T4)
   E. Potassium chloride

ANSWERS

1: A. *The initial phase of an attack with weapons of mass destruction is known as the crisis management phase, and the lead federal agency is the Central Intelligence Agency (CIA).*

2: A. *Diethylenetriamine pentaacetic acid (DTPA)*

3: E. *It is expected that state and especially federal response assets will be on the scene of a nuclear attack within hours or even minutes of an attack.*

4: B. *Potassium iodide*

REFERENCES

1. G-7 (Group of seven industrialized nations—United States, Japan, Germany, Britain, France, Italy and Canada), June 27, 1996. Declaration on Terrorism.
2. U.S. Senate, 104th Cong, 1st Sess, Part 1, October 31 and November 1, 1995 (hearings also held by the subcommittee on March 20, 22, and 27, 1996). Global Proliferation of Weapons of Mass Destruction, Hearings before the Permanent Subcommittee on Investigations of the Committee on Governmental Affairs.
3. U.S. Congress, Office of Technology Assessment (August 1993), Proliferation of weapons of mass destruction: assessing the risks. Office of Technology Assessment, Document OTA BP ISC 559. U.S. Congress, Office of Technology Assessment (December 1993), Technologies Underlying Weapons of Mass Destruction. Office of Technology Assessment, Document OTA BP ISC 115.
4. Henderson DA. The looming threat of bioterrorism. Science 1999;283:1279-83.
5. Shapiro RL, Hatheway C, Becher J, et al. Botulism surveillance and emergency response—a public health strategy for a global challenge. JAMA 1997;278:433-5.
6. Tucker JB. Historical trends related to bioterrorism: an empirical analysis. Emerg Infect Dis 1999;5(4):498-504.
7. Goldman M. The Russian radiation legacy: its integrated impact and lessons. Environ Health Perspect 1997;105:1385-92.
8. Kossenko MM. Cancer mortality among Techa river residents, and their offspring. Health Phys 1996;71:77-82.
9. Robertson JB. Toxicology of ionizing radiation. In: Marquis JK ed. A guide to general toxicology. 2nd ed. New York: S. Karger AG, 1989;141-56.
10. Maruyama Y, Feola JM. Relative radiosensitivities of the thymus, spleen, and lymphohemopoietic systems. In: Altman KI, Lett JT eds. Advances in radiation biology. Vol. 14. Relative radiation sensitivities of human organ systems. San Diego: Academic Press, 1987;1-82.
11. Monroy RL. Radiation effects on the lymphohematopoietic system: a compromise in immune competency. In: Conklin JJ, Walker RI eds. Military radiobiology. San Diego: Academic Press, 1987;113-34.
12. Mettler FA Jr, Modeley RD Jr. Medical effects of ionizing radiation. New York: Grune and Stratton, 1985.
13. Mickley GA. Can animals serve as useful models for research on the psychological effects of radiation exposure? In: Ricks RC, Berger ME, Berger, E, et al. eds. The medical basis for radiation-accident preparedness. III. The psychological perspective. New York: Elsevier, 1991;25-38.
14. Riches AC. Experimental radiation leukaemogenesis. In: Hendry JH, Lord BI eds. Radiation toxicology: bone marrow and leukaemia. Washington, DC: Taylor & Francis, 1995;311-34.
15. Wright EG. The pathogenesis of leukaemia. In: Hendry JH, Lord BI eds. Radiation toxicology: bone marrow and leukaemia. Washington, DC: Taylor & Francis, 1995;245-74.
16. Astakhova LN, Anspaugh LR, Beebe GW, et al. Chernobyl-related thyroid cancer in children of Belarus: a case-control study. Radiat Res 1998;150:349-56.
17. Rytomaa T. Ten years after Chernobyl. Ann Med 1996; 28:83-7.
18. Andrew FD, Lytz PS. Biochemical disturbances associated with developmental toxicity. In: Kimmel C, Buelke-Sam J eds. Developmental toxicology. New York: Raven Press, 1981;145-65.
19. Brent RL, Beckman DA, Jensh RP. Relative radiosensitivity of fetal tissues. In: Lett JT, Altman KI eds. Advances in radiation biology. Vol. 12. Relative radiation sensitivities of human organ systems. San Diego: Academic Press, 1987;239-56.
20. Cockerham LG, Prell GD. Prenatal radiation risk to the brain. Neurotoxicology 1989;10:467-74.
21. Otake M, Schull WJ. Radiation-related brain damage and growth retardation among prenatally exposed atomic bomb survivors. Int J Radiat Biol 1998;74:159-71.
22. Schull WJ, Otake M. Neurological deficit among the survivors exposed in utero to the atomic bombing of Hiroshima and Nagasaki: a reassessment and new direction. In: Kriegel H, Schmahl W, Gerber GB, et al. eds. Radiation risks to the developing nervous system. Stuttgart: Gustav Fischer Verlag, 1986;399-419.
23. Schull WJ. Effects of atomic radiation: a half century of studies from Hiroshima and Nagasaki. New York: Wiley-Liss, 1995.
24. Mole RH. Expectation of malformations after irradiation of the developing human in utero: The experimental basis for predictions. In: Altman KI, Lett JL eds. Advances in radiation biology. Vol. 15. Relative radiation sensitivities of human organ systems. San Diego: Academic Press, 1992;217-301.
25. Byelorussia and Chernobyl. The delegation of the Byelorussia SSR at the 45th session of the UN General Assembly: a review. Minsk Belarus: Minsk Belarus Publishers, 1991;6-52.
26. Dallas CE. Aftermath of the Chernobyl nuclear disaster: pharmaceutical needs in the republic of Belarus. Am J Pharm Ed 1993;57:182-5.
27. Segerstahl B. The costs. In: Segerstahl B ed. Chernobyl: a policy response study. New York: Springer-Verlag, 1991;59.
28. BEIR IV. Health risks of radon and other internally deposited alpha-emitters. Report of the Committee on the Biological Effects of Ionizing Radiations, Nation Research Council. Washington, DC: National Academy Press, 1988.
29. BEIR V. Health effects of exposure to low levels of ionizing radiation. Report of the Committee on the Biological Effects of Ionizing Radiations, National Research Council. Washington, DC: National Academy Press, 1990.
30. Hall EJ. Radiation and life. 2nd ed. New York: Pergammon Press, 1984.
31. Mettler FA Jr., Modeley RD Jr. Medical effects of ionizing radiation. New York: Grune and Stratton, 1985.
32. Fetter SA, Tsipis K. Catastrophic releases of radioactivity. Sci Am 1981;244:41-7.
33. Furchtgott E. Ionizing radiations and the nervous system. In: Galli GE ed. Biology of brain dysfunction. Vol. 3. New York: Plenum Press, 1975;343-79.
34. Mettler FA Jr, Modeley RD Jr. Medical effects of ionizing radiation. New York: Grune and Stratton, 1985.
35. Cerveny TJ, Cockerham LG. Medical management of internal radionuclide contamination. Med Bull U.S. Army Eur 1986;43:24-7.
36. Eisenbud M. Environmental radioactivity from natural, industrial, and military sources. 3rd ed. New York: Academic Press, 1987.
37. BEIR III. The effects on populations of exposure to low levels of ionizing radiation. Report of the Committee on the Biological Effects of Ionizing Radiations, National Research Council. Washington, DC: National Academy Press, 1980.
38. Mickley GA. Can animals serve as useful models for research on the psychological effects of radiation exposure? In: Ricks RC, Berger ME, Berger E, et al. eds. The medical basis for radiation-accident preparedness. III. The psychological perspective. New York: Elsevier, 1991;25-38.
39. Collins DL. Behavioral differences of irradiated persons associated with the Kyshtym, Chelyabinsk, and Chernobyl nuclear accidents. Mil Med 1992;157:548-52.
40. Mole RH. Expectation of malformations after irradiation of the developing human in utero: The experimental basis for predictions. In: Altman KI, Lett JL eds. Advances in radiation biology. Vol. 15. Relative radiation sensitivities of human organ systems. San Diego: Academic Press, 1992;217-301.
41. Baum A, Gatchel RJ, Schaeffer MA. Emotional, behavioral, and physiological effects of chronic stress at Three Mile Island. J Consult Clin Psychol 1983;51:565-72.
42. Giel R. The psychosocial aftermath of two major disasters in the Soviet Union. J Traumatic Stress 1991;4:381-93.

43. Havenaar JM, van den Brink W, Kasyanenko AP, et al. Mental health problems in the Gomel Region (Belarus). An analysis of risk factor in an area affected by the Chernobyl disaster. Psychol Med 1995;26:845-55.

44. Viinamäki H, Kumpusalo E, Myllykangas M, et al. The Chernobyl accident and mental well being—a population study. Acta Psychiat 1995.

45. Viel JF, Ckurbakova E, Dzerve, B, et al. Risk factor for long-term mental and psychosomatic distress in Latvian Chernobyl liquidators. Environ Health Perspect 1997;105:1539-44.

46. Chinkina OV. Psychological characteristics of patients exposed to accidental irradiation at the Chernobyl atomic-power station. In: Ricks RC, Berger ME, O'Hara FM eds. The medical basis for radiation-accident preparedness. III. The psychological perspective. New York: Elsevier, 1991;93-103.

47. Maisin JR. Acute radiation syndromes in man. In: McCormack PD, Senberg CE, Bücker H eds. Terrestrial space radiation and its biological effects. New York: Plenum Press, 1988;445-63.

48. Mettler FA Jr, Modeley RD Jr. Medical effects of ionizing radiation. New York: Grune and Stratton, 1985.

49. Young RW. Acute radiation syndrome. In: Conklin JJ, Walker RI eds. Military radiobiology. New York: Academic Press, 1987;165-90.

50. Severa J, Bar J. Handbook of radioactive contamination and decontamination. New York: Elsevier Science, 1991.

51. Aoyama M, Hirose K, Inoue H, et al. 30 years record of the radioactive fallout in Japan. J Radiat Res (Tokyo) 1989;30:11.

52. Clarke RH. Current radiation risk estimates and implications for the health consequences of Windscale, TMI and Chernobyl accidents. In: Crosbie WA, Gittus, JH eds. Medical response to effects of ionizing radiation. New York: Elsevier Science, 1989;103-18.

53. Archambeau JO. Relative radiation sensitivity of the integumentary system: Dose response of the epidermal, microvascular, and dermal populations. In: Lett JT, Altman KI eds. Advances in radiation biology. Vol. 12. Relative radiation sensitivities of human organ systems. San Diego: Academic Press, 1987;147-203.

54. Mettler FA Jr., Modeley RD Jr. Medical effects of ionizing radiation. New York: Grune and Stratton, 1985.

55. Fry FA. Doses from environmental radioactivity. In: Jones R, Southwood R eds. Radiation and health: the biological effects of low-level exposure to ionizing radiation. New York: Wiley, 1987;9-17.

56. Imanaka T, Seo T, Koide H. Radioactivity release from the Chernobyl-4 accident and its cancer consequences. J Radiat Res (Tokyo) 1988;29:80.

57. Khokhryakov VF, Belyaev AP, Kudryavtseva TI, Schadilov AE, Moroz GS, Shalaginov VA. Successful DTPA therapy in the case of 239Pu penetration via injured skin exposed to nitric acid. Radiation Protection Dosimetry 2003;105(1-4):499-502.

58. Thompson DF, Church CO. Prussian blue for treatment of radiocesium poisoning. Pharmacotherapy 2001;21(11):1364-7.

59. Spencer H, Lewin I, Belcher MJ, Samachson J. Inhibition of radiostrontium absorption by aluminum phosphate gel in man and its comparative effect on radiocalcium absorption. Int J Applied Radiation & Istopes 1969;20(7):507-16.

60. Fisher DR, Kathren RL, Swint MJ. Modified biokinetic model for uranium from analysis of acute exposure to UF6. Health Physics 1991;60(23):335-42.

19

Nuclear Power Plant Disasters

Wilfredo Rivera

NAME OF AGENT

Nuclear Power Plant Disaster

THEORETICAL AND SCIENTIFIC BACKGROUND

The first successful nuclear detonation took place in New Mexico in July 1945 as part of the "Manhattan Project" in the United States. Ten years later in June 1955, the first nuclear reactor was unveiled by the former Soviet Union in a town called Obninsk, 60 miles south of Moscow. Since the conception of the nuclear bomb and nuclear powered plants, terrorism associated with these has been a concern of governments and individuals all over the world. After the events on September 11, 2001, in the United States, the concern of a terrorist attack to nuclear power plants, with subsequent dispersal of radiation, has increased significantly.

Radiation dispersal can be achieved by several mechanisms. The ultimate dispersal method is by the detonation of a nuclear weapon (Chapter 18). This will result in explosive destruction along with the massive dispersal of radioactive material, depending on the magnitude of the bomb. The use of conventional explosives mixed with radioactive material is another type of dispersal mechanism (Chapter 17). The use of liquid radioisotopes to be dispersed in the water supply of certain cities has also been considered a possible threat although the amount of material needed to cause large-scale illness is so large that experts believe that this is not a feasible method for an event. The psychological implications of this type of threat are perhaps the most significant and may affect a large number of people in a given area (1,2). Alternatively, an attack on a fixed nuclear facility or on radioactive material in transit may disperse radioactive material in a local region and is considered a possibility in a terrorist attack (2).

TABLE 19-1 U.S. Nuclear Power Plants in Operation

STATE	NUMBER OF NUCLEAR PLANTS
Alabama	2
Arizona	1
Arkansas	1
California	2
Connecticut	1
Florida	3
Georgia	2
Illinois	6
Iowa	1
Kansas	1
Louisiana	2
Maryland	1
Massachusetts	1
Michigan	3
Minnesota	2
Mississippi	1
Missouri	1
Nebraska	2
New Hampshire	1
New Jersey	3
New York	4
North Carolina	3
Ohio	2
Pennsylvania	5
South Carolina	4
Tennessee	2
Texas	2
Vermont	1
Virginia	2
Washington	1

United States Nuclear Power Plants currently in operation as reported by the U.S. Nuclear Regulatory Commission as of December 2002.

TABLE 19-2	Nuclear Power Plants in Operation around the World as Reported by the Nuclear Energy Institute

COUNTRY	NUMBER OF NUCLEAR PLANTS
Argentina	2
Armenia	1
Belgium	7
Brazil	2
Bulgaria	4
Canada	14
China	7
Czech Republic	6
Finland	4
France	59
Germany	19
Hungary	4
India	14
Japan	54
Lithuania	2
Mexico	2
Netherlands	1
Pakistan	2
Romania	1
Russian Federation	30
Slovak Republic	6
Slovenia	1
South Africa	2
South Korea	18
Spain	9
Sweden	11
Switzerland	5
Ukraine	13
United Kingdom	27

Nuclear power plants are found in multiple locations around the world. The United States currently has over 100 commercial nuclear power reactors in operation as reported by the Nuclear Regulatory Commission (Table 19-1). Nuclear power plants of different types are also found in many other parts of the world (Table 19-2). The widespread distribution of these power plants enhances the concern of the threat of terrorism. Each nuclear power plant contains multiple sites where radiation could be released. The reactors contain radioactive material that could lead to radiation exposure to surrounding areas if not contained in the event of a meltdown. These nuclear power plant facilities also house storage facilities for spent fuel that can also provide a target for terrorists. Such facilities may vary from spent fuel pools to underground storage in containers that are more highly resistant to direct impact from munitions and from aircraft impacts akin to the attack on the World Trade Center in 2001.

Nuclear safety is a very high priority in all of these power plant facilities. Several incidents have occurred where power plant emergencies have occurred (Table 19-3). With each of these events, communicating risk to the public has become a critical feature of the response. A method for grading these incidents has become widely accepted. Figure 19-1 shows the International Nuclear Event Scale (INES), a tool created to communicate and report to the public in common terms when an event has happened in any nuclear power plant (Fig. 19-1). The scale is divided into seven levels with the lower ones described as incidents and the upper levels termed "accidents." Most events involving nuclear power plants in history have been described as incidents, and only a handful have met accident criteria. In this chapter we will focus on two main accidents, Chernobyl and Three Mile Island. The Chernobyl accident is considered the worst nuclear power plant accident in history because it had significant health effects, in both the immediate area surrounding the plant and other countries surrounding Chernobyl. Although controversy exists about the health effects of the Chernobyl accident, much of the literature supports that the effects on thyroid cancer and other diseases have been significant following the accident in the areas adjacent to the plant and also remote areas downwind from the accident (3–12).

TYPES OF REACTORS

Energy production by conventional and nuclear power plants is very similar. The difference is the substrate for the production of heat. Conventional power plants use fossil fuel, oil, gas, or coal to produce heat, which in turn is used to produce power. Nuclear power plants use different radioactive materials with a controlled reaction to produce heat, and this heat is used to produce power.

Nuclear power plants have been controversial since the beginning of the nuclear era. These issues and worries intensified after the September 11, 2001, attack on the landmark towers in New York City in the United States. Nuclear facilities have implemented multiple redundant systems to ensure their safety. In the United States, nuclear power plants are designed with the idea that the deeper nuclear material is placed in the structure, the safer the structure is. Failure of three specific barriers is needed before a release of radioactive material would occur. Fuel rods are lined by steel and buried inside the reactor with the reactor coolant system/pressure vessel that has steel walls about 9 inches thick. The containment building surrounds these structures and is constructed of concrete 3 to 5 feet thick. These facilities are designed to withstand the impact of hurricanes and airborne objects with very substantial force (13–16).

In 2002, a study based on a computer model found that the structures that house the nuclear reactor fuel (including the dry storage containers) will protect against the release of radiation even if they are struck by a large commercial jetliner (14). Sandia National Labs used an F-4 Phantom jet and hit a similar structure at 480 miles per hour. The jet was completely destroyed, and the maximum penetration to the concrete wall was 2.4 inches. Spent fuels are stored in different locations in dry storage canisters built and tested to withstand extremely severe impacts that include fire, hurricanes, earthquakes, and other extreme forces (14,17).

Throughout the world, several types of nuclear power plants are used for energy production. The most common types are *light water reactors*, which are divided into pres-

TABLE 19-3 Nuclear Power Plant Disasters in History

YEAR	LOCATION	EVENTS
1952 Dec 12	Chalk River, near Ottawa, Canada	A partial meltdown of the reactor's uranium fuel core resulted after the accidental removal of four control rods. Although millions of gallons of radioactive water accumulated inside the reactor, there were no injuries.
1957 Oct. 7	Windscale Pile No. 1, north of Liverpool, England	A fire in a graphite-cooled reactor spewed radiation over the countryside, contaminating a 200-square-mile area.
1976	Near Greifswald, East Germany	The radioactive core of reactor in the Lubmin nuclear power plant nearly melted down due to the failure of safety systems during a fire.
1979 March 28	Three Mile Island, near Harrisburg, Pennsylvania	One of two reactors lost its coolant, (so the radioactive fuel to overheat,) which caused a partial meltdown. Some radioactive material was released.
1986 April 26	Chernobyl, near Kiev, former USSR	An explosion and fire in the graphite core of one of four reactors released radioactive material that spread over part of the Soviet Union, Eastern Europe, Scandinavia, and later Western Europe. Thirty-one were claimed dead. Total casualties are unknown, but estimates run into the thousands. It is the worst such accident to date.
1999 September 30	Tokyo, Japan	Workers added seven times the required amount. Radiation was released to the surrounding areas. The three workers performing the operation were exposed to high levels of radiation and were treated. Thirty-nine workers were exposed in total.

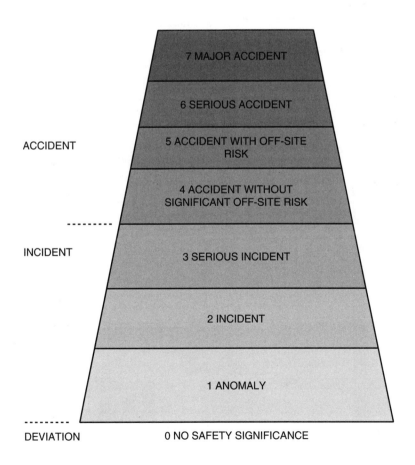

Figure 19–1. International nuclear event scale.

surized water reactors and boiling water reactors; heavy water reactors; and graphite-moderated reactors. Other types of reactors are used in experimental installations and submarines, but they are beyond the scope of this chapter. Pressurized water reactors (PWRs) and boiling water reactors (BWRs) are the two reactors currently used in the United States. PWRs keep water under pressure, but this water does not boil. The water from the reactor heats up the water in the steam generator, which in turn produces steam to power the turbine. These two never mix, so any radioactive materials stay in the reactor area (Fig. 19-2). With *boiling water reactors*, the water boils inside the reactor, which causes the turbines to revolve. The steam is converted back to water in the condenser and is pushed back to the reactor. The water is allowed to boil in the reactor, but the pressures are much smaller in this type of reactor than they are in PWRs (Fig. 19-3).

Another type of reactor is the RBMK, which is a Russian acronym for *Reactor Bolshoi Moschnosti Kanalynyi*; it uses a graphite moderator (Fig. 19-4). The world's first nuclear power plant in Obninsk was of this type. The coolant is boiling water, like the BWR. The Chernobyl reactor is a reactor of this type. The major advantage of these reactors is the massive amounts of power that can be achieved but its major disadvantage is that the core is so large that it is very difficult to control. After the Chernobyl accident the use of RBMK reactors was discontinued in the United States.

MAJOR NUCLEAR INCIDENTS

THREE MILE ISLAND, PENNSYLVANIA, 1979

The Three Mile Island station is located on 814 acres of an island near the state capital at Harrisburg, near Middletown, Pennsylvania. The reactor is a pressurized light water reactor (Fig. 19-2). The site consists of four reactors, and the ac-

cident occurred in the number two reactor. A combination of equipment malfunctions and human error led to a loss of coolant, which precipitated the emergency events. It remains the most significant accident at a U.S. nuclear power plant to date.

On March 28, 1979, at approximately 4:00 A.M. a failure was experienced in the secondary section of the plant. An undetermined failure caused the main pumps that run water to stop running. This in turn prevented the steam generators from removing heat. As a result, the turbine and then the reactor automatically shut down causing the pressure in the primary system to increase. The pressurizer relief valve opened to prevent the pressure to continue rising and become dangerous. This valve should have reclosed after a certain pressure was reached, but it never did, and there were no signals available to the operators to alert them of this situation. In addition to these occurrences, the emergency feedwater system was tested 42 hours prior to the accident. This test consists of closing a valve and then reopening it at the end of the test. This time, for an unknown reason, the valve was not reopened, which prevented the emergency water feeding system from functioning. After several minutes, this malfunction was discovered, and the valve reopened allowing cooling water to flow into the steam generators. The pressure in the primary system continued to rise, and voids, areas where no water is present, began to form in portions of the system where they were not supposed to be. Consequently, the water was redistributed and caused a false reading that the system was full of water. The operators then stopped pumping water in a system that needed water to cool down the fuel in the reactor because of this false reading in the instrumentation. As a result, the nuclear fuel overheated to the point where some of the long metal tubes or jackets that hold the nuclear fuel pellets (made of zirconium) reacted with the water and generated hydrogen. This hydrogen was released into the reactor containment building. Two days after the start of the events, some hydrogen remained, forming a "hydrogen bubble" above the reactor core. The concern at this point was that the

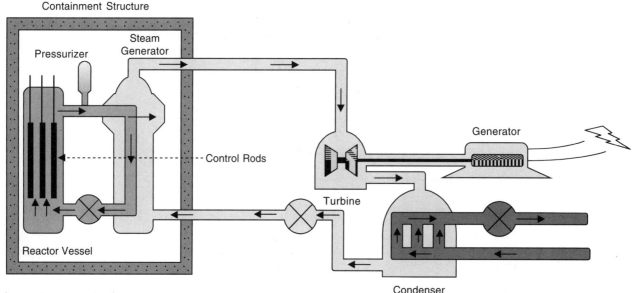

Figure 19–2. Pressurized water reactor.

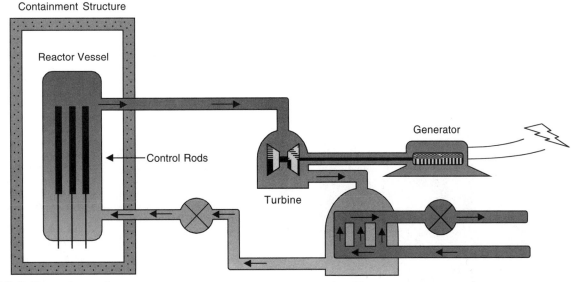

Figure 19–3. Boiling water reactor.

hydrogen could expand and interfere with the flow of cooling water through the core if the reactor pressure decreased. The bubble was reduced by degassing the pressurizer.

The primary damage to the reactor occurred two to three hours into the accident. Although the fuel did not melt through the floor beneath the containment (the classic idea of meltdown) or through the steel of the reactor vessel, a significant amount of fuel did melt inside the reactor. Radioactivity inside the reactor vessel increased dramatically, and some small leaks occurred in the coolant system. This caused the radiation levels in other parts of the plants to register as elevated, and some minimal release occurred to the environment. Shortly after, some water leaked to the basement of the reactor building. This water condensed in the walls passing through the concrete and layers of iron that became corroded (18).

Initially, it was believed that the main threat after the accident was the release of radioactive cesium and iodine. It was concluded that the main threat was the release of noble gases into the atmosphere with the main one being xenon-133 (19).

MANAGEMENT AFTER THE INCIDENT

The Three Mile Island incident has been described as a logistical failure with respect to the management of the accident. The information was leaked in the news and was not consistent from one agency to the other. The evacuation of people living in the vicinity of the plant including hospitals and patients was a major point in the discussions at the time. The county closest to the area, Dauphin, had a plan to evacuate a 5-mile radius around the plant. As days went by, the plans were expanded, and the radius was increased to 20 miles. Hospitals in the area began a massive effort to decrease admissions and to discharge patients who were not in critical condition (20,21).

At the same time, discussions began on how to supply potassium iodide (KI) to the people surrounding the area. At the time of the accident, there were enough doses of KI for a few thousand people but not nearly enough for the popula-

tion around the neighboring city, Harrisburg, Pennsylvania. After a massive effort, with the help of the U.S. Air Force and a pharmaceutical company, 237,000 family-sized bottles, 250,000 droppers, and 250,000 patient information sheets were assembled in a Harrisburg warehouse ready for distribution just 72 hours after the accident. No dose was given, and no bottles were ever distributed (20,21).

Several days after the accident was controlled it was determined that no need for massive evacuation was needed. This accident resulted in many changes for the Nuclear Regulatory Commission. One of the many lessons learned was that preparing for a possible nuclear accident is very complex and the multitude of agencies involved needs a centralized figure to direct all efforts.

CHERNOBYL, UKRAINE, 1986

The Chernobyl reactors are of the RBMK type (Fig. 19-4). Fourteen RBMK systems are still in operation in the former Soviet Union. There are four reactors at Chernobyl: Unit 4 reactor was destroyed in the 1986 accident; Unit 2 reactor was shut down five years later, after a serious turbine building fire; Unit 1 was closed in November 1996. Because of energy shortages, Unit 3 continued operation until December 2000 (22).

The Chernobyl power station is located in the Ukraine, one of the Soviet Union's most productive regions for agriculture. It is 130 km north of Kiev, capital of the Ukraine, with a population of more than 1,000,000 people. The town of Chernobyl is 12 km to the southeast of the plant. The town of Pripyat, with a population of more than 40,000, is immediately northwest of the plant. The plant is located close to the Pripyat River, which is a tributary of the Dnieper, the second largest river in southern Russia (23). A modest-sized concrete shell surrounded the reactor; however, multiple pipes for the cooling system passed through the shell, possibly weakening the structure.

On April 25, 1986, a scheduled service shutdown was started. The objective was to determine how long the decel-

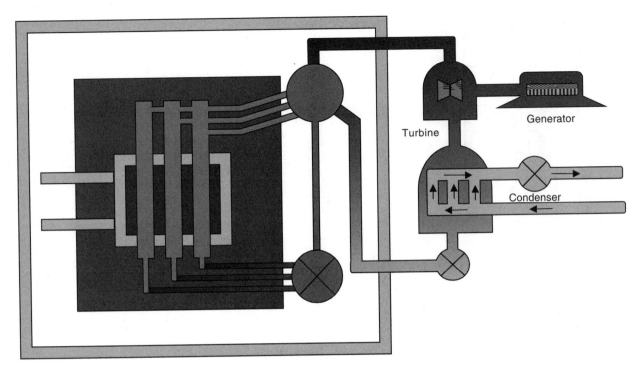

Figure 19–4. RBMK reactor.

erating turbines would spin and supply power to some of the reactor's emergency systems. Similar tests had already been carried out at Chernobyl and other plants, despite the fact that these reactors were known to be very unstable at low power settings. Operators disabled automatic shutdown mechanisms and withdrew most of the control rods for the purpose of the experiment. A series of nuclear chain reactions caused the reactor power output to drop. The operators reduced the flow of coolant to stabilize steam pressure. A feature known as "positive void coefficient," a feature of RMBK reactors, can produce a power surge if cooling water is lost. Because of the positive void coefficient, a huge power surge resulted. It is theorized that the reactor may have reached more than 1 million megawatts. It was originally designed to operate at only 3,200 megawatts (24).

As a result of the uncontrolled reaction steam, pressure was building up in the coolant water area, and the core temperature rose markedly. The fuel elements ruptured, bringing them in contact with water, which in turn caused more steam and increased the pressure. The steam pressure at the plant went to between 100 and 500 times the maximum levels it was designed for, and lifted a 1,000-ton cover plate, turned it on its side, and ripped open the reactor, leaving the hot core exposed to the environment (25). Air rushed in, coming in contact with the graphite and causing it to burst into flames. Experts dispute the character of this second explosion.

Ten days of efforts were needed to bring the disaster under control. Lead, sand, clay, and boron in excess of 5,000 tons were dropped in the area by helicopters to contain the fire. Authorities made no announcement of the disaster until two days later, resulting in delayed evacuation and possible increased problems in adjacent areas (22).

The accident destroyed the Chernobyl Unit 4 reactor and killed 30 people, 28 of whom died from radiation exposure. Another 209 individuals on site were treated for acute radiation poisoning; among these, 134 cases were confirmed, all of whom reportedly recovered. Nobody off-site suffered from acute radiation effects. However, large areas of Belarus, Ukraine, Russia, and beyond were contaminated in varying degrees.

It is estimated that all of the xenon gas, about half of the iodine and cesium, and at least 5% of the remaining radioactive material in the Chernobyl Unit 4 reactor core were released in the accident. Most of the released material was deposited close by as dust and debris, but the lighter material was carried by wind over the Ukraine, Belarus, Russia, and to some extent over Scandinavia and Europe. Most of the casualties were among the firefighters, including those who attended the initial small fires on the roof of the turbine building. All these were put out in a few hours.

After extinguishing the fire, the next task was cleaning up the radioactivity at the site so that the remaining three reactors could be restarted, and the damaged reactor could be shielded more permanently. About 200,000 people ("liquidators") from all over the USSR were involved in the recovery and cleanup during 1986 and 1987. It is estimated that this group may have received high doses of radiation at around 100 millisieverts (mSv). Some 20,000 of them received about 250 mSv, and a few received 500 mSv. Later, the number of liquidators swelled to over 600,000, but most of these later participants received only low radiation doses (22,23).

Many children in the surrounding areas were exposed to radiation doses sufficient to lead to thyroid cancers. These are usually not fatal if diagnosed and treated early

(5,6). Initial radiation exposure in contaminated areas was due to short-lived iodine-131; later cesium-137 was the main hazard (both are fission products dispersed from the reactor core). On May 2–3 (7 days after the accident), some 45,000 residents were evacuated from within a 10-km radius of the plant, notably from the plant operators' town of Pripyat. On May 4, all those living within a 30-km radius—an additional 116,000 people—were evacuated and later relocated. About 1,000 of these have since returned unofficially to live within the contaminated zone. Most of those evacuated received radiation doses of less than 50 mSv, although a few received 100 mSv or more (26).

In the years following the accident, 210,000 more people were resettled into less contaminated areas, and the initial 30-km-radius exclusion zone (2,800 km^2) was modified and extended to cover 4,300 km^2. Psychosocial effects among those affected by the accident are emerging as a major problem and are similar to those arising from other major disasters such as earthquakes, floods, and fires (1,23,27).

MANAGEMENT FOLLOWING THE CHERNOBYL INCIDENT

The Chernobyl Nuclear Power Station was equipped with a medical center with a wide array of instrumentation and personnel needed to treat patients. Most of the instruments used for detecting radiation were lost in the explosion, so the triage of patients was made based only on clinical signs and symptoms. The emergency medical plan for this type of accident in the Soviet Union specified three levels of care: rescue and first aid at the plant site; emergency treatment at regional hospitals; and definitive evaluation and treatment at a specialized center in Moscow (28).

Most of the patients were initially sent to Kiev for treatment. The government radiation disaster team arrived approximately 10 hours after the accident. Subsequently 129 seriously injured patients were transported to Hospital 6 in Moscow, an institution specializing in the treatment of radiation injuries (23). The magnitude of this accident required a large number of workers and hospital beds to treat the injured. Hundreds of workers were called to assist in the initial response, in addition to the more than 500 workers already in the plant including technicians, firefighters, and support personnel. The initial triage and decontamination was performed on site before transport to other facilities. Victims received large doses of radiation in addition to burns and traumatic injuries. Attempts were made to treat these patients with techniques that were not fully developed and were still undergoing research. Bone marrow transplantation was attempted in patients that received more than 6 Gy, which resulted in almost a 100% death rate. Of the 203 victims hospitalized, 30 died of different causes (28).

The third phase of medical response involved the arrival of medical teams from outside of the region. This phase was started after initial evaluation and definitive treatment, within days of the accident. Approximately 450 medical brigades were organized and sent to Chernobyl from all parts of the Soviet Union. More than 5,000 medical personnel were activated for this part of the treatment (28). The mission of these brigades was to evaluate and treat patients who were not significantly injured but who required management in one of the main treatment facilities in the surrounding area.

Potassium iodide was readily available for use during the accident. A total of 90,000 people received KI from the onsite personnel 1.5 hours after the accident; residents of Pripyat were given KI 6.5 hours after the accident; and the rest of the population within a 30-km radius received KI during the first days of May. The use of KI in nuclear incidents is discussed in more detail later in this chapter.

Due to increased winds and rain during the accident days, the spreading of radioactive material to adjacent areas was increased. The day after the incident (April 27), increased air radioactivity was detected in Poland (300 miles away from the accident). By 10 A.M. on April 28, all Polish monitoring stations reported air, soil, and water contamination, and a 24-hour emergency alert was initiated. Air samples showed over 80% of contamination being iodine isotopes. No confirmation of this incident was received in Poland until late on April 28. After soil, air, and water levels were taken, officials concluded that important threshold radiation levels (above 50 mSv) were exceeded. Given the fact that these towns were mainly agricultural centers and consumed most of its products, large-scale prophylaxis with KI was started in children 16 years of age and younger. Although some thyroid uptake was believed to have already occurred by the time prophylaxis could be started, stable iodine was still considered to be useful to protect against the continuing contamination resulting from Chernobyl (6). Because the cancer risk for adults was believed to be low, and because some side effects might be anticipated, iodide prophylaxis was not recommended for adults. The mass media was used to alert the population and to look for volunteers for the nationwide distribution. They banned the feeding of cows with fresh pasture, and children under 4 were provided with powdered milk for consumption until the levels in the atmosphere and soil were normal. People, especially children and pregnant and lactating women, were encouraged to eat a minimal amount of fresh vegetables. A total of 10.5 million doses of KI were given to children, with 90% of the under-16 group receiving the iodide tablets. In spite of the recommendations for adults not to receive iodine, 7 million doses were taken by adults.

ROLE OF POTASSIUM IODIDE

Radioactive fallout in the immediate vicinity of a nuclear reactor is introduced into the body predominantly through inhalation. Radiation is absorbed into the body fastest via this route of exposure. Particles then may be deposited in the soil, water, and vegetation, subsequently being ingested by humans and animals several days after fallout. For example radioiodines can appear in cow's milk within 5 to 10 hours of contamination of their fodder, with peak concentrations by 36 to 48 hours postingestion (3,11). Thus the issue of maintaining a supply of prophylaxis is important not only for those in the immediate area surrounding a reactor but also to the people in more distant communities near the reactor sites, who may be at risk of contamination from food and water.

Radioisotopes of iodine are produced in fission reactions, and after an accident in a nuclear reactor several of them will be released to the environment. There are 24 isotopes of iodine ^{117}I to ^{140}I all of which are radioactive except ^{127}I (11,29). Iodine-132 to iodine-135 are produced in greater yields than iodine-131, which has the longest half-life (approximately 8 days).

Different factors influence the absorption of radioactive iodine into the thyroid gland. These include dietary intake of iodine and previous thyroid disease (e.g., Grave's disease). The presence of food in the gastrointestinal (GI) tract also influences the rate of absorption into the bloodstream. After exposure, the iodine is absorbed into the blood and then taken up by the thyroid gland over a long period of time. One study demonstrated that radioactive tracer is measured in the neck approximately 3 minutes after oral administration of ^{131}I (11). In euthyroid subjects, a single ingestion of radioactive iodine results in a saturation plateau at 10% to 40% of the total iodine ingested with maximum accumulation reached by 36 to 48 hours (3,9,11).

Potassium iodide is a thyroid-blocking agent. The salt saturates the thyroid gland with stable iodine, which in turn will stop the absorption of further iodine hence blocking the absorption of radioactive iodine. The reports of blockade of thyroid absorption of radioactive iodine are varied in the literature. Some reports show that if KI is given 12 hours before the exposure to radioiodine, 90% blockade can be achieved; however, if it is given 24 hours before, there is only 70% blockade. Reports also vary from 98% blockade if prophylaxis is given at the same time of exposure to 60% blockade if prophylaxis is given after 3 hours to 40% blockade if it is given 8 hours after exposure, with the approximate time of blockade duration being 48 to 72 hours (3,9,11).

RESPONSE TO AN ACCIDENT

Nuclear power plants in the United States are mostly privately owned facilities that are required to adhere to strict regulatory measures imposed by different agencies. The Nuclear Regulatory Commission (NRC) is one of the agencies responsible for the regulation of U.S. commercial nuclear power plants. They are responsible for licensing and evaluating the different power plants across the nation. Licensing of a nuclear power plant facility requires that the safety of the plant be up to national standards and that an emergency plan is in place in each of these facilities. The Federal Emergency Management Agency (FEMA) has developed guidelines and plans in accordance with the NRC to give specific guidelines on how to respond to a nuclear power plant accident. These plans are state-specific and have specific guidelines depending on the magnitude of the incident or accident.

The NRC/EPA Task Force Report on Emergency Planning (NUREG 0396, EPA 52011-78-016) delineates and describes the different steps to be taken in case of a nuclear power plant accident. The risk area associated with a nuclear power plant accident is divided in two geographical areas designated Emergency Planning Zones (EPZs). These define the areas for which planning is needed to ensure that prompt and effective actions are taken to protect the health and safety of the public. These EPZs are in theory a circle centered on the power plant and may change depending on such characteristics as topography and specific landmarks. A short-term area or "plume exposure pathway" includes everything within a 10-mile radius of the power plant. This area's risk includes whole body injury from exposure to gamma radiation and other injury from inhalation of radioactive material.

The other EPZ is the long-term ingestion exposure pathway, which includes everything within a 50-mile radius of the power plant. The risks in this area are whole-body and thyroid injury from ingesting water and food supplies contaminated with radioactive materials. These general guidelines must be modified in each specific event. In the case of the Chernobyl accident, the ingestion exposure pathway extended well beyond 300 miles from the nuclear power plant site. This was demonstrated in the Polish exposures seen after the accident as explained in the previous section. For this reason, the exposure areas depend on the extent of the accident, the atmospheric conditions, and the specific conditions of the terrain in the different areas.

In the event of an accident, the response will be directed by a multitude of agencies. The initial response has to be within the power plant itself in that it must identify the accident and notify the local and state agencies of the fact that an accident has occurred. NUREG-065/FEMA-REP-1, an article describing nuclear power plant accident response from FEMA and the NRC, states that "Normally, the State emergency management organization will be the primarily responsible for the response planning required for the ingestion pathway EPZ" and that "an appendix to the State or local emergency plan must address the provisions that have been made to detect contamination, implementing procedures, prepare maps for secondary surveys, implement evacuation etc. as well as any requests for federal assistance."

Important parts of the emergency plan include public warning, emergency public information, evacuation, mass care areas, and resource management. In the event of a nuclear power plant accident, initial evaluation and care of workers and people living close to the plant is expected. A plan has to be in place for the evaluation and care of these immediate patients in conjunction with the management of the accident itself. The care of emergency personnel working in the relief efforts in the accident is also a crucial part of this emergency plan. Coordination with several local, state, and federal agencies must be in place for the undertaking of patient management and possible evacuation zones and routes for the immediate or plum EPZ. For the ingestion EPZ, other agencies and concerns must be undertaken to examine the possibility of evacuation or prophylaxis with potassium iodide.

The management of a nuclear power plant disaster needs the intervention of local, state, and federal agencies. Every location with a nuclear power plant has a plan in the event of an accident, as required by the NRC to be licensed. The medical management of these events will be as any other mass casualty event. The Radiation Emergency Assistance Center/ Training Site (REACT/TS) provides support to the U.S. Department of Energy, the World Health Organization, and multiple international agencies in the medical management of possible radiological accidents.

Each state and agency has designated a team of responders who, in the case of an emergency, will take over the management of the emergency site, and local plans must be identified in each area in order to be involved in the management of these cases.

SUMMARY

Nuclear power plant accidents are a very rare occurrence, and history has shown that nuclear power plants have generally been safe to operate. The two major power plant disasters in history are discussed here. One of these, the Chernobyl incident, had significant health implications to humans around surrounding areas. The major causative factor in the Chernobyl event is now believed to have been the faulty construction of a reactor that should not have been in operation in any part of the world (23,27). Because of the great number of power plants around the globe and the variety of designs, there is still a possibility of another accident of great magnitude happening. It is believed that the robust construction of the U.S. nuclear power plants will prevent these accidents, but debate still exists in the literature (2,16,30).

The release of radioactive material will be varied and specific to the reactor fuel being used in the specific plant. After an accident, the major concern is the release of radioactive isotopes that may travel for many miles and present a radiation hazard far from the immediate areas surrounding these power plants. The release of radioactive iodine from the site of the accident is still considered to be responsible for the increase in the incidence of thyroid cancer in Belarus (7,8,10–12). The cause of the increased intake of radioactive iodine in the population of Poland and areas surrounding Chernobyl downwind from the accident is believed to be a combination of factors including dietary intake and not necessarily the "cloud" of radioactive material (11,19). In this instance, the use of a thyroid-blocking agent may be effective in protecting the incorporation of radioactive iodine into various organs, especially the thyroid. The use of potassium iodide for this purpose is still debated in the literature, but it is widely stored for use in the event of a nuclear power plant incident (3,5,6,9,11,12,31,32).

Nuclear power plants are still considered a prime target for terrorists by many experts. In the United States, the strict requirements for construction and management of these plants should enable them to withstand many threats. The possibility of leakage of radioactive material to adjacent areas in the event of a terrorist attack cannot be excluded. For this reason, the regulatory commissions and government agencies are working diligently to make this threat negligible.

Some of the most important issues to remember are listed in Table 19-4.

TABLE 19-4	Key Features of Nuclear Power Plant Disasters

1. Pressurized water reactors (PWR) and boiling water reactors (BWR) are the two reactors currently used in the United States.

2. The emergency medical plan for a nuclear incident includes rescue and first aid at the plant site, emergency treatment at regional hospitals, and definitive evaluation and treatment at specialized centers.

3. The issue of maintaining a supply of potassium iodide (KI) prophylaxis is important not only for those in the immediate surroundings of a reactor but also to the people in more distant communities near the reactor sites, who may be at risk of contamination from food and water.

4. The risk area associated with a nuclear power plant accident is divided into two geographical areas designated Emergency Planning Zones (EPZs). They define the areas for which planning is needed to ensure that prompt and effective actions are taken to protect the health and safety of the public.

5. Important parts of the emergency plan include public warning, emergency public information, evacuation, mass care areas, and resource management.

RESOURCES

1. Nuclear Energy Institute Web site: http://www.nei.org
2. Nuclear Regulatory Commission (NRC) Web site: http://www.nrc.gov
3. Radiation Emergency Assistance Center/Training Site (REAC/TS) Web site: http://www.orau.gov/reacts/

QUESTIONS AND ANSWERS

1. **Which of the following statements is FALSE?**
   A. The first successful nuclear detonation took place in New Mexico in July 1945 as part of the Manhattan Project in the United States.
   B. The United States currently has over 1,000 operating commercial nuclear power reactors.
   C. Nuclear power plant accidents are a very rare occurrence, and contemporary designs have more safety features than their predecessors.
   D. Most events involving nuclear power plants in history have been described as incidents, and just a handful have met accident criteria.
   E. Throughout history, several nuclear power plant incidents have occurred, and most of these have not had any effect on the population, with no radioactive material having been exposed.

2. **Which of the following regarding the Chernobyl accident is FALSE?**

A. The Chernobyl accident is considered the worst nuclear power plant accident in history because it had significant health effects in the immediate area surrounding the plant and also other countries surrounding Chernobyl.

B. The Chernobyl accident killed 30 people, including 28 from radiation exposure. The main casualties were among the firefighters, including those who attended the initial small fires on the roof of the turbine building.

C. Nobody off-site from the Chernobyl accident suffered from acute radiation effects; 1.5 million residents were evacuated from within a 10-km radius of the plant.

D. The release of radioactive iodine from the site of the accident is still considered to be the responsible for an increased incidence of thyroid cancer in Belarus.

E. The most recent and authoritative UN report has confirmed that there is no scientific evidence of any significant radiation-related health effects to most people exposed to the Chernobyl disaster.

3. Which of the following statements is FALSE?

A. There are several types of nuclear power plants used for energy production around the globe.

B. Light water reactors are divided into pressurized water reactors and boiling water reactors.

C. Heavy water reactors and graphite-moderated reactors are the two reactors currently used in the United States.

D. The main threat after the Three Mile Island accident was the release of radioactive cesium and iodine.

E. RBMK is a Russian acronym for reactor *bolshoi moschnosti kanalynyi* and is a reactor in which its moderator is graphite. The world's first nuclear power plant in Obninsk was of this type.

4. Radiation dispersal can be achieved by several mechanisms. Which of the following statements is FALSE?

A. The ultimate dispersal method is the nuclear weapon.

B. The use of conventional explosives mixed with radioactive material is considered to be another type of dispersal mechanism.

C. The use of liquid radioisotopes to be dispersed in the water supply of certain cities is also considered a possible threat.

D. The amounts of liquid isotope material needed to create a successful terrorist water supply attack could be stored in an 8-ounce lead can.

E. An attack on a fixed nuclear facility or on radioactive material in transit may disperse radioactive material and is considered a possibility in a terrorist attack.

ANSWERS

1: *B. The United States currently has over 1,000 operating commercial nuclear power reactors.*

2: *C. Nobody off-site from the Chernobyl accident suffered from acute radiation effects; 1.5 million residents were evacuated from within a 10-km radius of the plant.*

3: *C. Heavy water reactors and graphite-moderated reactors are the two reactors currently used in the United States.*

4: *D. The amounts of liquid isotope material needed to create a successful terrorist water supply attack could be stored in an 8-ounce lead can.*

REFERENCES

1. Dew MA, Bromet EJ, Schulberg HC, et al. Mental health effects of the Three Mile Island nuclear reactor restart. Am J Psychiatr. 1987;144(8):1074-7.
2. Timins JK, Lipoti JA. Radiological terrorism. N Eng J Med. 2003;100(6):14-21; quiz 22-4.
3. Becker DV, Zanzonico P. Potassium iodide for thyroid blockade in a reactor accident: administrative policies that govern its use. Thyroid. 1997;7(2):193-7.
4. Goulko GM, Chumak VV, Chepurny NI, et al. Estimation of ^{131}I thyroid doses for the evacuees from Pripjat. Radiat Environ Biophys. 1996;35(2):81-7.
5. Kazakov VS, Demidchik EP, Astakhova LN. Thyroid cancer after Chernobyl. Nature. 1992;359(6390):21.
6. Nauman J, Wolff J. Iodide prophylaxis in Poland after the Chernobyl reactor accident: benefits and risks. Am J Med. 1993;94(5):524-32.
7. Ron E, Modan B, Preston D, et al. Thyroid neoplasia following low-dose radiation in childhood. Radiat Res. 1989; 120(3): 516-31.
8. Schwenn MR, Brill AB. Childhood cancer 10 years after the Chernobyl accident. Curr Opin Pediatr. 1997;9(1):51-4.
9. Verger P, Aurengo A, Geoffroy B, Le Guen B. Iodine kinetics and effectiveness of stable iodine prophylaxis after intake of radioactive iodine: a review. Thyroid. 2001;11(4):353-60.
10. Williams D. Thyroid cancer and the Chernobyl accident. J Clin Endocrinol Metab. 1996;81(1):6-8.
11. Zanzonico PB, Becker DV. Effects of time of administration and dietary iodine levels on potassium iodide (KI) blockade of thyroid irradiation by 131I from radioactive fallout. Health Phys. 2000;78(6):660-7.
12. Zarzycki W, Zonenberg A, Telejko B, Kinalska I. Iodine prophylaxis in the aftermath of the Chernobyl accident in the area of Sejny in north-eastern Poland. Horm Metab Res. 1994; 26(6):293-6.
13. Security effectiveness: independent studies and drills. In: Nuclear Energy Institute.
14. Deterring terrorism: aircraft crash impact analyses demonstrate nuclear power plant's structural strength. In: Nuclear Energy Institute; 2002.
15. Champlin RE, Kastenberg WE, Gale RP. Radiation accidents and nuclear energy: medical consequences and therapy. Ann Intern Med. 1988;109(9):730-44.
16. Helfand I, Forrow L, Tiwari J. Nuclear terrorism. Br Med J. 2002;324(7333):356–9.
17. Sprung JL, Ammerman DJ, Kosi JA, Weiner RF. Spent fuel transportation package performance study. In: Issues Report (NUREG/CR6768) U.S. Nuclear Regulatory Commission: Sandia National Laboratories; 2003.
18. Fact sheet on the accident at Chernobyl power plant. In: U.S. Nuclear Regulatory Commission; 2003.
19. Fact Sheet on the Accident at Three Mile Island. In: U.S. Nuclear Regulatory Commission; 2003.
20. Small WE. Mobilizing for Three Mile Island—the disaster that wasn't. Am Pharm. 1979;19(6):8-9.
21. Smith JS Jr., Fisher JH. Three Mile Island: the silent disaster. JAMA. 1981;245(16):1656-9.
22. Fact sheet on the accident at the Chernobyl Nuclear Power Plant. In: U.S. Nuclear Regulatory Commission; 2003.
23. Bonte FJ. Chernobyl retrospective. Semin Nucl Med. 1988; 18(1):16-24.

24. Marshall E. The lessons of Chernobyl. Science. 1986;233 (4771):1375-6.

25. Wilson R. A visit to Chernobyl. Science. 1987;236(4809):1636-40.

26. Perry AR, Iglar AF. The accident at Chernobyl: radiation doses and effects. Radiol Technol. 1990;61(4):290-4.

27. Kasper K. Chernobyl: facts and fiction. Health Phys. 2003;84 (4):419-20.

28. Linnemann RE. Soviet medical response to the Chernobyl nuclear accident. JAMA. 1987;258(5):637-43.

29. Gudiksen PH, Harvey TF, Lange R. Chernobyl source term, atmospheric dispersion, and dose estimation. Health Phys. 1989;57(5):697-706.

30. von Hippel FN. Revisiting nuclear power plant safety. Science. 2003;299(5604):201–3; author reply 201-3.

31. Balter M. France distributes iodine near reactors. Science. 1997;275(5308):1871-2.

32. Potassium iodide stockpile for nuclear accidents. JAMA 1990; 263(12):1632.

Explosives and Traumatic Terrorism

20

Types of Explosions and Explosive Injuries Defined

Richard Linsky and Adam Miller

The worldwide escalation of violence, both civilian and military, demands that medical personnel and first responders be prepared to deal with the consequences of bombings. Explosions serve terrorist goals well. They are dramatic and gain immediate public attention, creating chaos and mass hysteria. Bombings are not only meant to kill and maim, but to strike fear in those removed from the event itself. Despite widespread concerns regarding biological and chemical attacks, conventional and improvised explosive devices are by far the most commonly utilized terrorist weapons. According to FBI statistics, there were 12,216 bombings in the United States between 1980 and 1990, causing 1,782 injuries, 241 deaths, and almost $140 million of property damage. Between 1990 and 1994, there were 8,567 bombings and nearly 2,000 additional bombing attempts, the majority of which involved pipe-bomb-type devices (1). Suicide bombings in Israel are increasing exponentially, with 107 suicide bombings between 2000 and 2003 (2).

In most bombings, many more are injured than killed. For example, the 1993 bombing of the World Trade Center in New York City killed 6 but injured over 1,000. The truck bomb detonated outside the Murrah Federal Building in Oklahoma City in 1995 killed 168 and injured over 750. In 1998, the bombing of the U.S. embassy in Nairobi killed 253 and created a staggering 5,000 casualties. The large numbers of casualties generated can easily overwhelm any local medical system.

Explosions cause a unique form of barotrauma, known as primary blast injury, which affects principally the air-filled organs in the body. The violent forces created also cause all types of penetrating and blunt injuries, termed secondary and tertiary blast injuries, which are more familiar to medical personnel. The number of casualties and the severity of their injuries varies depending on the type of attack, size of the explosive charge, and whether located in a confined or open space (3). Improvements in prehospital trauma care and EMS systems have allowed more bombing victims to arrive at the medical center with signs of life (3). This chapter discusses types of explosive devices, blast physics, and the pathophysiology and management of blast-related injury, focusing on the organ systems most at risk.

TYPES OF EXPLOSIVE DEVICES

Many bombs manufactured by terrorists are relatively unsophisticated "improvised explosive devices," or IEDs, made using readily obtainable materials such as agricultural fertilizer or household cleansers. Recipes for such homemade bombs abound on the Internet. The pipe bomb, the most common type of improvised terrorist bomb, consists of low explosives inside a tightly capped piece of metal pipe, often wrapped with nails or scrap metal to cause even more harm. The Molotov cocktail is another easily constructed terrorist weapon that can cause considerable damage. Materials such as gasoline, diesel fuel, kerosene, ethyl or methyl alcohol, lighter fluid, or turpentine are placed in a glass bottle, which is thrown and breaks upon impact. A piece of cotton serves as a fuse, which is ignited before the bottle is thrown at the target (4).

More sophisticated explosive devices generally contain three basic elements: a trigger, a fuse, and the main charge. Various triggering mechanisms may be employed, including motion detectors, photoelectric cells, time switches, radiation triggers, and remotely controlled electronic signals. Once triggered, the fuse is activated and the main charge ignited.

Common *high* explosives include TNT, C4, PETN, and dynamite. High explosives can be mixed with plasticizers such as oil or wax to create soft, hand-malleable substances called plastic explosives, or plastique. Terrorists frequently employ plastic explosives because of their ease of concealment, and they have been the predominant weapons used in aviation-related terrorism incidents (5). Only 312 grams of the plastic explosive SEMTEX, connected to a battery and a barometric trigger mechanism, and small enough to be hidden inside a portable cassette player, was responsible for the destruction of Pan Am Flight 103 over Lockerbie, Scotland, in 1988.

An explosion is caused by the rapid chemical conversion of the main charge into a gas with resultant violent release of energy. Explosives are classified as "high" or "low," depending on the speed with which they release that energy. *Low* explosives, such as flash powder or gunpowder, release energy relatively slowly via a process called *deflagration*. The low explosives exert more of a pushing or heaving effect and are generally used as propellants.

By contrast, high explosives undergo *detonation* when initiated, an almost instantaneous transformation of the original explosive material into gases filling the same volume and therefore under extremely high pressure (6). The highly pressurized gases expand rapidly and compress the surrounding medium, generating a pressure pulse that is propagated as a blast wave in all directions. It is this instantaneous rise in pressure that gives high-explosive blast waves the unique characteristic of *brisance*, or shattering ability. The rapidity with which an explosive reaches its peak pressure is a measure of its brisance. Low explosives do not release energy fast enough to demonstrate brisance.

PATHOPHYSIOLOGY OF BLAST INJURY

Although the physics are complex, a blast wave has three basic components: an extremely short burst of increasing pressure, a longer phase of negative pressure, and a massive movement of air called the blast wind. An idealized blast wave is depicted in Figure 20-1. During the positive-pres-

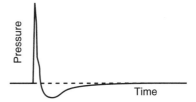

Figure 20–1. Idealized high-explosive blast wave as it passes over a fixed point in space.

sure phase, the blast front moves away from its point of origin at supersonic speeds. Under ideal conditions, the blast front is spherical and propagates outward equally in all directions. This positive-pressure phase, much more powerful than the negative phase, is responsible for the majority of the damage. The magnitude of the positive phase impulse, the *peak overpressure,* is the primary determinant of the severity of blast injury. The overpressure needed to cause blast injury to the lung is approximately 40 pounds per square inch (psi). More than half of all victims will suffer pulmonary damage with pressures of 80 psi or more; overpressures exceeding 200 psi are uniformly fatal (7).

The peak overpressure is governed largely by three factors: (a) the size of the explosive charge, (b) the distance from the detonation, and (c) the surrounding medium (air or water). The larger the charge, the greater the peak overpressure will be and the longer its duration. With the common high explosives used in civilian terrorist bombs, the duration of the positive-pressure impulse is 2 to 10 milliseconds (8). Small bombs that may be carried by hand or in a parcel may contain up to 30 pounds of explosives; car bombs may contain up to 500 pounds or more (9). The size of the truck bomb used in Oklahoma City in 1995 has been estimated to be about 4,000 pounds. The truck bomb that destroyed the Al Khobar Towers in Saudi Arabia in 1996 detonated with an estimated likely yield of more than 20,000 pounds of TNT-equivalent explosives. The 1998 bombing of the U.S. embassy in Nairobi was deadly but fairly small by comparison, equivalent to 3 metric tons of TNT. The 1993 World Trade Center bomb had the explosive power of about 2,000 pounds of TNT.

The peak overpressure at any given point is inversely proportional to the cube of the distance from the blast. As blast waves travel outward, their velocity and pressure fall off rapidly and eventually deteriorate into acoustic waves (10). As a result, casualties must be relatively close to the detonation, or the explosion must be of great magnitude, to make significant primary blast injury a likely finding in survivors (11). As a point of reference, an explosive charge equivalent to 20 kilograms of TNT that detonates more than 6 meters away from the body is unlikely to cause significant blast injury to the lung (7).

Because water is essentially incompressible, a blast wave will be transmitted with greater speed and intensity and over a longer range than the same blast wave in air (9). Underwater blast injuries are more prevalent at any given distance (12), and the lethal range of an underwater explosion is far greater than a similar open-air blast (13). The presence of reflecting or absorbing surfaces, such as walls or other people, will alter the peak overpressure. When reflected by a solid surface, a blast wave can be magnified many times the original incident pressure. Victims who are near walls, large solid objects, or corners can have injuries several times greater than what would be expected for any given blast pressure (14). A recent Israeli study reported that mortality was 8% in open-air terrorist bombings but 49% in enclosed-space bombings. Similarly, the incidence of primary blast injury in enclosed spaces was twice that of open-air bombings. Body armor may protect from penetrating injury but acts like walls surrounding the thorax and can potentiate the blast effect (15). Animal studies have shown that intrathoracic pressure is generally higher in those wearing ballistic vests (15). The negative-pressure phase of the blast wave follows immediately after the positive phase and lasts about 10 times as long. The mass movement of air away from the blast epicenter creates an area of low pressure, rarely exceeding −1 atmosphere. The suction effect generated reverses the direction of the blast wind and pulls debris into the area, causing additional damage and injury (9).

Although the ultimate clinical presentation depends on whether an explosion occurs in open or confined quarters, open air, or water, the pattern of injury inflicted on the body is relatively consistent (3). As a blast wave passes through the body, it causes damage by several different mechanisms: spalling, implosion, inertia, and pressure differentials (9). *Spalling* occurs at tissue interfaces when particles from a denser medium are thrown into a less dense medium as a blast wave passes through. In the lungs, for example, particles of liquid are spalled into the alveolar space, much as water is thrown into the air in an underwater explosion (9). Blast waves passing through organs containing pockets of gas, such as the middle ear or the sinuses, cause *implosion* of the air pocket, followed by a rebound expansion once the wave has passed. Because air is easily compressible by a passing blast wave but fluid-containing tissues are not, *pressure differentials* develop at such air-fluid interfaces, causing shear forces that tear and disrupt tissues. Lastly, the *inertia* imparted from the force of the blast wind may propel a victim against a stationary object, causing injury on impact (9).

CLASSIFICATION OF BLAST INJURIES

Injuries caused by explosives have traditionally been divided into primary, secondary, and tertiary blast injuries, and miscellaneous or quaternary injuries. *Primary blast injury* is a form of barotrauma, unique to explosions, which causes damage to air-filled organs: the lungs, the gastrointestinal tract, and the auditory system. *Secondary blast injury* refers to penetrating trauma caused by the acceleration of shrapnel and other debris by the blast wind. *Tertiary blast injury* is caused by the displacement of the body by the blast wind, with typical patterns of blunt trauma occurring on forceful impact with a solid object or the ground.

PULMONARY BLAST INJURY

The hallmark of primary blast injury is damage to the respiratory system, or "blast lung," and is manifested by varying degrees of pulmonary contusion and barotrauma. The extent of pulmonary pathology is directly proportional to the velocity of chest-wall displacement by the incoming blast wave (16), which in turn is dictated by the size of the explosive charge, distance from blast epicenter, orientation of the thorax in relation to the blast wave, and geography of nearby reflecting surfaces. Injury tends to be worse on the side of approach of blast waves in open air but is usually bilateral or diffuse when the victim is located in a confined space (17).

As a blast wave propagates through the chest, enormous pressure differentials are generated at interfaces between media of different densities (8,13) resulting in alveolar tears and vascular disruption. There is also evidence from rat lung models that subtle biochemical changes and free-radical-mediated oxidative stresses contribute to blast-induced injury (18,19). Pleural or subpleural petechiae are the mildest pathological findings (17,20). Higher energy stress waves conducted deeper into the lung can cause subpleural hemorrhage where the blast front first contacted the chest wall, as well as near the diaphragm and mediastinum, where reflections and summations of stress waves occur (7,21). Even more powerful blast impulses cause large parenchymal tears and stripping of small airway epithelium (22). Communication between the airways and the pleural space can lead to simple or tension pneumothorax, hemothorax, traumatic emphysema, and alveolo-venous fistulae, which, in the already compromised lung, will precipitate even more rapid respiratory failure. Unfortunately, the need for early positive-pressure ventilation to treat such patients with rapidly progressing respiratory failure can aggravate the situation, increasing the risk for both tension pneumothorax and air embolism (3).

Clinically, blast lung injury can appear very similar to a pulmonary contusion from blunt chest trauma but without associated rib fractures or chest wall injury (13,23). This is rarely seen in the absence of other secondary or tertiary explosion injuries. Like blunt pulmonary contusion, gas exchange is impaired at the alveolar level, and the degree of respiratory insufficiency depends on the extent of hemorrhage. Signs and symptoms of primary pulmonary blast injury may include dyspnea, difficulty completing sentences in one breath, rapid shallow respirations, poor chest wall expansion, cough, hemoptysis, decreased breath sounds, and wheezes.

SYSTEMIC AIR EMBOLISM

A dreaded complication of primary pulmonary blast injury is the development of arterial air embolism, thought to be responsible for most of the sudden deaths that occur within the first hour after blast exposure (24). The true incidence of systemic air embolism is unknown. Only those with clinical evidence of blast lung injury seem to be at risk, with a greater incidence following explosions in confined spaces (25).

Large blast impulses passing through the lung can cause hemopneumothoraces, traumatic emphysema, and vascular disruption (6). Air emboli result from the direct communication created between the traumatized pulmonary airspace and vasculature. Such communication can develop at any time after a blast injury, either directly from the blast or as a complication of therapy for respiratory failure (24). Normally, in a patient with spontaneous respirations, the airway pressure remains lower than the pulmonary venous pressure. After blast trauma, states of low pulmonary venous pressure (hypovolemia) or high airway pressure (positive-pressure ventilation, coughing, or tension pneumothorax) may cause the pressure gradient to reverse, allowing air to enter the pulmonary circulation (26-28) and to be systemically disseminated. One of the first animal studies linking air embolism with blast lung injury subjected a dog to a near-lethal air blast. Showers of carotid air emboli were detected for 30 minutes after injury (29). Animal experiments have also demonstrated coronary air emboli in rats dying immediately following a blast (9).

Obstruction from air bubbles may occur in any vascular bed. The passage of air bubbles causes a transient precapillary block and arterial spasm, dilatation, stasis, and ischemia (9). Air emboli to the heart or brain are thought to be the most common cause of rapid death solely caused by blast injury in immediate survivors (30-32). The introduction of as little as 2 milliliters of air into the cerebral circulation can be fatal (33,34). Likewise, as little as 0.5 to 1 milliliter of air injected into a pulmonary vein can cause cardiac arrest from coronary air embolism (35).

Clinical manifestations of systemic air embolism depend on the location of embolic occlusion and on the degree of resultant ischemia. Air embolism is often heralded by a rapid decompensation immediately following intubation and positive-pressure ventilation (36); such collapse is usually unresponsive to conventional resuscitation (37). Hemoptysis, suggesting communication between pulmonary blood vessels and the airway, was seen in 22% of cases of systemic air embolism in one large series (38). Other symptoms include blindness due to air in retinal vessels, focal neurological deficit or loss of consciousness following cerebral obstruction, and chest pain from coronary obstruction and myocardial ischemia. Air emboli to the skin may produce a reddish-blue mottling discoloration called livido reticularis. Tongue blanching and pharyngeal petechiae may be seen. An arterial blood gas sample may appear frothy with air bubbles, and EKG may reveal arrhythmias or ischemia (39). In those with lung trauma, the combination of hemoptysis and circulatory or CNS dysfunction immediately after initiation of positive-pressure ventilation is sufficient to make the provisional diagnosis of systemic air embolism (27).

GASTROINTESTINAL (GI) BLAST INJURY

Gas-containing abdominal structures are injured in a similar manner as the lungs (17), but such injuries are frequently occult and overshadowed by the more immediately life-threatening manifestations of pulmonary blast injury (24). Military studies have found that in open-air bombings, GI injury occurs with the same frequency as lung injury (40) and at lower pressures following blasts in enclosed spaces (41). Victims of underwater explosions seem to be at a much greater risk for GI injury, especially if treading water or partially submerged (39).

Blast injury tends to affect the colon more often than the small bowel, owing to the greater amount of air in the for-mer. Damage may range from edema to hemorrhage to frank rupture. Rupture is commonly delayed 24 to 48 hours, after stretching and ischemia have weakened the bowel wall (42). Tangential shear waves affecting the liver, spleen, and kidneys have been described, causing subcapsular petechiae, contusions, lacerations, or rupture (39,43). However, nonbowel or solid organ injuries seen following explosions are far more likely to occur from the effects of secondary or tertiary blast injury (8). Signs and symptoms of GI blast injury are nonspecific and include abdominal pain, nausea, vomiting, diarrhea, tenesmus, absent or decreased bowel sounds, rebound tenderness, guarding, or frank rectal bleeding.

AUDITORY BLAST INJURY

The ear is designed to amplify ambient sound waves, and the thin tympanic membrane is directly exposed to the surrounding air. It is not surprising that blast injury to the auditory system occurs much more commonly and at much lower overpressures than do pulmonary or GI blast injury. As a frame of reference, extremely loud acoustic waves, such as those generated at a concert, are generally less than 0.04 psi. Overpressures of at least 1 to 8 psi are needed to cause tympanic membrane rupture (44,45), whereas the threshold for lung injury is typically upward of 50 to 100 psi.

Blast waves are known to cause conductive, sensorineural, and mixed hearing defects. Conductive loss is usually caused by rupture of the tympanic membrane, although ossicular chain disruption may also be seen (24). Such defects are rarely found in isolation, however; most casualties will invariably suffer some degree of concomitant sensorineural hearing loss (46). Blast-related inner ear damage due to transient cochlear dysfunction can cause acute sensorineural hearing loss, often accompanied by tinnitus, which can be quite incapacitating in the moments following an explosion (24). Vertigo and balance disorders have also been described but are thought to be more likely secondary to blunt head injury than primary auditory damage (47).

Although tympanic membrane rupture is objective evidence of significant exposure to blast overpressure and was once thought to be an effective marker for occult pulmonary or GI blast injury, a recent Israeli study demonstrated no significant correlation. In fact, no patients with isolated tympanic membrane rupture later developed evidence of lung or GI pathology (48).

SECONDARY BLAST INJURY

Secondary blast injury, caused by shrapnel and displaced debris, is responsible for the majority of casualties resulting from an explosive event, partly because victims do not have to be close to the blast epicenter to be injured. In fact, blast winds channeled by an alleyway or corridor can be magnified substantially (49), causing significant secondary blast injury to those distant from the epicenter. Shrapnel injuries have been reported in 20% to 40% of blast victims, with an increased incidence in enclosed spaces (50). Injuries from all types of missiles have been described, although in the urban setting, glass has been the most common hazard (9). Terrorists often deliberately pack small metal objects such as nails, bolts, and screws around an explosive charge in an attempt to increase shrapnel injuries; military shell casings are specifically designed to fragment to achieve a similar goal. These irregularly shaped missiles are generally of high mass and therefore high kinetic energy. The kinetic energy is dissipated rapidly along wound tracts to produce severe tissue destruction (51). Such wounds are usually heavily contaminated. At missile speeds of 15 meters per second (m/s), skin may be lacerated; at speeds of 120 m/s and above, body penetration and significant tissue damage can occur (9). A detonation causing a peak overpressure of 5 psi, just strong enough to rupture half of exposed tympanic membranes, may generate a blast wind of up to 70 m/s (156 mph) (6), a speed that, although not sustained, can exceed that of most hurricanes (52). A blast wind sufficient to cause primary lung injury in a significant number of casualties may exceed 400 m/s (895 mph) (6). Most conventional military explosives can propel fragments with initial velocities reaching 1,500 m/s (53). Secondary blast injuries were a significant cause of morbidity in the Oklahoma City bombing; the Murrah Building's glass facade shattered and was propelled over an area of many city blocks. Similarly, in the 1998 U.S. embassy bombing in Nairobi, flying glass wounded people up to 2 km away (52).

TERTIARY BLAST INJURY

Tertiary blast injury is a feature of high-energy explosions and occurs when the individual becomes the missile. A high explosive blast wind may propel a 75 kilogram adult with an acceleration of close to 15 G's. Typical patterns of blunt trauma and deceleration injury are seen when casualties are thrown against a solid object or the ground. Blunt head injury is a leading cause of death in blast victims. Tertiary blast injury accounted for most of the pediatric casualties in the Oklahoma City bombing because children are lighter and more easily displaced by blast wind. There was a high incidence of skull fractures, closed head injuries, and long-bone fractures.

QUATERNARY (MISCELLANEOUS) BLAST INJURY

A variety of other blast-related injuries have been described. Ocular injuries from flying debris are very common after explosions. Injury can be extensive and can involve all tissues of the eye, the ocular adnexa, and the orbit, including simple corneal abrasions, lid lacerations, global rupture, retinal detachment, intraocular foreign bodies, and orbital fractures. Retinal air embolism is also a potential cause of visual disturbance. A review of ocular injuries sustained by survivors of the 1995 Oklahoma City bombing found an 8% overall incidence of ocular injury, with 71% of injuries occurring within 300 feet of the point of detonation. The Murrah Building's glass facade, shattered by the blast, accounted for two-thirds of all ocular injuries (54).

Musculoskeletal injuries will be seen in almost all blast casualties. Fractures may occur in any extremity, are often associated with extensive soft tissue injury, and are typically heavily contaminated. Traumatic amputations, thought to be due to bone-shattering blast waves and near-simultaneous high-velocity blast winds (55), are rarely seen in survivors. Only 1% to 2% of blast victims who survive will have a traumatic amputation, and its presence, evidence of exposure to extreme overpressures, is highly suggestive of other severe injuries (9). Crush injuries and rhabdomyolysis are among the most frequent injuries seen when explosions cause structural collapse, falling debris, and displaced heavy objects.

Cardiovascular injury following an explosion is usually secondary to lung damage or coronary air emboli. However, a vagally mediated direct blast effect, causing a triad of bradycardia, hypotension, and apnea, has been described in rat models. This response was attenuated after surgical vagotomy (56) and not seen at all following directed abdominal blasts (57). It has been postulated that this vagal reflex can contribute to those cases of shock seen immediately after an explosion (58). Other studies in rats demonstrated a variety of EKG disturbances from ventricular extrasystoles to ventricular fibrillation; all abnormalities reverted to sinus rhythm within minutes except in fatally injured rats (57).

Flash burns may result from the short-lived but intense blast heat, which can reach 3000°C (59). In the absence of secondary fires, such burns usually occur only in those closest to the blast and are generally superficial and confined to exposed areas of the body. Burns to the upper respiratory tract are uncommon with small bombs (3). Deeper or more extensive burns may occur if the clothes ignite. Fires occurring in enclosed spaces may cause carbon monoxide, cyanide, or particulate inhalation, further complicating the clinical picture. This was a particular problem in the 1993 bombing of the World Trade Center, when a large number of victims suffered from smoke inhalation.

Often overlooked, psychiatric problems are among the most common sequelae following explosions. One large series reported a 58% incidence of postevent psychological problems among males and 82% among females (60). A French study of 254 survivors of terrorist attacks (including 20 separate bombings) documented posttraumatic stress disorder in 10.5% of uninjured, 8.3% of moderately injured, and 30.7% of severely injured casualties; major depression was seen in 13.3% of all victims (61). One animal study has demonstrated blast-induced cognitive and memory deficits (62). A variety of biochemically mediated effects on the central nervous system suggest that direct neuronal blast injury could be responsible for some aspects of what is now considered to be posttraumatic stress disorder (63). Radiation exposure from a dirty bomb is also a potential complicating factor (see Chapter 17).

EPIDEMIOLOGY

Most of the injuries seen after high explosive detonations will be conventional blunt and penetrating trauma directly produced by the explosion and flying missiles. Soft tissue, orthopedic, and head injuries predominate in most larger series (64-69). A large Israeli series found that although primary blast injuries were not the most common type of injury overall, they were the most common *severe* injury seen in survivors of suicide bombings (3). Explosions in confined spaces are associated with a much higher incidence of primary blast injury, with more severe injuries and with a higher mortality rate in comparison with explosions in the open air. An Israeli study of 297 victims of four suicide bombings found a 7.8% mortality rate in open-air bombings, but a 49% mortality rate following bombings that occurred on a bus (an enclosed space). Similarly, the 77.5% incidence of primary blast injury following bus bombings was double the incidence in open-air bombings (48). Secondary blast injury also occurs with a higher incidence in enclosed spaces (50).

The spectrum of pediatric injuries seen after a bomb blast is poorly documented, and only limited data exist. The only large series describes the injuries seen in the 19 pediatric fatalities and 47 surviving casualties of the 1995 Oklahoma City bombing. The pediatric patients sustained a high incidence of cranial injuries, fractures, and traumatic amputations. Intraabdominal and thoracic injuries occurred frequently in the deceased but infrequently in survivors (70).

The number of fatalities seen after an explosion seems to be more closely related to the type of attack rather than to the amount and type of explosives used (71). Injuries observed among fatalities of Israeli suicide bombings include crush injury (38%), significant penetrating injury (25%), burns (15%), limb amputation (11%), and decapitation (5%) (3). One of the largest series to date, providing a study population of 3,357 casualties from 220 incidents worldwide, found that although head injuries predominated in both immediate (71%) and late (52%) fatalities, injury to the abdomen carried the highest specific mortality rate (19%) among immediate survivors (60).

Compared to other mechanisms of trauma, victims of explosive attacks sustain more severe injuries, utilize more hospital resources, require more surgeries and intensive care, and have longer hospital stays and higher in-hospital fatality rates. Also, the patient population as a whole tends to be younger, implying a greater loss of potential life years and longer disabled lives. This creates a burden not only on the health care system but also on society as a whole (72).

MANAGEMENT AT THE SCENE

Regardless of the mechanism of explosion-related injury, the basic principles of trauma care still apply. In the prehospital setting, the focus should be on casualty extrication, initiation of life support, appropriate triage and transport, and history gathering. However, in every case, scene safety must be addressed *first*; it is of critical importance to protect EMS personnel. Terrorist tactics often involve the use of secondary bombs positioned to harm first responders. Snipers or radiation exposure from dirty bombs can present additional potential hazards. In such situations, no one without protective equipment or hazmat training should be allowed to enter the scene. Most importantly, no attempts at victim rescue should begin until some assessment of structural stability has been made. The importance of this was never more tragically demonstrated than on September 11, 2001, when

the collapse of the World Trade Center Towers claimed the lives of countless EMS personnel.

Once the blast site is secure, any nonambulatory patients should be immediately extricated and delivered to a triage staging area. It is important to remember that victims who have auditory blast injury may not respond appropriately to triage. Lack of awareness of this fact may lead to incorrect evaluation and triage of those unable to hear commands (9). Multiple types of trauma will be seen, but most will be the familiar penetrating and blunt injuries. Such injuries are often dramatic and can overshadow the sometimes subtle presentation of primary blast injury. First responders must specifically seek evidence of primary blast injury (52). Those with immediate, severe respiratory insufficiency caused by blast effect have less of a chance of survival. The only chance for survival of such victims in the field is the availability of early advanced life support (3).

Establishing an airway is the critical first step. Victims with mild or moderate respiratory distress may benefit from the placement of an oral or nasal airway, but those with severe respiratory embarrassment or massive hemoptysis should be intubated, anticipating mechanical ventilatory support (24). In the Israeli experience, early control of the airway (with attention to cervical spine precautions) has been the treatment that has saved most victims after terrorist bombings, especially if they are unconscious (3). Ultimately, spontaneous breathing is preferred because positive-pressure ventilatory support can increase the incidence and severity of both pulmonary barotrauma and arterial air embolism (39,73). However, ventilatory support should never be withheld from casualties in respiratory distress. Special care should be taken in the intubated patient with evidence of pulmonary blast injury to avoid overvigorous ventilations and to keep the airway pressure as low as possible. Casualties with asymmetrically decreased breath sounds and shock should have immediate needle decompression. Some have advocated the prophylactic placement of bilateral chest tubes in all blast victims before intubation (8). Hypotension in the blast casualty may be caused by tension pneumothorax, hemorrhage from secondary blast injury or other wounds, intraabdominal hemorrhage, coronary air embolism, or vagal reflexes (24). Control of hemorrhage in the field is only possible if it is confined to external bleeding, and application of an extremity tourniquet should be performed only if direct pressure fails to control the bleeding (3). Resuscitation with intravenous fluids should be done cautiously in the blast victim because excessive volume replacement may contribute to the development of pulmonary edema (24).

Stabilization of fractures, spinal immobilization, and wound dressings are other important aspects of prehospital casualty management. In mass casualty settings, limb-to-limb splinting and the use of tapes to secure victims to stretchers will usually suffice if sufficient materials are otherwise lacking (3). Penetrating soft tissue wounds require little management at the scene other than controlling hemorrhage and covering the wound to avoid further contamination. Impaled objects should not be removed and should be stabilized manually or with bulky dressings. Multiple studies and military experience have shown that exertion after blast exposure can increase the severity of pulmonary blast injury; thus it is critical to minimize the physical activity of any ambulatory casualties (74,75).

On-scene medical providers can play an important information-gathering role. The magnitude of surrounding structural damage and how far away it extends from the blast epicenter can give clues as to the type and size of the explosive. An assessment of damaged objects near a particular casualty may yield a gross estimate of the overpressure experienced by that victim. Blast waves strong enough to rupture a tympanic membrane are capable of shattering automobile glass, snapping utility poles, and cracking brick walls (52,76). Craters indicate magnitudes capable of disintegrating objects. The relative location and orientation of the casualty, whether the blast occurred in an open or confined space, and the nearby presence of any reflecting surfaces are extremely important historical aspects. In general, the farther away from the detonation an individual was, the less likely that person is to have sustained a given type and severity of *primary* blast injury (52). This does not apply to *secondary* blast injury, however, because fragments can be propelled over long distances (11). The presence of fumes, smoke, or flames can indicate the possibility for inhalation injury or exposure to toxic or radioactive materials. Proper on-scene *triage* leads to better utilization of limited medical resources. The importance of accurate triage as a survival determinant for critically injured casualties has been well documented (60). The triaging officer should balance the flow of patients among different hospitals while ensuring that patients with significant blast injuries are transported to a trauma center, if available (77). Casualties with severe injuries will have a higher survival rate and lower morbidity if they are transported to a trauma center (3,69).

Helicopter transport of patients with suspected blast injury may worsen *barotrauma*, and marginal oxygenation will only worsen with altitude. Expanding pneumothoraces may occur. Prophylactic tube thoracotomy may be performed. The flight should take place at the lowest altitude possible, and the cabin should be pressurized to 5,000 to 8,000 feet (24). Air evacuation is a limited resource and may not be available during severe weather or when the civil authorities close off airspace as they did during 9/11.

Finally, it is important to remember that the scene of a terrorist bombing is also a crime scene, and all materials removed, including embedded foreign bodies, are potential forensic evidence.

MANAGEMENT AT THE HOSPITAL

The majority of traumatic injuries seen after explosions will be familiar to hospital personnel; thus only those aspects of care specific to blast injury are discussed here. The manifestations of secondary and tertiary blast injury will often dominate the clinical picture, and a high index of suspicion for occult primary blast injury must be maintained. Evidence of exposure to overpressure should be specifically sought. Unfortunately, there are no pertinent negative findings on physical examination that absolutely exclude life-threatening primary blast injury (52). Therapy is directed at the specific manifestations as well as avoiding iatrogenic injury.

On arrival to the hospital, casualties should be retriaged into urgent and nonurgent categories. Advanced trauma life support should be promptly initiated for the most urgent, with attention to the airway, breathing, and circulation.

The judicious use of diagnostics is essential in the mass casualty setting. A chest radiograph and arterial blood gas are helpful in the initial evaluation of pulmonary blast injury, but few other tests are useful in the early management of primary blast injury (39,78,79). Additional studies can be obtained as indicated for the evaluation of secondary, tertiary, and miscellaneous injuries (52).

Management of patients with severe blast lung injury is challenging because it is often complicated by shock and altered levels of consciousness (28). Primary pulmonary blast injury impairs oxygen diffusion, much like pulmonary contusions, and the degree of respiratory insufficiency that results will depend on the extent of hemorrhage. All victims with potential pulmonary blast injury should be initially given the highest fraction of inspired oxygen possible (52). The treatment then focuses on correcting the effects of barotrauma and supporting gas exchange. Pulmonary blast injury can cause delayed respiratory insufficiency, hours after an explosive event. Early chest radiography can provide a good estimation of the severity of injury (28) and may show the characteristic "butterfly" pattern of hilar-based fluffy infiltrates seen with pulmonary edema. Chest CT can also identify small pneumothoraces. In one Israeli study, all patients with blast lung injury had a rather fulminant clinical course that was evident soon after admission (48). Blast lung injury also tends to stabilize rapidly (24), and it is uncommon for the radiographic changes to worsen more than 6 hours after blast exposure. However, in severely injured patients, adult respiratory distress syndrome (ARDS) may develop within 24 to 48 hours (9). Lung injury developing later in the hospital course may be secondary to or aggravated by hypovolemic shock, sepsis, overly aggressive fluid administration, or aspiration (80). The severity of the primary blast lung injury seems to have a dominant effect on the later development of ARDS (28).

Early signs of impending respiratory failure include tachypnea and a falling P_aCO_2 level. Positive-pressure ventilation should not be withheld in such patients, but measures should be taken to decrease the risks of air embolism and additional barotrauma (24). The tidal volume, respiratory rate, and ratio of inspiratory to expiratory time should be set to maximize mean airway pressure and minimize peak airway pressure (24). Any time it is necessary to increase the pressures, it is important to be vigilant for worsening barotrauma and pneumothorax (9). Poorly compliant blast-injured lungs can be ventilated using techniques proven successful for pulmonary contusions and ARDS (81), including permissive hypercapnia, pressure-controlled inverse ratio ventilation, independent lung ventilation, and high-frequency jet ventilation (82). The actual mode used should be determined based on each individual's particular requirements, as all have been used successfully, and no specific mode has been found to be superior to another (3). Effective pneumothorax drainage and adequate mechanical ventilation should result in improved oxygenation during the first 24 hours in the majority of patients (28). Routine steroids and prophylactic antibiotics are not advocated (9).

The etiology of shock, if not the result of tension pneumothorax or profound hypoxia, must next be assumed to be the result of hemorrhage. If external and internal blood loss can be reasonably excluded, coronary air embolism with myocardial infarction and cardiogenic shock should be considered as a cause. Nitrates should never be given for EKG findings of ischemia or infarction, and thrombolytic agents are absolutely contraindicated (52). Arterial air embolism will only be seen in casualties with clinical evidence of pulmonary blast injury. Management of suspected air embolism begins with the administration of supplemental oxygen, which not only improves gas exchange but also promotes more rapid absorption of arterial air bubbles (24). A primary goal is to keep the airway pressure lower than the vascular pressure to minimize further risk of air emboli. This is generally the case in the spontaneously breathing patient. In the patient requiring positive-pressure ventilation, pressures and volumes should be kept as low as possible to maintain adequate oxygenation and ventilation. In lungs stressed by mechanical ventilation, air emboli have been demonstrated for hours to days after blast exposure (73,83).

Theoretically, if it is possible to determine which lung is injured, isolating that lung can stem the flow of gas into the circulation (27). Several techniques for selective lung ventilation have been described using double-lumen tubes, Univent tubes, and bronchial blockers, although such specialized tubes may not always be available and can be difficult to place in trauma situations. If only standard endotracheal (ET) tubes are on hand, right main-stem intubation can be accomplished with 99% success by advancing a normally placed ET tube distally; left main-stem intubation may be accomplished with 92% success by turning the patient's head 90 degrees to the right, rotating the ET tube 180 degrees and passing it distally. If cervical spine injury is a concern, an alternate method is to rotate a normally placed ET tube 90 degrees counterclockwise and then advance (84). Obviously, in those with bilateral lung injury, emboli may originate from either lung, and lung isolation is not an option. If lung isolation and resuscitation are unsuccessful, immediate thoracotomy may be needed to allow hilar clamping or isolation of the injured lung segment (27).

Measures may be taken to limit air embolism damage by positioning the victim's body appropriately. Trendelenberg positioning may keep air from entering the cerebral circulation. If unilateral lung injury exists, keeping the injured lung dependent to the left atrium can increase pulmonary venous pressure and prevent emboli from entering the coronary circulation. The definitive therapy for systemic air embolism is hyperbaric oxygen therapy (HBOT). Benefits of HBOT include improved tissue oxygenation, decreased intracranial pressure, decreased reperfusion injury, and reduced mortality among severely brain-injured patients (27). Prognosis is generally good if HBOT is started within 6 hours of the insult (85), but delays due to other management priorities should not discourage the use of hyperbaric therapy (27).

Nonemergent surgery in casualties with pulmonary blast injury or systemic air embolism should be delayed because general anesthesia in these patients is poorly tolerated. Regional or local anesthesia is preferred for those needing immediate surgery (86).

Fluid management in patients following blast injury is a major challenge. Preload must be maintained to prevent tissue ischemia, but fluid overload can cause pulmonary edema and worsen lung dysfunction. Early measurement of central venous and pulmonary artery wedge pressures may be helpful diagnostically and useful in guiding fluid management (52).

Despite the predominance of other injuries after blast exposure, major morbidity and mortality among immediate survivors is caused by delayed perforation of intestinal mural contusions. The initial approach to the casualty with gastrointestinal blast injury is not dissimilar to that of any other cause of abdominal trauma. Abdominal injuries are treated according to general surgical principles, including volume replacement and nasogastric suction. The most challenging aspect is the identification of intestinal injury and discrimination between those lesions destined for perforation or for spontaneous recovery.

Although it is very uncommon for blood loss from pulmonary blast injury to cause hypotension, shock commonly will result from blast injury or blunt trauma causing abdominal hemorrhage (24). Casualties with any evidence of shock and abdominal hemorrhage should proceed directly to laparotomy. In the patient without clear indication for laparotomy, but with otherwise unexplained hemodynamic instability, abdominal sonography may be used and can be particularly useful in mass casualty situations (52). CT scan of the abdomen, if available, can also provide detail for surgical decision making but does not always identify bowel injury well in the absence of pneumoperitoneum (87,88).

Successful treatment of soft tissue wounds depends on meticulous wound debridement, with excision of nonviable tissue and foreign material likely to cause infection, adequate drainage, and delayed closure (89). Treatment decisions are based on an estimation of the type and location of wounds, the amount of tissue disruption, and the patient's hemodynamic status. Any penetrating abdominal or thoracic wound in a hemodynamically unstable patient requires emergent operative intervention. Secondary blast wounds in general are extensively contaminated. Adequate debridement is mandatory, and deep wounds should not be closed acute. Delayed primary closure is more appropriate. Because of the high velocity of shrapnel, the superficial appearance of entry wounds can be quite deceptive, and all penetrating wounds to the chest or abdomen should be adequately explored. Tetanus prophylaxis and broad-spectrum antibiotics should be routinely given. Again, it should be emphasized that after a terrorist bombing, the forensic aspects of documentation must be considered (52); all foreign bodies removed are potential evidence and must be preserved.

Although auditory injury, in contrast to other blast-related trauma, has no devastating or life-threatening effects, eardrum perforation, hearing loss, and dizziness can interfere with daily activities and have a telling effect on quality of life (46). The ears should be examined for blast-induced TM perforation or ossicular chain disruption, as well as findings suggestive of basilar skull fracture, such as the presence of blood or cerebrospinal fluid. Ossicular damage may be associated with vertigo and dizziness, and it carries a high incidence of associated head injury.

Initial treatment of tympanic membrane rupture consists of removing debris from the auditory canal and irrigating the canal with antiseptic solution. Antibiotics or ear drops are generally not indicated. Most perforations involving less than a third of the TM surface should be left to heal spontaneously. Patients with larger perforations or ossicular chain disruption should be referred to an otolaryngologist for further outpatient management and tympanoplasty. Sensorineural deafness due to cochlear damage or ossicle dislocation may improve with time, although some will be left with chronic tinnitus, vertigo, or permanent hearing loss (90).

The presence of isolated TM rupture is objective evidence of exposure to overpressure but does not appear to be associated with delayed-onset or occult pulmonary blast injury, in contrast to traditionally held beliefs (91). Conversely, the absence of rupture makes pulmonary blast injury unlikely (80).

Only patients without respiratory or abdominal complaints, who have a normal chest radiograph and arterial blood gas, may be safely discharged from the emergency department after a reasonable period of observation. Hospital admission for observation is prudent in all others.

SUMMARY

Urban terrorism has become a reality, and the use of explosives is all too common. In general, a high-explosive detonation will cause many minor injuries and some significant injuries with which medical personnel lack familiarity. Blast waves impacting the human body cause a unique form of barotrauma, affecting the lungs, gastrointestinal tract, and ears. The violent forces generated by explosions will also cause familiar penetrating and blunt trauma. Understanding the mechanisms of injury, expected injury patterns, and treatment issues will have a significant impact on the survival of the victims.

QUESTIONS

1. Which of the following is FALSE?
   A. Primary blast injury primarily affects the solid organs of the body, such as the liver, kidneys, and spleen.
   B. Primary blast injury is a form of barotrauma.
   C. Recipes for homemade bombs abound on the Internet.
   D. High explosives can be mixed with plasticizers such as oil or wax to create soft, hand-malleable substances called plastic explosives, or plastique.
   E. The rapidity with which an explosive reaches its peak pressure is a measure of its brisance, or shattering ability.

2. Basic components of a blast wave include:
   A. A short burst of increasing pressure
   B. A shorter phase of negative pressure
   C. Minimal wind movement
   D. A + B
   E. A + B + C

3. As a blast wave passes through the body, it causes damage by the following different mechanisms:
   A. Spalling
   B. Implosion
   C. Inertia
   D. Pressure differentials
   E. All of the above

4. Which of the following is FALSE?
   A. Primary blast injury is unique to explosions.
   B. Secondary blast injury refers to penetrating trauma caused by the acceleration of shrapnel and other debris by the blast wind.
   C. Tertiary blast injury is caused by the displacement of the body by the blast wind, with typical patterns of blunt trauma occurring on forceful impact with a solid object or the ground.
   D. Pulmonary pathology from blast injuries is inversely proportional to the velocity of chest-wall displacement by the incoming blast wave.
   E. Inertia imparted from the force of a blast wind may propel a victim against a stationary object, causing injury on impact.

ANSWERS

1: *A.* *Primary blast injury primarily affects the solid organs of the body, such as the liver, kidneys, and spleen.*
2: *A.* *A short burst of increasing pressure*
3: *E.* *All of the above*
4: *D.* *Pulmonary pathology from blast injuries is inversely proportional to the velocity of chest-wall displacement by the incoming blast wave.*

■ Case Study

Terrorism And Explosive Trauma: The Colombian Experience

Nelson Téllez and Jenny Gil Almanza

Dedicated to the memory of Natalia Téllez, who takes care of us from above (1993–2003).

Colombia's Violent History

Colombian history has been marked by diverse manifestations of violence against individuals, groups, or at random in order to paralyze society and promote particular goals. The Spanish conquest in Central and South America took place following 1492, starting off a period of increasing violence in the region of Columbia. Multiple ethnic killings occurred in the conquest period and during the formation of early population centers by Spanish colonizers in what would become Colombia (92). Today, paramilitary organizations from the political right and guerrillas from the left act against the civilian population to take over territories that have strategic military value or natural resources (93). Terror has resulted in important demographic shifts as people move into the cities in search of greater security. The resulting transient communities are ripe with illnesses, poverty, prostitution, and violent crime (93). Many of these organizations force young people to join as "conscripts" to fight (94) or require them to perform prostitution. Many children are born as a result of this forced prostitution (95).

Although violence existed for many years in Colombia, many refer to a specific date as the start of the modern era of civil war. On April 9, 1948, Jorge Eliécer Gaitán, a political leader from the Liberal Party, was assassinated in a central street in Bogotá. This is considered the onset of a civil war between liberals and conservatives. Large numbers of victims have succumbed to this violence, and the world media has brought dramatic images of these tragedies to the world. There are several reports of forces moving into a town and killing men, women, and children. These individuals have sometimes left disfigured bodies, cut into pieces, behind as they left, perhaps even conducting a soccer match with a victim's head (96,97).

During the violence of the 1950s, guerrilla groups were formed that continue to exist in Colombia and contribute to the ongoing conflict. One such group constitutes the oldest continuously present guerrilla organization in the world, the Fuerzas Armadas Revolucionarias de Colombia (Armed Revolutionary Forces of Colombia; FARC). This organization has been declared a terrorist group by the Colombian state and other countries, and multiple killings of both the civil population and the authorities such as police, army, and intelligence have been attributed to them.

It is appropriate to recognize that the social situation in Colombia, although not excusing the extremely cruel activities by the subversive groups just described, undoubtedly contributes to the civil unrest. Over time, the more loosely affiliated paramilitary groups that formed in the 1970s and 1980s became highly organized and sophisticated as they began to cultivate, process, and traffic marijuana to meet the great demand for these products by the merchants of the United States and Europe. The first bands of modern *narcotraficantes* were created in Colombia, the leaders of which rapidly became wealthy and acquired large urban and rural properties for high prices, inflating the local economy. These same narcotic traffickers felt the need to protect themselves and their families, and so they surrounded themselves with small armies. These armed groups forced small land owners to leave their property and sell it at unrealistically low prices. As this continued to happen, the size of properties owned by the powerful drug *capos* (chiefs) began to swell to enormous proportions. Perhaps the most infamous narcotic king was Pablo Escobar, who even had a private zoo. The term "narcoterrorism" was first used to describe Escobar and his activities. Sizable communities in Colombia were forced to leave their homes, which contributed to the poverty of certain regions within the country. In addition, as much as 10% of the population has chosen to immigrate to other countries, particularly to Europe and the United States. This process, which started in the 1970s, reached its peak during the 1990s. There has been a very significant switch from marijuana to cocaine and heroin.

This panoramic view of Colombian history from its independence to the present day allows us to understand how terrorism developed in Colombia. In other parts of the world, terrorism has been fomented from foreign invasion or religious extremism. In Colombia, terrorism has been used by diverse groups of political and economic extremists, mostly based on illegal drug traffic.

During the years of Escobar, terrorism was used by several groups to achieve economic power and political control. Members of the society were frightened. They were eventually not willing to defend the state. The use of explosives has become especially prominent since the late 1980s. Many devices were exploded against strategic targets, such as politicians who were willing to openly oppose the illegal drug infrastructure and commerce. On November 27, 1989, a bomb was detonated in an airplane targeting a presidential candidate, using 5 kilograms of ammonium-based gelatin dynamite. All of the 107 occupants in this Boeing jet were killed (100). Specially designed scenarios were aimed at killing political leaders. On most of these occasions, civilian bystanders were killed as well. Particularly devastating were the situations in which cars were detonated with very large quantities of explosives near military and key governmental administrative buildings. Additionally, competing illegal drug trafficking groups launched attacks against each other. In general, the civilian bystanders were the ones most devastated by the violence.

One particularly cruel practice was to kidnap a family and require one of its members to drive a vehicle laden with large amounts of explosives up to police stations and other governmental buildings to be detonated. These acts of desperation were conducted under the threat that their families would be killed if they did not complete the mission. Another method used repeatedly has been to leave donkeys loaded with explosives along the road. When a soldier or police officer would come to move the animal, the charge would be detonated remotely. A particularly shocking case occurred in a small town outside of the capital city in May 2000 (101). In this instance, Elvia Cortez, a 53-year-old dairy farmer, was fitted with an explosive necklace collar, which had been loaded with gunpowder and a remote detonation device. Reportedly, the device was very sophisticated, operating by sensing her body temperature and requiring specialized equipment to defuse it safely. The collar exploded, killing her and an explosive technician who was trying to remove it. In 2003 the same method was used again; however, technicians were able to remove it successfully without detonation.

Another common explosive trauma technique in Colombia is the use of ammonium nitrate and food oil, known as ANFO (98). This substance is combined with homemade metallic objects to enhance the injurious impact. In Colombia, the transit of vehicles that distribute propane to homes is prohibited at certain hours because of the metal cylinders the fuel comes in. These cylinders on many occasions have been used to make charged bombs with ANFO.

The number of terrorist attacks in Colombia increased sharply from 1966 to 1999. These have been most common in the Andean region (see Table 20-1). Bogotá, which is also in the Andean region, is separated out in the table for the purpose of display.

TABLE 20-1 Fatal Victims of Terrorist Acts in Colombia by Region, 1993–2003

REGION	TERRORISTS KILLED	CIVILIANS KILLED	SOLDIERS AND POLICE KILLED	TOTAL DEATHS
Amazon	12	107	159	278
Andean (mountainous)	139	677	622	1,438
Atlantic	59	364	226	649
Orinoco	57	163	279	499
Pacific	4	29	38	71
Bogota (capital)	10	134	40	184
Medellin	21	151	37	209
Totals	302	1,625	1,401	3,328

Source: Revista Criminalidad, Centro de Investigaciones Criminologicas, DIJIN, Policia Nacional de Colombia, Numero 45, 2003.

The accuracy of police statistics is sometimes questioned because the data can be either increased or decreased by various factors. It is widely assumed that many cases of death by terrorism are not recorded. Deaths that occur during military operations are sometimes counted as terrorist deaths. Some authorities have been accused of attempting to increase the numbers of victims to make the opposition appear larger than it really is. Certain American authors allege that this practice of inaccurately reporting statistics has been used by politicians with respect to many historical events, including the fall of the Berlin wall, the fall of communism, the end of the Cold War, and the necessity to justify the wars in Iraq, Afghanistan, or Colombia (99,100).

Health services for victims of terrorism in Colombia are provided by various governmental agencies that answer directly to the president of Colombia. Survivors receive minimal economical assistance. There is no specific medical school training for attention to terrorism or disasters. Only since the tragedy of September 11, 2001, has there been special attention paid to biological and chemical warfare agents in Colombia. There have been no cases of such weapons being used, even in the guerrilla conflict. Colombian medical students receive only the standard teaching in microbiology and nothing about biological warfare agents. Trauma, however, has been emphasized in medical education in Colombia.

Colombian experience with explosive trauma

The spectrum of explosive injuries from terrorist acts is highly variable and depends on the specific circumstances of the event. Important factors include the type and quantity of explosive used, the detonation mechanism employed, and the location of the victim with respect to the explosion (Fig. 20-2).

As elsewhere, forensic pathologists generally evaluate fatal cases, which of course are the more severe injuries. Forensic physicians in Colombia have documented various types of shrapnel injuries, including both minimal injuries in survivors and fatal cardiac lesions. Many cases involved extensive destruction of the body in which advanced genetic techniques were required to identify the victim. Several fatalities have been described involving extensive cranioencephalic avulsions, either isolated or associated with penetrating trauma to the thorax, abdomen, and extremities. In other cases, lesions are lim-

Regions	1966–1970	1971–1975	1976–1980	1981–1985	1986–1990	1991–1995	1996–1999	Totals
Amazon	0	2	2	11	27	115	262	419
Andean	86	270	571	822	1,229	2,373	3,241	8,592
Atlantic	16	61	69	176	421	1,041	936	2,720
Bogota	25	90	404	445	463	415	271	2,113
Medellin	0	0	0	0	364	628	455	1,447
Orinoquia	1	0	18	10	125	318	510	982
Pacific	19	38	124	413	144	73	119	930
Totals	147	461	1,188	1,877	2,773	4,963	5,794	17,203

Figure 20–2. Territorial sections and according to the victims: civilian, soldiers, or perpetrators. (Adapted from Revista Criminalidad, Centro de Investigaciones Criminologicas, DIJIN, Policia Nacional de Colombia, Numero 45, 2003.)

ited to the thorax, involving vital organs. Still others involve injuries to abdominal organs and vessels.

Several incidents have occurred in Colombia that deserve special attention. There was a direct large-scale attack against a Colombian security installation, Departamento Administrativo de Seguridad (FBI equivalent in Colombia), which resulted in hundreds of victims in 1989 in Bogotá. This case involved a truck with a large load of dynamite that was detonated from a distant location. The explosion of a commercial airliner was mentioned previously, as was the "collar bomb," which also took the lives of the technician/rescuers. Another example in 2001 involved the use of a cadaver as a decoy placed in an abandoned vehicle charged with explosives, occurring in a town called Soacha, near the capital city of Bogotá. The explosives were detonated as the car was being investigated. Others died from carbon monoxide inhalation produced by the subsequent fire. During the presidential inauguration of August 7, 2002, a guerrilla attack occurred against the Presidential Palace, known as the Nariño House, resulting in 15 deaths, all of which were of bystanders outside of the executive compound. More recently, an exclusive social club in Bogotá was destroyed by the detonation of a vehicle loaded with explosives in February 2003. The case resulted in 36 deaths, some with very severe mutilations.

A final category of attacks are those that occur against industrial or commercial targets. Defense of this strategic national infrastructure results in tremendous costs to the government and citizens of Colombia. Very large oil spills have occurred with attacks against the principal oil pipeline in Colombia, from Caño Limón in the Arauca region (102–104). In July 1997 a helicopter transporting soldiers responding to such an attack was shot down with missiles, resulting in the death of all 22 persons on board the aircraft. Many of these victims were so mutilated that identification was possible only through DNA testing.

The terrorism that has gripped Colombia has been so great, and so pervasive, that it has had an overall negative social impact in the country. Society has been faced with these great challenges, along with an increase in many forms of violent crime. As these acts of terror persisted, indifference has developed among many ordinary citizens. This societal apathy provides an opportunity for insurgent groups to push the limits of terrorism to further extremes and to be rewarded their violent acts.

REFERENCES

1. Federal Bureau of Investigation Bomb. General Information Bulletin 96-1: 1996 bombing incidents. Washington, DC: U.S. Department of Justice, 1996.
2. IDF web site: http://www.israel-mfa.gov.il/mfa/go.asp?MFAH0i5d0, Suicide and other bombing attacks in Israel since the Declaration of Principles.
3. Stein M, Hirshberg A. Medical consequences of terrorism: the conventional weapon threat. Surg Clin North Am 1999;79(6).
4. Conventional Terrorist Weapons. United Nations Office on Drugs and Crime. http://www.unodc.org/unodc/terrorism_weapons_conventional.html.
5. Safeer HB. Aviation security research and development plan. NJ: U.S. Department of Transportation, Federal Aviation Administration, NJ, March 1992.
6. Stuhmiller JH, Phillips YY, Richmond DR. The physics and mechanisms of primary blast injury. Conventional warfare: ballistic, blast, and burn injuries. Washington, DC: Office of the Surgeon General of the U.S. Army; 1991:241-70.
7. Cooper GJ, Townend DJ, Cater SR, et al. The role of stress waves in thoracic visceral injury from blast loading: modification of stress transmission by foams and high-density materials. J Biomech 1991;24:273-85.
8. Mellor SG. The pathogenesis of blast injury and its management. Br J Hosp Med. 1988;39:536-9.
9. Gans L, Kennedy T. Management of unique entities in disaster medicine. Emer Med Clin North Am 1996;14(2):301-26.
10. Iremonger MJ. Physics of detonations and blast-waves. In: Cooper GJ, Dudley HAF, Gann DS, et al. eds. Scientific foundations of trauma. Oxford, England: Butterworth-Heinemann, 1997:189-99.
11. Bellamy RF, Zajtchuk R. The weapons of conventional land warfare. In: Bellamy RF, Zajtchuk R eds. Conventional warfare: ballistic, blast, and burn injuries. Washington, DC: Office of the Surgeon General of the U.S. Army, 1991;1-51.
12. Hill JF. Blast injury with particular reference to recent terrorist bombing incidents. Ann R Coll Surg Engl 1979;61:4-11.
13. Phillips YY. Primary blast injuries. Ann Emerg Med 1986;15:1446-50.
14. Boffard KD, MacFarlane C. Urban bomb blast injuries: Patterns of injury and treatment. Surg Ann 1993;25(part 1):29-47.
15. Phillips, YY, et al. Cloth ballistic vest alters response to blast. J Trauma 1988;28(1 Suppl):S149-52.
16. Axelsson H, Yelverton JT. Chest wall velocity as a predictor of nonauditory blast injury in a complex wave environment. J Trauma 1996;40(suppl 3):S31-7.
17. Mayorga MA. Pathology of primary blast overpressure injury. Toxicology 1997;121:17-28.
18. Elsayed NM. Toxicology of blast pressure. Toxicology 1997;121:1-15.
19. Gorbunov NV, Elsayed NM, Kisin ER, et al. Air blast-induced pulmonary oxidative stress: interplay among hemoglobin, antioxidants, and lipid peroxidation. Am J Physiol 1997;272:320-34.
20. Sharpnack DD, Johnson AJ, Phillips YY. The pathology of primary blast injury. In: Bellamy RF, Zajtchuk R eds. Conventional warfare: ballistic, blast, and burn injuries. Washington, DC: Office of the Surgeon General of the U.S. Army, 1991; 271-94.
21. Cooper GJ, Taylor DE. Biophysics of impact injury to the chest and abdomen. J R Army Med Corps 1989;135:58-67.
22. Cooper GJ, Maynard RL, Cross NL, et al. Casualties from terrorist bombings. J Trauma 1983;23:955-67.
23. Brismar BBL. The terrorist bomb explosion in Bologna, Italy, 1980: an analysis of effects and injuries sustained. J Trauma 1982;22:216-20.
24. Argyros GJ. Management of primary blast injury. Toxicology 1997;121(1):105-15.
25. Katz E, Ofek B, Adler J, et al. Primary blast injury after a bomb explosion in a civilian bus. Ann Surg 1989;209:484-8.
26. Chiu C-J, Golding MR, Linder JB, et al. Pulmonary venous air embolism: a hemodynamic reappraisal. Surgery 1967;61:816-9.
27. Ho AM-H, Ling E. Systemic air embolism after lung trauma. Anesthesiology 1999;90:564-75.
28. Pizov R, Oppenheim-Eden A, Matot I, et al. Blast lung injury from an explosion on a civilian bus. Chest 1999;115:165-72.
29. Mason WH, Damon EG, Dickinson AR, et al. Arterial gas emboli after blast injury. Proc Soc Exp Biol Med 1971;136:1253-5.

30. Phillips YY, Zajtchuk JT. The management of primary blast injury. In: Bellamy RF, Zajtchuk R eds. Conventional warfare: ballistic, blast, and burn injuries. Washington, DC: Office of the Surgeon General of the U.S. Army, 1991;295-335.

31. Clemedson C-J, Hultman HI. Air embolism and the cause of death in blast injury. Mil Surg 1954;114:424-37.

32. Gouze FJ, Hayter R. Air embolism in immersion blast. US Naval Med Bull 1944;43:871-7.

33. Michel L, Poskanzer DC, McKusic KA, et al. Fatal paradoxical air embolism to the brain. Complication of central venous catheterization. JPEN 1982;6:68-70.

34. Sinner WN. Complications of percutaneous transthoracic needle aspiration biopsy. Acta Radiol Diagn 1976;17:813-28.

35. Goldfarb B, Bahnson HT. Early and late effects on the heart of small amounts of air in the coronary circulation. J Thorac Cardiovasc Surg 1980;80:708-17.

36. Yee ES, Verrier ED, Thomas AN. Management of air embolism in blunt and penetrating thoracic trauma. J Thorac Cardiovasc Surg 1983;85:661-8.

37. Thomas AN. Air embolism following penetrating lung injuries. J Thorac Cardiovasc Surg 1973;66:533-40.

38. Swanson J, Trunkey DD. Trauma to chest wall, pleura, and thoracic viscera. In: Shields TW ed. General thoracic surgery. 3rd ed. Philadelphia: Lea & Febiger, 1989;463.

39. Huller T, Bazini Y. Blast injuries of the chest and abdomen. Arch Surg 1970;100:24-30.

40. Yelverton JT, Johnson DL, Hicks W, et al. Blast overpressure studies with animals and man: non-auditory damage risk assessment for simulated weapons fired from enclosures. Final report, Contract DAMD17-88-C-8141, U.S. Army Medical Research and Materiel Command, Ft. Detrick, MD.

41. Stuhmiller LM, Ho KM, Stuhmiller JH. JAYCOR analysis of blast overpressure injury data. Technical report, Contract DAMD17-93-C-3005, U.S. Army Medical Research and Materiel Command, Ft. Detrick, MD.

42. Paran H, Neufeld D, Shwartz I, et al. Perforation of the terminal ileum induced by blast injury: delayed diagnosis or delayed perforation? J Trauma 1996;40:472-5.

43. Harmon JW, Haluszka M. Care of blast-injured casualties with gastrointestinal injuries. Milit Med 1983;148:586-88.

44. Richmond DR, Yelverton JT, Fletcher ER, et al. Physical correlates of eardrum rupture. Ann Otol Rhinol Laryngol 1989;98 (suppl 140):35-41.

45. Garth RJN. Blast injury of the ear. In: Cooper GJ, Dudley HAF, Gann DS, et al. eds. Scientific foundations of trauma. Oxford, England: Butterworth-Heinemann, 1997;225-35.

46. Cohen JT, Ziv G, Bloom J, et al. Blast injury of the ear in a confined space explosion: auditory and vestibular evaluation. IMAJ 2002;4:559-62.

47. Kerr AG, Byrne JE. Concussive effects of bomb blast on the ear. J Laryngol Otol 1975;89(2):131-43.

48. Leibovici D, Gofrit ON, Stein M, et al. Blast injuries: bus versus open-air bombings—a comparative study of injuries in survivors of open-air versus confined-space explosions. J Trauma 1996;41:1030-5.

49. Yelverton JT. Blast biology. In: Cooper GJ, Dudley HAF, Gann DS, et al. eds. Scientific foundations of trauma. Oxford, England: Butterworth-Heinemann, 1997;200-13.

50. Wolf YG, Rivkind A. Vascular trauma in high-velocity gunshot wounds and shrapnel blast injuries in Israel. Surg Clin North Am 2002;82(1):237-44.

51. Almogy G, Makori A, Zamir O, et al. Rectal penetrating injuries from blast trauma. IMAJ 2002;4:557-8.

52. Wightman JM, Gladish SL. Explosions and blast injuries. Ann Emerg Med 2001;37:664-78.

53. Bellamy RF, Zajtchuk R. The physics and biophysics of wound ballistics. In: Bellamy RF, Zajtchuk R eds. Conventional warfare: ballistic, blast, and burn injuries. Washington, DC: Office of the Surgeon General of the U.S. Army, 1991;107-62.

54. Mines M. Ocular injuries sustained by survivors of the Oklahoma City bombing. Ophthalmology 2000;107(5):837-43.

55. Hull JB, Bowyer GW, Cooper GJ, et al. Pattern of injury in those dying from traumatic amputation caused by bomb blast. Br J Surg 1994;81(8):1132-5.

56. Ohnishi M. Reflex nature of the cardiorespiratory response to primary thoracic blast injury in the anaesthetized rat. Exp Physiol 2001;86(3):357-64.

57. Guy RJ. Electrocardiographic changes following primary blast injury to the thorax. J R Nav Med Serv 2000;86(3):125-33.

58. Irwin RJ, Lerner MR. Shock after blast wave injury is caused by a vagally mediated reflex. J Trauma 1999;47(1):105-10.

59. Marshall TK. Injury by firearms, bombs, and explosives: explosion injuries. In: Tedeschi CG, Eckert WG, Tedeschi LG eds. Forensic medicine, a study in trauma and environmental hazards. Vol. 1. Mechanical trauma. Philadelphia: WB Saunders, 1977;612.

60. Frykberg ER, Tepas JJ. Terrorist bombings, Lessons learnt from Belfast to Beirut. Ann Surg 1988; 208:569-76.

61. Abenhaim L. Study of civilian victims of terrorist attacks (France 1982–1987). J Clin Epidemiol 1992;45(2):103-9.

62. Cernak I. Cognitive deficits following blast injury-induced neurotrauma: possible involvement of nitric oxide. Brain Inj 2001;15(7):593-612.

63. Cernak I, Wang Z, Jiang J, et al. Ultrastructural and functional characteristics of blast injury-induced neurotrauma. J Trauma 2001;50(4):695-706.

64. Hadden WA, Rutherford WH, Merrett JD. The injuries of terrorist bombing: a study of 1532 consecutive patients. Br J Surg. 1978;65:525-31.

65. Mallonee S, Shariat S, Stennies G, et al. Physical injuries and fatalities resulting from the Oklahoma City bombing. JAMA 1996;276:382-7.

66. Frykberg ER, Tepas JJ, Alexander RH. The 1983 Beirut Airport terrorist bombing: injury patterns and implications for disaster management. Am Surg 1989;55:134-41.

67. Waterworth TA, Carr MJ. Surgery of violence: report on injuries sustained by patients treated at the Birmingham General Hospital following the recent bomb explosions. BMJ 1975;2:25-7.

68. Pyper PC, Graham WJ. Analysis of terrorist injuries treated at Craigavon Area Hospital, Northern Ireland, 1972–1980. Injury 1983;14:332-8.

69. Scott BA, Fletcher JR, Pulliam MW, et al. The Beirut terrorist bombing. Neurosurgery 1986;18(1):107-10.

70. Quintana DA, Parker JR, Jordan FB, et al. The spectrum of pediatric injuries after a bomb blast. J Pediatr Surg 1997;32(2): 307-10; discussion 310-11.

71. Hiss J. Suicide bombers in Israel. Am J Forensic Med Pathol 1998;19(1):63-6.

72. Peleg K, Aharonson-Daniel L, Michael M, et al. Patterns of injury in hospitalized terrorist victims. Am J Emerg Med 2003;21(4):258-62.

73. Weiler-Ravell D, Adatto R, Borman JB. Blast injury of the chest: a review of the problem and its treatment. Isr J Med Sci 1975;11:268-74.

74. White CS. Rationale of treatment of primary blast injury to the lung. Technical Progress Report DA-49-146-XZ-372 1968. Lovelace Foundation, Albuquerque, NM.

75. Yelverton JT, Viney JF, Jojla B, et al. The effects of exhaustive exercise on rats at various times following blast exposure. Technical report, DASA 2707, 1971b. Headquarters, Defense Nuclear Agency, Washington, DC.

76. Wright RK. Death or injury caused by explosion. Clin Lab Med 1983;3:309-19.

77. Shapira S, Shermer J. Medical management of terrorist attacks. IMAJ 2002;4:489-92.
78. Clemedson C-J. Blast injury. Physiol Rev 1956;36:336-54.
79. Harmon JW, Sampson JA, Graeber GM, et al. Readily available serum chemical markers fail to aid in diagnosis of blast injury. J Trauma 1988;28(suppl 1):S153-9.
80. Mellor SG. The relationship of blast loading to death and injury from explosion. World J Surg 1992;16:893-8.
81. Battistella FD. Ventilation in the trauma and surgical patient. Crit Care Clin 1998;14:731-42.
82. Sorkine P. Permissive hypercapnia ventilation in pts with severe pulmonary blast injury. J Trauma 1998;45(1):35-8.
83. Damon EG, Henderson EA, Jones RK. The effects of intermittent positive pressure respiration on occurrence of air embolism and mortality following primary blast injury. Technical report, DNA 2989F 1973, Headquarters, Defense Nuclear Agency, Washington, DC.
84. Kubota H, Kubota Y, Toyoda Y, et al. Selective blind endobronchial intubation in children and adults. Anesthesiology 1987;67:952-9.
85. Kindwall EP. Uses of hyperbaric therapy in the 1990s. Cleve Clin J Med 1992;59:517-28.
86. Hamit IU. Primary blast injuries. Indust Med 1973;42:14-21.
87. Fischer RP, Miller-Crotchett P, Reed RL. Gastrointestinal disruption: the hazard of nonoperative management in adults with blunt abdominal injury. J Trauma 1988;28:1445-9.
88. Sherck JP, Oakes DD. Intestinal injuries missed by computed tomography. J Trauma 1990;30:1-7.
89. Covey DC. Blast and fragment injuries of the musculoskeletal system. J Bone Joint Surg Am 2002;84-A(7):1221-34.
90. Roth Y, Kronenberg J, Lotem S, et al. [Blast injury of the ear]. Harefuah 1989;117(10):297-301. [Hebrew].
91. Leibovici D, Gofrit ON, Shapira SC. Eardrum perforation in explosion survivors: is it a marker of pulmonary blast injury? Ann Emerg Med 1999;34:168-72.
92. Friede J. La conquista del territorio y el poblamiento. En: Nueva historia de Colombia. Editorial Planeta, 1989.
93. Niño P. Las migraciones forzadas de población por la violencia en Colombia: una historia de éxodos, miedo, terror y pobreza. Scripta Nova. Revista electrónica de Geografía y Ciencias Sociales. Universidad de Barcelona (ISSN 11389788) 1999;45(33).
94. Vivanco JM. (Human Rights Watch). Citado por la Consultoría para los Derechos Humanos y el Desplazamiento, abril 21 de 2004.
95. Informe del Alto Comisionado de las Naciones Unidas para los Derechos Humanos sobre la situación de los derechos humanos en Colombia Naciones Unidas. Consejo Económico y Social, febrero 17 de 2004.
96. The Permanent Committee for Human Rights Defense (CPDH), Informe sobre la situación de derechos humanos en el eje cafetero. http://cpdh.free.fr/informes/informe_mayo _02.htm
97. Christus Rex Information Service, August 25, 1996. http://www.christusrex.org/www1/news-old/8-96/sm8-25-96.html. Accessed April 22, 2004.
98. Aguirre CM. Uso y aplicación de explosivos en operaciones al tajo abierto (Use and application of explosives in open mining). http://amsac.com.mx/mminero/septiembre/sep98a5.html. Accessed April 25, 2004.
99. Weineberg E. New York diary. Translated version by Aurelio Major and Rafael Vargas. El Malpensante 34, November 1 to December 15, 2001.
100. Wolfowitz and Khalizad, Defense planning guidance for the fiscal years 1994–1999. Cited by Weinberger E. New York 16 months later. Translated version by Margarita Valencia. El Malpensante 44, February 1 to March 15, 2003.
101. Condena de 32 años por collar bomba (Condemned to 24 years of prison for the collar bomb) ElPais.com. Septiembre 24 de 2002 http://elpais-cali.terra.com.co/historico/sep24 2002/NAL/ A224N2.html. Accessed April 25, 2004.
102. Selsky A. U.S. crew battles oil well fires caused by rebels in Colombia. August 15, 2003 Environmental News Network (AP). http://www.enn.com/news/2003-08-13/s_7468.asp. Accessed April 25, 2004.
103. Colombia—the pipeline war. Frontline World. Public Broadcasting System. November 2002. http://www.pbs.org/ frontlineworld/stories/colombia/. Accessed April 25, 2004.
104. Pederson DM. Fuel tank ignition prevention measures. Federal Register 1997;62(64): 16013-24. From the Federal Register Online http://www.epa.gov/fedrgstr/EPA-GENERAL/ 1997/April/Day-03/g8495.htm. Accessed April 25, 2004.

21

Structural Collapse, Extrication, Crush Syndrome, and Rhabdomyolysis

Adam H. Miller

In the new era since 9/11, our world faces not only the constant threats of natural disasters but also man-made tragedies. Health care providers, and the study of disaster medicine, must seek to understand these events and plan for their medical and surgical consequences. By coupling predisaster preparedness with the best available techniques in search, rescue, and health care, the best results can be achieved. This chapter looks at the importance of building structure design. It then continues with the medical consequences of these structural flaws when they are faced with natural and man-made disasters.

A review of the disaster literature suggests that some of the morbidity and mortality of past world events could have been prevented, particularly if structures were reinforced and medical intervention had been initiated more expeditiously. Whether it is from an earthquake or a bomb blast, loss of life may result either from the direct effect of trauma or the metabolic consequences of crushing weight upon the body. As we shall see, this excessive weight damages muscle and other tissues and results in various complications.

The development of firm guidelines for building construction and the improvement in the organization of urban search and rescue are the essential types of prevention required to ensure improved outcomes. Key medical features include renal failure, electrolyte disturbances, and the potential for loss of one or more limbs. Acute renal failure (ARF), a deadly consequence of rhabdomyolysis, is mostly preventable by timely rehydration therapy. Hyperkalemia and infection are the commonest causes of death in victims who survive the direct effect of trauma (1). In addition, fasciotomy can be limb saving if it is done in the early hours. Each of these features will be described.

BUILDING STRUCTURE AND THE RISK OF CRUSH INJURIES

Many papers have been written pertaining to natural and man-made disasters, including descriptions of earthquakes,

bombings, gas explosions, and derailments and collisions of trains, along with other types of trauma-related events (2–4). As building structures age, the risk of their collapse and injury to human life increases. This chapter explores several past events, which may provide insight that may be applicable to modern events.

The Turkish earthquake literature describes the primary mechanism of injury and death in earthquakes as attributable to the physical trauma from collapse of human-made structures (2). This literature points out the vulnerability of certain types of building structures. The most likely to collapse were the midrise, unreinforced masonry buildings (MUMBs) and the one-story adobe structures with soft ground floor construction. These buildings were typically designed with a ground floor intended for commercial use, incorporating large shop-front windows. The higher floors were used as residential apartments.

In the Turkish earthquake of March 13, 1992, the epicenter occurred 5 km (3 miles) east of the city of Erzincan, at the intersection of the North and Northeast Anatolian fault lines in response to movement of the Arabian, Anatolian, and Northeast Anatolian tectonic plates. Of the 526 mortalities, 92% were attributed to the MUMB collapses characterized by a ground floor collapse pattern. Being on the first floor was an important predictor of death. In addition, the Turkish literature looked at the disaster response effort, discussing a detailed account of local response, which included the city administration, the national response, and the substantial international participation, especially crews from neighboring cities and countries. There was typically a delay of more than 24 hours in the arrival of appropriate search and rescue personnel and equipment. This prolonged response contributed to a significant number of deaths, which otherwise may have been preventable with immediate rescue and medical response.

The literature on the Hanshin-Awaji Japanese earthquake of 1995 describes 14 patients who sustained crush injuries (3). They had been buried under collapsed houses for an average of 6.7 ± 5.7 (SD) hours (5–8). Victims who arrived at major treatment centers later (2 of the 6 victims), were more likely to have developed renal failure than those who were brought earlier. The major clinical problems encountered in the treatment of these patients included deciding whether to use the fluid resuscitation regimen to prevent ARF and determining whether there were clear indications for fasciotomy in an attempt to prevent the loss of limbs.

CRUSH SYNDROME

A syndrome associated with myoglobinuria was first described by Meyer-Betz in 1910 (28). However, it was recorded earlier in association with crush injuries after the earthquake in Messina, Italy, in 1909, and again later by Bywaters and Beall after observations of crush victims during World I (29,30). In the era since the London Blitz in World War II, the term "crush syndrome" has been applied to the ischemia-induced syndrome of myonecrosis, myoglobinuria, and renal failure.

In 1941, Bywaters described a syndrome of "being trapped under the rubble for hours." After release, patients developed "swelling and later muscle weakness in the injured limb, vasoconstriction and hypotension after several hours, decreased urine output, changes in urine sediment, hemoconcentration, hyperkalemia, acidosis, and persistence of loss of blood supply and gangrene in the affected limb even after correction of blood pressure" (9).

Crush syndrome is the general manifestation of a crush injury involving one or more limbs or abdomen under extreme pressure for a few hours. The prolonged pressure to the limb or abdomen leads to a breakdown of the integrity of the muscle cell membrane and derangement of cellular transport and occurs when individuals are trapped under fallen debris during earthquakes, bombings, and other disasters (1,10). This in turn may cause a syndrome of rhabdomyolysis and ARF, hyperkalemia, disseminated intravascular coagulation (DIC), cardiomyopathy, and other systemic manifestations, which may be fatal if not treated promptly and properly (11).

In crush syndrome, the damaged muscle cells lose the capacity to pump water out of cells by active transport, which is necessary to maintain their internal environment. When a myocyte exhausts adenosine triphosphate (ATP), its normal homeostatic, synthetic, and reparative functions deteriorate (12–13). The result is loss of sarcolemmal and cellular membrane integrity and leakage of intracellular contents. Prolonged pressure on a muscle group can produce intracompartmental pressures reaching up to 240 mm Hg. This interrupts the normal blood supply, cutting off essential nutrients for oxidative phosphorylation. In turn, too little ATP, which is essential for cells to live, is produced (14). Cell rupture releases potassium and muscle pigment, and then the body's water begins to move into this area of injury, known as "third spacing." Therefore, hypovolemia is a major problem. Along with the deposition of myoglobin from the injured muscles, the hypovolemia causes acute tubular necrosis (ATN) and acute renal failure. This can be mitigated by early administration of intravenous fluids. In addition, patients may

require acute dialysis therapy if ARF is severe. In fact, if kidney failure is present, death may result within a week if dialysis is not instituted (9).

Since the original description by Bywaters in 1941, crush injury has been examined extensively; in general, the clinical course and subsequent prognosis are significantly altered by multiple factors such as the severity of the crush injury, the timing of treatment, and the character of initial treatment provided to the victim. *Delivery of fluids to a victim of crush injury is the critical feature in the proper resuscitation of the patient.* Other interventions are often promoted including mannitol (15–17) and bicarbonate (15,16,18,19); however, animal and human data are not conclusive, and currently the literature in inconclusive.

The 1988 Armenian earthquake experience underscores the importance of fluid resuscitation, where hundreds of victims had delays to treatment of 24 to 48 hours (20). This holdup resulted in a large number of patients with renal failure and subsequently a very large demand for hemodialysis among these victims. The time to recovery is a significant factor in determining the success of extrication from collapsed structures (Fig. 21-1) (21).

Better et al. (21,22) reported that administration of an average of 12 L/day of fluid with sodium bicarbonate and mannitol to 75-kg adults successfully prevented renal failure in severe crush syndrome cases. In this report, the patients received initial infusion of fluid on site, and most were admitted to the hospital within 30 minutes where they were given massive fluid, sodium bicarbonate, and mannitol. In the Hanshin-Awaji earthquake paper (24), the intravenous fluids were given in conjunction with sodium bicarbonate during the initial few hours (to correct only metabolic acidosis) and low dose dopamine for several days to maintain urine output above 200 mL/hour without mannitol-alkaline diuresis.

Crush victims may have a variety of causes of renal failure, including acute dehydration or bleeding. Patients may have hypotension, prerenal azotemia, decreased urine output, and hemoconcentration. Conditions leading to shock should not be confused with crush syndrome because they have a different pathogenesis. Experience from earthquakes indicates that hypotension and hyperkalemia are the top two causes of death in the first day following rescue (3) (Fig. 21-2). Hypotension in patients with upper extremity crush syndrome usually cannot be explained solely by third spacing, so other sources of shock must be considered. Calculation of the *fractional excretion of sodium* (FE_{Na}) is a classic way to determine if the patient is simply dehydrated; in this case, the renal tubule conservation of sodium is maximized (Fig. 21-3). The ATN disrupts cell function; hence, sodium conservation is compromised leading to a high fractional sodium excretion. A low fractional sodium excretion can be misleading in ATN because of rhabdomyolysis. The creatinine level may be initially normal but rises rapidly after the rhabdomyolysis of crush injury. Acute renal failure from other causes may manifest with a more slowly rising creatinine. Metabolic acidosis, hyperphosphatemia, hypocalcemia, hyperuricemia, and a low fractional sodium excretion are more likely to be present in ATN secondary to rhabdomyolysis. Limb paralysis in a trauma victim may be from acute nerve trauma not necessarily related to rhabdomyolysis.

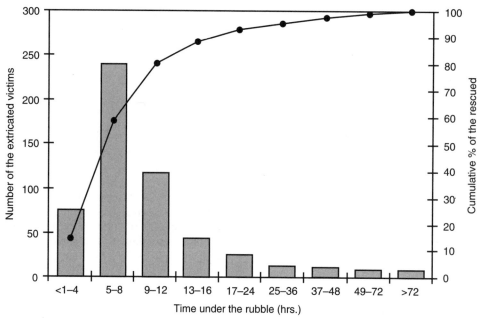

Figure 21–1. Proposed mechanism in the development of rhabdomyolysis in crush injury. (From Malinoski DJ. Crush injury and rhabdomyolysis. Crit Care Clin. 2004;20(1):171-92. With permission.)

MANAGING VICTIMS OF CRUSH INJURY: PREHOSPITAL CONSIDERATIONS

The first priorities after a catastrophic event is to minimize further injury resulting from collapse of unsafe buildings or other heavy objects and to extricate those who may still be buried. Retrieval of severely traumatized patients from difficult locations remains a complex science, which is studied and taught by emergency medical providers. The challenges associated with retrieval situations can be extreme (24–26).

A very important principle relating to the initial treatment of crush injury is the risk of acute deterioration and sudden death with release of pressure on the involved extremity. Extrication accelerates the muscle ischemia and edema. As soon as the compressive forces are released and blood flows through the injured area, the sequelae of crush syndrome begin. If extrication is prolonged, fluid replacement should begin as soon as prehospital personnel reach the victim. Aggressive fluid therapy should begin once a site is available to an intravenous line. If the victim is normotensive, isotonic saline can be infused at a rate of 1.5 L/hour (27). For patients in a shock state, fluid replacement should be instituted in a 3:1 ratio, where 3 L of isotonic saline are used for every 1 L of blood loss.

The hours spent trapped under the compressive forces of debris with crush injuries often leads to massive tissue and bone injury. Without access to fluids or nutrients, hypo-

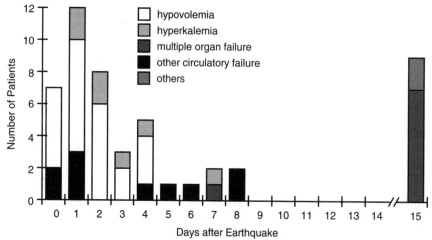

Figure 21–2. The causes of death in 50 patients with the crush syndrome following the Hanshin–Awaji earthquake. Deaths from hypovolemia and hyperkalemia were the most common in the early period, while sepsis leading to multiple organ failure was responsible for most of the late deaths. (From Oda J, Tanaka H, Yoshioka T, et al. Analysis of 372 patients with crush syndrome caused by the Hanshin–Awaji earthquake. J Trauma 1997;(42):470-6. With permission.)

(UNa/SNa)/(UCr/SCr) x 100

UNa—Concentration of sodium in the urine

SNa—Concentration of sodium in serum

UCr—Concentration of Creatinine in urine

SCr—Concentration of Creatinine in Serum

A fractional excretion of sodium of <1% indicates that the patient is likely to have hypovolemia or other "prerenal" causes of renal failure.

Figure 21–3. Calculation of the fractional excretion of sodium (FE_{Na}).

volemia, negative nitrogen balance, and inevitable ketosis ensue. Third spacing of fluids in affected limbs or abdomen is the consequence of rhabdomyolysis (Fig. 21-4). With hypovolemia and acidosis being present, circulating myoglobin has an ideal milieu for precipitation in the renal tubules.

HYPOVOLEMIA, RHABDOMYOLYSIS, AND RENAL FAILURE

The result of prolonged pressure to the limbs when individuals are trapped under the debris of earthquakes, bombings, and other disasters results in the compromise of myocyte integrity. After pressure is removed from a trapped limb, extracellular fluid enters damaged cells. A fluid volume equal to that of the entire extracellular space may enter damaged muscle within hours or days after injury (11,30). This type of hypovolemia, unlike acute blood loss, is due to fluid shifting to the interstitial spaces from the intravascular fluid space. At the same time,

potassium, phosphate, myoglobin, and other cell products leak from damaged muscle cells. This can be detected by measuring the plasma creatine phosphokinase (CPK) as early as the first hour (11). Severe hyperkalemia, exacerbated by low calcium, may result in sudden cardiac arrest. Lactic acid and other organic acids released into the extracellular fluid may cause acidosis (30). DIC may occur as a result of thromboplastin release. The myoglobin released from muscle cells damages renal tubules and, particularly in the presence of severe hypovolemia occurring at the same time, may cause ARF. The muscle mass of the body constitutes 40% of the total body weight, and with severe trauma it is possible to "third space" up to 12 L of fluid in muscle (31). The drop in mean arterial systemic pressure of 60 to 70 mm Hg can induce ischemic injury to the kidneys by resultant low perfusion states and decreased glomerular filtration rates (GFR) (10); acidosis and aciduria compound the effect of myoglobin on the kidney (32).

Rhabdomyolysis has many causes, which can be classified into hereditary and sporadic forms. The inherited disorders include the glycogen storage diseases, muscular dystrophy, and malignant hyperthermia. The sporadic forms are due to severe

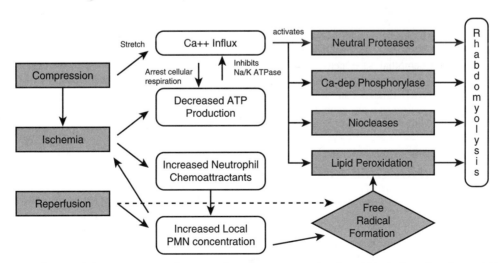

Figure 21–4. Number of rescued victims corresponding to various time strata under the rubble (*columns*) and cumulative percentage of the rescued renal victims by the function of time lapsed after the disaster (*line*). (From Sever MS. Lessons learned from the Marmara disaster: time period under the rubble. Crit Care Med 2002;30(11): 2443-9. With permission.)

physical exertion, crush or compression injuries, ischemia, metabolic depression, exogenous drugs and toxins, or combinations of these entities (33–36).

Rhabdomyolysis most typically results from the disruption of the muscle cell with release of myoglobin and other components. These components include serum glutamic oxalaoacetic transaminase (SGOT), lactate dehydrogenase (LDH), creatine phosphokinase, glucose, and potassium (37). Tubular deposition of pigment may obstruct the renal tubules and also dilate nephrons, leading to ATN. It is thought that the injurious agent is the iron molecule of the heme moiety in combination with free radical formation (38).

The prediction of patients most at risk of impending ARF in rhabdomyolysis after crush injury (soft-tissue) may be possible by obtaining a reduced venous bicarbonate concentration (VBC) of <17 mmol/L. This may result from tissue hypoperfusion with resultant tissue anoxia (39,40).

ARF in rhabdomyolysis can be mitigated most effectively by the initiation of early parenteral sodium chloride treatment aimed at increasing renal blood flow and decreasing the concentration of nephrotoxic pigments early after the release of the victim. Alkalinization of the urine was part of the preventive rehydration strategy described by several authors during the late 1980s (41,42). It had been proposed that sodium bicarbonate infusion could result in alkalemia and increased potassium excretion because sodium bicarbonate infusion exceeds the absorption capacity of the proximal tubules (15). In some cases, elevated serum creatinine levels returned to normal within 24 hours after initiating rehydration and increasing urine output (43). In other reports, hypertonic mannitol was successfully infused along with rehydration (16,44).

Normal saline combined with one vial of sodium bicarbonate can be infused. Some authors advocate adding hypertonic mannitol to the intravenous set. The urine output should be monitored. Therapy should be continued using half normal saline containing one to two vials of HCO_3 (44 mEq each vial) per liter, administering 3 to 6 L in the first day (11,15,44) and adding at least 25 g of mannitol (doses up to 1 g/kg have been tried) to decrease intercompartmental pressure and possibly prevent further renal damage. If the patient is not elderly or high-risk for overhydration, one may use higher quantities of intravenous fluid (16).

If urine output does not increase, remaining low in the face of adequate rehydration, and if plasma creatinine is rising, the patient should be considered for renal replacement therapy (RRT). Types of RRT include hemodialysis or peritoneal dialysis, performed temporarily or continuously as needed. If urine output increases, intravenous rehydration can be continued until the urine is clear and tests for urine myoglobin are negative. The usual time for this recovery is 48 to 72 hours (1).

COMPARTMENT SYNDROME AND INDICATIONS FOR FASCIOTOMY

Anyone who has had a limb or abdomen trapped under the ruin for a few hours (crush injury) or has a limb fracture is prone to develop a compartment syndrome and consequently crush syndrome. Compartment syndrome has been reported with trapping times of less than 1 hour (3). Extensive soft tissue injury is often sufficient to cause severe increases in compartment pressure and vascular compromise. Fracture is not mandatory for the compartment syndrome to develop (45). Abdominal injury by itself can result in crush syndrome (11).

Assessment of the local tissue crush may reveal a pale, swollen, tense extremity that is painful (43). Early diagnosis of compartment syndrome is very important because there is only a brief period of time when fasciotomy may save the muscle and nerves of the limb. Whitesides et al. (43) suggested "there is inadequate perfusion and relative ischemia when the tissue pressure within a closed compartment rises to within 10-30 mm Hg of the patient's diastolic blood pressure. Fasciotomy is usually indicated, therefore, when the tissue pressure rises to 40-45 mm Hg in a patient with a diastolic blood pressure of 70 mm Hg and any of the signs or symptoms of a compartmental syndrome." If the intracompartment pressure (ICP) is critically high for more than 8 hours using Whitesides' criteria, neuromuscular damage is irreversible (46).

When the victim has motor or sensory findings, or if the limb is very tight and tender with or without a fracture, then compartment syndrome probably exists. Confusion exists when the patient has none of the previously mentioned problems. In cases where symptoms or physical findings are not clear-cut, measuring the ICP will be very useful. The absence of clinical findings suggestive of the compartment syndrome has a negative-predictive value of over 97% (47).

PREPARING FOR THE FUTURE

First responders and other medical professionals must be familiar with the logistical, medical, and surgical issues related to disaster management of victims trapped under collapsed buildings and other structures. Much of the historical morbidity and mortality resulting from natural and man-made disasters could have been lessened, were it not for poor mobilization of rescue efforts.

Early rescue should focus on the management of hyperkalemia, hypovolemia, and circulatory collapse. In the days that follow, attention should shift to minimizing the consequences from acute muscle injury, especially the avoidance of acute compartment syndrome and aggressive management of sepsis.

Individual governmental agencies, universities, and other entities responsible for clinical education must coordinate their efforts to better prepare health care responders to disaster scenarios.

Communication networks must be developed to enable regional health systems to be aware of potential events requiring effective organization of crush victim rescue operations. Systems are needed to deploy resources to a disaster event site to provide a sufficient stream of supplies, such as intravenous fluids, intravenous setups, and fracture immobilization equipment. This type of infrastructure would be accountable for the updating of key databases, resource utilization, and educational information.

Several potential areas of focus of disaster response preparation include the following:

1. Education of laypeople to assist professionals with structural rescue, basic life support, and potential structural collapse in communities where large populations exist

2. Coordination with the local media to reinforce rescue and medical concepts pertaining to disaster preparedness including issues relating to rescue and prognosis in crush syndrome

3. Development in each community of practice scenarios relating to extrication of victims who are trapped under damaged building structures

4. Preparation of effective guidelines through scientific investigations to develop evidence-based guidelines and to determine "best practices" relating to rescue, communication, and medical issues dealing with crush syndrome

QUESTIONS AND ANSWERS

1. Which of the following is FALSE?
   A. The term "crush syndrome" has been applied to the ischemia-induced syndrome of myonecrosis, myoglobinuria, and renal failure after crush injuries.
   B. Prolonged pressure to the limb or abdomen leads to a breakdown of the integrity of the muscle cell membrane and derangement of cellular transport. This occurs when individuals are trapped under fallen debris during earthquakes, bombings, and other disasters.
   C. Crush syndrome may cause a syndrome of rhabdomyolysis and ARF, hypokalemia, DIC, cardiomyopathy, and other systemic manifestations that may be fatal if not treated promptly and properly.
   D. Delivery of fluids to a victim of crush injury is the critical feature in the proper resuscitation of the patient.
   E. The time to recovery is a significant factor in determining the success of extrication from collapsed structures.

2. Which of the following has been shown to prevent renal failure in severe crush syndrome cases?
   A. Administration of an average of 12 L/day of fluid with sodium bicarbonate and mannitol to 75-kg adults
   B. Calcium ethylrnrdiaminetetraacetic acid
   C. Sodium polystyrene sulfate
   D. High-dose dopamine
   E. Fluconazole

3. Crush victims may have a variety of causes of renal failure. These include each of the following, EXCEPT:
   A. Dehydration
   B. Hypotension
   C. Bleeding
   D. Hypertension
   E. Rhabdomyolysis

4. Which of the following is FALSE?
   A. ARF in rhabdomyolysis can be mitigated most effectively by the initiation of early parenteral sodium chloride treatment aimed at increasing renal blood flow and decreasing the concentration of nephrotoxic pigments early after the release of the victim.
   B. Anyone who has had a limb or abdomen trapped under the ruin for a few hours (crush injury) or has a limb fracture is prone to develop a compartment syndrome and consequently crush syndrome.
   C. Early diagnosis of compartment syndrome is very important because there is only a brief period of time when fasciotomy may save the muscle and nerves of the limb.
   D. A very important principle relating to the initial treatment of crush injury is the risk of acute deterioration and sudden death with release of pressure on the involved extremity.
   E. After crush injury, myoglobin released from muscle cells damages renal tubules and, particularly in the presence of severe hypovolemia, may cause proliferative glomerulonephritis.

ANSWERS

1: C. *Crush syndrome may cause a syndrome of rhabdomyolysis and ARF, hypokalemia, DIC, cardiomyopathy, and other systemic manifestations that may be fatal if not treated promptly and properly.*

2: A. *Administration of an average of 12 L/day of fluid with sodium bicarbonate and mannitol to 75-kg adults*

3: D. *Hypertension*

4: E. *After crush injury, myoglobin released from muscle cells damages renal tubules and, particularly in the presence of severe hypovolemia, may cause proliferative glomerulonephritis.*

REFERENCES

1. Atef-Zafarmand A, Fadem S. Disaster nephrology: medical perspective. Adv Renal Replacement Ther 2003;10(2):104-16.
2. Angus DC, Pretto EA, Abrams JI, et al. Epidemiologic assessment of mortality, building collapse pattern, and medical response after the 1992 earthquake in Turkey. Prehospital and Disaster Med 1997;12(3):222-31.
3. Oda J, Tanaka H, Yoshioka T, et al. Analysis of 372 patients with crush syndrome caused by the Honshin-Auaji earthquake. J Trauma 1997;42:470-5; discussion 475–6.
4. Shimazu T, Yoshioka T, Nakata Y, et al. Fluid resuscitation and systemic complications in crush syndrome: 14 Hanshin-Awaji earthquake patients. J Trauma. 1997;42(4):641-6.
5. MacLean GB, Barrett DS. Rhabdomyolysis: a neglected priority in the early management of severe limb trauma. Injury 1993;24:205-7.
6. Angus DC, Barbera JA, Kvetan V. Modern medical response to disasters. In: Carlson RW, Gehe MA, eds. Principles and practice of medical intensive care. Philadelphia: WB Saunders; 1993. pp. 25-48.
7. Better OS, Rubinstein I, Winaver J. Recent insight into the pathogenesis and early management of the crush syndrome. Semin Nephrol 1992;12:217-22.

8. Gabow PA, Kaehny WD, Kelleher SP. The spectrum of rhabdomyolysis. Medicine 1982; 61:141-52.
9. Bywaters EG, Beall D. Crush injuries with impairment of renal function. Br Med J 1941; 1:427; J Am Soc Nephrol 1998;9:322-32.
10. Michaelson M. Crush injury and crush syndrome. World J Surg 1992;16:899-903.
11. Better OS. The crush syndrome revisited. Nephron 1990; 55:97-103.
12. McArdle B, Verdi D. Myopathy due to defect in muscle glycogen breakdown. Clin Sci 1951;10:13-35.
13. Vesweswaran P, Guntupalli J. Rhabdomyolysis. Crit Care Clin 1999;15(2):415-28,ix–x.
14. Owen C, Mubarak S, Hargens A, et al. Intramuscular pressures with limb compression. N Engl J Med 1979;300:1169-72.
15. Homsi E, Barreiro MF, Orlando JM, et al. Prophylaxis of acute renal failure in patients with rhabdomyolysis. Renal Fail 1997;19:283-8.
16. Eneas JF, Schoenfield PY, Humphreys MH. The effect of mannitol-sodium bicarbonate on the clinical course of myoglobinuria. Arch Intern Med 1979;139:801-5.
17. Zager RA, Foerder C, Bredl C. The influence of mannitol on myoglobinuric acute renal failure: functional, biochemical, and morphological assessments. J Am Soc Nephrol 1991;2(4): 848-55.
18. Heyman SN, Greenbaum R, Shina A, et al. Myoglobinuric acute renal failure in the rat: a role for acidosis? Exp Nephrol 1997;5(3):210-16.
19. Moore KP, Holt SG, Patel RP, et al. A causative role for redox cycling of myoglobin and its inhibition by alkalinization in the pathogenesis and treatment of rhabdomyolysis-induced renal failure. J Biol Chem 1998;273(48):31731-7.
20. Angus DC, Barbera JA, Kvetan V. Modern medical response to disasters. In: Carlson RW, Gehe MA, eds. Principles and practice of medical intensive care. Philadelphia: WB Saunders; 1993. pp. 25-48.
21. Sever MS, Erek E, Vanholder R, et al. Lessons learned from the Marmara disaster; time period under the rubble. Crit Care Med. 2002;30(11):2443-9.
22. Better OS, Rubinstein I, Winaver J. Recent insight into the pathogenesis and early management of the crush syndrome. Semin Nephrol 1992;12:217-22.
23. Gabow PA, Kaehny WD, Kelleher SP. The spectrum of rhabdomyolysis. Medicine 1982;61:141-52.
24. Wilmink AB, Samra GS, Watson LM, et al. Vehicle entrapment rescue and pre-hospital trauma care. Injury 1996;27:21-5.
25. Mahoney PF, Carney CJ. Entrapment extrication and immobilization. Eur J Emerg Med 1996;3:244-6.
26. Miller BJ. The John Graham extrication prize: its history and importance. Aust N Z J Surg 1999;69:564-6.
27. Farmer C. Rhabdomyolysis. In: Civetta J, Taylor R, Kirby R, eds. Critical care. 2nd ed. Philadelphia: Lippincott; 1990.
28. Meyer-Betz F. Beobachtungen an einem eigenartigen mit Muskellahmungen verbunden Fall von Hamoglobinurie. Dsch Arch Klin Med 1910;101:85127.
29. Weeks RS. The crush syndrome. Surg Gynecol Obstet 1968;127:369-75.
30. Odeh M. The role of reperfusion-induced injury in the pathogenesis of the crush syndrome. N Engl J Med 1991;324:1417-22.
31. Chiu D, Wang HH, Blumenthal MR. Creatine phosphokinase release as a measure of tourniquet effect on skeletal muscle. Arch Surg 1976;111:71-4.
32. Better OS. Acute renal failure and crush injury. In: Bihari D, Neid G, eds. Acute renal failure in the intensive therapy unit. London: Springer-Verlag; 1990.
33. Rowland LP, Fahn S, Hirschberg E, et al. Myoglobinuria. Arch Neurol 1964;10:537-62.
34. Rowland LP, Penn AS. Myoglobinuria. Med Clin North Am 1972;56:1233-56.
35. Androecial VE. Acute renal failure. Boston: Martinus Nijhoff Publishing; 1984. pp. 251-70.
36. Koffler A, Friedler RM, Massry SG. Acute renal failure due to nontraumatic rhabdomyolysis. Ann Intern Med 1976;85:23-8.
37. Mars D, Treolar D. Acute tubular necrosis-pathophysiology and treatment. Heart Lung 1984:13:194-201.
38. Better OS, Stein JH. Early management of shock and prophylaxis of acute renal failure in traumatic rhabdomyolysis. N Engl J Med 1990;322:825-9.
39. Muckart DJ, Moodley M, Naidu AG, et al. Prediction of acute renal failure following soft tissue injury using the venous bicarbonate concentration. J Trauma 1992;33(6):813-17.
40. Santangelo M, Usberi M, Disalvo E, et al. A study of the pathology of the crush syndrome. Surg Gynecol Obstet 1982;154: 372-4.
41. Hamilton RW, Hopkins MB, Shihabi ZK. Myoglobinuria, hemoglobinuria and acute renal failure. Clin Chem 1989:35: 1,713.
42. Paller SM. Haemoglobin and myoglobin induced acute renal failure in the rat: the role of iron in nephrotoxicity. Am J Physiol 1988;255:F539.
43. Whitesides TE, Haney TC, Morimoto K, et al. Tissue pressure measurements as a determinant for the need of fasciotomy. Clin Orthop 1975;113:43-51.
44. Bywaters EG. 50 years: The crush syndrome. Br Med J 1990;301:1412-15.
45. McQueen MM, Gaston P, Court-Brown CM. Acute compartment syndrome: who is at risk? J Bone Joint Surg Br 2000;82: 200-3.
46. Whitesides TE, Heckman MM. Acute compartment syndrome: update on diagnosis and treatment. J Am Acad Orthop Surg 1996;4:209-18.
47. Ulmer T. The clinical diagnosis of compartment syndrome of the lower leg: are clinical findings predictive of the disorder? J Orthop Trauma 2002;16:572-7.

Part 2

All-hazards Preparedness for Terrorism

Planning Preparedness for Terrorism

22

Introduction to All-hazards Preparedness and Planning for Terrorism

Adam H. Miller, John Munyak, Raymond E. Swienton, Phillip L. Coule, and Karelene Hosford

INTRODUCTION

In this post–September 11 era, more horrific acts of terrorism will likely occur in the United States. Health care providers must be ready to respond and coordinate their actions. This chapter identifies basic definitions of commonly used terms, discusses the need for standardized education and training, provides an overview of disaster planning, and demonstrates the importance of good communication among all agencies and responders involved in disaster management. Furthermore, several essential elements vital to disaster preparation and response are reviewed in the context of an all-hazards approach.

PREPAREDNESS ESSENTIALS, HISTORIC EVENTS, AND CASE HISTORIES

There are many examples of terrorism events in or directly affecting the United States. The devastation resulting from the events of September 11, 2001, will never be forgotten. Historically, several different types of terrorism and attempts at utilizing weapons of mass effect are noted. There have been reports of failed attempts (1), numerous anthrax hoaxes (2,3), and actual attacks, such as the inoculation of salmonella into Oregon salad bars in 1984 (4), the New York City Trade Center bombing in 1993 (5), the release of sarin in Japan in 1994 (6) and again in 1995 (7), the Oklahoma City bombing in 1996 (8,9), and the U.S. embassy bombings in Kenya and Tanzania in 1998 (10).

Over the years, the increasing likelihood of the use of weapons of mass destruction (WMD) on large populations has been discussed in various official publications, from international government alerts to congressional hearings (8,18). The threat is real regarding the use of nuclear, biological, and chemical (NBC) agents and is due to the sheer number of weapons in the NBC arsenal worldwide, global security limitations, and changes in the political and overall socioeconomic status and stability of several countries (12). Although the threat of nuclear events is important, historically the use of chemical and biological agents is utilized more frequently (13,14). In addition to terrorist events and the military use of weapons, there are many examples of natural disasters including events requiring a national response, tornados in prone regions, devastating earthquakes worldwide (e.g., in Iran and Turkey), the severe flooding and forest fires in California, and the devastation from hurricanes in the Caribbean and the United States. Volcanic eruptions, such as that of Mount Saint Helens in 1980, also demonstrated that the risk of natural disasters is real in the United States and throughout the world. All of these events have a high potential for multiple injuries and fatalities, and they all have the potential to recur and create more havoc.

Mass casualty incidents (MCI) from events other than terrorism have identified and shaped the evolution of the disaster response in the United States. For example, when two commercial airliner crashes and a large military helicopter crash occurred over a 3-year period in Dallas, Texas, although not caused by terrorism, it significantly impacted the medical response approach in the Dallas-Fort Worth (DFW) area, as stated by Klein (15): "Working at a level 1 trauma center, we shared an attitude of complacency about disaster drills. We had a disaster plan, the available manpower, the experience, and the knowledge, and we felt confident that we could handle a local disaster. The knowledge we gained through three aircraft disasters proved to us that most of our perceptions were wrong" (15).

DEFINITIONS

Terminology such as "WMD," "MCI," and "all-hazards" are important to understand because they frequently have varied and broad definitions. Take the word "disaster," for instance. Its definition encompasses the loss of life, loss of property, loss of control, and many injured or killed. A disaster has been described as an emergency that disrupts normal community function and causes concern for the safety, property, and lives of its citizens (16). The Joint Commission on Accreditation of Healthcare Organizations (JCAHO) defines an emergency (disaster) as "a natural or manmade event that suddenly or significantly disrupts the environment of care; disrupts care and treatment; or changes or increases demands for the organization's services" (17). Depending on the readiness and sheer ability to handle a certain magnitude of an event, a disaster is practically defined as any event that exceeds the capabilities of the response. A "disaster" is present when *need exceeds resources*. "All-hazards" are a collection of various human-made and natural events that have the capacity to cause multiple casualties. "All-hazards preparedness" is the comprehensive preparedness required to manage the casualties resulting from possible hazards. Frequently, events exceed the quantitative or qualitative ability of the on-site responders or receiving hospitals to treat and transport the casualties involved. This is considered a "mass casualty incident" (MCI). The term "casualty" refers to a person who is ill, injured, missing, or killed as the result of an event. And the term "incident" is used when a significant event has occurred that requires scene and casualty management (18).

Many organizations, including emergency medical services (EMS), fire, municipal, and hospital, must be integrated to provide seamless patient care from the out-of-hospital to the hospital setting. This effort will involve lay individuals such as hospital administrators, local and state emergency planners, law enforcement personnel, poison centers staff, laboratory agencies staff, industry personnel, public health officials, safety officers, and medical specialists (19–22). A seamless integration requires an approach that is quite simple yet effective.

Planning

After the terrorist attack on the World Trade Center on September 11, 2001, the disaster management community's review of the incident identified areas of needed improvement. Among the difficulties encountered were poor communication, lack of standardized training, and inconsistent definitions of key terms, principles, and concepts including interagency jargon. The intended result of this retrospective analysis has enabled the disaster response community to remediate any such future catastrophe with better planning and ideally more favorable outcomes. The communication infrastructure must be designed with multiple levels of redundancy in order to accommodate for failure at one or more levels. Hospitals, state, and federal agencies must be able to communicate valuable information in spite of difficulties and demand on the system. During the World Trade Center disaster, communication among the Fire Department (FDNY), Police Department (NYPD), and EMS was interrupted because major equipment was located at World Trade Center tower number one. Similarly, vital organizations charged with the coordination of any disaster, such as the Office of Emergency Management (OEM), should not be located in a building that is a potential target for terrorist activities.

To utilize resources appropriately and effectively and distribute victims of a disaster, hospitals, EMS, and the locality (community, region, or state) must first clearly understand their own capabilities and capacities and then be able to assess rapidly the magnitude of the response needs. This is very important because the outcome of disasters is always significantly impacted by the local community's response during the initial phase of management.

Historically, the literature cites examples of categorizing the magnitude of a MCI using a system of MCI levels. Level I MCI is an emergency that is manageable with medical resources available within the locality but produces alterations in the normal delivery of medical care. This level designation implies that the capability exists for local EMS to provide adequate field triage and stabilization and for local health care facilities to provide adequate diagnosis and treatment. Level II MCI is an incident associated with significant numbers of casualties that exceed the normal medical response capability of the involved community. Routinely available multijurisdictional mutual aid and medical support are required and provide an adequate response to meet the demands of the incident. Level III MCI is a medical disaster that overwhelms the capabilities of routinely available local and regional resources, exceeds the capacity of available multijurisdictional medical mutual aid, and frequently necessitates state or federal support (23).

When a MCI is reported to the health care system, it communicates to the appropriate agencies and to the community that a certain amount or level of response is urgently needed and emergency preparedness plans should be put into motion. The goal in a MCI is to do the greatest good for the greatest number of potential survivors (16). This requires a coordinated plan to mobilize the responses from local, regional, and national sources in a predetermined manner. Whether or not a MCI has occurred depends on several variables. This would include the overall number of casualties, the severity and type of casualties, equipment demands, facilities capabilities and surge capacities, transportation requirements, scene safety such as hazardous materials team (hazmat) risks, secondary devices, and other items that increase the likelihood of causing more victims. Other issues include the continued functionality of the local community; the impact on clean water supply, power sources, and key roadways; the ability of the incident to remain static or the potential for spread; and the potential for a national threat, such as in the recent anthrax incidents.

Hospitals not within the immediate area of the disaster scene do not all have to be prepared to the same extent and at the same time. If appropriate communication exists among hospitals, OEM, and EMS, hospitals will then have the ability to scale the response based on the likelihood of patients being transported to any given hospital. It is imperative that effective communication be maintained among hospitals during a disaster. During the World Trade Center disaster in 2001, significant amounts of time, effort, and resources were expended in hospitals not located in the immediate vicinity of ground zero. Many hospitals were prepared but did not receive patients. Hospitals closest to the disaster site should care for the critically ill while distant hospitals could manage the walking wounded, for example.

Emergency management plans must address four phases of activities during a disaster: mitigation, preparedness, response, and recovery. The goal of mitigation planning is to lessen the severity and impact of a potential emergency. This process begins by identifying potential hazards, known as a hazard vulnerability analysis (HVA), that may affect an organization's operations such as a subway, hospital, or any building that may be at risk for natural or human-made disaster. During this phase, strategies are developed to support perceived vulnerabilities most likely to occur. Preparedness activities involve the construction of organizational capacity to manage the effects of an emergency. This includes but is not limited to resource inventory of supplies and equipment, advanced arrangements with vendors and health care networks, staff orientation and training, and organizational rehearsals or drills.

The response phase is the real-time confrontation with an event. The goal is to control the negative effects of the incident. Management must take steps to initiate the emergency plan, continually assess and reassess the situation, and frequently set new objectives. Occurring concurrently with the response phase are recovery activities. The main initiative is to restore essential services and resume normal activities with minimal delays. Issues such as loss of revenue, staff support, and community reaction are addressed.

Disaster planning should incorporate multiagency, multidisciplinary coordination and information sharing, evacuation procedures, and integration of unsolicited emergency responders and spontaneous civilian volunteers.

Additional disaster planning components to be addressed include the coordination of widespread search and rescue, triage, emergency medical care, casualty distribution, victim tracking, hazmat decontamination, security, restrictions of site access, and handling of the dead. Logistics to be addressed include support for emergency personnel (food, shelter, sanitation, etc.), public information dissemination, and mass media control, insight, and involvement.

At the institutional level, the development of an external and an internal emergency contingency plan should be considered. An external disaster is anything that indirectly affects the institution infrastructure. This type of an event in the health care arena mainly addresses how increased numbers of patients will be triaged, decontaminated, transported, and treated. An internal disaster includes conditions that affect a facility directly and may be an extension of an external emergency. This type of disaster carries the additional burden of not just caring for patients but also ensuring the safety of patients and staff.

Educational Needs

The mission of the U.S. health care system has been changed by acts of terrorism that have occurred. Although disaster preparedness has always been a focus within the health care community, recent events are serving to refocus this preparedness to a new level. Publications have reported opportunities for improvement in several areas. A 2001 survey suggested that 100% of hospitals surveyed were inadequately prepared for a biological incident and 73% were inadequately prepared for a chemical or nuclear event (24). In another survey of over 180 emergency departments, fewer than 20% of hospitals had plans for dealing with biological or chemical weapons events (25). The lack of preparedness suggests a lack of training, and this theory was supported in research that found inadequate training in our current educational process for the target groups who would be called on to deal with a WMD incident (16).

The need for a uniform, coordinated approach to mass casualty management is critical to all-hazards preparedness. This is best accomplished by standardized training that provides peer-reviewed, validated, didactic, and practical training for the responders to mass casualty events. In the emergency medicine literature, one model suggests a dual phase approach (2). Phase I must focus on the (a) identification of the needs, demands, and feasibility for MCI-related training, (b) determination of the barriers and challenges related to delivering MCI training, and (c) development of high-level educational goals and strategies to attain the identified goals. Phase II must focus on the (a) review of educational curricula for each of the target audiences and of the existing courses, (b) definition of levels of proficiency and development of associated behavioral objectives, (c) identification of recommendations for integrating WMD and other disaster content into initial and continuing education, (d) identification of recommendations for sustaining WMD and other disaster knowledge and skills, and (e) specification of techniques to ensure continuing proficiencies (16).

Several areas important to disaster management are traditionally absent or lacking in current health care provider education. These include casualty decontamination, regulatory and legal issues, media and communications, mass fatality management, personal protective equipment (PPE), and decontamination, as well as community, state, and federal resources. In addition, the behavioral aspects and overall psychological impact of disaster management must be addressed. The potential long-term psychological impact of disasters on responders and their careers is significantly related to the availability of proper psychological impact management. Communication is a key to managing the psychological impact. Effective communication methods and proper interactions with the media are therefore vital to operations during a disaster. Education and training programs need to be included in disaster planning. Community and hospital disaster planning is the foundation of an effective response to a MCI, and standardized preparedness methods and models are essential for maximizing success.

The positive impact in clinical skills delivery has been noted in several successful standardized training initiatives. At the citizen level, consider the impact on victim survival and the performance of cardiopulmonary resuscitation (CPR). At the health care provider level, nationally recognized and validated training programs such as Advanced Cardiac Life Support (ACLS) and Advanced Trauma Life Support (ATLS) over the past three decades have standardized the management of cardiac and trauma care, respectively. Furthermore, these courses have become a standard part of civilian and U.S. military medical training and continuing medical education (CME).

The American Medical Association (AMA) is leading a national and international initiative to meet this critical need in health care disaster preparedness through the implementation of a standardized training program. Under a federal appropriation managed by the Centers for Disease Control and Prevention (CDC), disaster management educational programs were initiated from all-hazards training programs developed by a variety of academic, state, and federal centers. These groups formed the National Disaster Life Support Educational Consortium (NDLSEC) that now consists of both international and domestic leaders in disaster management. The NDLSEC has designed a series of courses that includes Advanced Disaster Life Support (ADLS), Basic Disaster Life Support (BDLS), and Core Disaster Life Support (CDLS).

The National Disaster Life Support (NDLS) group of courses serves a broad target audience, which includes physicians, nurses, paramedics, emergency medical technicians (EMTs), pharmacists, veterinarians, physician assistants (PAs), nurse practitioners (NPs), laboratory technicians, law enforcement officers, city officials and planners, as well as other health care providers and nonmedical groups. The Core Disaster Life Support (CDLS) course is focused on the all-hazards preparedness needs of first responders, nonmedical personnel, and as an introduction to the topics for other health care provider types. Basic Disaster Life Support (BDLS) is a review of the all-hazards topics including natural and accidental human-made events, traumatic and explosive events, nuclear and radiological events, biological events, and chemical events. The Advanced Disaster Life Support (ADLS) training program is designed for the BDLS provider and consists of an intensive practicum 2-day course with training focused on skill development and reinforcement.

ELEMENTS

Education and training is critical to all aspects of disaster preparedness. Several elements in disaster management have been identified as areas in which performance improvement is needed. These essential elements are common to all aspects of disaster management and include detection, incident command, scene safety and security, assessment of hazards, support, triage and treatment, and evacuation and recovery (18). An introductory review of these essential topics will lay the foundation for assisting health care providers in assessing their own training and educational needs. These and many other topics will be further developed in detail in the following chapters.

Detection is awareness. Detection utilizes surveillance methods to audit or screen for patterns of illness or agent identification clues. During an incident, detection involves the recognition of a situation that will likely overwhelm the resources available to the on-scene providers or the receiving health care facilities. It may be from an obvious source such as damage sustained from a tornado or from a source more difficult to identify such as in the case of a biological agent release.

The Incident Command System (ICS) started as an approach to the problem of managing rapidly moving wildfires in the early 1970s. Originally, an interagency task force comprised of local, state, and federal representatives called FIRESCOPE (Firefighting Resources of Southern California Organized against Potential Emergencies) was formed. The original ICS concepts have been modified to all phases of disaster preparedness and management to facilitate an organized response to all-hazards. Standardization of terminology and a uniform system for coordination across agency and facility lines is the goal of ICS. Although several variations of the original ICS exist, the majority have the same key elements, including the unified incident command, planning, finance, logistics, and operations. The unified incident command section includes the incident commander and the staff that leads the component areas. Planning involves strategic assessment and component analysis. Finance is the administration component and involves the contracting and payment necessary to obtain the resources needed. Logistics is responsible for obtaining and providing all the personnel, equipment, supplies, and services to accomplish the mission. Operations are the implementation of event management at the scene or facilities involved in the incident. This coordinated scene effort reflects the multitude of agencies responsible for incident management such as fire, medical, law enforcement, and many others.

Safety and security are very important at every stage in disaster management. In the hospital or prehospital situation, many factors affect safety and security such as effective communication, scene access, hazard recognition, crowd control, and others. Assessing hazards is a key aspect of safety and security. Remember always that protection is more valuable than identification. Utilizing proper personal protective equipment (PPE) and applying sound principles of scene management that protect the responders will ultimately help victims and the general public. Maintaining an all-hazards approach to each incident is important.

Terrorism has expanded the scope of hazards that must be considered. The use of secondary devices, which are intentionally placed devices intended to detonate or cause further destruction or injuries after the initial event has occurred, are a significant threat to all scene response personnel. Some of the injured may be the event perpetrators who may still remain armed and represent a serious threat to those responding. In addition to these relatively new considerations, there is the multitude of usual hazards to consider such as downed power lines, fire, explosions, natural gas line ruptures, structural collapse, adverse weather, toxic fumes/smoke inhalation, and so on.

Support is having what is needed readily available to get the task completed. Providing support in this manner requires an effective ICS. Each responder must be able to assess and communicate effectively his or her own capabilities and capacities as well as size up the incident.

Triage is the sorting of victims based on the severity of injury and likelihood of survival. Historically, there is not any standardized system of triage universally accepted in civilian health care. The U.S. Department of Defense (USDOD) utilizes a standardized triage approach that has been effectively used in the setting of military operations for many years. In civilian health care, however, there are many triage models in existence that may have significant limitations. Some of them would be better defined as individual patient assessment tools because they are not effective at the initial sorting of patient groups. Others involve somewhat complicated scoring systems to quantitate severity that is difficult to apply in actual events. Terminology and color assignments to each group complicate the matter further and include immediate versus urgent, delayed versus nonurgent versus minimal, and different methods of victim identification tagging.

The NDLS program sponsored by the AMA is helping establish a standardized triage method appropriate to all victim scenarios (18). The objective is to modify and improve, over time, a triage system through appropriate research and evaluation while practically meeting the current need for a common triage system. The MASS Triage model, a modified version of standard military triage, is gaining widespread civilian acceptance. The MASS Triage model includes four areas: *move*, *assess*, *sort*, and *send*. These four action steps serve to group patients, assess them individually, identify need for immediate life-saving interventions, and determine transportation needs for the injured. Injury categories and color designation for victim group assignment are standardized for ease of use. A complete description of this system can be found in the NDLS Provider Manuals sponsored by the AMA (18).

The treatment of the injured victims begins at the incident scene and continues throughout the chain of care. The amount of treatment delivered depends on the resources and provider skills available. Terrorism can significantly affect the treatment delivery phase of disaster management. The ongoing threat of a secondary device may demand the immediate removal of the injured or the responders, thereby altering the typical treatment response phase. The sheer number of victims as well may alter the treatment delivered at the scene or a receiving facility. Many of the treatment algorithms of pediatric, cardiac, and trauma care apply to the treatment of victims of terrorism. However, there are many aspects of mass casualty management that may need additional algorithms. For example, several of the weapons of mass effect, such as nuclear, biological, and chemical, are not traditionally covered.

The evacuation of everyone from the scene is a primary focus of incident management. The transportation of the injured to appropriate health care facilities, establishing designated treatment areas, the safe removal and return to duty of response personnel, and the removal of the general public from the area are important. Terrorism superimposes additional complexities (e.g., a sniper, an unexploded ordinate, or unidentified secondary device) to the evacuation phase that may alter the evacuation effort.

Recovery begins immediately after the incident occurs and is the long-term objective and overall goal of MCI management (18). Minimizing the immediate as well as long-term impact of the event are the overall objectives. This involves many different areas including reestablishment of the local health care infrastructure, which may require the use of state or federal resources to accomplish. The immediate need for shelter and fresh water may be needed in the early recovery phase. During this phase, the psychosocial impact of the incident is important. The psychosocial impact on the victims, their families, responders, the public, and all personnel involved must be considered early and maintained long term.

SUMMARY

All-hazards planning and preparation for terrorism is a serious requirement of the health care delivery system in the United States. The horrific acts that have been committed and the threat of additional incidents validate this position. Standardized training and education is fundamental to effective preparedness. In this introductory chapter a number of essential principles and components of disaster management related to terrorism have been identified. Throughout the remaining chapters of this textbook, these and many related topics will be addressed in more detail.

REFERENCES

1. Henderson DA. The looming threat of bioterrorism. Science 1999;283:1279-82.
2. Anon. Bioterrorism alleging use of anthrax and interim guidelines for management—United States, 1998. MMWR Morb Mortal Wkly Rep CDC Surveill Summ 1999;48(4):69-74.
3. Keim M, Kaufmann AF. The anthrax hoax phenomenon: principles for emergency response to bioterrorism. Ann Emerg Med. 1999;34:177-82.
4. Torok Tj, Tauxe RV, Wise RP, et al. A large community outbreak of Salmonellosis caused by intentional contamination of restaurant salad bars. JAMA 1997;278:389-95.

5. NYCEMS. Terrorism hits home. Emerg Med Serv 1993;22 (5):31-41.

6. Okudera H, Morita H, Iwashita T, et al. Unexpected nerve gas exposure in the city of Matsumoto: report of rescue activity in the first sarin gas terrorism. Am J Emerg Med 1997:15:527-8.

7. Okumura T, Suxuki K, Fukuda A, et al. The Tokyo subway sarin attack: disaster management. Part 2. Hospital response. Acad Emerg Med 1998:5:618-24.

8. Mallonee S, Shariat S, Stennies G, et al. Physical injuries and fatalities resulting from the Oklahoma City bombing. JAMA 1996;276:382.

9. Hogan DE, Waeckerle JF, Dire DJ, et al. Emergency department impact of the Oklahoma City terrorist bombing. Ann Emerg Med 1999;34:160-7.

10. State Department web site. Available at: http//www.state.gov/www/global/terrorism/1998 report/sponsor.html.

11. G-7 (Group of seven industrialized nations—United States, Japan, Germany, Britain, France, Italy and Canada), Declaration on Terrorism, June 27, 1996.

12. U.S. Senate, 104th Cong, 1st Sess, Part 1, October 31 and November 1, 1995 (Hearings held by the subcommittee on March 20, 22, and 27, 1996). Global proliferation of weapons of mass destruction.

13. Tucker JB. Historical trends related to bioterrorism: an empirical analysis. Emerg Infect Dis 1999;5:498-504.

14. Shapiro RL, Hatheway D, Becher J, et al. Botulism surveillance and emergency response—a public health strategy for a global challenge. JAMA 1997;278:433-5.

15. Klein JS, Weigelt JA. Disaster management lessons learned. Surg Clin North Am 1991;71:257-66.

16. Waeckerle JF, et al. Executive summary: developing objectives, content, and competencies for training of emergency medical technicians, emergency physicians, and emergency nurses to care for casualties resulting from nuclear, biological, or chemical (NBC) incidents. Ann Emerg Med 2001;37:587-601.

17. JCAHO. Facts about the emergency management standards. Available at http://www.jcaho.org. Last accessed October 9, 2003.

18. Coule PL, Dallas CE, James JJ, et al. eds. Basic disaster life support (BDLS) provider manual. Chicago: American Medical Association, 2003.

19. Waeckerle JF. Disaster planning and response. N Engl J Med 1991;324:815-21.

20. Centers for Disease Control and Prevention. Biological and chemical terrorism: strategic plan for preparedness and response. Recommendations of the CDC Strategic Planning Workgroup. MMWR Morb Mortal Wkly Rep CDC Surveill Summ 2000;49: RR-4.

21. Lillibridge SR. Testimony presented to the Government Reform and Oversight Committee, Subcommittee on National Security. Washington, DC, September. 22, 1999.

22. Knouss RF. Testimony presented to the Government Reform and Oversight Committee, Subcommittee on National Security; Washington, DC, September 22, 1999.

23. Doyle CJ. Mass casualty incident integration with prehospital care. Emerg Med Clin North Am 1990;8:163-75.

24. Irwin RL. The incident command system (ICS). In: Auf der Heide E. ed. Disaster response: principles of preparation and coordination. St. Louis: Mosby, 1989;133-63.

25. Treat KN. Hospital preparedness for weapons of mass destruction incidents: an initial assessment. Ann Emerg Med 2001;38:562-5.

23

Scene Preparedness

Marc Eckstein and Ray Fowler

INTRODUCTION

Preparedness is the key to being able to respond safely and efficiently to terrorist incidents. Even though one certainly cannot plan for every possible contingency, certain fundamentals must be in place to maximize the effectiveness of the response and mitigation of this type of incident. This chapter discusses the key elements of scene preparedness that must be in place in order to minimize the resultant loss of life.

PREPAREDNESS ESSENTIALS

LOCAL CAPABILITY

The Emergency Medical Services (EMS) agency planning for terrorist events should know the capabilities of the local EMS system. In order to prepare for the potential "mass casualty" incident, the planner should have answers to these questions. How many EMS resources are available at any one time on a "normal" day? Of these resources, how many ambulances are available?

This local capability assessment is the first step in determining the overall needs of any particular system. If only a few ambulances are on the streets, how can scores of patients be transported from an event resulting from a terrorist incident? An example of such a capability assessment would be found in planning for a smallpox outbreak. The planner should, for example, identify a cadre of medical provider individuals who could serve in the role of "mass vaccinators," in coordination with the public health department. Such a cadre can be screened for their "prevaccination" appropriateness through various methods, such as Internet-based services (See www.smallpoxscreen.us) (1). Additionally, the American Medical Association (AMA) Center for Disaster Preparedness and Emergency Response maintains a database of providers that are trained in smallpox immunization skills

from their Advanced Disaster Life Support (ADLS) course (2). This database may be essential in the identification of a skilled workforce in the event of a smallpox outbreak.

MUTUAL AID

Most EMS provider agencies, especially smaller ones, typically have mutual aid agreements in place. These agreements serve to quickly augment the normal capacity of a system, both in terms of manpower and transport resources. Questions that the EMS agency preparing for a medical terrorism event must answer include: How many additional ambulances can be summoned? What is the estimated time to get these additional resources on-scene?

A mutual aid agreement usually stipulates that resources and personnel will only be provided if conditions permit (i.e., if the other agencies can spare some of their resources). Obviously, this will depend upon the scope and location(s) of the incident. For this reason, it is beneficial to have mutual aid agreements in place with multiple agencies. One important factor to consider in terms of the provision of mutual aid staffing and equipment is that all agencies typically account for their full-time and part-time personnel rosters. Full-time personnel commonly work part-time at other agencies and thus may be counted as a resource for a second agency (or more). Thus, personnel rosters may indeed show a larger number of personnel than are physically available to respond because an individual responder may be counted as a potential responder by more than one agency.

CALLBACK SYSTEM

Each system should have an internal system in place to augment its daily staffing with a callback/holdover system. In the event of a terrorist incident, which may generate a large number of patients, a system must be in place to recall off-duty personnel and augment resources with reserve apparatus. This callback system must be as automated as possible, with at least one backup method in place. Relying on off-duty personnel to call a single phone number for instructions is impracti-

226

cal because of the overwhelming number of calls that come in to individual(s) answering the phone. Additionally, out-of-service (or crowded) land-lines make a backup method of contact essential.

A functional callback system ensures the availability of additional personnel and activation of additional reserve equipment. Off-duty personnel must have specific, preauthorized standing orders that direct them where to go and to whom to report. The spontaneous response of numerous off-duty FDNY firefighters from their homes directly to the World Trade Center incident, for example, created a myriad of additional problems. "Chain of command and control" and accountability issues arose as additional manpower entered the "immediate danger to life and health" (IDLH) area without the knowledge of any supervisors. Also, responding individuals may have been placed at risk by not having the basic personal protective equipment (PPE) that the on-duty firefighters had.

INCIDENT COMMAND SYSTEM

Strict adherence to the incident command system (ICS) is essential to respond to a terrorist incident optimally (Fig. 23-1). The only way to fully incorporate the ICS into a terrorist incident is to utilize ICS appropriately in the daily operations of the EMS agency. One of the advantages of the ICS is its flexibility and adaptability. Therefore, the ICS should be used whether an incident involving 2 patients or 200 patients is being handled.

In establishing the ICS, it is imperative for the first-arriving resources to provide an accurate "size-up" of the scene. The estimated number of patients should be determined through standard triage sorting using a triage assessment system such as the MASS (Move-Assess-Sort-Send) triage method (Fig. 23-2) (2–4). This system, which utilizes standard military triage categories and is compatible with many civilian triage systems (such as START Simple Triage and Rapid Transport), allows first responders to rapidly identify the number of "Immediate,"

"Delayed," and "Minor" patients that must be managed, as well as the number of persons in the "Expectant" category that have been identified. By separating patients based on their ability to ambulate or move, patients are separated into categories based on the gross motor component of the Glasgow Coma Score (GCS). There is evidence that supports the gross motor component of the GCS as the most sensitive indicator of who will survive and who will not (2–6). One additional critical point is that triage is a dynamic process. Patients may change categories upon reassessment as patients initially identified in one group may improve or worsen. Additionally, Expectant patients should be upgraded to Immediate when resources become available to care for them.

Any identified or potential hazards must be delineated to allow incoming personnel to take the necessary precautions and don the appropriate PPE. This hazard assessment cannot be overemphasized enough. Secondary explosive events, such as the secondary bomb that was detonated at the Atlanta clinic bombing and the second plane crash into the World Trade Center, have shown that injury to emergency providers is of major concern. This risk is not just to the lives of the providers but also to the ultimate mitigation of the effects of the incident.

In addition to estimating the number of patients, a command post location and designation should be made. A location for the staging of incoming resources must be established. Instructions must be broadcast through appropriate channels regarding the safest approach to the incident. Important questions that must be immediately addressed include:

- Is a parking area nearby for apparatus to stage?
- Should the parking area be uphill from the event?
- Is the wind direction pertinent so that resources should approach from an upwind direction?
- Where will the responding agencies park, so that ingress and egress can be controlled carefully?

An individual must remain with each vehicle *with the keys to the vehicle* so that no responding unit blocks the egress of

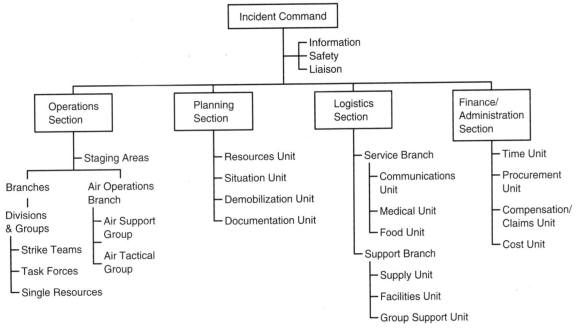

Figure 23–1. ICS organizational chart.

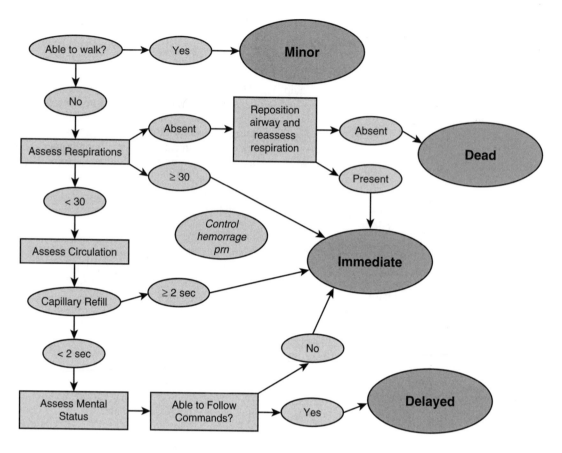

Figure 23–2. ICS organizational chart.

another vehicle when patient transport—or potentially expanding hazard—requires the movement of the vehicle. Finally, the command post location should allow for an expanding incident and for the arrival of additional agency/department representatives.

Establishing a unified command is essential for any terrorist incident. "Managers" from each key agency involved in such an incident must be designated. Invariably a need will arise for representatives ("agency reps") to be present from law enforcement, fire suppression, EMS, public health, federal agencies, and so on. The overall commander for the incident will depend on the type of incident. A multiple casualty shooting incident with the shooter still on-scene, for example, will typically have a law enforcement leader serve as the incident commander (IC), whereas a chemical weapons release would likely have a fire department officer serve as the IC.

SPECIALIZED RESOURCES

Larger EMS provider agencies, particularly those that are fire department-based, typically have the ready availability of a number of specialized resources. Some of these resources that may be needed for a terrorist incident include hazardous materials (hazmat) teams and equipment, decontamination (decon) teams and equipment, metropolitan medical response system (MMRS), Tactical Emergency Medical Support (TEMS), and so on. The greater the availability of these specialized resources on a regular

basis, the faster they can respond to such an incident. This faster response will make it easier to integrate these teams into an operation. This is because the individuals comprising these teams will regularly train with the other firefighters and agencies and will become accustomed to working within the same chain of command. Logistical issues such as unfamiliarity with the ICS, different types of PPE, different radio frequencies, different medical protocols, and different standard operating procedures (SOPs) make the integration of some of these specialized teams very problematic at a real incident.

MEASURES OF SUCCESS

How can the successful mitigation of a terrorist incident be measured? Three benchmarks by which to measure success in this area are useful:

1. No responder became a victim during the event.

2. Potentially salvageable patients received care in a timely manner.

3. The time elapsed from the time of alarm of the incident until the time of transport of the last Immediate patient was kept to a minimum.

Item 1 is self-explanatory. How do first responders, whether they are firefighters, emergency medical technicians, or law enforcement officers, avoid becoming victims? With proper training and constant reinforcement, first responders will maintain appropriate vigilance to suspect a terrorist incident every time they respond. This vigilance actually begins with properly trained dispatchers. If multiple calls are received by the dispatch center for "persons down," especially in an enclosed location (or a "high risk" location), it is incumbent upon the dispatch center to notify the first responders that multiple calls on this incident for multiple victims have been received, especially if callers are describing a particular constellation of signs and symptoms (such as one of the "toxidromes"). Such prompting by the dispatcher should advise the use of caution by the first responder and may result in a larger dispatch of multiple resources, including the closest hazmat squad to perform air sampling. This warning should prompt the first responders to consider donning the appropriate level of PPE as they approach the incident location.

The role of the call-taking and dispatch agency in community preparedness for terrorist events bears careful examination. Indeed, this agency is often the first contact of professionally organized resources with the event (though on-scene professional personnel, such as public safety individuals, may already be present). Thus, those preparing the community for potential terrorist events must be especially skilled in such areas as the interpretation of events that may have multiple victims. An example would be in setting to high priority those calls coming to the agency in which multiple victims have altered levels of consciousness and/or are experiencing various other emergency conditions, such as seizures. This would quickly give concern to the agency that a potential toxic exposure is ongoing, and thus appropriate warning would be quickly conveyed to responding agencies. Many agencies are utilizing computer-based syndromic surveillance for just this purpose: to identify conditions and situations in which multiple victims of various conditions must be identified (shortness of breath, for example), and to help prepare responding agencies for potential hazards (7).

In order for the first responders to avoid becoming victims, they must have received both the proper amount of training and the necessary PPE. What is the necessary training? One could argue that there is never "enough" training. This is particularly true for the "low frequency-high risk" incident, which is precisely what best describes a terrorist incident. Recognition of certain clues and "red flags" will increase the likelihood that the first responders will be judicious before rushing into an incident location and becoming victims themselves, thereby exacerbating the problem rather than helping to mitigate it.

The following are important "red flags" that should prompt concern on the part of the first responders to any emergency situation:

1. Multiple victims in relatively close proximity—The presence of multiple victims in close proximity suggests a chemical or vapor hazard, especially if the victims are inside a structure. These multiple victims close together are likely suffering the effects of the same hazard, and due caution must be exercised by the responder.

2. The incident location is a "high-risk" target—All first responders must be thoroughly familiar with all known high-risk locations in their areas. Some of these so-called high-risk locations include potential targets for terrorists. Such targets may include houses of worship, gathering places for political conventions, women's health care facilities, and sports arenas. Any call from such a location should prompt the highest level of vigilance on the part of the first responders.

3. Patients are reportedly exhibiting similar symptoms—Several patients with similar signs and symptoms suggest exposure to a single, common offending agent. Indeed, a common constellation of symptoms may suggest a "toxidrome," that is, exposure to an agent that produces predictable symptoms in the victims. While the agent's effects may be delayed or immediate, the rapid recognition of such a clinical pattern in the victims should prompt the first responders to exercise due caution, to don the appropriate PPE prior to approaching the scene, and to consider the appropriate therapy for the condition. The preparation of responders through initial and periodic retraining on this point cannot be overemphasized.

4. Potentially salvageable patients receive care in a timely manner—Even though taking the necessary precautions and establishing the ICS are fundamental aspects of responding to a potential terrorist incident, it has also been clearly recognized that minimizing all potential hazards can go too far, especially if it compromises the care of potentially salvageable patients. This type of excessive care might occur, for example, in response to a reported hazmat incident.

In the past, some fire departments had standard operating procedures for first-arriving companies at a suspected hazmat incident to merely provide an assessment or "size-up" of the incident, set up a perimeter, set up a command post up-wind of the incident location, and request the response of the hazmat team. Patients were ordered to shelter in place (i.e., where they were located at the moment).

It is now clear, though, that if the patients in such an event were exposed to a potentially toxic substance, this approach could result in preventable deaths. What is an "acceptable risk" for first responders to take? Certainly, stringing up yellow fire or police line tape around the incident and waiting for the "experts" to arrive will not help the victim in need of time-critical medical intervention (e.g., a patient exposed to nerve agent who could benefit from having an airway cleared and ventilation assisted). The initial IC may typically be a fire engine captain. This individual must weigh the "risks versus benefits" of going into the area known as the "immediate danger to life and health" (IDLH). If an engine company arrives on the scene of a potential vapor release inside a structure and people are down inside, it might be prudent to call for the appropriate additional resources, don PPE (self-contained breathing apparatus [SCBA] and Level B suits if available), make rapid entry, and extract Immediate yet viable patients. This rapid extraction typically must be done prior to definitive identification of the offending agent. However, a rapid extraction might permit those viable but nonambulatory patients to receive time-critical care and survive their exposures. Even if a particular antidote is not immediately available, the extraction of victims to a clean environment and out of the toxic one may allow improvement of some, if not all, symptoms.

Once removed from the IDLH area, victims must be properly triaged, as discussed earlier. Responding agencies must be trained well in advance in a rapid triage method which has been adopted by the agency (recall the MASS triage system mentioned previously and illustrated in Figure 23-2). Once patients are triaged, rapid decontamination should be performed (if appropriate, or if any doubt is present in the minds of the responders), and treatment and transport should be provided. An assessment should be made as to how long it took for the first and the last patient triaged to the Immediate category to receive treatment and to be transported. Such a time interval assessment will provide later some objective criteria for how successful the mitigation was of a terrorist incident.

For example, if 20 patients are triaged as Immediate, but too few ambulances are requested by responders, then avoidable delays in care will occur. Responders should be well-versed in advance with the knowledge that it is better to request too many resources and then cancel some of them than to keep requesting more as the incident expands, thereby "piecemealing" the response to the incident and possibly jeopardizing the lives of potentially salvageable patients.

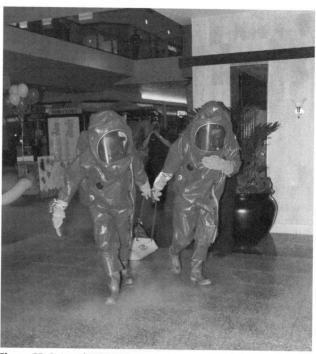

Figure 23–3. Level A PPE. Photo courtesy of Rick McClure, LAFD.

TREATMENT VERSUS TRANSPORT

Is treatment on the scene or rapid transport to a hospital (or alternative destination) the priority? The answer obviously depends upon the particular type of incident with which providers are confronted. If 30 patients are complaining of eye and throat irritation from an exposure that occurred inside a structure, and these patients have no obvious life-threatening symptoms and no worrisome toxidrome, then merely the act of moving these patients outside to fresh air should mitigate the majority of their symptoms if the offending agent was merely the release of an irritant chemical (e.g. pepper spray) inside a building. These patients do not require a "rush to transport" because these symptoms should resolve without any treatment other than perhaps local decontamination. In fact, the decision to delay transport might be prudent, since premature transport might needlessly tie up ambulances and crowd emergency departments with patients having self-limiting, minor symptoms. On the other hand, it is also clear that certain pulmonary irritants, such as phosgene, might present with worsening symptoms—indeed with frank pulmonary edema and death—many hours later. Thus, just because victims of potential inhalation injuries don't appear to have symptoms at the outset of exposure does NOT mean that the emergency provider should not refer these victims for further evaluation or observation.

Conversely, a terrorist incident involving the use of explosives may result in victims with various thermal, blunt, and penetrating injuries. These patients obviously require rapid transport to the appropriate facility, with only essential resuscitative and stabilizing treatment being provided on-scene.

An incident involving scores of patients exhibiting eye pain, miosis, rhinorrhea, shortness of breath, seizures, and excessive salivation should be presumed to be a nerve agent release until proven otherwise. Patients with moderate or severe symptoms must be treated with the proper antidote(s) on-scene, prior to transport. In this scenario, coordinating the timing of decontamination, triage, field treatment, and transport is essential to minimize the number of preventable deaths.

PROPER PPE

What is the proper level of PPE that an emergency responder should use? The levels of PPE are covered elsewhere in this text. However, given the current realities in the world and especially the concerns over the potential for terrorist incidents, first responders must now have ready access to higher levels of PPE than once thought. Some systems have trained single-function (non-fire suppression certified) paramedics to carry self-contained breathing apparatus to provide better personal protection in an IDLH area resulting from a terrorist-type incident.

Level A protection is carried only by hazmat personnel (Fig. 23-3). Level B protection, which involves a chemical suit with SCBA, may be carried by first responders. Level B protection may be donned quickly to perform rapid extraction of patients in the IDLH area (Fig. 23-4). In many cases, indeed in perhaps most cases, emergency medical providers may not have the protective suits mentioned above, and it is thus vital for the EMS response to be closely coordinated with the HAZMAT teams in the given area. Other options include some types of "escape masks" that are rapidly donned, but provide far less protection than SCBA or powered air-purifying respirators (PAPRs) (Figs. 23-5 and 23-6).

AVAILABILITY OF ANTIDOTES

Many EMS agencies have procured large quantities of specific antidotes to some weapons of mass destruction.

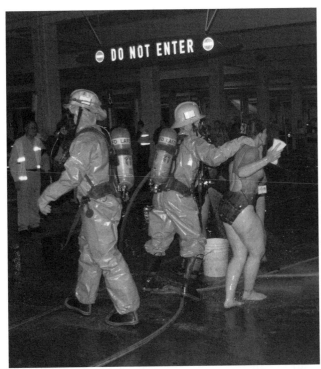

Figure 23–4. Level B PPE. Photo courtesy of Rick McClure, LAFD.

Some of these include atropine and pralidoxime auto injectors (to treat victims of nerve agent exposure) and amyl nitrite (to treat victims of cyanide exposure). If these antidotes are stored at a specific location in a "disaster cache," it is unlikely they will be of substantial benefit at a real incident. By the time the identification of the need for the antidote is made, a request goes out for the antidote, and the supply of antidote is located and transported to the site of the incident, few, if any patients will benefit. More importantly, those pa-

tients with severe exposures may suffer preventable deaths due to a delay in treatment. Still, providing these caches of medications and supplies may buy time until additional resources may be made available to the community.

Antidotes must be carried by all front-line emergency responder resources, especially paramedic resources. For example, each Los Angeles Fire Department (LAFD) paramedic ambulance carries 30 nerve agent antidote kits (each kit contains an atropine 2-mg and pralidoxime 600-mg autoinjector) and 20 amyl nitrite ampules (for cyanide poisoning). Additional caches of both antidotes are carried by all EMS field supervisors. Furthermore, each fire-fighter-emergency medical technician (EMT) carries a personal escape kit, which is a web belt that has 2 nerve agent antidote kits for personal use, along with an escape mask.

HOSPITAL NOTIFICATION

Ensuring proper scene preparedness without prospectively involving the hospital notification system in an overall preparedness program is a recipe for failure. Rapid and effective mitigation of a terrorist incident requires a responsive and adequately prepared hospital system. Hospital surge capacity issues, decontamination capabilities, and emergency department (ED) overcrowding issues are beyond the scope of this chapter. However, it is essential that a seamless system of obtaining hospital availability information and providing hospital notification be maintained and frequently tested.

Many major metropolitan areas now have a specialized computer system in place that interconnects each hospital's ED with the local department of health services, department of public health, and the local EMS provider agency or agencies. One such system, used in Los Angeles, is called the ReddiNet® system. This computer system connects all 81 paramedic-receiving hospitals in Los Angeles County with the Los Angeles County Department of Health Services (LACDHS) and the dispatch center of the LAFD. The ReddiNet® system provides the mechanism for hospital EDs to go on diversion for ambulances, trauma patients, internal disaster, and so on. It also requires each ED requesting diversion to enter the reason for the request, such as the lack of open ED beds, a lack of intensive care unit beds, lack of open operating rooms, and so on (Fig. 23-7).

The system also requires the ED to enter into the computer tracking system whether a preponderance of any specific symptoms or chief complaints in their ED has been detected, thus allowing biosurveillance to be performed by DHS. For example, a cluster of EDs requesting diversion due to a preponderance of patients presenting

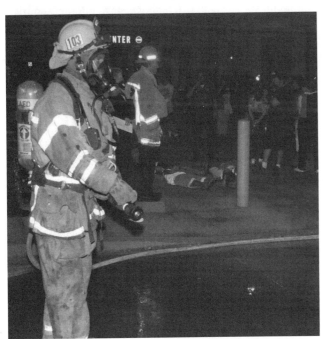

Figure 23–5. Self-contained breathing apparatus (SCBA). Photo courtesy of Rick McClure, LAFD.

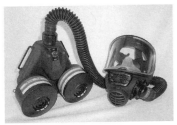

Figure 23–6. Powered air purifying respirator.

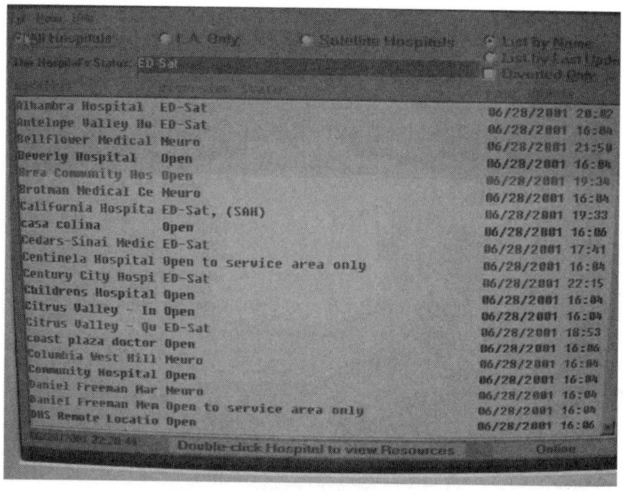

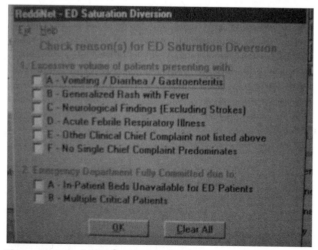

Figure 23–7. ReddiNet® hospital diversion screen.

with flu-like symptoms during the summer months would then raise sufficient concern to direct the epidemiologists from Public Health to respond to those EDs to examine the particulars of the cases and to identify any suspicious outbreaks that may represent bioterrorism (Fig. 23-8).

Early into the response to a potential terrorist incident, it is the responsibility of the first-arriving paramedic ambulance to assist with patient triage and establish communications with medical control. Every LAFD apparatus (fire engines and ambulances) has access to the ReddiNet® system, as does the dispatch center. This allows on-scene personnel the ability to determine hospital availability quickly. Central medical command facilities, monitoring similar software (EmSystem®), can provide assistance in the determination of hospital capacity as well. Future improvements of such computer-assisted technology will enable this system to be used to notify hospital notification of incoming patients. Currently, hospital notifications must be made verbally.

Again in Los Angeles, if 10 or more patients are found at a single incident, or if the incident is presumed to be terrorist-related, paramedics communicate directly with the communications center of the DHS, instead of their assigned base station. Communications personnel at DHS

can use land-line "hotlines" to query each receiving hospital as to the number of patients (for each triage category) that hospital can accommodate. Furthermore, this communications center can put out an alert via the ReddiNet® system to all hospitals that a large-scale incident has occurred and that hospitals should prepare to receive potentially large influxes of patients. EDs should have plans in place to clear their emergency departments quickly of the patients not experiencing life-threatening emergencies, activate the disaster mode for their hospitals, discharge stable patients, open their overflow area(s), and mobilize additional staff and equipment as called for in their disaster plans.

This warning can also prompt hospitals to prepare to perform decontamination on any patients who may have self-evacuated and were transported to the hospital via private means instead of by EMS. This notification can be vital if it prevents a contaminated patient from walking into an unsuspecting ED, thereby risking the health of the ED staff members and potentially shutting down that ED from receiving any further patients.

DISASTER PLAN PREPARATION AND DRILLS

The preparation of the internal disaster mitigation plan by any facility requires a multidisciplinary, thoughtful approach to determining what emergencies might befall a hospital, including internal ones, and planning for the optimal use of equipment and personnel to respond to those disasters. Such preparation includes the design of an internal emergency communications center (ECC), which should be in a central, hardened portion of the facility and be available to be established with momentary notice. The ECC must be provided with a comprehensive communications network that will bring together through multiple communications media (telephone, fax, Internet, courier, and others) that can reach all necessary internal and external services and agencies necessary to mitigate a disaster.

The disaster mitigation plan must be developed with careful attention to all potential internal and external disasters. This plan must include how to secure the ED in the setting of potentially enormous numbers of patients seeking care so that an orderly process may take place providing decontamination (if necessary), patient assessment, and emergency management based upon an agreed triage mechanism. All members of the hospital and physician staffs of the facility must be trained in the plan, must know their responsibilities in the setting of an emergency, and must be periodically updated and reminded of their duties.

Disaster drills are essential to determine the degree of preparedness for any agency or department. While these drills are certainly no substitute for the "real thing," they can provide an invaluable opportunity to both evaluate a system's degree of preparedness as well as to identify any potential weaknesses. Those preparing the details of these drills must remember that the more realistic the drill, the more effective it is likely to be.

Tabletop exercises, in general, assist managers, supervisors, and officers with ICS components and identify any potential conflicts regarding command and control issues

Figure 23–8. ReddiNet® rationale for diversion screen.

and the unified command process. Drills with actual volunteer "patients" are quite valuable. An ideal drill will provide a setting in which participants actually get to go through each step as the "incident" unfolds. Logistical issues such as the donning of proper PPE, accurate size-up of the emergency, requesting appropriate additional resources, establishing a command post, creating a staging area, setting up a decon area, and fulfilling each aspect of the ICS should be performed. Having personnel actually work in their proper PPE, including triaging victims, setting up treatment areas, and transporting to designated locations helps bring a sense of realism to the drill. Each participant quickly appreciates the limitations of working in various levels of PPE.

The results of the disaster drill should be studied. How quickly does it actually take to get a hazmat team on-scene? How quickly does it take to get a disaster medical cache on-scene? Did the front-line ambulances carry the various appropriate antidotes (e.g., nerve agent antidote kits), or are they only available in the disaster caches? If the antidotes were not available on front-line ambulances, how many patients might have been compromised by the delay in their definitive care in the case of an exposure to a nerve agent? The answers to these and many more important questions relative to disaster preparedness and assessment are key to success in the event of a real disaster.

DECONTAMINATION

Decontamination (decon) has become a necessary focus for many of the individuals planning for the response by emergency agencies to terrorist incidents. Important questions for each potentially involved agency include how extensive a decon is necessary, and who is trained to perform decon?

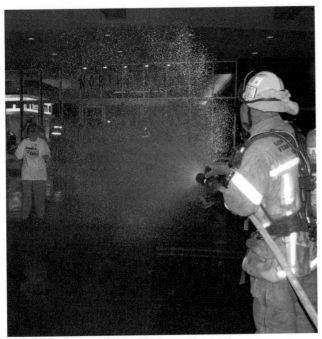

Figure 23–9. Gross decontamination with firefighters donning Level B protection. Photo courtesy of Rick McClure, LAFD.

In the past, only those individuals trained and certified as hazmat technicians or specialists were responsible for performing decon. However, certain types of terrorist incidents may require that the decon be done very quickly so that time-critical medical care and transportation may be provided.

One must be mindful that the longer decon takes, the longer the delay for the patient to receive medical care becomes. Many fire departments have developed standard operating procedures whereby first responder fire engines and fire trucks can provide gross decon. This gross decon provides an optimal use of resources, since the firefighters, serving as first responders, already have a water supply and a very short response time to the incident. By donning Level B protection, or at a minimum donning firefighting "turnout" gear with SCBA, firefighters can safely provide gross decon in most instances (Fig. 23-9).

By merely having patients remove their clothing, it is generally estimated that some 80% to 90% of all contaminants are removed from the patient, perhaps even more when the exposure is a vapor hazard (2). When the removal of clothing is followed with a gross decon with water, most decon requirements are satisfied for most terrorist incidents. Performing secondary or more detailed and thorough decon runs the risk of delaying medical treatment and transport to the point of compromising patient care. If a given patient is still ambulatory after removing all clothing and undergoing initial and secondary decon, it may be argued that such a patient does not have a significant exposure that poses an immediate threat to life. Conversely, subjecting a nonambulatory patient to such rigorous decon may delay life-saving care. EMS personnel with the proper training and expertise must guide the IC to provide just the proper amount of decon necessary, if any, for the victims of the incident.

PREPAREDNESS HISTORIC EVENTS AND CASE HISTORIES: A LOS ANGELES PERSPECTIVE

As of the writing of this chapter, Los Angeles (thankfully) has not suffered a major terrorist incident. Many large-scale disasters have been experienced, both natural and human-made (earthquakes, wildfires, riots, etc.). Many disaster drills have been conducted, including at least two large-scale, multiagency drills that simulated a terrorist incident and involved volunteer "patients." The following describes one such recent drill, dubbed "Operation Dark Cloud."

THE SCENARIO

Two individuals posing to work in a community shopping center selling helium-filled balloons release a vapor of an unknown gas into the mall on a busy day. No one suspected anything unusual since the balloons were normally filled from helium contained in two large cylinders. The initial dispatch is for a single fire engine to investigate the "unknown chemical problem." Upon arrival, this engine company encounters scores of people quickly exiting the mall. They immediately request additional resources, including a full hazmat response, don their Level B protection with SCBAs, and make entry into the mall. There they encounter approximately 50 patients, of whom 15 appear to be Immediate, with no obvious signs other than respiratory distress. They perform rapid extraction of the most critical patients, excluding those tagged as "apneic."

The key elements of this drill were as follows.

1. This engine company quickly recognized an expanding incident, possibly resulting from terrorism, donned the proper PPE, and performed rapid extraction of the sickest patients.

2. The second engine company on-scene assisted to perform gross decon of the patients.

3. The first chief officer on the scene requested the appropriate number of fire resources, ambulances, field supervisors, hazmat teams, and expanded the ICS.

4. A unified command was established, and a medical branch was set up with one division for each of the two exits from the mall where patients were presenting.

5. After undergoing decon, patients were triaged and tagged. (The use of tags is essential with any multiple casualty incident, especially a terrorist incident. These tags not only quickly identify the severity of each patient but also identify whether they have been decontaminated.)

Perhaps even more important than any particular drill are the "lessons learned". No matter how well or how poorly a drill is performed, there are always lessons learned that must be addressed so that all those who participated and those who may be involved in a real incident in the future can learn from any mistakes that were identified and key issues that were addressed.

PREPAREDNESS CHECKLIST TABLE AND SUMMARY

As the unfolding of the events of September 11, 2001 tragically demonstrated, a plan for every possible scenario cannot be maintained. However, by planning ahead, performing an accurate systems analysis and capability review, maximizing training and education, providing proper PPE, and conducting realistic drills, the effects of not only a terrorist incident, but any type of incident that can potentially generate large numbers of casualties, can be minimized for the greatest benefit of the populations being served (Table 23-1).

REFERENCES

1. Fowler RL, LaChance R. www.smallpoxscreen.us. University of Texas Southwestern, 2003.
2. Advanced disaster life support. National Disaster Life Support Publications, American Medical Association; 2004.
3. Basic disaster life support. National Disaster Life Support Publications, American Medical Association; 2004.
4. Core disaster life support. National Disaster Life Support Publications, American Medical Association; 2004.
5. J Trauma. 1995 Jan;38(1):129-35.
6. Ann Emerg Med. 2001 Nov;38(5):541-8.
7. Personal Communication, Mr. Jerry Overton and Dr. Joe Ornato, Richmond, VA.

SUGGESTED READINGS

1. Christen HT, Maniscalco PM. The EMS incident management system. Upper Saddle River, NJ: Prentice Hall; 1998.
2. Kuehl A, ed. Prehospital systems and medical oversight.

TABLE 23-1 Preparedness Summary Checklist Table

ITEM	RESPONSIBILITY	ADDITIONAL DUTIES
Dispatch	Identify potential terrorist incident and advise dispatched resources. Establish scene safety. Provide concise size-up. Don proper PPE.	Notify and dispatch additional, specialized resources as necessary. Request additional resources.
First on-scene	Make entry if appropriate. Perform rapid extraction of critical, viable patients. Don proper PPE.	Perform gross DECON, if necessary.
Next-arriving companies	Assist with rapid patient extraction. Assist with triage, don proper PPE.	
First ALS resource on-scene	Assist with triage. Establish medical communications.	
First chief officer on-scene	Provide more detailed size-up. Request additional resources. Expand ICS.	Establish ICS designation. Set up command post and staging locations.
Next arriving chief officer	Establish unified command and request multiple agencies.	Request specialized resources (MMRT, Public Health, FBI, Bomb Squad, etc.).

24

Hospital Preparedness

Kathy J. Rinnert and Daniel C. Keyes

INTRODUCTION

Terrorist-related events have been increasing over the last decade (1). Coping with them is an ever-changing, dynamic process. In response to these domestic and international threats, the United States has developed programs designed to promulgate domestic counterterrorism response capabilities at all levels of government. These programs, especially at the local level, have been problematic in their implementation and virtually untried in their effectiveness. Hospitals play a pivotal role in this process as the principal sites for triage, diagnosis, stabilization, treatment, and disposition of the victims of terrorist events. However, government reports and the medical literature have identified hospitals as a weak link in domestic terrorism preparedness (2–5).

The Joint Commission on Accreditation of Healthcare Organizations (JCAHO), in the January 2001 Comprehensive Accreditation Manual for Hospitals, requires hospital emergency management to function as an integrated entity within the scope of the broader community. The revised emergency management standards (EC. 1.4) emphasize the need for a common language among emergency agencies, compatible intra-and interagency command structures, and an approach that incorporates all-hazards, including common events and also atypical disaster scenarios such as terrorist events.

BARRIERS AND CHALLENGES TO HOSPITAL PREPAREDNESS

The health care community is exceedingly complex and fractionated. There are a bewildering array of providers, including physicians, nurses, emergency medical services (EMS) personnel, and others. Similarly, the sites for health care delivery vary widely and may include physician offices, clinics, urgent care centers, public health departments, and visiting nurse agencies. Hospitals provide a multitude of services as well. Such fractionation may act as a barrier in efforts to unify and organize the medical community.

Unique challenges that may hinder hospital preparedness include unfunded legislative and regulatory mandates, competition between institutions, diminishing reimbursements, workforce shortages, aging physical plants, competing institutional priorities, absence of disaster preparedness funding, and lack of guidance for counterterrorism efforts (6).

A realistic medical counterterrorism plan should incorporate the resources of all hospital facilities within a community. Such factors as bed capacity, complexity of medical services, workforce sophistication, and mutual aid and contractual agreements may define roles and responsibilities for individual hospital facilities within the context of a community-based response to a terrorist incident. Hospital administrators, physician and nursing leaders, and other health care decision makers must be prepared for the pivotal role they will play in the stabilization and treatment of victims, who may number in the thousands.

PHASES OF EMERGENCY MANAGEMENT

The JCAHO has adopted the Federal Emergency Management Agency's (FEMA) four-phase organizational model for emergency management and disaster readiness. The model defines the four phases of emergency management as mitigation, preparedness, response, and recovery.

Mitigation refers to actions taken before an event to prevent or reduce the impact to life and property. *Preparedness* refers to the activities, actions, procurements, planning, training, and interjurisdictional cooperation designed to increase response readiness to identified hazards within the community. *Response* refers to the mobilization of resources to meet the needs of the community in response to an emergency event. *Recovery* refers to returning the community to its pre-event condition.

PHASE 1: MITIGATION

The first phase of emergency management, mitigation, refers to activities to lessen the severity and impact of a terrorist event. Mitigation begins by identifying potential hazards that may affect the organization or the demand for its services. This is followed by a vulnerability analysis of risk for such an event and finally the implementation of a strategy to address these areas of vulnerability. Mitigation efforts serve as the basis for all other activities relative to emergency management.

Hazard Identification

The first task associated with mitigation efforts is the *identification of potential emergency events* that can reasonably be expected to occur within a given community or hospital facility. All-hazards planning begins with the creation of a comprehensive list of all possible disasters. Potential hazards may be grouped into three categories: natural events, technological failures, and human threats. *Natural* hazards are defined by the location of the community. Examples include hurricanes, tornadoes, severe thunderstorms, earthquakes, tidal waves, temperature extremes, drought, flood, wildfire, landslide, volcano, and seasonal or sporadic disease spread. *Technological* hazards are disruptions in public service and determined by the population density and socioeconomic conditions of the surrounding community. Examples include *utility failure,* such as water, sewer, electricity, natural gas, steam, fuel, communications, and information systems; *transportation failure,* such as rail, subway, airplane, shipping, and trucking; and *structural disruption,* such as buildings, roadways, and bridges. The age of the municipality, its rate of growth, and its geographical location help identify these hazards. *Human* hazards can include both intentional and unintentional acts. Examples include civil disturbances, hostage situations, bomb threats, VIP situations, hazardous materials spills, mass casualty incidents, and explosive, chemical, biological, and radiological threats.

Vulnerability Analysis: Probability, Magnitude, and Resources

The JCAHO requires that response plans identify "direct and indirect" effects that hazards may have on the hospital. *Hazard vulnerability analysis* (HVA) is the second step in mitigation efforts. Based on the probability and magnitude of hazards, resource allocations may need to address prevention *activities.* When assessing the *probability* of an event, issues to consider may include geography, weather variations, disaster patterns, demographics, migration patterns, topography, endemic and seasonal disease patterns, local businesses, national landmarks, and high-profile events. The *magnitude* of an event may be determined by considering the human impact, the property impact, and the business impact.

The assessment of *resources* for handling the event involves an estimate of the hospital's capacity such as numbers of beds, number of respiratory ventilators, number of decontamination suits, and capability such as the service acuity level and sophistication of personnel, advanced technological resources, and advanced training. Resources can

be *internal,* such as bed capacity, workforce capability, currency of training status, insurance, and availability of backup systems, and *external,* including health care facilities, private business, mutual aid, vendor supply agreements, and so on. Most HVA templates focus on "common" hazards to establish priorities for protective countermeasures. Each category of vulnerability—probability, magnitude and resources—is described in semiquantitative terms: low, moderate, high, or not applicable (7,8).

Hospitals themselves may become terrorist targets. Contemporary ethical standards dictate that institutions of health and rescue be protected against attack. Precisely because it is considered unethical to attack such a facility, they are at high risk for becoming a target of terrorism. Hospital preparedness efforts must take this grim reality into account and search for vulnerabilities. Potential interventions include target hardening (distance, physical barriers, firewalls); security visibility (signage, security patrols, surveillance cameras); controlled vehicular and pedestrian access (traffic separation, selective searches, use of passkeys, "smart" entry portals, video monitors); and employee awareness (education, training, drills).

Tools to Assess Hospital Preparedness

Several hospital questionnaires exist. One example is the AHRQ-HRSA Bioterrorism Emergency Planning and Preparedness Questionnaire for Healthcare Facilities, which is currently for bioterrorism only but is likely to be expanded to include other major forms of terrorism preparedness (33). The Hospital Emergency Analysis Tool (HEAT) is used by the Navy Medicine Office of Homeland Security and documents the status of 100 critical preparedness factors (32). These tools help not only in assessing the status of a health care facility but also can provide direction to administrators and physician and nursing leaders.

The Emergency Operations Plan

The final step in mitigation involves the *emergency operations plan* (EOP). This document describes how the hospital intends to behave during an event, bringing hospital services and departments into one incident-focused organization. The EOP requires annual revision based on changes in the local community, newly identified vulnerabilities, and on the lessons learned from exercises and drills. Many templates for EOPs exist in health care (11,12). The EOP must take into account the requirements of regulatory and accreditation agencies, professional standards, and current best practices of emergency planning. This plan addresses four key issues: (a) *life safety* refers to the protection of personnel, patients, visitors, and the public from injury and life threats; (b) *property protection* refers to the prevention or limitation of structural damage; (c) *continuity of operations* refers to protection of critical hospital functions; and (d) *environmental protection* refers to the prevention or limitation of adverse effects on vegetation, animals, land, air, and water.

The basic EOP defines command and control, lines of communications, life safety, property protection, community outreach, recovery and restoration, and administration and logistics. Departments should be assigned roles that closely mimic their typical operations. During a disaster event, operations may be limited to only mission-critical activities.

Based on the HVA, all high-risk events will have an *hazard-specific appendix* in the EOP that defines the relevant mitigation, preparedness, response, and recovery activities. *Standard operating procedures* delineate the major activities common to all emergency responses. These include command and control, communications, personnel, supply procurement, and mutual aid.

PHASES 2 AND 3: PREPAREDNESS AND RESPONSE

The second phase of emergency management, *preparedness,* refers to the activities designed to increase response readiness to vulnerabilities. *Response,* the third phase of emergency management, refers to the mobilization of resources to meet the hospital's and community's needs during an incident. Comprehensive preparedness and response for hospitals encompasses 22 critical elements (13–17) (Table 24-1). Although an in-depth discussion of each element is beyond the scope of this chapter, an overview of the important aspects is presented.

Incident Command

The incident command system (ICS) is that portion of the EOP that relates to the authority structure and control of personnel, facilities, equipment, and communications during an event. The ICS remains operational until the requirements for its operation no longer exist. It unfolds in a modular fashion and is scalable, depending on the type and size of an incident.

Five management sectors are described for ICS: Command, Operations, Planning, Logistics, and Finance. *Command* responsibilities are an executive function designed to develop, direct, and maintain a viable organization and to coordinate with other entities. The highest level of authority rests with the incident commander (IC), who, in turn, is supported

TABLE 24-1	Critical Elements of Preparedness and Responses
Incident command	Bed availability/surge capacity
Interagency coordination	Pathology laboratory
Response	Security
Treatment logistics	Supplies
Decontamination	Equipment
Morgue capabilities	Services
Epidemiology/surveillance	Facility management
Personnel management	Contingencies
Mental health resources	Education and training
Communications systems	Exercises
Media/public information	Demobilization

by the public information officer, the safety officer, and the liaison officer. These individuals assist and advise the IC relative to issues concerning the media, safety, and external agencies. Policy, objectives, and priorities are set by Command. *Operations* identifies the doers in the organization, where the real work of incident control is accomplished. Operations carry out directions of the Command sector. The *Planning* sector provides past, present, and future information about the incident. Real-time incident reports are utilized to support the Command and Operations sectors. The Operations and Planning sectors work together to meet established incident objectives. The *Logistics* sector identifies and obtains all personnel, equipment, supplies, and services required for the incident. Operations and Planning sectors then manage these resources. Finally, the *Finance* sector is a staff function responsible for the financial management and accountability of the incident. Extensive resources are available to assist in preparing a hospital ICS (17–19).

The Hospital Emergency Incident Command System (HEICS) is a preexisting plan that can be adapted to individual hospitals. HEICS is free of charge and has been adapted by many U.S. hospitals. Many of the components are available on the Internet, and conferences exist to orient new users and assist them in adapting the system to their health care facility (19). It provides an authority structure and job descriptions designed for hospitals, incorporating many of the principles already discussed. HEICS provides for an incident commander who is supported by at least four chiefs, operating over sections: Logistics, Planning, Finance, and Operations. The program has a preformatted organizational chart and job descriptions that can be applied to an individual hospital. A glossary of terms is provided so all participants communicate with a common language.

Interagency Coordination

Hospitals are key participants in the response to terrorist events and so must work seamlessly with local government officials, emergency managers, law enforcement, fire/rescue services, emergency medical services, public health officials, and other health care providers.

Interagency coordination may be seen as occurring along three simultaneous axes (15). One axis involves the *sequential* response that is conducted in the region where the threat occurs, from event identification, law enforcement, hazardous materials response, on-scene triage, prehospital care and transportation, hospital services, and ultimately recovery. A second axis, which is often forgotten in planning and response, involves the *parallel* coordination of other organizations, facilities, or providers that offer similar services as the hospital, such as other hospitals, outpatient clinics, and physician offices. The third axis involves the coordination of *remote* resources separated from the incident either in time or distance. Mutual aid agreements that delineate the role and responsibility for each agency will assure a consistent, coordinated, graduated response.

Response

Response begins with event recognition. The rapidity of recognition depends on the type of weapon utilized, the event location, and the method of dispersal. Explosive and incendiary events become manifest immediately, chemical events typically unfold over minutes or hours, and biological events will usually become evident only after an incubation period of days, weeks, or even months. Biological attacks, in particular, require regionwide surveillance, unusual event reporting, laboratory analyses, and sentinel case investigation.

The first priority in a terrorism attack is to secure the hospital physical plant and to protect personnel, current patients, and visitors. Another priority is to establish sites for victim reception and identification. Simple, rapid identification processes that facilitate ongoing and continuous patient tracking are most desirable. Use of encoded wrist bands, such as those widely used in industry (bar codes, infrared, radio frequency) are under evaluation for use in mass population settings. If victims are contaminated, decontamination and securing of valuables will be necessary.

The participants in the regional health care community should agree on a simple, unified system for patient classification and a way to standardize the initial treatment irrespective of which hospital receives the patient. The equitable and rational distribution of all patients dictates the use of all capable treatment facilities. Medical protocols consistent with current medical standards are utilized for each case. The various chapters in this book provide a solid foundation for such preparation.

Treatment Logistics

Treatment logistics involve placing patients with similar levels of exposure and symptomatology in the appropriate treatment setting. Predesignated locations within or near the hospital may be utilized if bed capacity is limited or absent. Military models for alternative health care facilities may provide ideas for the civilian medical community (20). The accessibility of regional and federal resources for additional hospital bed capacity should be determined early in the event. Community assets, such as sports arenas, school gymnasiums, hotels, or places of religious worship, may serve as holding or observation areas. Such facilities are especially appropriate for those who require minimal care. The public should be informed of the purpose of these treatment sites and where to find them. All treatment sites must provide a safe environment as well as privacy and hygiene. Self-care within individuals' private dwellings, such as homes, apartments, and hotels, is sometimes an option.

Decontamination

Health care facilities must possess a decontamination area, supplies, and adequately trained personnel (Chapter 29). The location of the decontamination unit may be internal or external to the hospital; however, it should be readily available and not disrupt routine operations. *Internal* decontamination facilities have the advantage of providing protection from inclement weather. Disadvantages include the risk of allowing contaminated patients to enter the hospital, the need for specialized vapor and ventilating systems, and a limitation in the numbers of patients it may accommodate. *External* decontamination facilities prevent contaminated patients from entering the hospital and allow for large patient volumes. Disadvantages include difficulty in controlling weather extremes and lighting conditions and inherent delay in setup.

The management of decontamination effluent is a difficult issue because most hospitals do not possess the ability to store contaminated wastewater. Although the discharge of contaminated water into sewer systems is technically in violation of the Comprehensive Environmental Response, Compensation, and Liability Act (CERCLA), there are indications that the inspector general of the Environmental Protection Agency (EPA) may not pursue legal action against response agencies that violate this act during disaster response.

The EPA and Occupational Safety and Health Administration (OSHA) both have regulations that help protect personnel dealing with hazardous substances and emergency response operations. Hospital planners are encouraged to review pertinent EPA, OSHA, and JCAHO requirements. Recent documents and articles in the medical literature discuss pertinent regulations, training requirements, and team selection, as well as decontamination equipment and evidence collection (21–23).

Morgue Capabilities

Disasters have the potential to produce catastrophic numbers of fatalities (24). Management of mass fatalities is discussed in greater detail in Chapter 43. If the incident involves criminal intent and victim contamination, this poses additional layers of complexity for pathologists, medical examiners, coroners, and morgue personnel. Effective planning and response must address these key issues:

1. Scalable capacity and capability
2. Protection of personnel
3. Victim identification
4. Determination of the manner and cause of death
5. Collection of forensic evidence
6. Death notification
7. Disposition of victim remains

Epidemiology/Surveillance

Epidemiology identifies, defines, and tracks an incident. Surveillance is discussed in greater detail in Chapter 30.

Personnel Management

The most important asset for an effective disaster response lies with the hospital personnel. A plan is required to notify on-duty personnel of a disaster event. In addition, a mechanism for the staged (staggered) recall of off-duty personnel, or those with unique job functions, must be clearly delineated.

Staff augmentation is addressed in a variety of ways, including extending the work hours for those presently on duty and calling in supplemental staff. It should be recognized that many health care workers hold a second job at another health care facility. This two-hat syndrome means that some employees may not be able to respond to the hospital's emergency request for additional personnel. In addition, it is acknowledged that the fear and uncertainty generated by a terrorist event may cause some employees not to respond to requests for work because family care issues may take precedence. Hospital leadership should consider alternative sources for personnel such as the Red Cross, Salvation Army, visiting nurse agencies, and physician offices. Other resources may include hospital personnel from adjacent, uninvolved states or regions or the federal medical assets including the Disaster Medical Assistance Team (DMAT). All nonemployee health care personnel must provide proof of licensure and be credentialed by the hospital prior to a disaster event.

Mental Health Resources

Mental health counseling is an important aspect of preparedness, response, and recovery from disaster events (25). These services should be made available to victims, health care personnel, emergency responders from all disciplines, and the community at large. This topic is discussed in greater detail in Chapter 40.

Communications Systems

Communications problems are among the most commonly cited shortfalls during any disaster response. These failures arise from the unreliable nature of wire-based and cellular telephones and the incompatible radio frequencies when using hand-held radios. In addition to these significant hardware problems, many communications failures occur as a result of people problems. There must be an agreed-upon terminology that is mutually understood by all parties (16). Health facility communications methods are discussed in detail in Chapter 31.

Media/Public Information Management

Disasters create a demand for public information. Planned and structured arrangements for communication throughout the incident are critical components of hospital and community preparedness. Assistance with media issues using a comprehensive risk communications plan is available from the Department of Health and Human Services (26). Interaction with various elements of the media is discussed in Chapter 32.

Bed Availability/Surge Capacity

Surge capacity encompasses the need for additional patient beds and also available space for triage, management, vaccination, decontamination, friends and relatives, or for those victims waiting to be seen. If alternative sites for patient care are being used, it is important to consider the personnel, medications, and equipment that will be necessary to care for patients in these areas. The legal capacity to deliver health care under situations that exceed authorized capacity should be considered in planning (27).

Augmentation of hospital bed capacity may be accomplished by expedient discharge of patients, cancellation of elective admissions or surgeries, transfer of patients to hospitals out of the disaster area, and placing additional beds in private rooms or hallways. Expansion to sites remote from the hospital requires extensive preplanning and may include school auditoriums, sports arenas, or hotels. Alternatively, open land or large parking lots may be turned into temporary field hospitals.

One option to assist with surge capacity is the Modular Emergency Medical System (MEMS) of the U.S. Department of Defense. This program provides a strategy to allow local health care facilities to respond to a large-scale incident (28). The system includes four modules, all managed under a unified command structure. The components include the Acute Care Center (ACC), the Neighborhood Emergency Help Center (NEHC), the Community Outreach (CO) module, and the Casualty Transportation System (CTS). Initial intake of patients into the system is through the NEHC, and a tiered-care approach is used to distribute minimal care victims to the CO, moderate care patients to the NEHC, patients needing hospital care to the ACC, and intensive care patients to existing medical facilities. Because the system is modular, it is both robust and scalable. Transfer of patients between sites is accomplished by the CTS.

The equitable and appropriate distribution of casualties among all available medical facilities by on-scene prehospital care providers and the use of broadcast public service announcements indicating which hospitals are nearing capacity will often avert the need for individual hospitals to invoke surge contingencies. However, this is not always possible, as in the case of chemical or biological casualties in which most patients are likely to choose the destination hospital independent of EMS.

Pathology Laboratory

Clinical and anatomical pathology testing are critical. The diagnosis of the sentinel (first) case and the collection of evidence may involve hospital laboratory personnel and staff. In the limited, moderate-sized incident, the process for test ordering, specimen collection and identification, and processing should not differ from routine practice. Some facilities may choose to utilize color-coded patient identification bands, specimen labels, and requisitions so as to expedite the throughput for these samples. Test volumes may temporarily increase as the first victims arrive at the facility. To facilitate early diagnosis, the laboratory may designate these assays as a priority, perhaps limiting or temporarily suspending the testing of nonaffected patients.

Novel toxicology and microbiological tests may be necessary to arrive at a diagnosis, and close coordination with local public health officials will facilitate proper epidemiological surveillance and investigative activities. Confirmatory testing by appropriate public health laboratories may be needed, and secure specimen transport procedures must be assured. If the agent in question requires special culturing techniques, or is especially dangerous, procedures must be in place to assure proper specimen collection, handling, and transport to the closest appropriate laboratory facility.

Security

Security is a vital aspect of preparedness and response. A guide for security-enhancing activities that are aligned with the five color-coded Homeland Security Advisory System (HSAS) levels has been developed by the U.S. Fire Administration's (USFA) Emergency Management and Response-Information Sharing and Analysis Center (EMR-ISAC). This document offers specific recommendations for security of information, facilities, personnel, and operations (29). Of paramount importance is the facility's coordination of these activities with local law enforcement agencies and security firms. During terrorist events, medical facilities may become targets of attack.

Hospital security planning and response must address perimeter management, personnel security, patient security, and resource security. *Perimeter management* (external traffic flow) involves controlling access to the facility and the surrounding hospital properties by vehicles and foot traffic. The use of monitored barricades at driveways and intersections serves to limit vehicular access. Cordoned walkways and locking of all hospital exits and entrances, with officers positioned at predetermined entry points, provide scrutiny for ambulatory traffic. Movement and activities of people within the facility (internal traffic flow) should be monitored by periodic security sweeps. Prior to the event, picture identification badges are distributed to all mission-critical *hospital employees and staff*. Specific points of entry should be designated for employees only. Separate patient access sites are located away from employee entrances. Security officers may use voice amplification devices, and media broadcasts may be used to discourage loitering and direct patients and employees to specific and separate access points. *Patient security* may involve the use of scanning portals or wand devices. If the incident involves the potential for contamination, all officers on the perimeter should wear PPE. *Resource security* involves procedures to protect supplies, hazardous materials, and equipment from tampering and diversion. Access to the facility from emergency vehicles and supply trucks must be closely monitored so these areas are not the source of an incursion.

Supplies and Equipment

It is recognized that the adequacy of existing hospital supplies and equipment may be problematic because current economic restrictions and storage limitations promote just-in-time inventories. Also, supplies and equipment may differ widely depending on the nature of the incident. Therefore it is not practical to cache a vast inventory of every potential supply item or equipment that may be needed. It is necessary, however, for every facility to maintain a 24-hour supply of all reasonably expected supplies and equipment, to allow for the rapid treatment of the first wave of casualties.

Several principles guide hospitals to ensure that adequate supplies and equipment are available for novel or large-volume incidents. These include inventory control, procurement, and donations. Prior to an event, an inventory must be determined and scrupulously maintained. Tracking of infrequently used supplies and pharmaceuticals is necessary to address shelf life and stock rotation. Automatic notification systems may identify when items are nearing reorder thresholds. During an event, it is necessary to track supplies and equipment from request through use. Acquisition methods are best established in advance of an incident. Vendor agreements for rapid resupply and shared inventory agreements with adjacent medical facilities are essential. Solicited and unsolicited donations in all forms may come from businesses and individuals. Such offers may include clothing, money, mobile phones, medical supplies, pharmaceuticals, and equipment. Guidelines for the tracking, use, return/disposal, and acknowledgment of these resources are necessary.

Services

During protracted or high-volume incidents, a modification in staffing patterns may be necessary. This may involve an increase in the numbers of staff, a prolongation in the work shift, and a need for overnight staff housing. At the same time, patient throughput and census may drastically increase. These events will likely increase the utilization of food, housekeeping, laundry, maintenance, and security. Managers and employees in each hospital department must be involved in the planning and response to disaster incidents so as to be able to meet the increase in service needs.

Facility Management

Effective event planning and response require that basic utilities to the hospital complex continue uninterrupted. Electricity, fuel, water, sewer, telephone systems, and air and water filtration systems are critical assets that must remain operational. Because terrorists may choose to target hospitals and their critical assets, these systems must be secured and monitored. Redundancy in each of these utilities is mandatory, and in the event of primary failure, secondary systems should be immediately available. Disaster exercises should test both the security and the operation of redundant contingencies.

Contingencies for the potential use of chemical and biological agents should address the safe storage, handling, and disposal of hazardous waste materials. In particular, the containment and disposal of runoff from decontamination activities should be determined in concert with local officials. The Agency for Toxic Substances and Disease Registry (ATSDR) provides a three-volume series of resources for health care providers in regard to the handling of hazardous materials (30). The National Institute for Occupational Safety and Health (NIOSH) has published a document on the protection of buildings from airborne chemical, biological, or radiological attacks (31). A number of government and regulatory bodies (CDC, OSHA, EPA, and JCAHO) provide hospitals with additional guidance. Professional organizations such as the American Society for Healthcare Engineers (ASHE), the American College of Healthcare Architects (ACHA), and the National Fire Protection Association (NFPA) are other sources of assistance.

Contingencies

Contingencies are activities that (a) predict potential disruptions or shortfalls in mission-critical supplies, (b) prevent delays or disruptions in supply lines and bed capacity, and (c) procure needed assets via novel alternative routes. Maintaining a sufficient number of hospital beds may involve moving the patients to an adjacent treatment area on the same floor (horizontal evacuation) or to another floor (vertical evacuation). In extreme situations, an incident may require that patients be completely removed from the hospital. Specific circumstances that require an evacuation must be clearly defined, and policies and procedures for carrying out these plans must be developed. Afterward, nursing and ancillary staff must be trained in the necessary procedures, followed by drills or exercises to ensure response readiness. Once evacuation is begun, methods to transport and track the location of both patients and staff must be used.

Communicable diseases may require the quarantine, isolation, or sheltering-in-place of individuals or groups of patients. Most medical facilities are limited in the number and types of isolation beds. Identifying specific disease entities and activating mass isolation, quarantine, or sheltering-in-place plans must be done preemptively.

Effective contingency planning must anticipate the potential for partial or total disruption in the supply chain for medical/surgical supplies, pharmaceuticals, cleaning supplies, maintenance supplies, linens, and food services. Memorandums of understanding between the hospital and vendors to provide necessary supplies are encouraged. Other hospitals may experience similar shortages and may be relying on the same local vendors for resupply of scarce resources.

Education, Training, and Exercises

Effective response to terrorist events is built on a foundation of knowledgeable, trained, and practiced local health care professionals. The education of health care providers and the development of drills and exercises is discussed at length in Chapter 33. Health care providers must learn of potential terrorist weapons, be able to diagnose unusual disease patterns or clinical findings, and know how to practice appropriate surveillance, reporting, and treatment. *It is critical that medical personnel be trained to protect themselves* from contamination, so they do not also become victims.

Exercises are conducted to evaluate an organization's capability to execute its response or contingency plan. The personnel, plans, procedures, facilities, and equipment must be exercised and tested on a regular basis. The exercise process is a continuous process that includes planning, training, exercising, and evaluation (32,33) (Fig. 24-1). Various exercise types are listed in Table 24-2 (33).

TABLE 24-2	Exercise Types
Seminars	Functional exercises
Workshops	Full-scale exercises
Tabletop exercises	Command post exercises
Games	Operations center exercises
Drills	Case studies

The three most commonly utilized exercise models are the tabletop, functional, and full-scale exercises. The *tabletop exercise* usually involves senior staff, elected officials, and other key staff with emergency management responsibilities gathering in an informal conference room setting to discuss simulated emergency situations. This type of exercise is intended to stimulate discussion of various issues concerning a hypothetical situation and the plans, policies and procedures or systems for response and recovery efforts. Participants focus on coordination, assignment of responsibilities, postevent mitigation priorities, and similar issues. The *functional exercise* is designed to test individual capabilities, multiple functions, or activities within a function. Exercise activities are usually under a time constraint, and an evaluation or critique is normally held at the end of the exercise. The functional exercise usually takes place in an operations center, field environment, or a combination of the two. A typical functional exercise might be designed to test and evaluate the evacuation and relocation of a hospital's emergency department. The *full-scale exercise* is used to evaluate the operational capabilities of emergency management systems. Actual mobilization of personnel and resources is required to demonstrate coordination, response, and recovery capability. This is the largest and most complex of the three types of exercises and may involve the participation of response agencies at the local, state, regional, and federal levels. A typical full-scale exercise involves multiple hospitals, the fire service, emergency medical services, law enforcement, city emergency planners, and public health.

Drills are utilized to develop, test, and maintain responder skills in a single emergency response procedure or task. For example, the hospital decontamination team may participate in a drill on donning, use, and doffing of PPE.

Demobilization

Demobilization describes a variety of actions that transition command, planning, operations, logistics, and finance functions back to normal operations. During demobilization, departmental functions are assessed, consumed resources and assets are accounted for, assets are returned to their original location, documentation is completed, and incident review and debriefing are conducted. Rapid return to normal operations will allow the hospital to be ready for either a secondary event or another unrelated incident. Rehabilitation of facilities, equipment, and personnel is also conducted at this stage, so as to promote completion and closure.

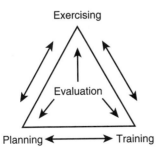

Figure 24–1. Exercise process as a component of hospital preparedness.

PHASE 4: RECOVERY

The fourth and final phase of emergency management, recovery, refers to the mobilization of support operations that work toward returning the facility and the community to its pre-event condition. These activities and processes are directed at restoring essential services and resuming normal operations.

Finance

Hospitals should seek financial reimbursement from government agencies for unrecoverable costs associated with providing care under disaster conditions. Effective pre-event documentation of all resources and assets may serve as a baseline for comparison with postevent conditions, which may improve reimbursement levels. Accurate and detailed records describing patient care activities during the event may include personnel, equipment, supplies, pharmaceuticals, and acuity levels. These may often be remunerated via standard medical billing processes. If prolonged hazard abatement, restoration activities, or damage/loss hampers the resumption of normal operations, loss of revenue may be claimed and financial relief may be sought. Preservation of records is essential because billing reimbursement, liability, malpractice, and insurance claims often require records retention for specific time frames.

Facility Recovery

Facility recovery involves inspection of the physical plant, hazard removal and abatement, and decontamination. Declarations that the facility is structurally sound and hazard free by qualified agencies may be necessary to restore public confidence. Disposal of solid waste, garbage, and decontamination runoff should adhere to local sanitary regulations so as to maintain environmental integrity. Materials and patient belongings contaminated with infectious biological agents must be sanitized and preserved for legal evidence. A complete inventory of consumables and resupply, salvage of damaged assets, servicing of utilities and equipment, and physical plant restoration and renovation may also be necessary.

Personnel and Psychological Considerations

Critical incident stress debriefing should be offered to anyone involved in the response. In addition, facilities should offer group and individual counseling services, family support programs, and employee assistance programs (Chapter 40). All employees involved in the response should be enrolled in a health surveillance program. Because some chemical and biological exposures may result in delayed or chronic effects, surveillance may continue for years. Government agencies such as the ATSDR may assist facilities with these ongoing surveillance activities.

All personnel should participate in after-action assessments. These incident reviews consist of the objective analysis of pertinent response information to produce "lessons learned." Based on these lessons, modifications in procedures, assignments, equipment, training, and personnel may contribute to improved response capability for future events.

SUMMARY

Hospital preparedness involves a concerted effort by administrators and physician and nursing leaders to plan for a wide spectrum of possible disaster situations. Various prepackaged systems exist that can assist a hospital administration with the development of a disaster plan.

Disaster preparedness is not a onetime activity. To be truly effective, readiness requires a rigorous and ongoing commitment of time, personnel, and resources. Done correctly, the process of mitigation, preparedness, response, and recovery requires a collaborative effort within the hospital and also from many facets of the community including law enforcement, fire service, emergency medical service, hospitals, public health, city officials, emergency managers, and business/industry.

Hospitals must work to achieve consensus within the community. There should be effective collaboration among the different health care systems and public health agencies in order to organize and strengthen counterterrorism measures. If readiness efforts are not cooperative, widespread, and comprehensive, institutions working in isolation are not likely to reduce community morbidity and mortality during a terrorist event (Table 24-3).

TABLE 24-3 Hospital Preparedness Summary Table

HOSPITAL PREPAREDNESS SUMMARY TABLE

1. Utilize the four-phase model for emergency management to assure a comprehensive approach, including: mitigation, preparedness, response, and recovery.
2. Define where you currently stand; perform a hazard vulnerability analysis (HVA). Consider the use of existing hospital survey tools.
3. Do not plan in isolation; coordinate with police, fire, EMS, public health, city officials, emergency planners, and business.
4. Maximize efficiency and economies of scale by planning in concert with all hospitals within the community.

■ Case Study

Hospital Preparedness for Disaster: The Israeli Experience

Moshe Michaelson, Gila Hyams, and Daniel C. Keyes

Introduction

It will be no surprise to the reader that in recent years, Israeli physicians, nurses, and EMS personnel have gained a large body of experience dealing with caring for the victims of suicide bombings. The first such bombing in Israel occurred in 1993. There have been almost 10,000 people injured in these bombing attacks since then. With the start of the current wave of violence in 2002, referred to as the Al Aqsa intifada, the violence has been particularly intense. As a result of these more recent 145 suicide bomber attacks, 307 Israelis have died and 2,235 were injured (35).

One organization, Hamas, is attributed with the largest proportion of the bombings. The late Salah Shehada, a former Hamas leader, described in an interview the sophisticated approach used for planning these attacks. The strategic methodology begins by video surveillance of potential targets. After several sites are selected, logistical coordinators, explosive experts, and transportation specialists design the attack. Subsequently, a committee selects the target and a bomber is recruited who is psychologically prepared to carry out the suicidal explosive event (36). The objective of each attack is to kill and injure as many individuals as possible, and the improvised devices are carefully prepared with shrapnel. The attackers seek out crowds in markets, cafés, and other such venues to increase the number of casualties from the blast.

To respond to this wave of explosive terrorism, the government and the health care community together have forged a sophisticated system of response, involving the preparation of personnel at the hospital and prehospital levels and the enhancement of equipment and infrastructure. The discussion that follows provides a brief description of a typical hospital response plan.

The Israeli System of Hospital Response

A *mass casualty incident* (MCI) is defined as a situation in which the need for treatment exceeds the resources. In such a critical situation, the most important shortage of resources is typically personnel (doctors and nurses) and equipment. An analogy may be made between a MCI and a military ambush. In both, a crisis occurs rapidly, without forewarning, and when least expected. In both of these situations, the most effective solution is an "automatic response." This rapid, coordinated response takes a lot of planning and exercise before it becomes truly automatic. The key to success in an MCI is prior preparation and the development of realistic drills.

A *limited mass casualty* (LMC) event refers to the situation in an individual hospital that receives a smaller, more controlled volume of patients following an event, such as when patients are divided among several hospitals. With a properly functioning EMS system, each hospital receives a more limited number of patients through on-scene triage and allocation of victims to various hospitals. This type of allocation is especially possible in the case of explosive or other trauma terrorist events, but it may be more difficult for large chemical terrorism events, for example, in which large numbers of victims are expected to bypass EMS. When it is properly executed, an efficient distribution of the wounded among acute care facilities allows for the optimal care of victims. The actual number of victims that defines an LMC event depends on the size of the specific receiving hospital and the emergency department (ED), but may typically be on the order of 20 to 25 patients in a larger institution. In the Israeli setting, a more specific definition of LMC has evolved: *If the number of victims is suffi-*

ciently small that all patients can be triaged within the ED itself, this is considered an LMC. Limiting the number of victims sent to each hospital is important because in such an LMC all victims can be treated on the usual aggressive scale that occurs in a typical trauma center. The expectant category of triage is usually not necessary in an LMC because all of the necessary hospital resources are applicable to each of the victims, no matter how seriously ill they are upon presentation. An experienced hospital administrator makes the determination of whether a specific incident qualifies as an MCI or LMC. This decision will impact various aspects of the hospital response, including which personnel are called in to the hospital.

Hospital Preparation

One of the first steps in preparation for *MCIs* is to write guidelines. The most important feature of this plan is the organization of the hospital to deliver critical medical treatment. The treatment given in an MCI is not the usual care provided on a daily basis in a hospital but rather the *minimal acceptable* intervention that is readily available. Guidelines are then adapted for use in every hospital into written standing orders and even into specific medical orders.

In Israel, the Ministry of Health (MOH) undertakes the coordination of guideline development. The Emergency Division of the MOH creates guidelines that must be applied to every acute care hospital. There is a specific committee for each type of mass casualty, including trauma, chemical, and biological. These MOH committees design template guidelines for use by hospitals. After final approval by the MOH, the guidelines are then distributed to the administration of each health care facility. They then create guidelines for their institution, usually through the establishment of a hospital disaster committee. These individual hospital plans are then sent back to the MOH, who gives them final approval. The MOH also mandates annual drills for each hospital that are carried out in conjunction with the Home Front branch of the Israeli Defense Forces. These drills are compulsory and financed by the Ministry of Health. The Emergency Division of the Ministry of Health develops educational programs to teach guideline implementation.

Hospital Guidelines

Each hospital administration appoints a chair and key staff members to participate on a hospital mass casualty committee. Typically one individual is in charge of each type of disaster, including chemical, biological, trauma, and nuclear events. In larger hospitals, one nurse is employed full time to coordinate disaster preparedness. Due to the typical methodology used to injure the public, the Israeli philosophy is that trauma is the basis of all MCI. Other types of disaster build on the trauma experience and modify their plans according to the type of incident. A chemical incident, for example, would require very different triage, decontamination, and treatment approaches than would an explosive trauma event (Chapter 1).

Guidelines should be simple, clearly expressed, and allow flexibility so individual hospitals can adjust to their own conditions. Some basic characteristics of guideline development merit special attention. These include triage, equipment, documentation, operations, and medical treatment.

Triage

Effective triage is the key to success in MCI. Various techniques of triage have become popular in recent years, but ultimately patients are divided into three groups: (a) the *immediate group*: patients who need urgent attention in order to sustain life or to prevent serious disability; (b) the *delayed group*: patients who can wait for further evaluation without serious threat to life or disability; (c) the *expectant group*: patients who are so critically injured that even in a normal situation they have little chance of survival.

It may seem intuitive that the physician in charge (PIC) of an MCI should perform triage directly on arriving patients. However, experience has taught that it is preferable for the PIC *not* to perform triage directly. This is because it is too easy for the PIC to lose the critical global perspective of the event. This role is usually performed by a physician (not the PIC) working in tandem with a nurse.

After triage, victims are sent to different sites based on their category. This allows for allocation of most doctors and nurses to the area of greatest need, the immediate group. The immediate patient group is best located in the ED so treatment can be initiated as soon as triage and decontamination (if necessary) are completed.

Equipment

As the number of casualties becomes large, a shortage of equipment develops. As such, a surplus should be stored in advance. The storage room should be in close proximity to the ED, locked, and properly secured (Fig. 24-2). The system used in Israel consists of medical supply carts clearly marked so they can be transferred to the appropriate site in the ED. There is a checklist for each cart and for all equipment. A label posted on the wall of the ED matches the label on the cart so it may be placed in the appropriate predetermined location, allowing for a very rapid and orderly distribution of equipment. The list of equipment, medical supplies, and the specific sites for lo-

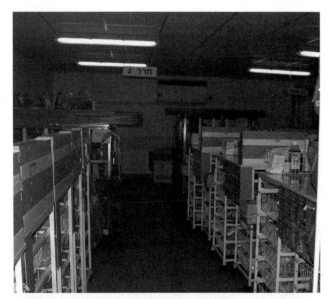

Figure 24–2. Storeroom for equipment used in mass casualty incidents. The facility is located near the ED. Signs on each cart match signs posted in the predetermined location where the equipment in that cart will be needed.

cating them should be decided in conjunction with the entire staff. In larger hospitals there is one nurse in charge of conducting a thorough review of the available equipment on one day each week. This includes ensuring that medications are not expired and are in proper condition.

Documentation

During mass casualty situations, proper identification and documentation is often quite difficult. It is important to develop special documentation for use specifically in this type of incident. Charts should be numbered in advance. Each arriving patient is given a file with a number. The patient is identified by number only. Misidentification is greatly lessened by this approach. Unconscious patients are also photographed with a digital camera. Experience in explosive terrorism has dictated that *documentation templates*, which prompt each nurse and physician to document specific critical information, should be used for MCI. Otherwise documentation is incomplete and inaccurate. The use of "open charts" and free-form documentation is not effective.

Surgical Infrastructure and Personnel

During a traumatic MCI, the number of functioning operating theaters is constant and so are the number of surgeons, nurses, and surgical support staff. Personnel are also needed for treatment at the units and wards where patients are admitted. In an MCI, inefficient use of these facilities may occur unless careful selection is implemented. A guideline should be created for prioritizing types of surgery, which surgeries must be performed acutely, and which can be safely delayed. The immediate operations should be just those that are lifesaving. Examples include patients with hemodynamic instability, torso injuries, or patients with major vascular injuries. All other surgeries should be delayed until the MCI ends and no other patients are expected to arrive. If these procedures are not followed, the operating room may become overwhelmed with nonemergency interventions, and inevitably patients who require lifesaving procedures will not receive the proper and immediate attention.

Nursing trauma case managers keep a checklist to track each patient by place and name. The checklist verifies that each patient has a name tag, the vital signs are recorded, results of the Focused Assessment with Sonography for Trauma (FAST) scan are noted, chart documentation has been completed, and each patient is accompanied by a nurse or physician prior to leaving the ED. The *nursing coordinator* also keeps a dynamic checklist, to ensure overall integrity of the departmental flow. This ensures that personnel are in their proper position, the equipment is properly relocated after a patient leaves, and all key elements have been completed prior to a victim leaving the ED for the operating room (OR) or other destinations.

Treatment

The guidelines for treatment in everyday trauma are those established in Advanced Trauma Life Support (ATLS). With any treatment, only the essential, immediate care should be administered during the actual MCI. One relies more on physical examination during these incidents than radiographic evaluation or tomographic (CT) scans. All other radiographs are delayed until after the immediate phase of the MCI is over. Bedside FAST ultra-

TABLE 24-4	Characteristics of the Hospital Disaster Information Center

1. Distinct separate location: A place separate from the ED but in the hospital that will interface directly with relatives and others. This site should include private rooms and also have access to telephones and a computer link.
2. Publicized telephone numbers: Special telephone numbers are publicized in the media for the public to call to obtain information.
3. Personnel: The information center should be run by social workers who can provide counseling to families as well as information.
4. National hospital information link: A computerized regional linkage allows information about the victims to be available to all hospitals, so families do not have to go from hospital to hospital looking for their loved ones. This is done through the use of a shared computer network.

sound studies are particularly useful as a diagnostic tool to exclude bleeding in the peritoneal cavity because they are portable, efficient, and do not require extensive time in the radiology department.

Trauma MCIs are multidimensional in nature. *Victims of explosive injuries often have a combination of burns and of blunt and penetrating trauma, creating a unique pattern of injury.* In an LMC, all of these patients receive full-body CT. All x-rays are kept as hard copy and not just as computer screen images because the surgeons in the OR usually will need to look again at the radiographs.

Information Center
During an MCI, there is an important demand from the public for information. This will result in two major challenges: overloading of the phone system and crowding of the hospital with people looking for their relatives. To minimize the effect of these two events, an information center must be established. The characteristic features of the information center are listed in Table 24-4.

Initiation of Emergency Response and Staff Notification
Verification of an event and recruitment of personnel are important aspects of an MCI. All reports of incidents are verified simultaneously with the start of staff call-in. This is usually done by one of three methods: communication with Magen David Adom ambulance dispatch, contact of the police, or monitoring the dispatch radio. Simultaneous with the verification, preparations in the ED are begun.

All employees of the hospital have pagers issued by the hospital. There is a specific group designated for ED personnel. An preselected group of responders are called to come in to the hospital first. Triage emergency physicians, surgeons, and nurses from the ER are on this list. In an MCI, one nurse calls the predetermined group of core responders. As people arrive, a check-in list is created. Those who will stay and participate in the care of victims are given written instructions that remind them of the expectations of the post they will occupy (Table 24-5).

If too many staff members arrive, some are selected to leave and return later. Most often, sufficient staff is already present in the hospital at the outset of an event, so only a few additional personnel must be called in for assistance. Although it is sometimes asserted that often too many staff members present to the hospital immediately after an MCI, this has not been the Israeli experience. The general rule is that more people are called than are actually required because it is easier to downscale an event than ramp up the response after starting.

TABLE 24-5	Review Card Given to Arriving Hospital Personnel Prior to the Arrival of Victims

SIDE A: IMPORTANT INSTRUCTIONS

1. You must first check in with the head nurse.
2. You will be assigned to a specific post. Wait there until your patient arrives.
3. When a patient arrives, put an ID tag (prepared in advance) on the patient's hand and forehead.
4. Take vital signs and write them on the documentation. Sign all MD orders that are completed.
5. Make sure blood sample tubes for blood bank are signed by MD and properly identified with patient's number.
6. Undress the patient completely, then cover.
7. Put belongings into a bag and label with patient's number.
8. Upon completion of ED treatment, the patient must be accompanied by an MD and nurse to the next site (e.g., the operating room).
9. After completing the care of a patient, return all equipment to its proper location.
10. Wait for the next patient.

SIDE B: ATLS THRESHOLDS FOR NOTIFYING A PHYSICIAN, AND SO ON.

After the return to normal levels of care, emergency staff members gather initially for a debriefing session to discuss how the events unfolded and how departmental operations could be improved in the future. This discussion is recorded, and planners are able to use these ideas for updating and improving the existing plan.

The Israeli approach has been modified over the years, and it can be assumed that future adaptation will also be necessary. The basic principle remains the same: The health care response in a terrorist event is absolutely critical in improving the outcome of the victims. Planning, exercises, and reviewing the successes and failures for each incident are fundamental aspects to improving the care provided to the victims of such events.

REFERENCES

1. Federal Bureau of Investigation. Counterterrorism Threat Assessment and Warning Unit. Counterterrorism Division. Terrorism in the United States 1999. Web site: www.fbi.gov/publications/terror/terror99.pdf. Accessed April 15, 2004.

2. Hospital preparedness: most urban hospitals have emergency plans but lack certain capacities for bioterrorism response. United States General Accounting Office Report to Congressional Committees (GAO-03-924). Washington, DC, August 6, 2003.

3. HHS bioterrorism preparedness programs: states reported progress but fell short of program goals for 2002. United States General Accounting Office Report to Congressional Committees (GAO-04-360R). Washington, DC, February 10, 2004.

4. Treat KN, Williams JM, Furbee PM, et al. Hospital preparedness for weapons of mass destruction incidents: an initial assessment. Ann Emerg Med 2001;38(5):562-5.

5. Wetter DC, Daniell WE, Treser CD. Hospital preparedness for victims of chemical or biological terrorism. Am J Public Health 2001;91(5):710-16.

6. Barbera JA, Macintyre AG, DeAtley CA. Ambulances to nowhere: America's critical shortfall in medical preparedness for catastrophic terrorism. Belfer Center for Science and International Affairs Discussion Paper (BCSIA) 2001-15, Executive Session on Domestic Preparedness Discussion Paper (ESDP) 2001-07. John F. Kennedy School of Government, Harvard University, October 2001. Web site: http://bcsia.ksg.harvard.edu/BCSIA_content/documents/Ambulances_to_Nowhere.pdf. Accessed April 15, 2004.

7. McLaughlin, SB. Hazard vulnerability analysis. Healthcare Facilities Management Series, American Society for Healthcare Engineering (ASHE) of the American Hospital Association (AHA). Chicago, February 2001.

8. Hospital Capability Assessment for Readiness. Healthcare Association of Hawaii (HAH), Honolulu, 2001. Web site: http://www.HAH-Emergency.net. Accessed April 15, 2004.

9. AHRQ-HRSA Bioterrorism Emergency Planning and Preparedness Questionnaire for Healthcare Facilities. Web site: http://www.ahrq.gov/about/cpcr/bioterr.pdf. Accessed April 22, 2004.

10. Emergency Analysis Tool (HEAT). U.S. Navy Medical Office of Homeland Security. Web site: http://www.eaicorp.com/pubs/DVATX%20Article%20JEM.pdfHospital. Accessed April 22, 2004.

11. Emergency Management Program Guidebook. VHA Center for Engineering and Occupational Safety and Health in conjunction with the VHA Emergency Management Strategic Healthcare Group, Emergency Management Academy. Washington, DC, February 2002. Web site: http://www1.va.gov/emshg/apps/emp/emp.htm. Accessed April 15, 2004.

12. Preparedness for health care professionals and facilities. U.S. Department of Health and Human Services, Health Resources and Services Administration (HRSA). Web site: http://www.hrsa.gov/bioterrorism/preparationandplanning/healthcare&facilities.htm. Accessed April 15, 2004.

13. Emergency management in the new millennium. Joint Commission on Accreditation of Healthcare Organizations (Oakbrook Terrace, IL). Special Issue, Joint Commission Perspectives 2001;21(12).

14. Macintyre AG, Christopher GW, Eitzen E, et al. Weapons of mass destruction events with contaminated casualties: effective planning for health care facilities. JAMA 2000;283(2):242-9.

15. Schultz CH, Mothershead JL, Field M. Bioterrorism preparedness. I. The emergency department and hospital. Emerg Med Clin North Am 2002;20:437-55.

16. Auf der Heide E. Principles of hospital disaster planning. In: Hogan, Burstein ed. Disaster medicine. Philadelphia: Lippincott, Williams, & Wilkins, 2002.

17. Barbera JA, Macintyre, AG. Medical and Health Incident Management (MaHIM) system: a comprehensive functional system description for mass casualty medical and health incident management. Institute for Crisis, Disaster and Risk Management, George Washington University. Washington, DC, October 2002. Web site: http://www.gwu.edu/~icdrm/publications/MaHIM%20V2%20final%20report%20sec%202.pdf. Accessed April 15, 2004.

18. National Incident Management System (NIMS), Department of Homeland Security, (Washington, DC), March 1, 2004. Web site: http://www.dhs.gov/interweb/assetlibrary/NIMS-90-web.pdf. Accessed April 15, 2004.

19. Hospital Emergency Incident Command System (HEICS). 3rd ed. The San Mateo County Health Services Agency, June 1998. Web sites: http://www.emsa.cahnet.gov/Dms2/HEICS98a.pdf. (Vol. 1). http://www.emsa.cahnet.gov/Dms2/HEIC98b.pdf (Vol. 2). Accessed April 15, 2004.

20. An alternative health care facility: concept of operations for the Off-Site Triage, Treatment, and Transportation Center (OST3C) mass casualty care strategy for a chemical terrorism incident. U.S. Army Soldier and Biological Chemical Command (SBCCOM), Chemical Weapons Improved Response Program Health and Safety Functional Group. Aberdeen Proving Ground, MD, March 2001. Web site: http://hld.sbccom.army.mil/cwirp/cwirp_concept_ops_ost3c_download.htm. Accessed April 15, 2004.

21. Recommendations for hospitals: chemical decontamination, staff protection, chemical decontamination equipment and medication list, evidence collection. California Emergency Medical Services Authority, June 3, 2003.

22. Hick JL, Hanfling D, Burstein JL, et al. Protective equipment for health care facility decontamination personnel: regulations, risks, and recommendations. Ann Emerg Med 2003;42(3):370-80.

23. Hick JL, Penn P, Hanfling D, et al. Establishing and training health care facility decontamination teams. Ann Emerg Med 2003;42(3):381-90.

24. Guidelines for mass fatality management during terrorist incidents involving chemical agents. U.S. Army Soldier and Biological Chemical Command (SBCCOM), November 2001.

25. Holloway HC, Norwood AE, Fullerton CS, et al. The threat of biological weapons: prophylaxis and mitigation of psychological and social consequences. Ann Emerg Med 1997;278(5):425-7.

26. U.S. Department of Health and Human Services. Communicating in a crisis: risk communication guidelines for public officials. Washington, DC: Department of Health and Human Services, 2002. Web site: http://www.riskcommunication.samhsa.gov/RiskComm.pdf. Accessed April 15, 2004.

27. JCAHO. Health care at the crossroads: strategies for creating and sustaining community-wide emergency preparedness systems. Oakbrook Terrace, IL, 2003. Web site: http://www.jcaho.org/news+room/news+release+archives/emergency+preparedness.pdf. Accessed April 15, 2004.

28. U.S. Army Soldier Biological Chemical Command. Modular emergency medical system: expanding local healthcare structure in a mass casualty terrorism incident. Aberdeen Proving Ground, MD, January 2002.

29. Fire and Emergency Services Preparedness Guide for the Homeland Security Advisory System. United States Fire Administration (USFA), Emergency Management and Response-Information Sharing and Analysis Center. Emmitsburg, MD, January 2004.

30. Managing Hazardous Materials Emergencies. Department of Health and Human Services, Agency for Toxic Substances and Disease Registry (ATSDR). Atlanta, GA, 2001. Web site: http://www.atsdr.cdc.gov/mhmi.html. Accessed April 15, 2004.

31. Guidance for protecting building environments from airborne chemical, biological, or radiological attacks. National Institute for Occupational Safety and Health (NIOSH). DHHS publication no. NIOSH2002-139. Cincinnati, OH, 2002. Web site: http://www.cdc.gov/niosh/bldvent/pdfs/2002-139.pdf. Accessed April 15, 2004.

32. Exercises. Department of Health and Human Services, Centers for Disease Control and Prevention. Atlanta, GA, 2003. Web site: http://www.phppo.cdc.gov/PHTN/2003DLSummit/TabletopEx-Skowronski.ppt. Accessed April 15, 2004.

33. Dunaway WM. Strategies for incident preparedness: a national model. National Bioterrorism Civilian Medical Response Center (CiMeRC). Philadelphia, 2003. Web site: http://www/cimerc.org/content/projects/strategies_for_incident_preparedness/sip/pdf. Accessed April 15, 2004.

34. Harel A. Shin Bet: 145 suicide bombers since the start of the intifada. April 28, 2004. Web site: http://www.haaretzdaily.com/hasen/pages/ShArt.jhtml?itemNo=213532&contrassID=2&subContrassID=1&SubContrassID=0. Accessed April 28, 2004.

35. Moore M, Ward-Anderson J. Suicide bombers change Mideast's military. Washington Post Foreign Service, Sunday, August 18, 2002, p. A01. Web site: http://www.library.cornell.edu/colldev/mideast/rantisx.htm. Accessed April 28, 2004.

25

Community Public Health Preparedness

Scott F. Wetterhall and Darren F. Collins

INTRODUCTION

For a mere 37 cents, the first wide-scale intentional attack with a biological agent began in the autumn of 2001. With the image of a double-breasted eagle affixed to a hand-lettered envelope, the bundled anthrax spores traversed a vast and complex postal system that can optically scan, date stamp, and automatically route over 500 million pieces of mail each day. In September 2001, the postal service began delivering a pathogen to communities that were ill prepared to recognize and respond to this novel threat.

Following discovery of a single case of inhalational anthrax in Florida, the outbreak quickly evolved to include multiple sites along the East Coast, prompting the need for unprecedented coordination across local, state, and federal agencies and collaboration between unfamiliar partners—law enforcement and public health. The media, seeking fresh items for an ever shortening news cycle, used opinions from any available spokesperson—including many who were not qualified scientifically to comment—and created an atmosphere in which one public health official described as being "under siege" (1). Who was exposed to anthrax, and when and how, were initially unknown. The medical community felt frustrated as screening and treatment guidelines changed abruptly, often with inadequate notice from public health officials. Postal workers felt they were getting second-class treatment, compared with Senate staff workers. Firefighters, lacking clear guidance for handling suspicious package calls, were running out of the personal protective equipment (PPE) used when handling unknown substances. Hundreds of unwieldy items—suspicious packages, boxes of powdered detergent, floor sweepings, and other items submitted by the police and public health officials—arrived at public health laboratories, straining their storage capacity and taxing their staff with long hours of duty as they tested them for the presence of anthrax. Businesses altered their mail-handling procedures. Ordinary citizens worried about opening their own mail. Only when no new cases of anthrax had appeared, over the course of several weeks, could we begin to presume that the outbreak was over.

All of these challenges reflect components of community public health preparedness. Preparedness is a collective effort involving the entire spectrum of society—individuals, community groups, businesses, government agencies, and elected officials. In this chapter, we will explore what comprises community preparedness, first by understanding how the response community is organized and then by illustrating the special role that selected preparedness partners contribute. Although current national and state efforts appropriately emphasize an "all-hazards"[1] approach to planning and response (2), we believe that events involving biological threats have unique characteristics that justify their closer examination. Thus, we will concentrate on the special challenges that biological events present to the preparedness and response community. We will examine in particular the special role that local public health agencies play in detecting and responding to an intentional attack with a biological agent. We conclude by providing a checklist for community public health preparedness.

PREPAREDNESS ESSENTIALS

ORGANIZATION OF EMERGENCY RESPONSE

Despite the emergence of global threats, including new and exotic diseases, all emergency response is local. In most states, the local political jurisdiction retains responsibility for emergency preparedness and response. Elected officials often vest this authority in a local emergency management agency, which has responsibility for coordinating the actions of local government agencies. Mutual-aid agreements (agreements for one jurisdiction to provide

---

[1] Preparedness planning efforts should enable the local community to address all threats—nuclear, chemical, biological, and other disasters, regardless of whether they are intentional or naturally occurring.

personnel and equipment temporarily to another jurisdiction) originated as a means for fire departments to enhance their response capacity and are becoming more common among emergency medical, law enforcement, and other agencies. When the disaster response outstrips local resources or involves multiple jurisdictions, the local emergency manager seeks assistance and coordination at the state level. If any domestic incident overwhelms the resources of state and local authorities, the governor may seek federal assistance, which is usually coordinated by the federal Department of Homeland Security (DHS).

For situations involving public health, a similar network of state and federal support exists. Local health departments, if faced with a widespread disease outbreak, may seek assistance from their state health department. State health departments may seek federal support, including consultation, personnel, and material, depending upon the event. The Centers for Disease Control and Prevention (CDC), when requested by state and local health officials, provides technical advice and personnel on a regular basis to state and local health departments. The DHS, in collaboration with CDC, manages the Strategic National Stockpile, a cached collection of antibiotics, vaccines, antidotes, and medical equipment for rapid delivery.

Since September 2001, the organization and responsibility of federal resources has evolved rapidly, and continues to evolve. With creation of the Department of Homeland Security and the President's issuance of Homeland Security Presidential Directive 5 (HSPD-5), the federal government mandated creation of a National Response Plan (NRP) whose purpose is "to enhance the ability of the United States to prepare for and to manage domestic incidents by establishing a single, comprehensive national approach" (2). The NRP frames the management of incidents into a "life-cycle" of domains: awareness, prevention, preparedness, response, and recovery. These domains reflect the grouping of activities that the government feels will need to be fulfilled to manage effectively any domestic incident (2).

The NRP recognizes that "state and local levels of government have the primary responsibility for funding, preparing, and operating the services that initially respond to an incident" (2,3). At the same time, the plan mandates that "consistent approaches to domestic preparedness as well as...incident management...must reach to all levels of domestic incident management, from the highest echelons of the Federal government to the individual field-level responders" (2).

The NRP applies to state and local authorities who request federal assistance; state and local authorities who accept federal grants, contracts, or other assistance; and private and nongovernmental entities that partner with the federal government around domestic incident management activities. Thus, community public health preparedness must now be viewed within the context of this overarching plan.

One significant new requirement is adoption, by all federal agencies, of the National Incident Management System (NIMS), a component of the NRP, which is designed to provide a "consistent nationwide framework within which Federal, State, and local governments and the private sector can work...together...[to address]...domestic incidents, regardless of their cause, size, or complexity"

(2). The Incident Command System (ICS), from which NIMS is derived, is a robust management tool that evolved from fighting forest fires in Southern California during the 1970s. Incident management organizes its efforts around five critical functions: command, planning, operations, logistics, and administration/finance. The management principles (common terminology, span of control, communications, and coordination) of incident command readily support the "all-hazards approach" currently being fostered under the NRP.

Because NIMS is required, this system will be adopted at all levels of the response community—among federal, state, and local government agencies, as well as within the private sector. Hospitals, under requirements for accreditation by the Joint Commission on Accreditation of Healthcare Organizations (JCAHO) (4), must adopt an incident management system for community preparedness and disaster management. Many hospitals are adopting the Hospital Emergency Incident Command System (HEICS), developed in California in 1992 (5). Since agencies and entities that are subject to the NRP will be required to participate in NIMS, we can increasingly expect local community preparedness to be framed within the context of federal guidelines and requirements. Community planners must be aware of this shift in orientation.

UNIQUE CHARACTERISTICS OF BIOTERRORIST EVENTS

Bioterrorism is the intentional use of a pathogen or biological product to cause harm to humans and other living creatures, to influence the conduct of government, or to intimidate or coerce a civilian population (6). Bioterrorism is fundamentally different from natural disasters, accidents, and civil or political incidents, the other types of events and range of contingencies that the NRP covers (2). Bioterrorism also has characteristics that distinguish it from other terrorist or criminal acts. Unlike nuclear or chemical incidents, an attack with a biological agent may evolve slowly, avoid early detection, and provide few clues to its likely geographical scope and duration (7,8). Bioterrorism is a form of "asymmetric" warfare, whereby a relatively "small" event (such as the 22 cases of anthrax nationwide in 2001) can produce widespread changes in a population's beliefs, behaviors, and practices. If the attack is with an agent capable of secondary spread—such as smallpox or pneumonic plague—the event can generate fear and anxiety well beyond its initial locus.

THE PREPAREDNESS AND RESPONSE COMMUNITY

The response community comprises a diverse group of individuals, private entities, public agencies, and others (Table 25-1). The core partners include traditional public safety agencies (fire and rescue, law enforcement, emergency medical services), health care organizations, public health agencies, elected officials, and other government agencies. Enhancing community preparedness requires creation and support of sustainable relationships among all members.

TABLE 25-1	The Community Public Health Preparedness and Response Community

Local emergency management	Local public health agency
Fire and rescue	State health department
Law enforcement	State emergency management
Emergency medical services	Centers for Disease Control and Prevention
Hospitals	Federal Bureau of Investigation
Infection control practitioners	Red Cross
Physicians	Business community
Mental health services	Community volunteers

Fire and Rescue Services

Although fire department personnel would play a primary role in the response to a chemical event, their role in a biological event is less pronounced. In the event of a covert or unannounced attack with a biological agent, there may be no "scene" to which firefighters can respond.

Fire departments will, however, have a significant role in responding to the public's concerns about "suspicious packages." In the wake of the first case of confirmed human anthrax illness in October 2001, public safety officials found themselves deluged with calls from a panicky public worried about spilled powders and other substances encountered at work or received through the mail. Fire services should interact closely with public health officials and the law enforcement community in responding to perceived threats, particularly those posed by "suspicious packages" that their residents report receiving.

Fire departments, in collaboration with local public health agencies, need to adopt standardized protocols for responding to suspicious packages. Between April 1997 and June 1999, local emergency responders treated more than 13,000 victims, often by having victims remove their clothing and be decontaminated with bleach solutions (9). Following the 2001 anthrax outbreak, local emergency responders throughout the United States responded to frequent calls for suspicious packages. Despite CDC recommendations that hand washing with soap and water, not gross decontamination with bleach solutions, was usually adequate, these inappropriate responses continued.

The protocol for evaluating suspicious packages should coordinate the efforts of firefighters, local law enforcement, the Federal Bureau of Investigation (FBI), and local public health. If local law enforcement, in consultation with the FBI, determines that there is a credible threat (e.g., presence of threatening letter), then fire and rescue personnel should work with law enforcement to have the specimen delivered for testing to the state public health laboratory. Local public health is responsible for follow up with the victim, including assessment of exposure and need for antibiotic prophylaxis, depending upon the laboratory test results. Such multiagency coordination is critical to avoid repeating past mistakes of inappropriate treatment.

Law Enforcement

During a terrorist event, the NRP designates the Attorney General, acting through the FBI, as having primary federal responsibility for coordinating law enforcement efforts. The NRP recognizes that "the laws of the U.S. assign primary authority to the Federal government to prevent and respond to acts of terrorism" (3). At the same time, local officials preserve authority and command over critical emergency operations. The NRP acknowledges that "the laws of the U.S. assign primary authority to the State and local governments to respond to the consequences of terrorism; the Federal government provides assistance, as required" (3).

When a bioterrorist attack occurs, law enforcement and public health staff must work closely together, often under rapidly evolving circumstances with much uncertainty. If the two agencies have not previously worked together, multiple potential conflicts may arise. Both sectors seek to protect the public's health, but they differ in the focus of their investigations: The role of law enforcement is to identify the perpetrator; public health seeks to identify those exposed or ill. Procedures for handling evidence, for example, the need for a documented "chain-of-custody" may be unfamiliar to public health officials and hence a cause for concern to law enforcement officials worried about compromising their investigation.

The standards to which the respective investigations are held are different: the public health investigation must produce interventions that are scientifically valid and, more importantly, prevent further illness and disease; the law enforcement investigation must meet constitutional standards and other legal challenges in order to achieve a successful conviction (10).

Information sharing will be critical to the success of both investigations, but actual practices may create tension and misunderstanding. Public health officials generally support open sharing of information with their co-investigators. The exception is that of personally identifiable medical information, which health officials do not disclose for legal or ethical reasons. Law enforcement personnel, however, will seek individual's medical information if it is deemed relevant to their investigation. Meanwhile, law enforcement will not be willing to share information with health officials if they feel its disclosure will jeopardize the safety of confidential informants or will enable a suspect to escape.

These differences in philosophy, culture, and practice between law enforcement and public health illustrate the critical importance of having strong, preexisting relationships and a genuine understanding of the respective roles each partner plays. CDC and a U.S. Attorney's Office, recognizing this need, have developed a "forensic epidemiology" course to foster communication and understanding between the two response sectors (11). The course presents case studies that require law enforcement and public health officials to work collaboratively to identify mutual solutions for solving the cases.

Hospitals and Other Heath Care Organizations

Hospitals will be responsible for treating the victims of a bioterrorist attack and may administer vaccines or antibiotics to those exposed but not yet ill. With this paramount role in community preparedness and response, hospitals and other health care organizations face formidable challenges: personnel issues—a nationwide nursing shortage and localized shortages of critical medical specialists; structural changes—a decrease in the number of hospitals during the past two decades; budget constraints—diminishing state-based Medicaid reimbursement and the rising number of uninsured patients; and the competitive pressures that foster new business models for sustaining fiscal solvency (4). All of these influences have contributed to a hospital system ill prepared to provide the sustainable surge capacity that a biological attack would require.

Hospitals need to transition from a facility-based approach to disaster drills to one that reflects their larger role within the community. They need to engage more fully with other preparedness and response partners. JCAHO encourages this transformation, with the new requirement that one of a hospital's annual preparedness exercises be community-based.

In many communities, hospitals and public health agencies lack an effective working relationship (4,12). Structural issues frame these differences. Hospitals focus on provision of care for individuals, whereas public health agencies emphasize population-based strategies (e.g., vaccination programs, disease investigations, restaurant inspections). Hospitals rely upon private funding sources, while public health requires public support (4,13). Public health agencies can facilitate improvements in relationships by encouraging collaboration with their hospitals around improving public health surveillance, fostering interagency communications, and training of hospital care providers (4).

Physicians

The physician plays a key role in community preparedness. An astute physician may be the first to identify that a biological attack is taking place, as was the case in Florida with the first anthrax case in 2001. Physicians need to be familiar with the clinical manifestations, diagnostic tests, and treatment regimens for the major biological agents. They must understand how their hospital ICS operates, and they should participate in hospital drills and community exercises.

The relationship between practicing physicians and the local public health agency is a critical one (14). Without strong relations, delays in recognition and response to a bioterrorist attack may occur. Physicians need to know the local health agency is monitoring the health of the community, and they need to know how to contact their local health agency on a 24/7 basis. During a rapidly evolving outbreak, the local health agency may be the primary source for treatment guidelines. The credibility of the health agency's recommendations can be sustained by having preexisting relationships with the community physicians.

Mental Health

Providing for the mental health needs of disaster victims, their families, and emergency response workers is an essential function of emergency management. Mental health issues following biological events and other forms of terrorism may differ from those seen in other disasters. Unlike other disasters that may produce immediate and physically horrific results, biological events may create the loss of one's notion of community safety—and thereby produce deep human fears about uncontrollable evil (15).

Psychological responses following a biological terrorist attack include anger, panic, fear of contagion, scapegoating, social isolation, demoralization, and loss of faith in social institutions. A critical first step is an effective risk communications plan, with the identification of credible and trusted spokespersons who can provide accurate and frequent assessments of what is known and what is not known as events unfold (16).

Medical personnel must anticipate that a biological attack may produce contagious somatization—breathing difficulties, tremors, sweating, feelings of anxiety, and labile moods (17). Such symptoms may compel persons to seek care at health care facilities, further stressing the already overworked health care system. Medical responders need to be able to recognize symptoms of anxiety, depression, and dissociation and provide timely, appropriate treatment.

We need to prepare for these and other threats to the community's psyche, first by recognizing that restoration of mental health following a biological event may be a prolonged process. Acute stress disorder may be common among both victims and responders. With appropriate treatment, however, including emphasis on the normal recovery process—talking to others, getting rest and respite, and returning to normal routines—recovery may be facilitated. Local preparedness to protect the mental health of our community begins with inviting all mental health practitioners—government agencies, academic centers, and individual counselors and care givers—to participate in the public health planning process. The provision of mental health services during a disaster must be fully integrated into and coordinated with other public health responses.

Public School System

The public school system, with its extensive ties to the community, is an important partner in community preparedness. Schools may serve as distribution centers for vaccines and antibiotics, shelter persons rendered homeless by a tornado or flood, or provide counseling and information following a terrorist attack. Schools are assuming larger roles in providing counseling and psychological support in the face of terrorist attacks (e.g., the recent Washington, D.C., sniper attacks) (8). School counselors represent a public partner in our mental health response plan.

Schools need to be integrated into any community-based preparedness planning effort. Local emergency management and public health agencies must recognize that the public health school system needs a seat in the local emergency operations center—to facilitate communications, operations, planning, and resource allocation. School officials need to become familiar with their roles and responsibilities under the local incident command structure. In anticipation of their role, schools need to engage in training and exercise programs that test their response capabilities. Public health agencies should encourage and foster the school system's participation in community preparedness.

Media

Although often viewed as adversaries, the news media represent critical community partners in preparedness and response. As with police, fire, and emergency services, the media should be considered first responders. During an emergency, the public relies almost exclusively upon the media for information; the response community communicates with the public through the media. Hence, public officials must heed the advice to "go out with the news quickly, no matter how inconvenient" (16). A priority should be having a well-rehearsed risk communications plan, with prepared materials (e.g., fact sheets on the pathogens) and procedures for coordinating messages among all government agencies and elected officials. The plan should include strategies to use alternative media venues, to prepare messages in languages other than English, and to tailor messages to specific groups who may be at increased risk (1,17).

Public health officials were not prepared for the media onslaught following the anthrax outbreak (1,4,12,18). Without credible public health officials available to provide context and commentary during the early stages of the 2001 anthrax outbreak, the media sought any available "expert," thereby spawning uncertainty and loss of confidence in the public health system (4,18). We need to engage the news media in the emergency preparedness planning process and be prepared to use the media for timely, accurate, and sensitive dissemination of critical information (4,19).

Community Volunteers

Recruiting sufficient numbers of community volunteers during a bioterrorist attack is a daunting and formidable task. If mass vaccination for smallpox were implemented, for example, we estimate that providing services, over a period of 5 days, in a county whose population is 700,000 residents would require 5,000 to 7,500 persons to staff neighborhood clinics. Volunteers need to be rapidly recruited, credentialed, and trained; liability issues must be addressed. Few communities have developed viable strategies to mobilize a large and reliable group of volunteers.

Preparedness involves enlisting the support of community organizations (19). The federal government has created the Citizens Corps (20) initiative to help localities coordinate volunteer activities, thereby making their communities better prepared to respond to emergencies. Components include an expanded Neighborhood Watch Program, a Medical Reserve Corps (to engage volunteer health professionals), a Community Emergency Response Team (to promote partnering between emergency response officials and the community they serve), and Volunteers in Police Service (to provide support to law enforcement following a disaster). Federal grants have been awarded to communities to develop these programs, which hopefully will provide successful models for adoption by other communities.

Business Community

The National Response Plan recognizes the essential role that the private sector plays, as owner of 85% of the national infrastructure, in mitigating the physical and economic effects following a disaster. Businesses are encouraged to perform risk assessments, develop contingency plans, and take actions to improve their state of readiness.

Business Executives for National Security (BENS), a nationwide, nonpartisan organization, employs the expertise of its members to enhance the nation's security by collaborating with federal, state, and local governments. BENS has developed a primer on preparedness to assist businesses in developing contingency plans (21). Their Business Force Initiative, piloted in New Jersey and now active in Georgia, uses the expertise of the business community to strengthen homeland security. In Georgia, BENS is assisting state and local health departments in developing procedures for dispensing the Strategic National Stockpile.

ROLE OF PUBLIC HEALTH IN PREPARING FOR AND RESPONDING TO A BIOTERRORIST ATTACK

As we noted earlier, bioterrorist attacks differ from other attacks using weapons of mass destruction. The medical community and public health system will be the first to detect and respond to the attack, particularly if the release is unannounced. Health officials, sharing authority with public safety officials, will coordinate the public response to save lives and prevent disease. While law enforcement officials, particularly the FBI, coordinate the law enforcement investigation, hospitals and physicians will provide treatment for ill persons. Concurrently, public health will be attempting to identify persons at risk of illness, marshal resources (e.g., vaccines or antibiotics, depending upon the pathogen) to prevent or ameliorate illness among exposed persons, and identify and remove (or remediate) the source of exposure. Detection and response are the two critical and unique functions that public health must fulfill during a bioterrorist attack.

Detection

Monitoring the health of the population is an essential public health service, one that must be performed daily and is not limited to attempts to detect bioterrorist events. Officials monitor the status of the population through public health surveillance—the ongoing collection, analysis, interpretation, and use of data about health events to prevent illness and death. The key attribute of a successful public health surveillance system for bioterrorism is the timely detection of threats. Early awareness will enable the public health and medical community to provide antibiotic prophylaxis, vaccinations, and treatment, thereby reducing morbidity and mortality.

Routine notifiable disease surveillance. Routine surveillance for infectious diseases is conducted at the state and local level, where physicians, hospitals, laboratories, and others are required by state law or regulation to report the occurrence of certain infections (called notifiable diseases because of their required notification) to health authorities. States participate in the National Notifiable Disease Surveillance System, which allows use of common definitions and enables sharing of data among states and with CDC. The primary purpose of this surveillance system is to identify outbreaks of illness. Typically, outbreaks are detected by analyzing a cluster of notifiable disease reports at a local or state health department and investigating their origin. Alternatively, astute clinicians who witness something unusual may notify health authorities and thereby generate an investigation.

Active surveillance. The notifiable disease surveillance system is regarded as a "passive" system because it relies upon a physician or health care provider to initiate notice. As such, this system frequently misses illness in the community, primarily because the physician fails to report the events to the health department. To overcome this shortcoming, health departments will implement "active" surveillance, when warranted, by actively calling hospitals and providers looking for specific cases.

Syndromic surveillance. Syndromic surveillance is the use of indicators of illness that may allow outbreak detection even earlier than traditional means. In the past five years, investigators have enthusiastically implemented syndromic surveillance systems, using a diverse set of indicators: for example, work and school absenteeism, purchase of certain medications, 911 calls, symptom complexes (e.g., fever and rash), and Internet use of a health care information site. Others are developing analytical tools and models that can sift through large quantities of electronic data, seeking clusters that may represent outbreaks.

Although many researchers remain optimistic that syndromic surveillance will provide a more sensitive and wider window of time for early response (22), others are skeptical. Criticisms include the inability to detect small and geographically dispersed clusters (as with the 2001 anthrax outbreak); the drain on health department staff as they repeatedly respond to false leads (which results from having a system that is sensitive enough to detect the exceedingly rare bioterrorist event); and the failure to demonstrate that syndromic surveillance has real value—that is, it outperforms usual methods of outbreak detection. Most agree that, in the event of an attack, the tangible benefit from having an existing syndromic surveillance system will be its help in rapidly assessing the extent of the outbreak. The system can be used to gather a quick snapshot of disease activity in the surrounding community (23), which will be invaluable information for planning purposes.

Laboratory support. Regardless which surveillance or detection system is used, a robust system that can provide rapid 24/7 laboratory diagnostic support serves as the critical foundation of all monitoring systems. One of the earliest steps in an outbreak investigation is "confirming the diagnosis," which typically relies upon laboratory confirmation. Few health officials would feel comfortable implementing vaccination or antibiotic prophylaxis programs in the absence of a laboratory-confirmed diagnosis. CDC has supported the Laboratory Response Network, a joint program with the Association of Public Health Laboratories and the FBI, with additional laboratories that are equipped with reagents to test for the most important pathogens (13). CDC places high priority on developing additional rapid diagnostic tests, thereby improving detection and response.

Response

The public health response to a bioterrorist event may include investigating cases, tracing contacts, and assuring provision of medical treatment and prophylaxis. The best response will be one in which public health officials are working in concert with all response partners and are openly sharing intelligence, information, and resources.

During a bioterrorist attack, the health department will be operating under a system of incident command. Organizing the public health response in this fashion will facilitate interaction with other response sectors; moreover, use of the incident management system will be required (beginning in October 2005) to receive federal assistance. Many local health departments, which vary considerably in staff size and population served (13), however, have limited experience in operating under an incident command system.

Organization of local public health under incident command. A local public health agency will need to organize its emergency response activities under an incident command system. Figure 25-1 illustrates the system employed by the DeKalb County, Georgia, Board of Health. This ICS structure has the standard five major functions: command, operations, planning, logistics, and finance and administration. A public information officer (PIO), safety officer, and liaison officer provide staff support to the incident commander.

The operations function comprises the unique functions that public health officials will perform to respond to a bioterrorist attack. The epidemiology unit has primary responsibility for investigating the outbreak, identifying persons who are at risk for illness, and halting the epidemic by interrupting disease transmission. Unit staff will work closely with law enforcement personnel throughout the investigation.

The case investigation unit is responsible for investigating persons who are "suspected cases" and assuring appropriate collection of information and laboratory specimens to properly classify their conditions. Case investigators may examine patients, identify potential contacts of cases (for communicable diseases such as smallpox or pneumonic plague), review medical records, and ensure that appropriate laboratory specimens are collected and tested. Investigators provide information to the surveillance and contact tracing sections.

When the disease under investigation is transmissible from person to person, the contact tracing unit attempts to identify all persons who may have been exposed to ill persons and ensure that they receive in a timely fashion either preventive measures (chemoprophylaxis or vaccination) or,

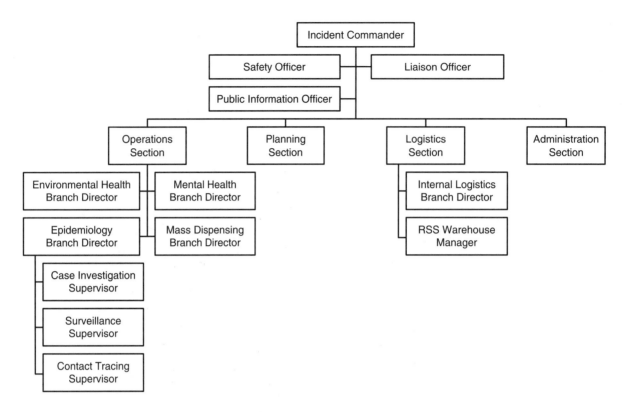

Figure 25–1. Organization of a local public health agency under an incident command structure during a public health emergency, with branches of Operations and Logistics sections.

if ill, diagnosis and appropriate treatment. Contact tracers work in the community with lists of persons who meet the definition of "contact" (for example, with smallpox, a contact is a household member or anyone with three or more hours of face-to-face contact with the "case-patient") provided from interviews with the case-patient. Some contacts may be readily identified and reached (e.g., close family members); others may be far more challenging (e.g., strangers with whom the encounter was in a public place). Contact tracers provide information to the surveillance section and the mass dispensing branch.

The surveillance unit monitors the occurrence of new cases of illness by checking with health care facilities and by receiving reports from physicians and other providers. Depending upon the outbreak, surveillance staff may ask hospitals to report any occurrence of patients meeting the criteria for reporting possible patients (e.g., patients admitted to the hospital with respiratory failure) (24), or they may assign health department staff to review hospital records. The surveillance unit also receives lists of persons (i.e., contacts) who have received any prophylactic treatments (medications or vaccinations), since these persons are at increased risk for illness, depending upon how timely the prophylactic measures were implemented.

The mass dispensing branch is responsible for providing preventive measures to exposed persons (antibiotics or vaccinations and health education). This branch receives from the contact tracing section lists of persons who need prophylactic treatment. Alternatively, if the exposure involves an environmental or occupational exposure (e.g., the Brentwood postal workers in Washington,

D.C.), the list of eligible persons may come from a different source (in this example, the employer). Depending upon the magnitude of the outbreak, the branch may set up dispensing clinics in existing health department facilities, or it may enlist schools to provide multiple sites to treat large numbers of persons. Mass dispensing includes registering clients, providing health education, performing any necessary medical screening (e.g., allergies to antibiotics, pregnancy testing), providing preventive treatment, and ensuring that mechanisms for appropriate follow-up are in place.

The environmental health branch oversees issues of environmental safety. The nature of the agent and the mode of attack will determine this branch's scope of effort. Under some circumstances, the environmental health branch will have few activities. With the 2001 anthrax attack, however, environmental cleanup unexpectedly blossomed into a large and complex issue that required considerable effort and prompted new guidelines for addressing this issue (25).

Although routine mental health services are provided by an agency separate from our board of health, we have directly incorporated, under an arrangement with our local mental health agency, the mental health branch functions into our operations function. A representative of the local mental health agency will work with the public and private community to ensure that mental health services are available for the following groups: patients; family members of patients; contacts of the patient (if the disease is communicable); providers (health care workers, public safety workers, public health personnel, and others); and the community (through coordination with the public information officers).

PREPAREDNESS CHECKLIST TABLE AND SUMMARY

Community preparedness is an ongoing process that requires trusting relationships and collaboration among all response sectors. This checklist recognizes the foundation that these relationships represent and highlights the critical needs that must be met, such as trained staff and redundant communications systems for notification and dissemination of information. The checklist also highlights specific actions that should be taken by various members of the response community.

- Collaborative working relationships exist across local, state, and federal governmental and nongovernmental agencies.
- Agencies understand legal basis of emergency response, including provisions in the NRP.
- Agency roles and responsibilities during an emergency are clearly defined.
- Agencies perform exercises using ICS.
- Interoperable and redundant methods of communications among all response partners are in place.
- Standardized protocols exist for handling suspicious packages.
- Public health understands how evidence in law enforcement investigations is handled.
- Hospitals plan to increase surge capacity, obtain additional staff, and provide emergency credentialing.
- Hospitals participate in community-wide exercises.
- Hospitals can conduct active surveillance for specified diseases and conditions.
- Physicians know how to contact their local and state health departments on a 24/7 basis.
- Physicians report unusual illnesses or clusters to health department on a timely basis.
- Physicians participate in community exercises.
- Health care providers can recognize and treat symptoms of stress.
- Mental health services can be provided to patients, their families, contacts of cases, and response personnel.
- Mental health operations are integrated into the ICS of local public health.
- Schools can provide facilities, staff, transportation, and security during a community emergency.
- A communications strategy is in place, including the identification of spokesperson(s) who have media training.
- Opinion leaders in the community (including faith-based organizations) are identified.
- Predeveloped materials, including fact sheets and press releases, are available.
- Individuals who can translate information into multiple languages have been identified.
- Protocol to triage phone calls and a system to handle the influx of large numbers of calls have been developed.
- Programs have been established to identify, recruit, and train volunteers.
- Business community participates in the creation of an emergency preparedness plan.
- Businesses have developed individual contingency plans.
- Public health can implement disease surveillance systems with hospitals and community physicians.
- Adequate laboratory capacity will be available to test specimens and samples in a timely manner.
- Public health can operate under incident management system.
- Staff members are trained to conduct epidemiologic investigations and contact tracing.
- Methods are established for organizing treatment centers for providing vaccines and antibiotics.
- Method is in place for rapidly distributing treatment guidelines to the medical community.
- Senior leadership supports preparedness planning activities.

RESOURCES

The following Internet sites provide additional information for enhancing community public health preparedness.

1. The National Association of County & City Health Officials (NACCHO) is the national nonprofit organization representing local public health agencies. For information on their bioterrorism and emergency response programs, visit http://www.naccho.org/project63.cfm.

2. Center for Risk Communication. The Center for Risk Communication is a pioneer in the development and use of advanced communication methods based on decades of university-level behavioral-science research and practice. Web site: http://www.centerforriskcommunication.com/home.htm

3. Heartland Centers for Public Health Community and Capacity Development – St. Louis University School of Public Health. The Heartland Center for Public Health Preparedness (HCPHP) is part of the national network of centers established through joint collaboration of Centers for Disease Control and Prevention, NACCHO, and the Association of Schools of Public Health. Web site: http://www.slu.edu/centers/heartland/

4. Public Health Foundation—TrainingFinder. TrainingFinder is a comprehensive database of nationwide learning opportunities for professionals who protect the public's health. Web site: http://www.train.org/DesktopShell.aspx?tabid=93

5. The Center for Biosecurity is an independent, nonprofit organization of the University of Pittsburgh Medical Center. The Center works to prevent the development and use of biological weapons. Web site: http://www.upmc-biosecurity.org/

6. The RAND Corporation is a nonprofit institution that helps improve policy and decision making through research and analysis. For information about their health and healthcare research, visit http://www.rand.org/research_areas/health/

7. Center for Infectious Disease Research & Policy – University of Minnesota. The center's mission is to prevent illness and death from infectious diseases through epidemiologic research and the rapid translation of scientific information into real-world practical applications and solutions. Web site: http://www.cidrap.umn.edu/

8. The Center for Law and the Public's Health at Georgetown and Johns Hopkins Universities. The Center seeks to enhance the visibility and effectiveness of law as a tool for the promotion of the public's health. Web site: http://www.publichealthlaw.net/

REFERENCES

1. Casani J, Matuszak DL, Benjamin GC. Under siege: one state's perspective of the anthrax events of October/November 2001. Biosecurity and bioterrorism 2003;1:43-45.

2. National Response Plan, initial plan. 2004. Available at: http://www.nemaweb.org/docs/national_response_plan.pdf [Accessed April 26, 2004].

3. CONPLAN. United States Government Interagency Domestic Terrorism Concept of Operations Plan, January 2001. Available at: http://www.fbi.gov/publications/conplan/conplan.pdf [Accessed April 26, 2004].

4. Joint Commission of Accreditation of Healthcare Organizations. Health care at the crossroads: strategies for creating and sustaining community-wide emergency preparedness systems. Available at: http://www.jcaho.org/news+room/press+kits/emergency+prep.htm [Accessed April 20, 2004].

5. San Mateo County Health Services Agency, Emergency Medical Services. HEICS: the hospital emergency incident command system (vol. 1). 3rd ed. June 1998. Available at: http://www.emsa.cahwnet. gov/Dms2/HEICS98a.pdf [Accessed April 26, 2004].

6. Gostin LO, Sapsin JW, Teret SP, et al. The Model State Emergency Health Powers Act: planning for and response to bioterrorism and naturally occurring diseases. JAMA 2002;288;622-8.

7. Wetterhall SF. Responding to bioterrorism. Ethn Dis 2003;13 [suppl]:S3-58-62.

8. Stein BD, Tanelian TL, Vaiana ME, et al. The role of schools in meeting community needs during bioterrorism. Biosecurity and bioterrorism 2003;1:273-81.

9. Cole LA. Bioterrorism threats: learning from inappropriate responses. J Public Health Management Practice 2000;6:8-18.

10. Butler JC, Cohen ML, Friedman CR, et al. Collaboration between public health and law enforcement: new paradigms and partnerships for bioterrorism planning and response. Emerg Infect Dis 2002;8:1152-6.

11. Goodman RA, Munson JW, Dammers K, et al. Forensic epidemiology: law at the intersection of public health and criminal investigations. J Law Med Ethics 2003;31:684-700.

12. Inglesby T. The state of public health preparedness for terrorism involving weapons of mass destruction: a six month report card. Congressional testimony before Committee on Government Affairs, April 18, 2002. Available at: http://www.upmc-biosecurity.org/pages/resources/hearings/inglesby_01.html [Accessed April 20, 2004].

13. Salinsky E. Public health emergency preparedness: fundamentals of the "system." National Health Policy Forum Background Paper, George Washington University. Available at http://www.nhpf.org/index.cfm?fuseaction=SearchCatalogue&iissueid=10 [Accessed April 21, 2004].

14. Gerberding JL, Hughes JM, Koplan JP. Biological preparedness and response: clinicians and public health agencies as essential partners. JAMA 2002;287:898-900.

15. Hall MJ, Norwood AE, Ursano RJ, Fullerton CS. The psychological impacts of bioterrorism. Biosecurity and bioterrorism 2003;1:139-44.

16. Mullin S. New York City's communications trials by fire, from West Nile to SARS. Biosecurity and bioterrorism 2003;1:267-72.

17. DiGiovanni C. Domestic terrorism with chemical or biological agents: psychiatric aspects. Am J Psychiatr 1999;156:1500-5.

18. Gursky E, Inglesby TV, O'Toole T. Anthrax 2001: observations on the medical and public health response. Biosecurity and bioterrorism 2003;1:97-110.

19. Glass TA, Schoch-Spana M. Bioterrorism and the people: how to vaccinate a city against panic. Clin Infect Dis 2002;34:217-23.

20. Federal Emergency Management Agency. Citizen Corps: programs & partners. Available at: http://www.citizencorps.gov/programs/ [Accessed April 21, 2004].

21. Business Executives for National Security, Metro Atlanta Branch. Getting ready: company primer on preparedness and response planning for terrorist and bioterrorist attacks. 2004. Available at: http://www.bens.org/images/GettingReady_042304.pdf [Accessed April 26, 2004].

22. Sosin DM. Syndromic surveillance: the case for skillful investment. Biosecurity and bioterrorism 2003;1:247-53.

23. Reingold A. If syndromic surveillance is the answer, what is the question? Biosecurity and bioterrorism 2003;1:77-81.

24. Bresnitz EA, DiFerdinando GT. Lessons from the anthrax attacks of 2001: the New Jersey experience. Clin Occup Environ Med 2003;2:227-52.

25. Inglesby TV, O'Toole T, Henderson DA, et al. Anthrax as a biological weapon, 2002: updated recommendations for management. JAMA 2002;287:2236-52.

26

Mass Gathering Preparedness

Carl Menckhoff and Michael Shaw

INTRODUCTION

The classic definition of a mass gathering is a group of greater than 1,000 people (1–4), although the vast majority of the literature deals with groups exceeding 25,000. In this chapter we define a mass gathering as a group of people who have come together in a particular location for a specific purpose for a period of time that may range from a few hours (in the case of a sporting event or concert) to a few weeks (in the case of the Olympic Games).

Mass gatherings are extremely common all around the world. In the United States alone, 165 million people attend NBA, NFL, and NCAA events (5,6) and 5.5 million attend NASCAR events (6,7), only a fraction of the mass gatherings that occur each year. Only a relatively small body of literature covers this topic, however, and it has just been over the last 15 years that more has been written on the subject. Weaver stated in 1989 that there are "few data from which to plan emergency medical needs for public events and no recognized standards or guidelines for providing emergency medical services at mass gatherings" (3,8). The majority of what has been published is descriptive papers of various events, and not until recently has there been an attempt to define the medical planning needed for mass gatherings (9–13).

Whenever a large group of people gather, there is a risk for catastrophe. The responsibility for public health protection falls squarely on the event planners. The concerns of all parties, from public utilities, public safety, and hospitals to the event attendees, are best addressed during the planning of the event.

This chapter outlines the necessary steps in preparing and implementing medical care for a mass gathering as well as the essentials of planning for mass casualties and terroristic events. The roles of local fire, police, and emergency medical services (EMS) are described, and the groundwork for planning is discussed. There are also a multitude of variables, often uncontrollable, which must be taken into account. Many of these, such as environmental hazards and physical and ecological barriers, are also described.

EVENT PLANNING

The first step in planning an event involves assembling the *event planning committee,* which should occur well in advance and involve the event coordinator, designee from public safety, the local fire department official, and the medical director. In the initial meeting, the chain of command should be established as well as how information will be transmitted.

The *event coordinator* heads up the committee. Through this person, key information regarding the logistics and financial support for the event should be readily available. Either the local police department or a private security company will likely supply the *public safety* component of the event. The role of this organization is defined later as we discuss each stratum individually. *Fire protection* will likely fall under the auspices of the local fire marshal. Medical coverage concerns will be relegated to the person designated as the medical director. Together this committee will deliberate to form the basis for the preparedness plan.

The role of the local law enforcement agency or the employed private security company needs to be clearly defined. They should be in control of access to the event and involved in the development of the disaster plan. Crowd control is an essential area that will fall under their jurisdiction. Access to and from the event will, at times, be difficult due to masses of people, and preplanned entry and exit routes for emergency vehicles must be secured. Public safety should also be available if the need arises to control unruly patients or crowds.

The local fire service will have a vested interest in fire safety for any event, especially an indoor one. The structure of the established fire response system needs to be taken into account when developing the disaster plan. The local fire marshal will be able to supply information regarding the planned response to the event location and should be made aware of any potential fire hazards caused by the event, numbers of expected spectators, and planned access routes to and from the event. The fire department must be aware of hazardous materials such as pyrotechnics as well as chemicals that may be present in large quantities for cleaning or special effects. The fire department will need to know who will be in charge of the event and negotiate the role of their department in the event of fire or mass casualty incidents.

Many fire departments utilize the incident command system (ICS), which offers a defined structure of who will be in charge of the scene at a mass causality incident. In this system, a command center is established. Large events with an established disaster plan risk adding to the chaos if the role of the event staff is not clearly defined beforehand. The medical director should negotiate a position in the command center as the medical consultant and coordinate the use of the established medical event staff with the incoming medical response from the local EMS agency and fire department first responders.

During the initial meeting with the event coordinator, the financial support for the medical team needs to be defined. Events held for profit should have resources available; nonprofit functions may not. Some hospital groups provide the medical support for events for an equivalent value in advertising. If resources are not available or are insufficient, donations from sponsors should be sought out. Medical supply companies or medical equipment companies might be willing to donate supplies or loan equipment for little more than advertisement at the aid station. The opportunity for local hospitals or community groups to show support for community events will encourage their involvement. Another option, which has not been commented on much in the literature, is to provide fee-for-service care.

The event medical director has many aspects to consider in planning for a mass gathering. Details include staffing, finance, communications, and logistics. Additionally, aspects of the event, such as estimated attendance, the type of event, weather, and the presence of drugs or alcohol, must be considered. Many of these variables cannot be predicted or controlled accurately but must be planned for as their presence becomes evident.

EVENT SITE PLANNING

The characteristics of the planned event site need to be clearly defined. Will the event be indoors or outdoors? If the event is planned for indoors, items such as access routes significantly change. Indoor event planners need to consider ventilation in case of fire or the dispersion of hazardous chemicals by terrorist attack. Evacuation plans for the building need to be reviewed and incorporated into the disaster plan. Locations of the established first aid stations need to be defined in indoor arenas early in the planning sessions because they often cannot be moved. How will patients be taken to the aid stations when the seats are filled? Planned routes of travel need to be laid out and protected by security.

Outdoor events, conversely, allow for the movement of the aid stations to fit the need of the particular event. Outdoor events aid stations should be located within a walking distance of 5 minutes for the average anticipated spectator or at least no further than 1/8 mile apart (9). In outdoor events, barriers of both an environmental and physical nature exist and are subject to change with the influx of spectators as well as the weather. Once easily traveled paths may become blocked by masses of people or by water from overflowing streams and ditches during heavy rainfall. Once again, safe passage for

emergency personnel needs to be planned early and protected by security. The area where medical care is provided needs to be clearly defined. What about the people in the parking lot? Will medical personnel be responsible for the participants in the event and the event support staff or the spectators only? This needs to be discussed in the initial planning session. If medical personnel will be responsible for the support staff, the medical teams need to be represented when the first of the staff arrive and stay there until the last of the cleanup crew has gone for the day. If they are responsible for the parking lot, an aid station may need to be positioned there as well.

Once the venue for the event is defined, the next appropriate measure is to visit the location. Detailed maps should be created paying close attention to environmental and physical barriers to passage. Potential hazards should be noted. For example, events occurring near wooded areas could pose hazards like snake bites or bee stings, and for indoor events, the concern for fire safety and ventilation becomes more important. Vital information can be attained from those who have provided care at the event during its prior engagements as to how the crowd tended to gather, the demographics of the attendees, and the numbers of requests for medical assistance. This information will be helpful in estimating the placement of aid stations and the needed level of coverage, including the number of aid stations and supplies that may be needed.

An article by Nordberg describes a general classification system for events. This classification system uses somewhat broad strokes to describe the general event venue and crowd activity and geographical layout. Class I events include those where the spectators all have seats and are generally stationary. Sporting events and concerts that have a short time period, in terms of hours in which they occur, are examples. Class II events consist of mobile crowds of people, who themselves may also participate in the event. These events occur over a period of time defined by days. Examples of these types of events would be Mardi Gras in New Orleans and the World's Fair. Class III events are smaller in terms of crowd size but cover a large geographical area. Marathons and road bike races represent these types of events (14).

CROWD DEMOGRAPHICS

The demographics of the crowd play an important role in planning for medical coverage. Some events may attract a wide demographical cross section, whereas others may attract a narrower segment of the population. For example, a visit by the pope (15–18) will attract an older population, in general, and a hard rock concert will bring an entirely different subset of people (19). Sporting events will attract spectators of all ages and physical abilities. Having knowledge of these typical crowds that specific event types attract can help predict the types of medical issues that might arise. One should be able to predict that mosh pit activity (where participants are hurled around inside a ring of participants) will likely be present at certain popular rock concerts, resulting in increased medical utilization rates (MUR) (20) and a higher percentage of trauma. Political events have their own inherent issues and pose the increased risk of a terrorist attack. High-ranking political officials often attend these types of events and come accompanied by their own medical staff and security. These VIPs need to be known as early as possible, and how their staff will fit into the overall medical care picture needs to be well defined. Some papers in the literature have attempted to define the "mood" of the crowd (6). This seems like a logical parameter to define; however, the mood often develops after the beginning of an event.

At Woodstock in 1994, for example, the mood changed significantly over the course of the multiple-day event (6,21,22). It started out as aggressive as people were trying to stake out their territories. After the rains, however, people began to help each other, and there was much more of a sense of community.

LEVEL OF SERVICE AND STAFFING

The next item to consider is the level of service that medical personnel will provide. The event coordinators may dictate this or it may be left for medical people to decide. This topic has spurred much debate in the literature. It seems clear, however, that there must be, at the very least, the input of a physician and usually one on site during the event itself (23). Also, regardless of the level of care, all possible efforts must be made to provide defibrillation to cardiac arrest victims within 5 minutes (10). This may be accomplished through the use of AEDs or carefully placed advanced life support (ALS) units.

The options for level of service provided can be divided into three broad categories: basic, intermediate, and advanced. Basic level service consists of basic-level EMTs and first responders. With this level of service, the care provided is limited to the provision of basic first aid, CPR, wound care, and it excludes the dispensing of medications. A physician medical director is required to develop protocols for treatment, disposition of patients, and quality improvement review. There should be provisions made for the presence of an ambulance on site or on call for those patients who require transport off site. Intermediate-level service should provide EMTs and nurses who possess the proper license to administer IV fluids and utilize some advanced airway devices. The physician may be present at the main aid station or may include these therapies in the protocols developed for this level of service. If the physician is not on site, there must be provisions made for the field crews to contact an online medical control physician. The therapies provided for in the protocols, especially with regard to dispensing medications, will be dictated by the limits set by the individual state boards of EMS. The question of who will be allowed to disposition patients must be clarified. Will the nurses and EMTs be allowed to release patients to the event or to home, for instance (24)? The option for an on-site ambulance still remains open at this level of service, but with advanced skills being performed on site, one would be preferred. An advanced-level service requires the continuous presence of a physician at the main aid station. Field crews should consist of paramedics, RNs, and physicians. The protocols developed are only limited by the physician's license. This system allows for on-site treatment of minor illness and injury and the potential for the patient to be released back to the event. On-site immediate ambulance transport should be provided with at least one ambulance on site at all times. Quality improvement review of this system should be more rigid, and all dispositions should be overseen by a physician.

Several reviews have analyzed the number of staff needed for adequate coverage of mass gatherings. One, adopted by the American College of Emergency Physicians, states that there should be one EMT/nurse team per 10,000 attendants and at least one physician per 50,000 people (9).

One common misperception of many event planners is that the local EMS service will be capable of supplying adequate coverage to the planned event without special arrangements. This expectation often falls short of what is required because the local EMS system could be easily overwhelmed or not immediately available when the call goes out. To prepare for an event adequately, a specific level of care at the event must be established and developed in conjunction with the local EMS organization. Once the level of service has been determined, the infrastructure can proceed in development. The event medical director should serve as the on-site physician or the lead physician at the event if multiple physicians will be present. All members of the medical team should have the appropriate licensure and malpractice coverage. Protocols and/or standard operating procedures should be developed and supplied to all providers of medical care at the event. These should include a standard method of providing a disposition for patients. Whether the level of service is basic life support (BLS) or ALS, the goal should be to provide rapid and efficient quality medical care. Many patients seen for medical attention can be treated and released back to the event.

The level of care is often dictated by what is locally available and what the event planners can afford. A basic structure that can be easily modified to fit the particular need of a specific event and will work for either an ALS or BLS system is described here. This structure centers on a base station, which will serve as the center where the highest level of medical care will take place and the center for communications. The base station should house the on-site physician, the communication center, all supplies needed at the event, and the most sophisticated treatment center that can be put in place. It should be adequately equipped to initiate treatment for all medical emergencies including cardiac and respiratory emergencies and provide the basics of advanced trauma life support. This should include advanced airway equipment and the necessary tools to treat acute traumatic injuries. When providing care at smaller events, this is likely all that will be needed.

The staffing of this station should consist of the physician and two to three support persons (EMTs or nurses). This will allow for adequate medical care at the center with some ability to respond away from the center to treat patients in the crowd or retrieve patients to the treatment center. In situations where increased coverage is needed, the base station should house all terminal supplies in sufficient quantity to restock satellite stations. When the need for expanded coverage is required to minimize response times, the decision to utilize roving units or fixed position secondary stations must be made. It is recommended that if spectator density is the limiting factor in response times, roving units on foot, on bicycle, or in a golf cart should be utilized. When the event is to cover a large geographical area, secondary stations may be more appropriate because they can provide basic medical care up to and including some basic procedures. This will allow simple treatments to be provided with minimal disruption to the individual patient's participation in the event. The care at these stations should be limited to short treatments such as sutures and minor wound care and tetanus prophylaxis and dispensing of medications. Treatments that may require longer to provide and may require a short period of observation and reevaluation can be initiated at the secondary station, and then the patient may be moved to the base station where a final disposition can be made by a physician. The base station should serve as the point from which all patients are transported away from the event unless the nature of the emergency prohibits it. This scheme will reduce the confusion often associated with locating a single patient in a crowd of thousands and provides the need to maintain a single route of entry and exit for emergency vehicles.

This setup is a useful base model to use because it lends itself to expansion or downsizing according to the size of the event for which coverage is needed. Frequently the same organization will be called on to provide medical coverage for multiple events of various sizes and types. The system can be further expanded to include multiple base stations when there is a physical barrier that is impassable such as a race track, which may require a base station on either side of the track. As the system expands, there will be the need for a runner to resupply secondary stations and retrieve supplies from an offsite location as needed. The secondary stations should be staffed by two to three people, which will allow for a member of the team to be dispatched to an individual in the crowd while leaving someone at the station. Response from a secondary station may be accomplished either on foot or in a golf cart, depending on the physical layout of the event. The medical event staff should be assembled and briefed weeks prior to the start of the event. They should be trained on the protocols and standard operating procedures that will be used. The arrival times for the medical team should be well defined, and an assembly point should be established from where teams can pick up supplies and be dispatched to the secondary stations. The base station serves this function well. A uniform dress code should be established that will allow medical personnel to be easily identified. Provisions for the medical team should include parking passes, appropriate tickets or passes to the event, and food coupons.

COMMUNICATIONS

Communication during a mass gathering is a crucial point that must be well delineated and ideally have some degree of redundancy. The failure of communication can destroy even the most well-planned event coverage. In the event of a disaster, communication among the medical staff will need to be intergrated to all other aspects of the public safety model. The broad availability of cellular service has improved this aspect of event coverage significantly. The communications center should be the base station, which should have the capability of communicating with all aspects of public safety including the local fire department, local EMS, police or security, and event administration as well as individual medical staff. This is often best accomplished through the use of two-way radios or cellular phones with similar capabilities. Hard line or cellular service should also be available at the base station. The physical layout should be defined during the initial event planning in such a way that the crowd can be divided into specific locations in order to narrow the search area for any specific individual during the event. All calls for assistance from the crowd should be coordinated through the base station, which will

then in turn dispatch the appropriate medical team. Even if a spectator reports an emergency to one of the secondary stations, the base station should be notified prior to the initiation of a response.

DOCUMENTATION

Provision of medical care at an event is not without liability. Thus there is a need for adequate documentation of all patient encounters. The documentation of any medical care provides medicolegal protection as well as an avenue of data collection and allows for reporting of the service provided back to the event coordinators. If fee for service is to be used, the level of documentation should allow for optimized billing and reimbursement. A method of documenting patient encounters must cover the scope of potential patient complaints without being overburdening on the individual provider. The person requesting an aspirin certainly does not require a full history and physical exam (H&P) like the patient presenting with chest pain. The patient requesting aspirin likely only requires name, age, sex, complaint, allergies, and his or her function at the event. The patient with chest pain will need a full H&P similar to what would be done in the emergency department. The form developed must be simple to fill out but provide adequate medical documentation of the complaint, exam, assessment, and treatment given. Refusal-of-care forms and AMA forms must also be established and in place at the event (10). Basic discharge instructions should also be provided for those treated at the event, and there will need to be a system of quality improvement review to improve care for future events and for risk management purposes.

POSTEVENT ANALYSIS

After the event is over, all the medical records should undergo analysis and the information should be compiled. The event coordinators will appreciate a postevent report, including the number of patients treated, the types of medical complaints encountered, the treatment provided, and the disposition of the patients. This postevent analysis serves many functions. It provides information for future event coverage of similar venues, allowing for minor adjustments in staffing and equipment needed. The event coordinators will be able to better appreciate the role of the medical team at their event, keeping in mind that many people who would otherwise have had to leave the event to seek medical attention were able to remain and continue to participate. Data collection will also serve as an invaluable research tool allowing for publication of the experience gained at the particular event. Finally, the data will be useful as the primary tool for quality improvement review of the coverage provided. Letters thanking those who have participated in the medical coverage of the event, either physically or financially, should be sent in an effort to encourage their support in the future. Letters from patients treated at the event should be forwarded to the event coordinators. All of these postevent efforts will serve to justify the presence of the medical team and solidify its position at future events.

PREPAREDNESS HISTORIC EVENTS AND CASE HISTORIES

Much can be learned from prior events. A review of the literature (Table 26-1) makes evident that medical usage rates (MURs) vary widely, from 3 patients per 10,000 (PPTT) in a 5-year review of concerts in Southern California (19) to 347 PPTT at the 1989 Special Olympics (9). Seventy percent of events reviewed had an MUR ≤70 PPTT. Multiple factors need to be taken into account when trying to predict MURs, such as type and duration of event, attendance, mobile versus seated, indoor versus outdoor, weather, physical plant, alcohol and drug usage, and age and mood of the crowd.

Several of these factors have been shown to correlate with higher MURs (6):

1. Drug and alcohol use
2. Hot weather
3. Being outdoors
4. Crowds being mobile rather than seated
5. Rock concerts (vs. classical music)

Although many other variables may intuitively point toward higher MURs, the reported data have been inconclusive.

In a review of the literature describing mass gatherings during which mass casualty incidents or terroristic events have taken place (25-27), there have been several success stories. What is evident is that although the majority of medical care at mass gatherings will involve taking care of spectators and participants, it is crucial to have a mass casualty plan that can be activated if necessary. This plan should ideally be based on "daily routine doctrine," whereby the disaster plan puts into effect an escalation of existing treatment protocols (27).

TABLE 26-1 Summary of Mass Gathering Events

EVENT	LOCATION	DATE	NUMBER OF PEOPLE	PPTT	VARIABLES AND SPECIAL FACTORS	REFERENCE
Glastonbury fair	UK	1971	150,000	77	Widespread use of drugs and alcohol	6,28
Summer Olympics	Munich	1972			Eight Arab terrorists in Olympic tracksuits forced their way into the Israeli Olympic Village compound. 11 Israeli athletes, 1 German police officer, and 5 terrorists dead.	25
Rock concert at Watkins Glen	NY	1973	600,000	6	High drug use	6,29
Rock festival	Vermont	1973	35,000	69	Widespread use of drugs and alcohol	6,30
NFL season	Denver	1978 10 games	720,000	4	Higher usage during earlier, hotter part of the season	6,31
Rock concert	Toronto	1980 August	30,000	163	High drug usage	32
Golf tournament, "The Open"	UK	1981–1990	1,568,833	51	Ten-year review. Emphasized good communications with the chief marshal, police, and ambulance services	33
Worlds Fair	Knoxville, TN	1982 October	11,000,000	23		6,34
Rock Concert US Festival	San Bernardino, CA	1982 September	410,000	64	Day 1: Punk rock—55 PPTT Day 2: New wave—50 PPTT Day 3: Contemporary rock—105 PPTT Low drug use overall. Older crowd on day 3	6,35
Summer Olympics	Los Angeles, CA	1984	3,450,000	16	Highest MUR (21) at outdoor events with mobile spectators and a crowd capacity of <30,000	25,36,37

TABLE 26-1 Summary of Mass Gathering Events *(continued)*

EVENT	LOCATION	DATE	NUMBER OF PEOPLE	PPTT	VARIABLES AND SPECIAL FACTORS	REFERENCE
Live Aid Concert	Philadelphia, PA	1985 July	90,000	33		38
College football, basketball, and concerts	NY	1980–1986			Crowd size has only a minor influence on patient volume	6,39
College football	AZ	1983–1986	1,264,341	3	No change in MUR pre and post EtOH ban, although extensive alcohol and drug smuggling	6,40
World Exposition	Vancouver	1986 October	22,100,000	39		41
Golf tournament	Advance, NC	1987 May	80,000	22	4 days	42
Papal visit	San Antonio, TX	1988			200 encounters, 90% heat related. Temperature (T)=100–106° F	6,15
Winter Olympics	Calgary, Canada	1988	1,800,000	15.2		43
Air show	Ramstein, Germany	1988			Airplane fell into spectator enclosure: 45 dead; over 500 injured. Mass casualty plan activated and all survivors treated, triaged, and evacuated within 96 minutes	26
Boating	PA	1988			Three Rivers Regatta accident: Formula 1 boat collided with shore, injuring 24 spectators (50% pedestrians). All patients triaged and evacuated in 32 minutes	27
Outdoor music festival	UK	1989	75,000	62	Three-day event held on private farm in England. Predicted 6,000; 75,000 arrived. Insufficient toilets and water. Gastroenteritis outbreak	6,44
Special Olympics	Galveston, TX	1989	777 athletes	347		33
Indianapolis 500 NASCAR event	Indianapolis, IN	1983–1990	400,000 per year	3.5	Average for 8 races	33,45,46
Royal Adelaide Show	Adelaide, Australia	1991 9 days	140,000	91	Usage rates correlated best with variations in temperature rather than attendance	6,47
Super Bowl	Tampa, FL	1991	70,000	185		48
Papal visit	Denver, CO	1993	500,000		Changing weather played a big role. Tmax 89° F during the day. Dropped to 56° F at night. Spectators cooled with hoses during the day were shivering at night.	6,16,17
Rock concert	Bryam Township, NJ	1993	54,000	15	Outdoor	49
Rock concert	Woodstock, NY	1994	350,000 (estimated)	143	Rain, with 30° F drop during concert	6,21,22
Papal visit	New York City	1995	130,000	4	In Central Park; T=50-60°F and scattered showers	18

TABLE 26-1 Summary of Mass Gathering Events *(continued)*

EVENT	LOCATION	DATE	NUMBER OF PEOPLE	PPTT	VARIABLES AND SPECIAL FACTORS	REFERENCE
Papal visit	New York City	1995	75,000	19	At Aqueduct racetrack; T=85°F and no water sold inside racetrack	18
College football		1995	485,989	11	Review of seven home games. Alcohol banned. Hot and humid	50
AIDS ride 3	CA	1996			Seven-day event. 2,650 riders; 25,379 medical treatments. One day T=107°F with 70% of cases heat related	6,51
Chicago Concert Series	Chicago, IL	1996	250,000	12	High rate of drug and alcohol use. When patients asked, half admitted to using some drug	52,53
Democratic National Convention	Chicago, IL	1996	30,000	16	Field hospital saw 12, 37 at convention site	54
Summer Olympics	Atlanta, GA	1996	19,000,000 calculated	23	July 27 bombing killed 2 and injured 110. Heat-related illness most common among spectators. No significant change in local hospital ED visits over baseline	55,56,57, 58
Concerts	Southern California	1993–1998	4,638,099	3	Max MUR 71 PPTT at a music festival at an outdoor pavilion where a riot broke out. Rock concerts had 2.5 times the overall patient load of nonrock concerts.	19
Millennium Eve celebration	Oxford, UK	1999			Temporary ED set up in smaller hospital closer to millennium festivities. Only 9 patients seen in temporary ED; 342 in main ED	59
Thunderdome Rave party	Antwerp, Belgium	1999	14,000	70	81% of patient contacts related to intoxication	60
Rock Concert	Washington, DC	1999			Lightning strike. Bystander CPR initiated <1 min. Found to be asystolic. Intubated after a couple more minutes by an emergency physician. Pulse was restored and pt. Arrived in ED <10 min after lightning strike with purposeful movements	61
Rock concert	Washington, DC	1999	186,000	82.9	Mosh pit experience. Moshing accounted for 37% of injuries	20
Solar eclipse	Cornwall, UK	1999			Used telemedicine to connect nurse-run minor injury units to a major hub ED; 4.6% of patients required a telemedicine consult	62
Royal Adelaide Show	Adelaide, Australia	1995–2001	4,316,404	17	63 show days, >7,000 patients. Positive correlation between temperature and MUR	63
Rock Concert Festival	Taipei	2001	50,000	6		6,64
Masters Golf Tournament	Augusta, GA	2000–2002	150,000 (estimated)	92	Actual attendance numbers are not released. Estimate of 50,000 each Masters with 1,379 total patient encounters for 3 years	Author

PREPAREDNESS SUMMARY

Mass gatherings provide a unique set of circumstances for the planning and provision of medical care. Due to the multiple variables involved, no one individual plan can be applied to all events. The approach, however, should be consistent, encompassing all of the aspects discussed in this chapter (Tables 26-2, 26-3, 26-4; Fig. 26-1). Ultimately, having a comprehensive plan for routine medical care and disaster scenarios is the best way to ensure a medically uncomplicated event and prevent unnecessary morbidity.

RESOURCES

1. American College of Emergency Physicians. Provision of emergency medical care for crowds [paper].
2. NAEMSP. Mass gathering medical care: the medical director's checklist [booklet].
3. NDMS web site: http://ndms.dhhs.gov/.
4. Local DMAT teams.
5. FEMA web site: http://www.fema.gov/.
6. Red Cross web site: http://www.redcross.org/.
7. U.S. Department of Homeland Security web site: http://www.dhs.gov/dhspublic/.
8. Local EMS.
9. Poison Control web site: http://www.aapcc.org/. Telephone: 1-800-222-1222.

TABLE 26-2 Timeline for Preparation

Prior to event tasks	12 mos.	10 mos.	8 mos.	6 mos.	5 mos.	4 mos.	3 mos.	2 mos.	1 mo.	1 wk.	1 d.
Contact event coordinators	X										
Assemble event planning committee	X	X									
Meet with planning committee		X	X								
Develop plan for medical coverage			X	X							
Assign medical director	X										
Secure malpractice insurance				X							
Recruit volunteers	X	X	X	X	X	X	X	X	X	X	
Order uniforms/shirts						X					
Visit site		X			X					X	X
Develop map of site		X			X						
Acquire communication system	X	X									
Test communication equipment										X	X
Acquire equipment and supplies	X	X	X	X	X	X	X	X	X	X	X
Set up for event										X	X

TABLE 26-3 Supply List

EQUIPMENT AND SUPPLIES	MAIN STATION	SECONDARY STATION	JUMP BAG
Stretchers or beds	X		
Portable suction	X	X	
Cardiac monitors/defibrillator	X		
AED	X	X	
Oxygen	X	X	
Cooling fans	X		
Warming blanket	X		
Laryngoscope set	X	X	X
ET tubes, 3.5 – 8.0	X	X	X
Oxygen supplies	X	X	X
Nebulizer sets	X	X	X
Oral airways	X	X	X
Backup airway device	X	X	X
Ambu bags (adult and pediatric)	X	X	X
End tidal CO2 detector	X	X	X
IV fluids: D5W, saline, LR	X	X	X
IV supplies	X	X	X
Bandages (Band-aids, Kerlex, etc.)	X	X	X
Splinting material	X		
Suture—assorted	X		
Suture trays	X		
Steri-strips	X	X	
Irrigation saline	X	X	X
Sphygmomanometer	X	X	X
Stethoscope	X	X	X
Thoracostomy tray	X		
Spine boards	X	X	
Cervical collars	X	X	X
Golf carts	X	X	
Tents for secondary stations	X		
Tables	X		
Jump bags		X	
Prescription pads	X		
Patient encounter forms	X	X	X
AMA forms	X	X	X
Glucose monitor	X	X	X
Handheld cautery	X		
Woods lamp	X		

TABLE 26-3 Supply List *(continued)*

EQUIPMENT AND SUPPLIES	MAIN STATION	SECONDARY STATION	JUMP BAG
Fluorescein strips	X		
Pulse-ox monitor	X		
Extra batteries	X		X
Clipboards	X	X	X
Epistaxis trays	X		
Cool packs	X	X	X
Otoscope	X		
Disaster triage tags	X	X	X
Pens	X	X	X
Pillows	X		
Ring cutter	X		
Coolers	X	X	
Soap	X	X	X
Sheets	X	X	
Eye irrigation	X	X	X
Oral rehydration fluids	X	X	
Suction tubing and tips	X	X	
Tape	X	X	X
Thermometer	X	X	
Towels	X	X	X
Pocket mask	X	X	X
IV poles	X	X	
Blankets	X	X	
Burn dressing			
Lock box for narcotics	X		

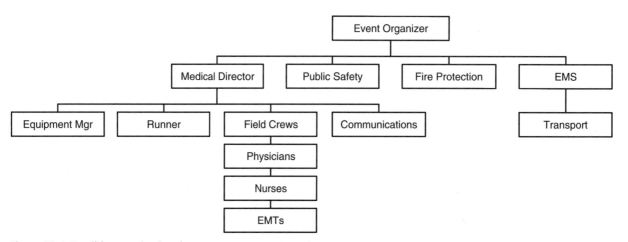

Figure 26–1. Possible organizational structure.

TABLE 26-4	Medication List		
MEDICATIONS	**MAIN STATION**	**SECONDARY STATION**	**JUMP BAG**
Aspirin	X	X	X
Tylenol	X	X	X
Motrin	X	X	X
Morphine	X		
1% lidocaine with and without epi	X	X	
Maalox	X	X	
Benadryl (IV, PO, IM)	X	X	X
Epinephrine 1:1000 and 1:10,000	X	X	X
Topical antibiotic ointment	X	X	X
Phenergan (PO, IM, IV, PR)	X	X	
Prednisone (IV, PO)	X		
Albuterol (nebulized, MDI)	X	X	X
1% hydrocortisone cream	X	X	X
Silver sulfadiazine	X	X	X
Xeroform gauze	X	X	
Atropine	X	X	X
IV lidocaine	X	X	X
Sodium bicarbonate	X	X	X
Calcium chloride	X	X	X
Fosphenytoin	X		
Dopamine	X		
Furosemide	X		
Metoprolol	X		
Adenosine	X		
Insulin	X		
D50	X	X	X
Imodium	X	X	
Versed	X		
Midriatic solution	X		
Valium	X		
Tetanus toxoid	X	X	
Activated charcoal	X		
Sunscreen	X	X	X
Sunburn lotion	X	X	X
Insect repellant	X	X	X

REFERENCES

1. Sanders AB, Criss E, Steckl P, et al. An analysis of medical care at mass gatherings. Ann Emerg Med 1986;15:515-9.
2. Rose WD, Larid SL, Prescott JE, et al. Emergency medical services for collegiate football games: A six and one-half year review. Prehospital and Disaster Med 1992;7:157-9.
3. Parrillo S. Medical care of mass gatherings. In: Hogan D, Burstein JL eds. Disaster medicine. Philadelphia: Lippincott, Williams, and Wilkins, 2002;274-8.
4. De Lorenzo RA. Mass gathering medicine: a review. Prehospital Disaster Med 1997;12:68-72.
5. Levitin HW. Providing medical care at mass gatherings. Lecture at the 1999 Scientific Assembly: ACEP, October 13, 1999.
6. Milsten AM, Maguire BJ, Bissell RA, et al. Mass-gathering medical care: a review of the literature. Prehospital Disaster Med 2002;17(3):151-62.
7. Grange JT, Baumann GW. The California 500: Medical care at a NASCAR Winston cup race event. Ann Emerg Med 1999;34(4):abstract.
8. Weaver WD, Sutherland K, Wirkus MJ, et al. Emergency medical care requirements for large public assemblies and a new strategy for managing cardiac arrest in this setting. Ann Emerg Med 1989;18:155-60.
9. Calabro JJ, Krohmer JR, Rivera EJ, et al. Provision of emergency medical care for crowds. ACEP EMS Committee, American College of Emergency Physicians, 1995-96.
10. Grange JT. Planning for large events. Curr Sports Med Reports 2002;1:156-61.

11. Jaslow D, Yancey A, Milsten A, for the NAEMSP Standards and Clinical Practice Committee. Mass gathering medical care: the medical director's checklist. National Association of EMS Physicians, 2000.

12. Jaslow D, Yancey A, Milsten A. Mass gathering medical care. Prehospital Emerg Care 2000;4:359-60.

13. Leonard RB. Medical support for mass gatherings. Emerg Med Clin North Am 1996;14(2):383-97.

14. Nordberg M. EMS and mass gatherings. Emerg Med Ser 1990;19(5):46-56.

15. Gordon D. The pope's visit: mass gatherings and the EMS system. EMS 1988;17(1):38-44.

16. Paul HM. Mass casualty: pope's Denver visit causes mega MCI. JEMS 1993;18(11):64-8, 72-5.

17. Schulte D, Meade DM. The papal chase. The pope's visit: A "mass" gathering. Emerg Med Ser 1993;22(11):46-9, 65-75, 79.

18. Federman JH, Giordano LM. How to cope with a visit from the pope. Prehospital Disaster Med 1997;12(2):86-91.

19. Grange JT, Green SM, Downs W. Concert medicine: spectrum of medical problems encountered at 405 major concerts. Acad Emerg Med 1999;6(3):202-7.

20. Janchar T, Samaddar C, Milzman D. The mosh pit experience: emergency medical care for concert injuries. Am J Emerg Med 2000;18(1):62-3.

21. Dress JM, Horton EH, Florida R. Music, mud and medicine. Woodstock '94: A maniacal, musical, mass-casualty incident. Emerg Med Serv 1995;24(1):21,30-2.

22. Florida R, Goldfarb Z. Woodstock '94: Peace, music and EMS. JEMS 1994;19(12):45-50.

23. Parillo SJ. Medical care at mass gatherings: considerations for physician involvement. Prehospital Disaster Med 1995;10:273-5.

24. McDonald CC, Koenigsberg MD, Ward S. Medical control of mass gatherings: can paramedics perform without physicians onsite? Prehospital Disaster Med 1993;8(4):327-31.

25. Feiner B. EMS at the 1984 Olympics. Emerg Med Serv 1984;13(2):16-19.

26. Seletz JM. Flugtag-88 (Ramstein Air Show Disaster): an army response to a MASCAL. Milit Med 1990;155:152-5.

27. Vukmir RB, Paris PM. The Three Rivers Regatta accident: an EMS perspective. Am J Emerg Med 1991;9(1):64-71.

28. Blandford AG, Obst CD, Dunlop HA. Glastonbury Fair: Some medical aspects of a rock music festival. The Practitioner 1972;209:205-11.

29. James SH, Calendrillo B, Schnoll SH. Medical and toxicological aspects of the Watkins Glen rock concert. J Forens Sci 1975;20:71-82.

30. Osler DC, Shapiro F, Shapiro S. Medical services at outdoor music festivals. Clin Ped 1975;14(4):390-5.

31. Pons PT, Holland B, Alfrey E, et al. An advanced emergency medical care system at National Football League games. Ann Emerg Med 1980;9(4):203-6.

32. Chapman KR, Carmichael, FJ, Goode JE. Medical services for outdoor rock music festivals. Can Med Assoc J 1982;126:935.

33. Hadden WA, Kelly S, Pumfort N. Medical cover for 'The Open' golf championship. Br J Sports Med 1992;26(3):125-7.

34. Gustafson TL, Booth AL, Fricker RS, et al. Disease surveillance and emergency services at the 1982 World's Fair. AJPH 1987;77(7):861-3.

35. Ounanian LL, Salinas C, Shear CL: Medical care at the 1982 US Festival. Ann Emerg Med 1986;15(5):520-27.

36. Baker WM, Simone BM, Niemann JT, et al. Special event medical care: The 1984 Los Angeles summer Olympics experience. Ann Emerg Med 1986;15:185.

37. Weiss BP, Mascola L, Fannin SL. Public health at the 1984 summer Olympics: The LA county experience. Am J Public Health 1988;78:686.

38. Mariano JP: First aid for live aid. J Emerg Med Serv 1986;11:47.

39. De Lorenzo RA, Gray BC, Bennett PC, et al. Effect of crowd size on patient volume at a large, multipurpose, indoor stadium. J Emerg Med 1989;7:379-84.

40. Spaite DW, Meislin HW, Valenzeula TD, et al. Banning alcohol in a major college stadium: Impact on the incidence and patterns of injury and illness. College Health 1990;39:125-8.

41. Weaver WD, Sutherland K, Wirkus MJ, et al. Emergency medical care requirements for large public assemblies and a new strategy for managing cardiac arrest in this setting. Ann Emerg Med 1989;18:155.

42. Leonard RB, Petrilli R, Noji EK, et al. Provision of emergency medical care for crowds. Disaster medical services of ACEP. ACEP publication, 1989-90.

43. Thompson JM, Savoia G, Powell G, et al. Level of medical care required for mass gatherings: the VX Winter Olympic Games in Calgary Canada. Ann Emerg Med 1991;20(4):385-90.

44. Chambers J, Guly H. The impact of a music festival on local health services. Health Trends 1991;23(3):122-3.

45. Bowdish GE, Cordell WH, Bock HC, et al. Using research analysis to predict volume at the Indianapolis 500 mile race. Ann Emerg Med 1992;21(10):1200-3.

46. Bock HC, Cordell WH, Hawk AC, et al. Demographic of emergency medical care at the Indianapolis 500 mile race (1983-1990). Ann Emerg Med 1992;21(10):1204-7.

47. Flabouris A, Bridgewater F. An analysis of demand for first-aid care at a major public event. Prehospital Disaster Med 1996;11(1):48-54.

48. Carlson L. Spectator medical care. Learning from the super bowl. The Physician and Sports Medicine 1992;20:141.

49. Foster TM. EMS meets grunge: EMS coverage of Lollapalooza 1993. JEMS 1993;18(12):47-51, 53.

50. Shelton S, Haire S, Gerard B. Medical care for mass gatherings at collegiate football games. Southern Med J 1997;90(11):1081-3.

51. Friedman LJ, Rodi SW, Krueger MA, et al. Medical care at the California AIDS ride 3: Experiences in event medicine. An Emerg Med 1998;31(2):219-23.

52. Erickson TB. Drug use patterns at rock concerts hold key to trends. Emerg Med News 1996;10.

53. Erickson TB, Koenigsberg M, Bunney EB, et al. Prehospital severity scoring at major rock concert events. Prehospital Disaster Med 1996;12(3):195-9.

54. Binder LS, Willoughby PJ, Matkaitis L. Development of a unique decentralized rapid-response capability and contingency mass-casualty field hospital for the 1996 Democratic National Convention. Prehospital Emerg Care 1997;1(4):238-45.

55. Center for Disease Control and Prevention—MMWR: prevention and management of heat related illness among spectators and staff during the Olympic Games—Atlanta, 6-23 July 1996. JAMA 1996;45(29):631-3.

56. Stiel D, Trethowan P, Vance N. Medical planning for the Sydney Olympic and Paralympic Games. MJA 1997;167:593-4.

57. Ellis JM. EMS at the Olympics. Emerg Med Services 1996;53-5.

58. Wetterhall SF, Coulombier DM, Herndon JM, et al. Medical care delivery at the 1996 Olympic Games. JAMA 1998;279(18):1463-68.

59. McGuire LC, Bell AZ. Developing an enhanced minor injury unit for support of urban festivities. Eur J Emerg Med 2001;8:193-7.

60. Suy K, Gijsenbergh F, Baute L. Emergency medical assistance during a mass gathering. Eur J Emerg Med 1999;6:249-54.

61. Milzman DP, Moskowoitz L, Hardel M. Lightning strikes at a mass gathering. South Med J 1999;92(7):708-10.

62. Wootton R, McKelvey A, McNicholl B, et al. Transfer of telemedical support to Cornwall from a national telemedicine network during a solar eclipse. J Telemed Telecare 2000;6:182-6.

63. Zeitz KM, Schneider D, Jarrett D, et al. Mass gathering events: retrospective analysis of patient presentations over seven years. Prehospital Disaster Med 2002;17(3):147-150.

64. Kao WF, Kuo CC, Chang H, et al. Characteristics of patients at a Taipei summer rock concert festival. Zhonghua Yi Xue Za Zhi (Taipei) 2001;64(9):525-30.

27

Federal, State, Regional, and Local Resource Access and Utilization

David W. Gruber

INTRODUCTION

An act of terrorism is by nature a surprise event that shocks any medical system. People, equipment, and finances will be stretched to capacity in many ways, and the ability of a medical system to maintain a concentrated effective effort may wane with time if the system is not initially prepared and refreshed on a regular basis.

During an acute incident of terrorism (e.g., explosive event), staffing may be inadequate or inappropriate, or staff members may be victims of the incident. During a chronic episode (e.g., infectious disease), responders may become exhausted or themselves become secondary victims, thereby reducing the ability of the medical system to sustain the required level of response. Supplies may be short, unavailable, or inaccessible, and resupply may be impossible. Equipment may not be appropriate for a response, or responders may be unable to reach response sites with the equipment. Planners may have missed certain needs or may have used faulty assumptions. An absence of effective command, control, and communications may negate the ability for a logistically capable system to provide an adequate response. Every level of medical organization—first responder, first receivers, single medical facility, local system, regional or state program, or federal effort—is stressed by the preparedness for, and response to, an act of terrorism or mass casualty incident.

This chapter will provide an overview of the federal, state, regional, and local resources available to the medical system that aid in the medical preparation for and response to terrorism. Since the boundaries of these resources may blur and their use may overlap, this chapter will also address the integration of the different levels of resources (federal, state, regional, and local). And since medical responders at these different levels are responsible for different aspects of response, this chapter will address the four areas of the Disaster Management Cycle: mitigation, preparedness, response, and recovery.

The objective is to provide planners with a shopping list of resources and assistance during preevent efforts, and to ensure that responders are aware of the resources and assistance available during and after their response to an act of terrorism. Since the list of resources is extensive, the chapter will recommend basic, intermediate, and advanced resources to allow the user to incorporate necessary assets progressively.

PREPAREDNESS ESSENTIALS

THE EMERGENCY PREPAREDNESS AND RESPONSE TRIAD

The Emergency Preparedness and Response Triad (the Triad) depicts three critical components that deal with the preparation for and response to an act of terrorism or mass casualty incident. The components of the Triad are emergency management, health care delivery systems, and public health systems (Fig. 27-1).

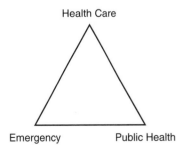

Figure 27–1. The Emergency Preparedness and Response Triad.

The health care delivery system includes hospitals, Emergency Medical Services (EMS), federally qualified health centers (FQHC), facilities related to care for the aging (long-term care), psychological treatment facilities, and other medically related organizations. This is the category most associated with the medical response to terrorism. Integration of this component with the public health system and with emergency management organizations provides a complete approach to readiness and response. When preparing for a medical response to terrorism or any public health emergency, all three components must individually plan how they would respond to such an event. However, it is just as important for individual plans to complement each other in order to ensure a complete and integrated response to a disaster.

THE DISASTER MANAGEMENT CYCLE

The Emergency Preparedness and Response Triad is applied to a cycle of events surrounding a public health emergency, act of terrorism, or mass casualty incident. This cycle, designated the Disaster Management Cycle (DMC), depicts the phases of an incident, emergency, mass casualty event, or disaster from prevention through recovery. The cycle is divided into four phases (Fig. 27-2). Although depicted as sequential, there may be overlap or jumping of phases and concurrent activities that simultaneously address different phases. The following describes the objectives and activities that occur within each phase.

Preparedness is the phase during which governments, organizations, and individuals develop plans to save lives, minimize disaster damage, and enhance disaster response operations. Preparedness measures include preparedness plans; emergency exercises/training; warning systems; emergency communications systems; evacuation plans and training; resource inventories; emergency personnel/contact lists; mutual aid agreements; and public information/education.

Response includes those activities that provide emergency assistance for casualties, reduce the probability of secondary damage, and speed recovery operations. Response measures include activating public warning; notifying public authorities; mobilizing emergency personnel/equipment; providing emergency medical assistance; manning emergency operations centers; declaring disasters and evacuating; mobilizing security forces; initiating search and rescue; and activating emergency suspension of laws.

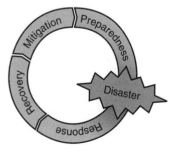

Figure 27–2. The Disaster Management Cycle.

Recovery includes those activities that continue until all systems return to normal or better. Recovery measures, both short and long term, include returning vital life-support systems to minimum operating standards. It encompasses damage insurance/loans and grants, temporary housing, long-term medical care, disaster unemployment insurance, public information, health and safety education, reconstruction, counseling programs, and economic impact studies. Information resources and services include data collection related to rebuilding, claims processing, and documentation of lessons learned.

Mitigation is the elimination or reduction in probability of the occurrence of a disaster, or the lessening of the effects of unavoidable disasters. Mitigation measures include building codes, vulnerability analyses updates, tax incentives and disincentives, zoning and land use management, building use regulations and safety codes, allocations and interstate sharing of resources, preventive health care, and public education. Information resources and services important in mitigation activities include GIS-based risk assessment, claims history, facility/resource identification, land use/zoning, and building code information. Use of modeling/prediction tools for trend and risk analysis is also important (1).

The medical preparation and response to terrorism may take place during any phase of the Disaster Management Cycle.

THE EFFECTS OF DISASTER MANAGEMENT CYCLE TEMPO ON MEDICAL PREPAREDNESS AND RESPONSE

The tempo of the DMC will frequently determine the availability and use of resources. For example, during the preparedness phase, in the absence of an infectious disease outbreak, a hospital may have the needed months to construct adequate isolation facilities. However, an outbreak of SARS might accelerate this same hospital into the response phase prior to isolation facility completion, and the same hospital may have only days to prepare itself for numbers of highly contagious patients. Likewise, a public health system may be able to adequately vaccinate a number of health professionals for smallpox during the preparedness stage of the cycle and, as part of the response phase, would be able to accelerate this process to include additional health professionals and first responders. However, the ability to effectively mass vaccinate millions in a timely fashion is a significant challenge.

Tempo control of the DMC is the most critical component of the preparedness for and response to any act of terrorism, public health emergency, or mass casualty incident. Access and use of appropriate resources at the appropriate time is a means of tempo control.

Traditionally, many medical planners focused only on the prehospital and hospital components of the response phase of the DMC. This focus understandably occurs for two reasons. First is the degree of comfort and expertise that medical professionals have in these areas. For example, fire and law enforcement first responders may depend on the medical community to treat the victims of an incident so that they may focus on the causes and effects of medical emergencies (i.e., hazmat incidents, fires, criminal actions, or search and rescue). The second reason that medical planners key on prehospital and hospital issues is the traditional stovepipe of programs. Until recently, cross-pollination of ideas, interaction of different preparedness and response communities, and integration of horizontal and vertical preparedness and response plans has been the exception rather than the rule. Fortunately, there is a shift in this paradigm. So while medical planners continue to focus on prehospital and hospital components, they now are expected to integrate these components into a holistic view of preparedness and response and to be subject matter experts for these components for others who plan for the DMC. This integration is occurring across all areas. The result is a tremendous amount of resources and assets available to the medical response to terrorism.

RESOURCES

Resources related to the medical response to terrorism are available in all phases of the DMC, and the most efficacious medical response to terrorism or mass casualty incident will take advantage of as many resources as possible. These resources fall into four general categories: governmental, partnerships/associations/volunteer organizations, academia, and commercial.

GOVERNMENTAL RESOURCES

Governmental resources are available at federal, state, and local levels and may support all phases of the DMC. This chapter will later address specific programs; however, as an overview, major federal resources are available through the Centers for Disease Control (CDC), U.S. Department of Justice Office for State and Local Domestic Preparedness (ODP), Federal Emergency Management Agency (FEMA), Health and Human Services (HHS) Health Resources and Services Administration (HRSA) and Agency for Healthcare Resources and Quality (AHRQ), and the U.S. military, specifically the U. S. Army Medical Research Institute of Infectious Diseases (USAMRIID). The Federal Bureau of Investigation (FBI), the Central Intelligence Agency (CIA), the National Domestic Preparedness Consortium, the National Health Professions Preparedness Consortium, and the National Disaster Life Support Educational Consortium (NDLSEC) have courses and background materials supporting planning and intelligence related to the medical response to terrorism. The NDLSEC is a collaborative effort of federal, state, and academic centers with financial support from the Centers for Disease Control and Prevention (CDC). The overarching goal of the NDLSEC is to standardize emergency response training nationwide and strengthen our nation's public health system. The resources listed in various forms provide for planning, training and exercise, equipment, funding, and response. (Note: Many programs listed now fall under the Department of Homeland Security; however, it is best to associate them with the organizations listed.)

The federal government, through Homeland Security Presidential Directive 5, has developed the National Incident Management System (NIMS) to provide interoperability between the federal, state, and local levels. A specific program supporting the medical response to terrorism is the Hospital Emergency Incident Command System (HEICS). HEICS is a hospital disaster management system that is based on the general disaster incident command system (ICS). Although HEICS is an Orange County, California, product, this system has become a model for most hospital incident management organizations. HEICS features a flexible management organizational chart that allows for the customized hospital response to a crisis to include the organized division of tasks and a realistic span of control for managers. The San Mateo County Emergency Services Agency provides information and download of the HEICS's project and plan on their web site (2).

The National Oceanic and Atmospheric Association (NOAA) provides weather and environmental information that could provide insight into deployment of terrorist weapons of mass destruction (i.e., plume dispersion, temperature, humidity), and the climatic conditions that responders would operate under during the medical response to an incident (3).

In the area of response, governmental teams are available for deployment to an affected site. These include CDC epidemiological investigation teams; CDC Strategic National Stockpile (SNS) Technical Advisory Response Units (TARU) to assist in state and local deployment of the SNS; FBI investigative teams; National Guard Civil Support Teams (CST), and the U.S. Marine Corps Chemical Biological Incident Response Force (CBIRF) both able to assist local, state, or federal agencies by providing capabilities for (a) agent detection and identification, (b) casualty search, rescue, and personnel decontamination, and (c) emergency medical care and stabilization of contaminated personnel. This book addresses governmental partnership teams later in this chapter.

State governmental resources vary in scope, responsibility, and comprehensiveness; however, there are some general resources available through state programs. State statues significant to the medical response to terrorism may address the emergency powers of the health response system (emergency powers acts), the role and responsibilities of the health system within a state's emergency management structure, and the cross-credentialing and mutual aid agreements. State emergency management plans are critical in defining how a state will organize and respond to a major incident, as well as the responsibilities of different organizations within these plans. State emergency management organizations will manage and operate a state's Emergency Operation Center (EOC). Within the state EOC, state health departments generally represent the medical community. However, the scope, guidance and responsibilities of individual state health departments vary greatly. One specific role of a state health department is as a conduit of CDC and HRSA policy and procedures to a state's constituents. Other key resources provided by state health departments include isolation and quarantine procedures, biological specimens transfer protocol, and pharmaceutical and medical stockpile distribution.

Depending on a state's organization, the departments of energy, environment, and agriculture and state's attorney general's office may play roles in the medical response to terrorism. Few states are organized identically; however, these listed departments are sources for information on communicable disease, nuclear/radiological incidents, water-borne threats, agricultural and animal-related terrorist events, and generalized counterterrorism. In addition to providing information, experts from these departments should be considered important resources in medical planning and response. Also at the state level, the FBI's Joint Terrorism Task Forces (JTTF) are sources of intelligence that can assist the medical community. Sixty-six JTTFs made up of federal, state, and local law enforcement members are located throughout the country. These teams share international, national, and local terrorism information and intelligence and serve as conduits of information to state agencies.

Major funding sources that provide states with funds specifically related to the medical planning and response to terrorism include federal grant money from CDC, HRSA, and ODP. These funds may be allocated by the state or passed through to localities for distribution. State subsidies vary greatly across the country with possible sources from specifically designated terrorism funding, health services funding, and EMS funding. In general, most states rely on FEMA funding to provide recovery assistance after a major incident, although some may have an emergency fund for this purpose.

Local governmental resources, normally from a health department, are limited. An exception is the federal contributions directly to localities funded by the Metropolitan Medical Response System (MMRS). The primary focus of the MMRS program is to develop or enhance existing emergency preparedness systems to respond effectively to a public health crisis, especially a weapons of mass destruction (WMD) event.

In March 2003, the MMRS joined FEMA and other programs from the Departments of Health and Human Services, Energy, and Justice to become the Emergency Preparedness and Response Directorate of the new Department of Homeland Security (4).

OTHER ORGANIZATIONS

Partnerships

There are formal partnerships significant to mass casualty response operations. Most noteworthy are those associated with the National Disaster Medical System (NDMS) operating under Operations Branch of the Response Division of the Federal Emergency Management Agency, U.S. Department of Homeland Security. The NDMS is a public/private partnership that provides emergency health care services and definitive medical care to disaster victims when state and local resources are overwhelmed. At the national level, the partnership includes Department of Defense, FEMA, HHS, and Veterans Administration (VA). The VA's role in NDMS is one of coordination of various NDMS areas throughout the United States. There are three circumstances under which the NDMS may be activated:

■ In response to an overseas military contingency

■ In response to a direct request to the Secretary of HHS for major medical assistance

■ After a Presidential declaration of a disaster under the Federal Response Plan

Specific Response Teams

Disaster Medical Assistance Teams (DMAT) are a volunteer group of medical and paramedical professionals who have prepared themselves to assemble rapidly as a self-sufficient medical response unit. This group, capable of mobilization and deployment within 24 hours of notification, is composed of physicians, nurses, and rescue and support staff, who can provide acute emergency and primary care to an affected population. Team members are trained to deliver medical and surgical care and to stabilize victims at a disaster site until they can be evacuated to a receiving hospital. A DMAT is also equipped to provide primary care services in cases where communities may have lost their health care facilities.

Disaster Mortuary Assistance Teams (DMORT) provides mobile morgue operations, forensic examination, DNA acquisition, remains identification, search and recovery, scene documentation, medical/psychology support, embalming/casketing, family assistance center, antemortem data collection, postmortem data collection, records data entry, database administration, personal effects processing, coordination of release of remains, provision of a liaison to United States Public Health Service (USPHS), provision of communications equipment, and safety officers and specialists.

Veterinary Medical Assistance Teams (VMAT) include veterinarians, technicians, and support personnel with small animal, large animal, exotic, livestock, and wildlife experience.

The Community Emergency Response Team (CERT) program helps train people to be better prepared to respond to emergency situations in their communities. When emergencies happen, CERT members can give critical support to first responders, provide immediate assistance to victims, and organize spontaneous volunteers at a disaster site. CERT members can also help with nonemergency projects that help improve the safety of the community. The CERT course is taught in the community by a trained team of first responders who have completed a CERT Train-the-Trainer course conducted by their state training office for emergency management or by FEMA's Emergency Management Institute (EMI), located in Emmitsburg, Maryland. CERT training includes disaster preparedness, disaster fire suppression, basic disaster medical operations, and light search and rescue operations (5).

The Center for Mental Health Services (CMHS) through an interagency agreement with FEMA via the Emergency Services and Disaster Relief Program supports immediate, short-term crisis counseling, and ongoing support for emotional recovery for the victims of disasters. CMHS staff helps to ensure that victims of presidentially declared disasters received immediate, short-term crisis counseling, as well as ongoing support for emotional recovery. CMHS collaborates with FEMA to train state mental health staff to develop crisis counseling training and preparedness efforts in their States.

The Comprehensive Hazmat Emergency Response - Capability Assessment Program (CHER-CAP) is offered by FEMA to assist local communities and tribal governments in obtaining a greater understanding of hazmat risks, identifying planning deficiencies, updating plans, training first responders, and stimulating and testing the system for strengths and needed improvements. CHER-CAP is a technological hazards component geared toward building more prepared communities throughout our nation.

CHER-CAP's purpose is to:

- Identify opportunities for plan revisions
- Identify communication needs
- Identify resource needs
- Improve coordination
- Comply with training requirements
- Clarify roles and responsibilities
- Improve individual performance
- Serve as a Train-the-Trainer initiative for additional jurisdictions
- Test plans and systems in a comprehensive hazmat exercise
- Motivate public and private officials to support emergency programs
- Increase general awareness of proficiency and needs
- Improve federal–state–tribal and government–local-industry emergency management relationships (6).

The Radiation Emergency Assistance Center/Training Site (REAC/TS) has provided support to the U.S. Department of Energy, the World Health Organization (WHO), and the International Atomic Energy Agency (IAEA) in the medical management of radiation accidents. A 24-hour emergency response program at the Oak Ridge Institute for Science and Education (ORISE) sponsored by REAC/TS trains, consults, or assists in the response to all types of radiation accidents or incidents. The center's specially trained team of physicians, nurses, health physicists, radiobiologists, and emergency coordinators is prepared around-the-clock to provide assistance on either the local, national, or international level (7).

Associations

Associations capable of assisting in the medical response to terrorism include profit and nonprofit, medical and nonmedical, professional and nonprofessional. These associations may contribute to different phases of the DMC.

Medical associations provide information and preparatory guidelines that can assist in mitigation and preparedness phases of the DMC. National medical associations in this category include the American Medical Association (AMA), Association for Professionals in Infection Control and Epidemiology (APIC), American Pharmaceutical Association, Advisory Committee on Immunization Practices (ACIP), College of American Pathologists (CAP), American Nursing Association (ANA), Pediatric Infectious Disease Society (PIDS), National Emergency Medicine Association, National Association of EMS Physicians (NAEP), National

Association of Emergency Medical Technicians (NAEMT), and National Mental Health Association (NMHA).

The NDLSEC in partnership with the AMA developed the National Disaster Life Support (NDLS) training program to better prepare health care professionals and emergency response personnel throughout the nation for all-hazards mass casualty events.

Public health-oriented associations include the Association of State and Territorial Health Officials and the National Association of County and City Health Officials. Hospital, Long Term Care (LTC), and primary care associations at the state and local levels are frequently strong partners in preparation and response to mass casualty incidents and should be consulted during planning stages.

Volunteer Organizations

Volunteer organizations provide a source of manpower and expertise that augment in-place medical responders.

The Red Cross provides disaster preparedness and response programs that support medical disaster response efforts. In addition to providing disaster planning to the community at-large and training and educating volunteers for disaster response, the Red Cross disaster relief effort focuses on the provision of shelter, food, and health and mental health services to address basic human needs. The Red Cross also feeds emergency workers, handles inquiries from concerned family members outside the disaster area, provides blood and blood products to disaster victims, and helps those affected by disaster to access other available resources (8).

The Salvation Army provides trauma counseling to individuals and families, identification and registration information for locating victims and providing information and communication to inquiring family and friends, mobile feeding of hot meals to victims and relief personnel on-site, and facilities for preparation and service of meals to victims and relief personnel (9).

Radio Amateur Civil Emergency Services (RACES) is a public service provided by a reserve (volunteer) communications group within government agencies in times of extraordinary need. Traditional RACES operations involve emergency message handling on Amateur Radio Service frequencies. These operations typically involve messages between critical locations such as hospitals, emergency services, emergency shelters, and any other locations where communication is needed.

RACES is administrated by a local, county, or state civil defense agency responsible for disaster services. RACES is a function of the Federal Communications Commission (FCC) Auxiliary Communications Service (ACS), sometimes known as DCS (Disaster Communications Service), ECS (Emergency Communications Service), ARPSC (Amateur Radio Public Service Corps), among others. FEMA provides planning guidance and technical assistance for establishing a RACES organization at the state and local government level (10).

First Aid/EMS volunteer organizations exist in varying forms depending on location. Due to this variance, the engagement of these volunteers will occur in different ways. This paragraph serves only as a reminder to include these organizations during the planning for and response to a mass casualty incident.

The National Voluntary Organizations Active in Disaster (NVOAD) goal is to coordinate the planning efforts by many voluntary organizations responding to disasters. NVOAD is not itself a service delivery organization. Instead, it upholds the privilege of its members to provide relief and recovery services independently, while expecting them to do so cooperatively. As such, it may serve as a coordinating organization for the medical planning and response to a major incident.

There are various businesses and business groups that volunteer goods and services in preparation for and during disaster response. Some of these goods and services are directly applicable to medical operations. Some are represented by organizations (i.e., Business Executives for National Security (BENS)) and others contribute individually. All should be considered during planning, response, and recovery operations.

Academia and Training Organizations

In 2000, CDC established a national system of Academic Centers for Public Health Preparedness (A-CPHP) to strengthen state and local workforce capacity to respond to bioterrorism and to support CDC's prevention programs in general. As of September 2003, 22 academic centers link schools of public health with state, local, and regional health departments to support bioterrorism preparedness and address public health infrastructure needs. In addition to these academic centers, CDC has designated Specialty and Advanced Practice Centers. The centers are listed here. For additional information regarding the A-CPHP program, access the CDC Internet site, http://www.cdc.gov/programs/bio.htm, or the individual centers' web sites.

The Academic Centers at the Schools of Public Health are University of Alabama-Birmingham, Columbia University, Emory University, Harvard University, Johns Hopkins University, University of California-Berkeley, University of California-Los Angeles, Saint Louis University, State University of New York-Albany, Tulane University, University of Iowa, University of Illinois at Chicago, University of Medicine and Dentistry of New Jersey, University of North Carolina-Chapel Hill, University of Michigan, University of Minnesota, University of Oklahoma, University of South Carolina, University of South Florida, University of Texas, University of Pittsburgh, and University of Washington.

Specialty Centers

CDC specialty centers are Dartmouth Medical College, Johns Hopkins and Georgetown University-Center for Law and the Public's Health, Saint Louis University-Center for the Study of Bioterrorism and Emerging Infections, University of Findlay (Ohio)-National Center of Excellence for Environmental Management, University of Georgia-Center for Leadership in Education and Applied Research in Mass Destruction Defense, University of Louisville-Center for Deterrence of Biowarfare and Bioterrorism, and Texas

A&M University-National Emergency Response and Rescue Training Center.

Advanced Practice Centers

The advanced practice centers are Dekalb County Board of Health-Georgia, Denver Health-Colorado, Monroe County Health Department-New York, Westchester County Health Department-New York, and Lawrence-Douglas County-Kansas. The Center for Domestic Preparedness (CDP) in Anniston, Alabama, offers specialized advanced training to state and local emergency responders in the management and remediation of incidents of domestic terrorism, especially those involving chemical agents and other toxic substances. CDP is a division of the Office for Domestic Preparedness (ODP) in the Office of Justice Programs, U.S. Department of Justice (DOJ). CDP serves as a member of the National Domestic Preparedness Consortium, which was established by DOJ's Office of Justice Programs/Office for Domestic Preparedness to provide expertise and training to the state and local emergency response community.

COMMERCIAL RESOURCES

The increase in federal funds aimed at countering threats of bioterrorism has resulted in an increase in commercial initiatives focused on this area. Numerous companies at the national and international levels are attempting to augment a core of defense, medical, pharmaceutical, and security businesses and consultants that had entered this sector prior to bioterrorism becoming a multibillion dollar in-vogue industry. The scope of this industry is too large to discuss in detail except to note there are specialists in training, equipment, planning, and information technologies all aimed at supporting the battle against health emergencies. The expertise of these specialists varies considerably as does the quality, appropriateness, and usefulness of their products.

PREPAREDNESS CHECKLIST TABLE AND SUMMARY

The following tables provide specific resources and assistance for the medical response to terrorism, which, for activities in support of this response, are consistent with the Emergency Preparedness and Response Triangle. Resources are identified for each phase of the Disaster Management Cycle and arranged according to the categories described earlier (governmental, partnerships/associations/volunteer organizations, academia, and commercial). These resources are then assigned either Basic, Intermediate, or Advanced levels to assist planners and responders in identifying which resources should be considered of most interest and which might be resources that supplement basic practices. As a result, the user should be able to initially address core capabilities and then build on this core toward a more advanced response design (Tables 27-1 to 27-4).

| TABLE 27-1 | Mitigation Resources for the Medical Response to Terrorism | | | |

CATEGORY	ORGANIZATION AND INTERNET ADDRESS	ACTIVITY CODE	ACTIVITY	LEVEL
GOVERNMENT				
Federal	Federal Emergency Management Agency (FEMA) www.fema.gov	P, F, I,T,C	Functions as specific area devoted to all-hazards/terrorism mitigation, funding for mitigation projects.	Basic
Federal	United States Army Medical Institute of Infectious Disease (USAMRIID) www.usamriid.army.mil	I,T	Supplies information on agents of CBRN and their effects, treatment protocols, latest research on WMD issues.	Basic
Federal	The Centers for Disease Control (CDC) www.bt.cdc.gov	P,F,I,T	Gives information on agents of CBRN and their effects, treatment protocols, SNS and mass vaccination programs, medical system/public health funding.	Basic
State/Local	Office of Emergency Management www.fema.gov/fema/statedr.shtm	P,I,C	Provides state information on mitigation coordination and activities.	Basic
Local	Metropolitan Medical Response System (MMRS) www.mmrs.fema.gov	T,R,E,C	Coordinates activities related to equipment associated with CBRNE agents. Although a federal program, contact should occur with the local MMRS.	Basic
Federal	Health Resources and Services Administration (HRSA) www.hrsa.gov	P,F,I	Offers mass vaccination support, medical system funding.	Intermediate
Federal	Agency for Healthcare Resources and Quality (AHRQ) www.ahcpr.gov	P,I	Provides assessment tools for clinical care delivery and public health.	Intermediate
Federal	Office for Domestic Preparedness (ODP) www.ojp.usdoj.gov/odp	T,I,F	Presents training for mitigation activities especially associated with chemical and toxic agents.	Intermediate
Regional	FBI Joint Terrorism Task Force (JTTF) www.fbi.gov/terrorinfo/ counterrorism/partnership.htm	I,C	Provides filtered intelligence and information regarding potential terrorist events.	Intermediate
Federal	Central Intelligence Agency www.cia.gov	I	For those without security clearance, offers general information associated with WMD; with security clearance and need-to-know, furnishes information associated with potential terrorist activities.	Advanced

TABLE 27-1	Mitigation Resources for the Medical Response to Terrorism *(continued)*

CATEGORY	ORGANIZATION AND INTERNET ADDRESS	ACTIVITY CODE	ACTIVITY	LEVEL
PARTNERSHIPS/ ASSOCIATIONS/ VOLUNTEER ORGANIZATIONS				
Federal/State/ Local	Comprehensive Hazmat Emergency Response-Capability Assessment Program (CHER-CAP) www.fema.gov/library/cher_cap.shtm	P,T,I	Identifies deficiencies and recommends improvements associated with hazmat risks.	Basic
Federal/State/ Local	Radiation Emergency Assistance Center (REAC) www.orau.gov/reacts	P,T,I	Provides advice on all issues related to radiation accidents and incidents.	Basic
Federal/State/ Local	Red Cross www.redcross.org/home	P,I,C	Provides disaster education and planning guidance.	Basic
Federal/State/Local	Community Emergency Response Team Program (CERT) www.citizencorps.gov/programs	P,T	Trained CERT members provide community training associated with mitigation programs.	Intermediate
Federal/State/Local	Center for Mental Health Services (CMHS) www.mentalhealth.org/cmhs/ EmergencyServices/default.asp	P,T	Promotes the development of crisis counseling teams.	Intermediate
ACADEMIA				
Federal	Center for Domestic Preparedness (CDP) www.ojp.usdoj.gov/odp/docs/ fs-cdp.htm	P,T	Offers specialized training for state and local responders to incidents of domestic terrorism.	Intermediate
Federal/State/Local	Academic Center for Public Health Preparedness www.phppo.cdc.gov/owpp/CPHPLocations.asp	T,I	Makes available research and educational material associated with disaster mitigation.	Advanced
COMMERCIAL				
State/Local	Risk Communication Services	P,I	Can provide mitigation risk communications, and public awareness materials and campaign services.	Basic

Activity Codes: P, Planning; T, Training, Education, Exercise; F, Funding; I, Information; R, Response Teams; E, Equipment; C, Coordination.

TABLE 27-2 Preparedness Resources for the Medical Response to Terrorism

CATEGORY	ORGANIZATION AND INTERNET ADDRESS	ACTIVITY CODE	ACTIVITY	LEVEL
GOVERNMENT				
Federal	Federal Emergency Management Agency (FEMA) www.fema.gov	P,T,I,C	Provides publications for all-hazards planning, provides direct advice through federal and regional FEMA representatives. Source for Federal Emergency Response Plan.	Basic
Federal	The Centers for Disease Control (CDC) www.bt.cdc.gov	P,T,I,F	Provides literature, publications, and planning documents focused on the planning for a biological incident; however, recent efforts are also focused on chemical, explosive, and radiological/ nuclear preparations. Specific planning for mass vaccinations and deployment of the SNS. CDC will coordinate site visits and exercises associated with the SNS and supply funding for bioterrorism preparedness, training, and equipment. Sponsor of Forensic Epidemiology Course.	Basic
Federal	Office of Domestic Preparedness (ODP) www.ojp.usdoj.gov/odp	P,T,I,F	Provides training, funds for the purchase of equipment, support for the planning and execution of exercises, technical assistance and other support to assist states and local jurisdictions plan for the response to terrorism.	Basic
State/Local	San Mateo Emergency Medical Services Agency www.emsa.cahwnet.gov/dms2/heics3.htm	P,T	Provides plans and programmatics for the Hospital Emergency Incident Command System (HEICS).	Basic
State/Local	Offices of Emergency Management www.fema.gov/fema/statedr.shtm	P,T,I,C	Offers varying levels of support and focus depending upon organization; it is, however, the focal point for all-hazards preparedness efforts in states and localities. Provides and defines Emergency Support Functions (ESF) specific to a state or locality to include ESF #8 Health and Medical Services.	Basic
Local	Metropolitan Medical Response System (MMRS) www.mmrs.fema.gov	P,R,E,C	Develops plans in the MMRS localities specific to WMD response within their own jurisdiction and may provide mutual aid to surrounding jurisdictions.	Basic
Federal	United States Army Medical Institute of Infectious Disease (USAMRIID) www.usamriid.army.mil	T,I	Provides educational material and medical training on subjects directly related to a WMD event.	Basic

TABLE 27-2 Preparedness Resources for the Medical Response to Terrorism *(continued)*

CATEGORY	ORGANIZATION AND INTERNET ADDRESS	ACTIVITY CODE	ACTIVITY	LEVEL
GOVERNMENT				
Federal	Health Resources and Services Administration (HRSA) www.hrsa.gov	T,F,I	Provides planning assistance, conference, and funding support for planning and response to terrorist activities	Intermediate
Federal	Agency for Healthcare Resources and Quality (AHRQ) www.ahcpr.gov	T,I	Supplies staffing models for hospital bioterrorism readiness, conferences on subjects related to bioterrorism, and hospital preparedness.	Intermediate
Regional	FBI Joint Terrorism Task Force (JTTF) www.fbi.gov/terrorinfo/ counterrorism/partnership.htm	I,C	Distributes information/intelligence associated with terrorist activities.	Advanced
PARTNERSHIPS/ ASSOCIATIONS/ VOLUNTEER ORGANIZATIONS				
Federal/State/ Local	Center for Mental Health Services (CMHS) www.mentalhealth.org/cmhs/ EmergencyServices/default.asp	T,I	Trains state mental health staff to develop crisis counseling training and preparedness efforts for mass casualty incidents.	Basic
Federal/State/ Local	Comprehensive Hazmat Emergency Response-Capability Assessment Program (CHER-CAP) www.fema.gov/library/cher_cap.shtm	P,T,I	Through direct interaction, helps communities to understand hazmat risks, identify planning deficiencies, update plans, train first responders, and stimulate and test the system for strengths and needed improvements.	Basic
State/Local	Association of State and Territorial Health Officials (ASTHO) www.astho.org National Association of City and County Health Officials (NACCHO) www.naccho.org	P,T,I	Assists state health agencies to develop comprehensive, coordinated bioterrorism programs and plans through collaboration with the CDC, and other local, state and federal partners.	Intermediate
Federal/State/ Local	Radiation Emergency Assistance Center (REAC) www.orau.gov/reacts	P,T,I	Provides courses in handling radiation emergencies and information related to radiological incidents.	Intermediate
Federal/State/ Local	Red Cross www.redcross.org/home	P,T,I,C	Provides nonmedical disaster planning assistance in support of all-hazard planning.	Intermediate
State/Local	Hospital, primary care, long-term care associations	T,I,C	Depending on organizational relationships, may provide coordination of membership and information dissemination during mass casualty incidents.	Intermediate/ Advanced

TABLE 27-2 Preparedness Resources for the Medical Response to Terrorism *(continued)*

CATEGORY	ORGANIZATION AND INTERNET ADDRESS	ACTIVITY CODE	ACTIVITY	LEVEL
Federal/State/ Local	Community Emergency Response Team (CERT) program www.citizencorps.gov/ programs/cert.shtm	T,I,C	Trains CERT members to give critical support to first responders, provide immediate assistance to victims, and organize spontaneous volunteers at a disaster site.	Advanced
State/Local	National Voluntary Organizations Active in Disaster (NVOAD) www.nvoad.org	P,C	Coordinates the efforts of volunteer organizations responding to disasters in the planning stages to ensure cooperative efforts during an actual event.	Advanced
ACADEMIA				
Federal	Center for Domestic Preparedness (CDP) www.ojp.usdoj.gov/odp/docs/ fs-cdp.htm	P,T,I	Offers specialized advanced training to state and local emergency responders in the management and remediation of incidents of domestic terrorism, especially those involving chemical agents and other toxic substances.	Basic
Federal/State/ Local	Academic Center for Public Health Preparedness (A-CPHP) www.phppo.cdc.gov/owpp /CPHPLocations.asp	T,I	Provides education and training for preparing the public health community for WMD events.	Intermediate
COMMERCIAL				
		E,C	Numerous companies and consulting services are available for training, planning, education, and exercise support.	Intermediate /Advanced

Activity Codes: P, Planning; T, Training, Education, Exercise; F, Funding; I, Information; R, Response Teams; E, Equipment; C, Coordination.

TABLE 27-3	Response Resources for the Medical Response to Terrorism

CATEGORY	ORGANIZATION AND INTERNET ADDRESS	ACTIVITY CODE	ACTIVITY	LEVEL
GOVERNMENT				
Federal	Federal Emergency Management Agency (FEMA) www.fema.gov	R,E,I,C	Provides urban search and rescue (USAR) teams, mobile telecommunications, operational support, life support, and power generation assets for the on-site management of disaster and all-hazard activities; coordinates federal disaster relief efforts. Linkage to the National Disaster Medical System (NDMS).	Basic
Federal	The Centers for Disease Control (CDC) www.bt.cdc.gov	R,E,I,C	Distributes SNS to states and localities with TARU, provides epidemiologic investigative teams, provides/assists in epidemiologic and laboratory analysis of WMD agents, and provides mass vaccination materials and support.	Basic
State/Local	Offices of Emergency Management www.fema.gov/fema/statedr.shtm	I,C,R,E	Directs and coordinates state and local emergency response efforts, liaise with federal and regional partners.	Basic
Local	Metropolitan Medical Response System (MMRS) www.mmrs.fema.gov	R,E,C	Provides response to WMD and hazmat incidents using MMRS equipment and trained teams.	Basic
Regional	Federal Bureau of Investigation (FBI) www.fbi.gov/terrorinfo/counterrorism/partnership.htm	R,I	Conducts criminal investigation of WMD events, as well as sampling and entry operations in coordination with state and local responders.	Basic
Federal	U.S. Marine Corps Chemical Biological Incident Response Force (CBIRF) www.cbirf.usmc.mil	R,E	Provides mass decontamination of WMD incidents using CBIRF equipment and manpower.	Intermediate
PARTNERSHIPS/ ASSOCIATIONS/ VOLUNTEER ORGANIZATIONS				
Federal/ Volunteer	Disaster Medical Assistance Teams (DMAT) http://teams.fema,gov/dmat/about/ndms.html/#dmat	R,I,E	A component of the NDMS; provides medical and paramedical professionals operating as a self-sufficient medical unit deployable with equipment within 24 hours of notification.	Basic
Federal/ Volunteer	Disaster Mortuary Assistance Teams (DMORT) www.dmort.org	R,I,E	A component of the NDMS; provides morgue operations, forensics, record keeping, scene documentation, and coordination of remains. processing and release.	Basic

TABLE 27-3 Response Resources for the Medical Response to Terrorism *(continued)*

CATEGORY	ORGANIZATION AND INTERNET ADDRESS	ACTIVITY CODE	ACTIVITY	LEVEL
ORGANIZATIONS				
Federal/ Volunteer	Veterinary Medical Assistance Teams (VMAT) www.vmat.org	R,I,E	A component of the NDMS; provides veterinarians and veterinary technicians trained in the treatment, handling, and care of normal and exotic animals.	Basic
Federal/State/ Local	The Red Cross www.redcross.org/home	R,I,E	Provides nonmedical disaster assistance to include facilities, supplies, and support to responders and victims during incident response.	Basic
State/Local	Hospital, primary care, long-term care associations	C	Provides coordination of membership and information dissemination during mass casualty incident planning.	Intermediate
State/Local	Radio Amateur Civil Emergency Services (RACES) www.races.net	R,E	Provide emergency radio message handling on Amateur Radio Service frequencies to include messages between hospitals, emergency services and shelters and other critical locations.	Basic
Federal/State/ Local	Radiation Emergency Assistance Center (REAC) www.orau.gov/reacts	I	At the REAC, equipped to perform medical and radiological triage, decontamination, diethylenetriaminepentaacetic acid (DTPA) chelation therapy, diagnostic and prognostic assessments of radiation-induced injuries, and biological and radiological dose estimates. Can be used as a remote information source during disaster response.	Intermediate
Federal/State/ Local	Community Emergency Response Teams (CERT) program www.citizencorps.gov/programs/cert.shtm	R,C	Provides support to first responders, immediate assistance to victims; organizes spontaneous volunteers at a disaster site.	Intermediate
State/Local	The Salvation Army www.salvationarmyusa.gov	R,E	Provides mobile feeding of responders and victims and assists family members in finding relatives and friends.	Intermediate
ACADEMIA				
Federal/State/ Local	Academic Center for Public Health Preparedness (A-CPHP) www.phppo.cdc.gov/owpp /CPHPLocations.asp	T,I	Provides education and training for responding to the public health community for WMD events.	Intermediate

TABLE 27-3	Response Resources for the Medical Response to Terrorism *(continued)*

CATEGORY	ORGANIZATION AND INTERNET ADDRESS	ACTIVITY CODE	ACTIVITY	LEVEL
COMMERCIAL				
		E	Numerous companies may provide supplies for purchase and, at times, free of charge. Preplanning with business organizations is recommended to ensure appropriate and timely commercial response. Planners should contact pharmaceutical and medical supply companies in advance to ensure resupply during a mass casualty incident.	Basic/ Intermediate/ Advanced

Activity Codes: P, Planning; T, Training, Education, Exercise; F, Funding; I, Information; R, Response Teams; E, Equipment; C, Coordination.

TABLE 27-4	Recovery Resources for the Medical Response to Terrorism

CATEGORY	ORGANIZATION AND INTERNET ADDRESS	ACTIVITY CODE	ACTIVITY	LEVEL
GOVERNMENT				
Federal	Federal Emergency Management Agency (FEMA) www.fema.gov	R,E,F,C	Provides financial assistance through the Public Assistance Program a federal disaster grant assistance program for the repair, replacement, or restoration of disaster-damaged, publicly owned facilities and the facilities of certain private nonprofit (PNP) organizations. Linkage to federal recovery assets.	Basic
State/Local	Offices of Emergency Management www.fema.gov/fema/statedr.shtm	R,E,C	Directs and coordinates state and local recovery efforts, liaise with federal and regional partners.	Basic
Local	Metropolitan Medical Response System (MMRS) www.mmrs.fema.gov	R,E,I	Provides decontamination and hazmat cleanup subsequent to a WMD event.	Basic
PARTNERSHIPS/ ASSOCIATIONS/ VOLUNTEER ORGANIZATIONS				
Federal/ Volunteer	Disaster Mortuary Assistance Teams (DMORT) www.dmort.org	R,I,E	A component of the NDMS; provides morgue operations, forensics, record keeping, scene documentation and coordination of remains processing and release.	Basic

TABLE 27-4	Recovery Resources for the Medical Response to Terrorism *(continued)*

CATEGORY	ORGANIZATION AND INTERNET ADDRESS	ACTIVITY CODE	ACTIVITY	LEVEL
COMMERCIAL				
Federal/ Volunteer	Veterinary Medical Assistance Teams (VMAT) www.vmat.org	R,I,E	A component of the NDMS; provides veterinarians and veterinary technicians trained in the treatment, handling and care of normal and exotic animals.	Basic
Federal/State/ Local	Center for Mental Health Services (CMHS) www.mentalhealth.org/cmhs/ EmergencyServices/default.asp	R,I	Provides trained crisis counseling teams to assist in the psychosocial consequences of a terrorist or mass casualty event.	Basic
Federal/State/ Local	The Red Cross www.redcross.org/home	R,E,C	Provides nonmedical disaster assistance to include facilities, supplies and support to responders and victims during incident response.	Basic
State/Local	The Salvation Army www.salvationarmyusa.gov	R,E,C	Provides food and shelter for victims and assists family members in finding relatives and friends.	Intermediate
COMMERCIAL				
		E,F	Numerous companies and services are available to provide supplies for purchase and at times free of charge. Preplanning with business organizations is recommended to ensure appropriate and timely commercial response.	Basic/ Intermediate/ Advanced

Activity Codes: P, Planning; T, Training, Education, Exercise; F, Funding; I, Information; R, Response Teams; E, Equipment; C, Coordination.

REFERENCES

1. U.S. Government. Disaster help [online]. Available from: https://disasterhelp.gov/portal/jhtml/search/search_dhelp.jhtml. Accessed August 20, 2004.
2. San Mateo County Emergency Services Agency. HEICS III [online]. Available from: http://www.emsa.cahwnet.gov/dms2/heics3.htm. Accessed August 20, 2004.
3. U.S. Government. National Oceanic and Atmospheric Agency [online]. Available from: http://www.noaa.gov/index.html. Accessed August 20, 2004.
4. U.S. Government. Metropolitan Medical Response System. [online]. Available from: http://www.mmrs.hhs.gov. Accessed August 20, 2004.
5. U.S. Government. Citizen Corps [online]. Available from: http://www.citizencorps.gov/programs/cert.shtm. Accessed August 20, 2004.
6. U.S. Government. FEMA library [online]. Available from: http://www.fema.gov/library/cher_capf.shtm. Accessed August 20, 2004.
7. Oak Ridge Institute for Science and Education. REAC/TS [online]. Available from: http://www.orau.gov/reacts/intro.htm. Accessed August 20, 2004.
8. American Red Cross. Red Cross [online]. Available from: http://www.redcross.org/home. Accessed August 20, 2004.
9. The Salvation Army. Salvation Army [online]. Available from: http://www1.salvationarmy.org. Accessed August 20, 2004.
10. RACES Webring. Radio Amateur Civil Emergency Service [online]. Available from: http://www.races.net. Accessed August 20, 2004.

Equipment Preparedness for Terrorism

28

Personal Protective Equipment

Joshua G. Schier and Robert S. Hoffman

INTRODUCTION

A hazardous substance (HS) may be defined simply as any substance that is potentially toxic to living systems (1). A more technical definition of a HS, as defined by the U.S. Occupational Safety and Health Administration (OSHA), is any substance designated or listed under (A) through (D) of this definition, exposure to which results or may result in adverse effects on the health or safety of employees:

> [A] Any substance defined under section 101(14) of CERCLA (Comprehensive Environmental Response, Compensation and Liability Act or CERCLA, also known as Superfund); [B] Any biologic agent and other disease causing agent which after release into the environment and upon exposure, ingestion, inhalation, or assimilation into any person, either directly from the environment or indirectly by ingestion through food chains, will or may reasonably be anticipated to cause death, disease, behavioral abnormalities, cancer, genetic mutation, physiological malfunctions (including malfunctions in reproduction) or physical deformations in such persons or their offspring. [C] Any substance listed by the U.S. Department of Transportation as hazardous materials under 49 CFR 172.101 and appendices; and [D]

> Hazardous waste (2). Hazardous waste is defined as: [A] A waste or combination of wastes as defined in 40 CFR 261.3, or [B] Those substances defined as hazardous wastes in 49 CFR 171.8 (2).

These criteria are extensively used in the classification of appropriate personal protective equipment regulations developed by OSHA. These standards developed by OSHA can provide guidance for employees who are handling or controlling a HS release (2). There is no formal interpretation of the applicability of these guidelines specifically for patient decontamination that is health care facility (HCF) based (2). See OSHA's web site at http://osha.gov for access to and further clarification of these criteria.

A HS release from a terrorism event may be an agent with the potential for significant lethality such as sarin nerve gas, or it may be simply an unanticipated byproduct of the event itself such as airborne dirt and debris from a collapsed building (3). There are a wide variety of potential agents with hazardous effects that could be released either intentionally or unintentionally (as a byproduct of combustion or structure collapse) that further complicates the situation (2). The wide variety of potential terrorist agents and scenarios in which these agents could be used substantiates the need for clearly developed recommendations and guidelines for personal protection.

The disregard of appropriate personal protective equipment (PPE) as well as adequate decontamination procedures (discussed in Chapter 29) may result in injury or death not only to the rescuer but also to surrounding persons (4–6). Secondary contamination of support staff and treating personnel may occur through physical contact of the patient, the patient's secretions, and even sharing the same breathing space (4–6). Furthermore, the improper utilization of PPE may result in harm to the user as demonstrated in Israel during the 1991 Gulf War (7). Several reports documenting fatalities were attributed at least in part solely to the use of gas masks (no HS was released) (7,8). Thirteen people suffocated to death due to mishandling of gas masks in one report (7). Three other postoperative patients died after developing complications related to the use of full-fitting gas masks during the first missile attack on Israel in 1991 (8).

PPE needs may vary considerably with the individual terrorist event. Factors in determining appropriate PPE include time and location of victim encounter by rescue personnel (first responders vs. emergency department staff), nature of HS (biological vs. chemical), unexpected hazards (burning PVC pipe from a fire), and available equipment. Some medical personnel will require the ability to perform sophisticated procedures such as endotracheal intubation or establishment of intravenous access. Certain levels of protection (A, B) may greatly complicate the completion of these tasks and have to be considered in the overall emergency response plan. This chapter reviews definitions of PPE and the current established recommendations for use in various situations.

PREPAREDNESS ESSENTIALS

A HS must gain entry to the body in order to cause toxicity. The two major ways chemical agents gain entry to the body is through the mucosa of the oral and respiratory tracts and by absorption through the skin (9). Biological agents also may gain entry through these pathways. Although consumption of HSs in foodstuffs or drinking water is well reported (10) and may result in toxicity, this pathway is not relevant for this chapter. The proximity of pulmonary blood to capillary membranes needed for gas exchange in the lungs provides a unique opportunity for rapid absorption of an inhaled toxin. As a result, there is considerable effort targeted to protection of the respiratory tract. Successful protection for medical personnel responding to a terrorist event depends on a careful assessment of known and unknown exposure risks and implementation of an integrated approach to respiratory and dermal protection.

The principles of respiratory protection are fairly simple. Either people can protect themselves by breathing air from a source other than the ambient atmosphere (self-contained air or oxygen supply) or they can breathe the ambient air after it has passed through some type of filter to remove the HS. Both applications are used today in different situations; however, the latter has been the more common historical and practical approach.

There are numerous obstacles to overcome when designing masks that provide effective respiratory protection. Some of the major factors that contribute to tolerability include resistance to breathing, external dead space of the equipment, and weight of the mask (11,12). Many nuclear/biological/chemical (NBC) type masks increase inspiratory resistance by four to five times that of normal (11). Compensatory changes in increased work of respiration include prolonged inspiratory time, decreased peak inspiratory flow, and de-

creased minute ventilation (due to reduced tidal volume, respiratory rate, and mildly increased CO_2) (11,12). A gas mask's internal volume (approximately 300 to 500 ml, depending on size) becomes external dead space that increases inhaled CO_2 concentrations (11). Ventilation must therefore be adjusted to maintain normal P_aCO_2 (11). The considerable variation in brain stem responsiveness to elevated P_aCO_2, along with the other mentioned factors, may interfere with adequate ventilation (11). Exercise increases demand for oxygen, which may worsen the limiting factors just mentioned and further interfere with ventilation (11,12).

Respirators are generally uncomfortable to wear for many other reasons. Psychophysiological responses commonly present as anxiety, respiratory distress, or hyperventilation (11). People with higher baseline amounts of anxiety have an increased likelihood of psychophysiological effects (11). This may ultimately result in impaired performance while wearing the mask or, worse, removal of the mask during an actual NBC attack (11). It is also important to reemphasize that these psychophysiological responses, the inherent obstacles to appropriate ventilation just mentioned, and increased levels of stress and anxiety (i.e., during a chemical attack drill) may be synergistic in their effects to cause harm to the patient while wearing the mask (7,8). Although there are inherent problems with respiratory protective devices (RPDs), they may indeed be lifesaving if utilized correctly in an appropriate situation.

Respirators are broadly classified into two different categories. An air-purifying respirator removes contaminants from the surrounding air (13). An atmosphere-supplying respirator (ASR) provides air from a completely different source other than from the surrounding atmosphere (13). Further classification is possible based on the type of adhesion to the face or type of alternate air source (if not from the surrounding air) (11). The covering that serves as a barrier to the surrounding atmosphere and serves as a framework to which air-purifying components can be attached covers the respiratory inlet (13). These coverings can be either tight-or loose-fitting barriers (13). Tight-fitting coverings (or face pieces) are generally made of a flexible substance such as neoprene, rubber, or silicone (13). The elastic material making up the bulk of many of these coverings is generally made of butyl rubber because silicone rubber and perfluorocarbon rubber is either permeable or fragile (9). Face-pieces commonly cover the mouth and nose only (quarter mask), cover the nose and entire chin (half mask), or cover from the hairline to below the chin (full face-piece) (13) (Fig. 28-1).

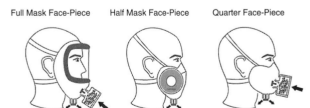

Full Mask Face-Piece   Half Mask Face-Piece   Quarter Face-Piece

Figure 28–1. Types of Tight-Fitting Respirators by Face-Piece. Adapted from: Bollinger NJ, Schultz RH. NIOSH guide to industrial respiratory protection. National Institute of Occupational Safety and Health. Washington DC, September 1, 1987 Publication No. 87-116. Web site: http://www.cdc.gov/niosh/87-116.html. Accessed October 22, 2003.

Loose-fitting coverings include a wide variety of protective materials including hoods, helmets, suits, and blouses (13). A hood is a lightweight product that covers only the head, neck, and shoulders (13). A helmet generally refers to a hood with some sort of firm headgear attached (13). A blouse covers the torso down to the waist (13).

Air-purifying respirators can be broadly classified into particulate filtering, vapor and gas removing, and powered or nonpowered. Particulate filtering respirators generally use a fibrous material to trap the particles desired (13). The efficacy for a certain type of particulate mask depends on both particle and mask fiber velocity, composition, shape, electrical charge, and size (12). These masks are generally used for dusts, fumes, and mists (13). Many types are also effective at blocking transmission of respiratory droplets containing biological agents such as the virus that causes severe acute respiratory syndrome (SARS) and the mycobacterium that causes tuberculosis (14).

The removal of a HS by vapor- and gas-removing masks occurs by a filter container inserted into these masks. Elimination from inspired air occurs inside the filter container by inactivation through reaction by chemicals inside the filter. For example, the "hypo helmet" of 1915 removed chlorine through a reaction with sodium thiosulfate inside the filter (9), adsorption to some substance such as activated charcoal, absorption to another specific material, catalysis, or a combination of methods (9,13). Adsorption refers to the ability of the filter material (commonly referred to as the sorbent) to attract and hold the agent through physical and chemical attraction (13). Effective sorbents have large surface areas to enhance adsorption (up to 1,500 m^2/g) (13). Activated charcoal is one of the most commonly used sorbents (9,13). Activated charcoal can also be impregnated with certain chemicals such as chromium and silver salts or copper oxide (9,13). This can increase the protection afforded by these masks through enhanced selective binding of a specific toxin (9,13). Catalysis refers to the utilization of a chemical to influence a chemical reaction. An example is the use of manganese oxide in a filter cartridge to speed the reaction between carbon monoxide and oxygen to make carbon dioxide (13). Absorption is similar to adsorption, except that it occurs much faster, absorbents tend to have smaller surface areas, and molecular space penetration is deeper (13). The modern C2A1 filter canister uses a pleated white filter (for aerosol removal), a layer of ASZ (impregnated with zinc) charcoal, and then a final filter to remove charcoal dust before allowing filtered air to exit the canister and be inhaled into the lungs (9). Protective masks all employ a filter layer that does not allow passage of particles and aerosols with a size greater than 3 micrometers (9). The effectiveness of all of these cartridges are commonly targeted toward specific types of agents such as organic vapors or acid gases and therefore they cannot always be safely used interchangeably (13).

These filters themselves can be inside canisters or cartridges. The major difference between the two is only due to sorbent volume (and subsequently greater adsorptive capacity). Canisters have greater volume and are often used with full face-piece coverings, commonly known as gas masks (13). Cartridges are smaller, have less sorbent, and are usually used on quarter, half, as well as full face-piece coverings (13). They are referred to as chemical cartridge respirators (CCRs) (13). Cartridges and canisters may protect against particulates as well (13).

Gas masks and CCRs can be powered or nonpowered. The term generally refers to a device that forces ambient air through the filtering device (13). Advantages of this device include cooling of the facial skin and decreased work of breathing. Disadvantages include the need for an electrical power source and potentially shorter life of the filter (because normal airflow through a nonpowered filter is only during inspiration) (13).

Atmosphere-supplying respirators (ASRs) can be classified into two major groups: self-contained breathing apparatus (SCBA) and supplied-air respirators (SARs). Each has its own unique set of advantages and disadvantages from each other as well as from the air-purifying respirators (APRs) category. Atmosphere-supplying respirators provide air from a source other than the ambient atmosphere. SCBA has the advantage of allowing increased mobility because the wearer carries a container of stored air with them. SCBA systems can be closed circuit or open circuit. A closed-circuit system utilizes 100% oxygen in a breathing bag. Oxygen is inhaled from the breathing bag through a one-way valve into the lungs. Exhalation occurs through a one-way valve, the oxygen/carbon dioxide mixture passes through a carbon dioxide scrubber that removes the carbon dioxide, and the oxygen returns to the breathing bag to be inhaled again. As oxygen is metabolized, additional oxygen is added to the breathing bag from a compressed oxygen source.

An open-circuit system is one where compressed air is inhaled through a regulator and the exhaled air is discharged into the ambient atmosphere (13). Open-circuit systems may be "demand" or "pressure demand," and these terms generally refer to the negative- or positive-pressure environment inside the suit and the regulator piece (13). Demand-type mechanisms utilize an admission valve that only opens and supplies breathing air during inhalation (13). During exhalation, the valve closes (13). This system tends to create more of a negative-pressure system and is probably only as effective as many APRs (depending on the face-piece) (13). This characteristic makes these systems inappropriate for environments that are immediately dangerous to life and health (IDLH) (13). Pressure-demand systems utilize a similar system with the exception of a spring, which tends to hold the admission valve partially open at most times thereby providing a tendency toward a positive-pressure environment (13). Closed-circuit systems have longer use times, typically from 1 to 4 hours, whereas open-circuit systems have much larger workloads and subsequently less service time (30 to 60 minutes) (13).

Supplied air respirators generally come in two major types: air-line respirators and hose masks. In an air-line respirator, compressed air is delivered through a hose under pressure from some external and generally stationary source. These respirators can be demand, pressure-demand, or continuous (airflow is controlled by a control valve or separate opening rather than a regulator valve). Hose masks receive their air supply by hose directly to the mask's respiratory opening and may or may not have a blower (13).

Combinations of different types of protective mechanisms are possible as well. Supplied-air/air-purifying respirators allow greater mobility than supplied-air respirators alone but carry the disadvantage of less protection when not connected to a supplied-air source (13). A combination supplied-air-SCBA respirator can be used in an IDLH atmosphere, assuming there is both a primary and auxiliary air source in case of failure of one (13). These systems primarily use the supplied-air source first, only relying on the SCBA system in case of emergency or air-line failure (13).

There are numerous advantages and disadvantages to each of the systems. Air-line respirators can be used for long periods of time and generally are more comfortable to the wearer (13). However, mobility is severely restricted by the length of the connecting air hose, and oxygen supply depends on uninterrupted airflow through the hose (13). Hose masks may also be used for long periods, are easy to use, and relatively inexpensive but have the same limitations when it comes to breathable air being supplied by a long hose (13). Furthermore, these masks are generally not certified for use in IDLH environments (13). SCBA systems are expensive to purchase and maintain, extremely bulky, require more training for effective functioning, and have relatively short amounts of service time before needing resupply. They do, however, afford significantly more protection than most other types because they are closed systems.

Other design characteristics of many of today's respirators intended for chemicals and poisonous gases come mainly from World War I innovations (9). These design characteristics include preventing exhaled air (with water vapor) from fogging lenses, separate one-way inlet and outlet valves (to minimize respiratory effort), and a movable diaphragm (to allow voice communication) (9). Most modern gas masks have a smaller, second mask referred to as a nose cup, which is an individual unit that requires individual insertion (9,11). It lies between the main mask and the wearer's midface (9,11) and has two major functions: It minimizes dead space ventilation and provides further protection against potential hazardous substances (9,11).

Dermal protection is the second vital component of protection for medical personnel responding to victims of a terrorist attack. There are two major design types of chemical protective clothing that will protect the wearer against NBC warfare. The first type is a uniform that is impermeable to most if not all molecules. Very few materials possess these abilities, with butyl rubber or certain types of plastics being exceptions (9). The protective impenetrability qualities of these suits are at the cost of preventing water vapor and air passage, which results in an unacceptable loss of inherent body-cooling ability (9). The alternative design is to use fabrics that are permeable to molecules but pretreated with certain protective chemicals (9). These treated fabrics can trap most harmful molecules (9). An example is the battle dress overgarment, utilized by the U.S. military, which is protective against chemical agent vapors, liquid droplets, biological agents, toxins, and radioactive alpha and beta particles but not against x and gamma radiation (9). Vinyl overboots are used to protect soldiers' combat boots against harmful agents (9). Gloves are the last component of a uniform and may severely interfere with tactile ability and agility (9).

There is currently a wide variety of commercially available protective equipment, each of which has detailed information on protective capability against certain agents. This equipment is not without inherent hazards of usage. Generally, full chemical protective gear (suit, mask, boots, gloves, etc.) predisposes the wearer to dehydration and overheating

(9). A full uniform can also add 9 to 14 pounds of additional weight (9). These suits can trigger numerous biopsychological responses, such as anxiety, dizziness, confusion, muscle cramps, and shortness of breath as well as real heat-related responses (15,16). Maintenance of adequate hydration status before suit utilization as well as after is extremely important. These uniforms are designed for soldiers entering into a battlefield environment where large releases of agents probably have occurred or for workers responding to large industrial releases of known toxins. The degree of protection afforded by these clothes will probably not be warranted for medical personnel responding to a terrorism event or hospital-based health care personnel treating victims of such an event after transport.

The degree of dermal protection will also vary depending on the individual wearer's role in the terrorist response. A first responder entering a confined space where an unknown but deadly agent was released will be required to wear a high level of protection. In this situation, level A would probably be the most appropriate protection. Medical personnel distant from the site of release, however, will only be exposed to an agent that is on or in the patient and his or her clothes (17–19). The concentration of agent will therefore be diluted in amount and potency (17–19). When these facts are taken into consideration, the same level of protection worn by the first responder may not necessarily be needed for all other health care workers (HCWs).

The protective ability of chemical-resistant clothing is usually measured by permeation rates of the agent after direct application to the fabric (17,19). This situation is probably not applicable to the HCW for the dilution and limited contact factors mentioned previously (17,19). This suggests that a lesser degree of protection is needed and therefore less costly materials may be adequate. A wide variety of commercially available protective clothing is available with a similar variety in cost (17,20).

Appropriate PPE for medical personnel will vary depending on when the victim encounters the health care system. Ideally, decontamination of patients should be done outside the hospital, preferably close to the scene (but at a safe distance from the event). Afterward, patients can be transported by emergency medical personnel to hospitals for further treatment. Unfortunately, transportation of patients to medical facilities does not always happen in this manner. Several events in recent history have illustrated very clearly that a significant number of patients may present directly to a HCF without any prior decontamination or treatment (21). Secondary contamination of treating medical personnel may also occur when inappropriate or no PPE is utilized by HCWs (22). These affected HCWs, now patients, may further worsen the situation by consumption of additional resources and depletion of the available skilled workforce (22). These events are discussed in further detail to help illustrate several important principles in personal protection in the section "Preparedness Historic Event and Case History."

PPE for personnel responding to a hazardous substance release is classified into four basic categories (Table 28-1). Level A protection is designed to maximize respiratory, eye, and skin protection. It includes a National Institute of Occupational Safety and Health (NIOSH) approved positive-pressure full face-piece self-contained breathing apparatus (SCBA) or positive-pressure SAR with escape SCBA

TABLE 28-1 NIOSH Guidelines for Personal Protection

LEVEL OF PROTECTION	INCLUDES	SCENARIO
Level A	1. NIOSH-approved positive pressure full-face-piece SCBA* or positive-pressure SAR[†] with escape SCBA* 2. Encapsulating chemical-protective suit 3. Chemical-resistant inner and outer gloves 4. Steel-toe chemical-resistant boots 5. Additional outer disposable suit, gloves, and boots [††]*Optional: Coveralls, long underwear, and a hard hat*	1. Agent is known and ambient concentrations known to be significant 2. Agent is known and normal work functions carry a significant exposure risk (splash, immersion, spray, volatilization) to an agent that can be absorbed transdermally 3. Agent is a known or suspected significant hazard to the skin 4. Surrounding conditions necessitating level A protection are not excluded
Level B	1. NIOSH-approved positive-pressure, full-face-piece SCBA* or positive-pressure SAR[†] with escape SCBA* 2. Hooded chemical-resistant clothing (overalls and long-sleeved jacket, coveralls, one- or two-piece chemical-splash suit; disposable chemical-resistant overalls) 3. Chemical-resistant inner and outer gloves 4. Steel-toe and steel-shank chemical-resistant boots. [††]*Optional: A hard hat, face shield, and exterior chemical-resistant disposable boot covers*	1. Agent is known and requires significant respiratory protection but less skin protection 2. Atmosphere contains less than 19.5 % oxygen 3. Vapors or gases incompletely identified, but dermal hazards or significant transdermal absorption potential not suspected
Level C	1. Full-face or half-mask APR[§] 2. Hooded chemical-resistant clothing (examples are overalls; two-piece chemical-splash suit; disposable chemical-resistant overalls) 3. Chemical-resistant inner and outer gloves [††]*Optional: Coveralls, steel-toe and steel-shank chemical-resistant boots, chemical-resistant disposable boot covers, hard hat, escape mask, and face shield*	1. Skin contact with identified agent(s) is non-hazardous and significant transdermal absorption does not occur 2. Agent type and ambient concentration are known to be completely removed by an APR[§] 3. Criteria for use of an APR[§] present
Level D	1. Coveralls along with steel-toe and steel-shank chemical-resistant boots [††]*Optional: safety goggles, disposable chemical-resistant boot covers, face shield, hard hat, escape mask, and gloves*	1. No known hazard 2. Potential exposure to hazardous substances only occurs outside of normal work activities

*Self contained breathing apparatus
[†]Supplied air respirator
[††]Usage of the optional items may be needed depending on the specific situation
[§]Air-purifying respirator

(23,24). A completely encapsulating chemical-protective suit, chemical-resistant inner and outer gloves, steel-toe chemical-resistant boots, and an outer additional disposable suit, gloves, and boots are part of the required uniform (23,24). Coveralls, long underwear, and a hard hat are optional items to be used if applicable (23,24). Level A protection is required by OSHA when certain environmental conditions are present. These include the following conditions: (a) the agent is identified and the highest protection is required for protection based on ambient concentrations of implicated vapors, gases, or particulate matter or when normal work functions carry a significant exposure risk (splash, immersion, spray, volatilization) to an agent that can be absorbed transdermally; (b) substances that are a known or suspected significant hazard to the skin; or (c) surrounding conditions necessitating level A protection have not been excluded and are in poorly ventilated or confined areas (23).

Level B protection includes maximum respiratory precautions while including lesser degrees of protection for

TABLE 28-2 Preparedness Checklist Table and Summary

CRISIS PHASE	CRITICAL ITEMS
Pre-event planning	1. Identify health care worker (HCW) groups likely to be on the front line and requiring PPE (first responders, emergency department personnel, decontamination teams, security, etc.) 2. Perform a risk-based assessment analysis for each of these groups' PPE needs 3. Examine existing supplies of PPE readily available (interhospital or interagency agreements should be established in the case of overwhelming demand) 4. Perform a regular review of available literature and recommendations to make revisions as necessary 5. Establish regular personnel training, such as fit testing and practice drills to increase efficiency and familiarity 6. Establish an emergency contact system to alert team members to report to assigned stations
Management	1. Alternate personnel to relieve first-line HCW to avoid fatigue-related errors 2. Contact poison control centers and local/state health agencies to share information 3. Early activation of preestablished interhospital or interagency sharing agreements in case of rapid depletion of existing PPE stores
Recovery	1. Establishment of postevent workgroups consisting of representatives from each area to discuss problems encountered and future PPE needs

the skin. Uniform requirements include a NIOSH-approved positive-pressure, full face piece SCBA, or positive-pressure SAR with escape SCBA, hooded chemical-resistant clothing (overalls and long-sleeved jacket, coveralls, one- or two-piece chemical-splash suit, disposable chemical-resistant overalls), chemical-resistant inner and outer gloves along with steel-toe and steel-shank chemical-resistant boots (23,24). A hard hat, face shield, and exterior chemical-resistant disposable boot covers are optional depending on the situation (23,24). Level B protection is required during the following conditions: (a) a hazardous substance is identified (type and concentration) and is known to require significant respiratory protection and less skin protection; (b) the atmosphere contains less than 19.5% oxygen; and (c) vapors or gases are present (incomplete identification only) but are not suspected to be harmful to the skin or have significant transdermal absorption potential (23). These conditions generally involve agents with significant risk via inhalation pathways but not through skin, which are not adequately protected against through use of APRs (23). The surrounding environment is usually one that is IDLH (23).

When the type of agent as well as the ambient agent concentration is known, level C protection is usually adequate, which still includes significant respiratory protection, usually in the form of an APR (23,24). Uniform requirements include a full-face or half-mask APR, hooded chemical-resistant clothing (examples are overalls, two-piece chemical-splash suit, disposable chemical-resistant overalls), and chemical-resistant inner and outer gloves (23,24). Optional items that may also be used, depending on the situation, are coveralls, steel-toe and steel-shank chemical-resistant boots, chemical-resistant disposable boot covers, hard hat, and escape mask and face shield (23,24). Level C PPE is adequate for the following conditions: (a) if skin contact with the particular identified agent(s) is known to not result in harmful effects and if transdermal absorption is known

to be insignificant; (b) if the type and concentration of the involved substances are known to be completely removed by an APR; or (c) if criteria for use of an APR is met (23).

Level D protection is generally understood to be consistent with an everyday work uniform. It may include a variety of components but is not designed to offer any significant protection. It should include, at the minimum, coveralls along with steel-toe and steel-shank chemical-resistant boots (23,24). Other optional items that can be employed include safety goggles, disposable chemical-resistant boot covers, face shield, hard hat, escape mask, and gloves (23,24). Level D PPE should be used when there is no known hazard or if any potential exposure to hazardous substances only occurs outside of normal work activities (23).

Advantages and disadvantages of the various levels of PPE are relatively obvious. When compared to levels C and D, levels A and B PPE tend to be more expensive, are bulkier to work in, require more training, are tolerated for shorter periods of time, and are more expensive (both to purchase and to maintain) (24). The decision to employ a level of protection will depend on the individual scenario. The PPE guidelines mentioned previously are for responders to HS releases (2). These guidelines generally apply to those involved in management and control of the HS release (2). OSHA has further clarified the issue by defining an emergency response as "a response effort by employees from outside the immediate release area or by other designated responders (i.e., mutual aid groups, local fire departments, etc.) to an occurrence which results, or is likely to result, in an uncontrolled release of a hazardous substance" (2). These guidelines apply to "emergency response operations for releases of, or substantial threats of releases of, hazardous substances without regard to the location of the hazard" (2).

These guidelines do not necessarily, nor directly, extrapolate to health care facility (HCF) decontamination teams (assuming the point of release is not at the HCF) or to health professionals caring for exposed patients at the HCF. This is due to several reasons including distance between the point of release and the HCF as well as different exposure risks (contact with a patient rather than direct containment, confinement, and control activities) (17,18). There is a high likelihood of patients presenting to a HCF directly without prior decontamination or medical personnel evaluation and stabilization (21,24). The HCF must be prepared to receive and treat these patients adequately, which might include decontamination if appropriate (Table 28-2). The question of how to approach these patients has been a controversial one. In the past, OSHA guidelines have been interpreted to necessitate level B PPE for hospital-based decontamination teams (25). Some facilities have established decontamination teams equipped with level B PPE based on individual community hazards necessitating a higher level of protection (24). A growing body of evidence supports level C PPE as being adequate for HCF decontamination teams as long as the point of release is not at the HCF itself (17,18,24,26,27). Air-purifying respirators should contain filters effective against organic vapors at a minimum as well as contain a high-efficiency particulate air (HEPA) filter cartridge (24). Availability of additional types of filters, such as acid gas filters for chlorine, as well as others, will offer greater flexibility in dealing with HSs (24).

NIOSH has recognized the unique problems facing first responders in developing effective respiratory protection for a situation when dealing with an unknown agent. They have instituted programs to test SCBA of various makes and models to ensure protection against all possible chemical, biological, radiological, and nuclear (CBRN) agents (28). The first approved respirators for first responder use against CBRN agents were posted on their web site in June 2002 (29). Models approved include Spiromatic Models 9030, 6630, and 4530 manufactured by Interspiro USA (29). This approval means that these masks should be expected to provide protection against CBRN exposures for firefighters and other responders to such an event (29). Interim recommendations for the selection and use of protective clothing and respirators against biological agents have been developed and are also available at their web site (30). These recommendations include using a NIOSH-approved, pressure-demand SCBA with level A dermal protection if certain information is unknown or if the event is uncontrolled (30). These situations include type of airborne agent(s) and dissemination method, if dissemination via an aerosol-generating device is still occurring or if it has stopped but there is no information on exposure concentrations or time interval of dissemination (30). A NIOSH-approved pressure–demand SCBA with level B dermal protection may be used if the suspected bioaerosol is no longer being produced or if other coexistent concentrations present a splash hazard (30). If an aerosol-generating device was not utilized to induce a high airborne concentration or dissemination was through a device such as a letter or package that can easily be contained, a full face-piece respirator with a P100 filter or powered APR with a HEPA filter can be used, assuming proper fit-testing has been performed (30). The reader is encouraged to check back frequently with OSHA's and NIOSH's web sites for the most current information.

PREPAREDNESS HISTORIC EVENTS AND CASE HISTORIES

In 1995 a Japanese cult named Aum Shrinyoko released dilute sarin nerve gas in the Tokyo subway system (21). Fortunately there were very few fatalities; however, several important lessons were learned from this event. The majority of persons (361 people, or >70% of total people) presenting after these attacks arrived at the hospital by foot, taxi, or through transport by a passing Good Samaritan (21). These people had not received any medical treatment at the scene, nor had they received any form of evaluation by skilled medical personnel. Perhaps most importantly, they had not undergone any form of decontamination or an evaluation to determine if decontamination was even needed. The normal emergency medical response, which should have included all of these steps followed by a controlled transport of these patients to a HCF, did not occur. The lesson learned from this experience is that HCFs can expect to receive a significant number of patients arriving by means other than emergency medical response systems. Hospitals also need to plan for primary evaluation and decontamination of large numbers of patients at the HCF itself.

Secondary contamination of other people, but perhaps more importantly responding medical personnel, is therefore a real concern. This problem was also illustrated in the Tokyo sarin attacks in the receiving hospital (22). More than 200 HCWs developed various signs and/or symptoms after contact with victims (22). Although hospital staff used gloves and masks, no chemical-resistant clothing was available (22). Fortunately, none of the affected HCWs developed serious illness or even required treatment; however, the potential for a worse outcome existed (22).

In 2000 a series of nosocomial poisonings in HCWs occurred in Georgia after several HCWs became secondarily contaminated by an organophosphorous (OP) compound after being exposed to a patient who had ingested the compound in a suicidal gesture (4). Three hospital staff members became ill with OP poisoning after being exposed to this patient in different ways (4). The patient did not receive adequate decontamination and was placed in a small, poorly ventilated hospital room (4). Health care workers did not wear adequate PPE, and all manifested signs and symptoms consistent with OP poisoning (4). The first HCW came into direct contact with patient secretions and required mechanical ventilation and antidotal therapy (4). The second and third HCWs shared the same breathing space as the patient, one of whom required antidotal therapy and the third required supportive care and observation only (4).

The World Trade Center (WTC) attacks of 2001 demonstrated that not all terrorist events require expensive high-level PPE. The collapse of the WTC towers resulted in significant airborne concentrations of dirt, dust, and other particulate matter. Although no exotic biological or chemical agent was used, there still was a need for basic respiratory protection against airborne debris (3).

SUMMARY

For medical personnel, effective protection against CRBN agents begins with adequate planning by the appropriate health agency or hospital itself before the terrorist event occurs. First responders should be afforded the widest variety of personal protection because the agent used and subsequent risks will probably be initially unknown. Health care facilities should be prepared to treat large numbers of patients who have not received any prehospital medical treatment or decontamination. Health agencies and HCFs should institute appropriate PPE protocols and provide adequate training programs for these protocols. The level of personal protection needed may vary not only for the agent used but also in regard to the role of the HCW encountering the patient (i.e., is this a first responder or an emergency department HCW triaging an already decontaminated patient?). If conditions are unknown and an agent with significant toxicity is suspected, medical personnel should take a conservative approach and utilize a higher level of protection than may be ultimately needed until the specifics of the threat are better characterized. Policies and guidelines should emphasize the possibility of secondary contamination of HCW from inadequate PPE. The consequences of a failure to recognize these basic issues and address them appropriately may ultimately result in a disaster for the exposed patients as well as treating medical personnel.

RESOURCES

Although the basic principles of dermal and respiratory protection remain the same, current information and guidelines for appropriate PPE to protect against CRBN agents are constantly being revised and improved with the development of new products. Use this chapter as a reference for utilizing or developing appropriate PPE guidelines but also check the current literature for the most up-to-date changes and additions.

The OSHA and the NIOSH web sites maintain up-to-date information on recommendations and guidelines for PPE: http://www.osha.gov and http://www.cdc.gov/niosh. NIOSH's review process for approved respiratory protection equipment against CRBN agents is ongoing. Check back frequently for additions to the site as well as modifications to existing regulations.

An area of interest within NIOSH that may provide additional information is the National Personal Protective Technology Laboratory. Its web site is found within the general NIOSH web site at http://www.cdc.gov/niosh/npptl/default/html.

A comprehensive text on the military aspects of PPE is the *Textbook of Military Medicine: Medical Aspects of Chemical and Biological Warfare*. The chapter on chemical defense equipment provides a thorough discussion on mili-tary-grade PPE for the battlefield but also presents a history of the development of PPE over the last century. This text is available online at http://www.vnh.org/MedAspChemBioWar/index.html.

Additionally, NIOSH has prepared a document discussing the different classifications of respirators along with detailed information about certain modifications on these different types. This document can be found on their web site at http://www.cdc.gov/niosh/87-116.html.

REFERENCES

1. Kales SN, Polyhronopoulos GN, Castro MJ, et al. Injuries caused by hazardous materials accidents. Ann Emerg Med 1997;30:598-603.
2. Occupational Safety and Health Administration. Hazardous waste operations and emergency response. Washington, DC: Occupational Safety and Health Administration; 29 CFR 1910.120. Web site: http://www.osha.gov/pls/oshaweb/owadisp.show_document?p_table=STANDARDS&p_id=9765. Accessed October 9, 2003.
3. Prezant D, Kelly K, Jackson B, et al. Use of respiratory protection among responders at the World Trade Center site—New York City, September 2001. MMWR 2002; 51:6-8.
4. Geller RJ, Singleton KL, Tarantion ML, et al. Nosocomial poisoning associated with emergency department treatment of organophosphate toxicity—Georgia, 2000. MMWR 2001; 49:1156-8.
5. Horton DK, Berkowitz Z, Kaye WE. Secondary contamination of ED personnel from hazardous materials events, 1995–2001. Am J Emerg Med 2003;21:199-204.
6. Nozaki H, Hori S, Shinozawa, et al. Secondary exposure of medical staff to sarin vapor in the emergency room. Intensive Care Med 1995;21:1032-5.
7. Hiss J, Arensburg B. Suffocation from misuse of gas masks during the gulf war. BMJ 1992;304:92.
8. Rivkind AI, Eid A, Weingart E, et al. Complications from supervised mask use in post-operative surgical patients during the Gulf War. Prehospital Disaster Med 1999; 14:107-8.
9. O'Hern MR, Dashiell TR, Tracy, MF. Chemical defense equipment. In: Sidell FR, Takafuji ET, Franz DR eds. Textbook of military medicine: medical aspects of chemical and biological warfare. Washington, DC: TMM Publications, 1997;361-96.
10. Patel M, Schier J, Belson M, et al. Recognition of illness associated with exposure to chemical agents—United States 2003. MMWR 2003;52:938-40.
11. Arad M, Epstein Y, Krasner E, et al. Principles of respiratory protection. Israel J Med Sci 1991;27:636-42.
12. Louhevaara VA. Physiological effects associated with the use of respiratory protective devices. Scand J Work Environ Health 1984;10:275-81.
13. Bollinger NJ, Schultz RH. NIOSH guide to industrial respiratory protection. National Institute of Occupational Safety and Health. Washington DC, September 1, 1987, Publication No. 87-116. Web site: http://www.cdc.gov/niosh/87-116.html. Accessed October 22, 2003.
14. NIOSH-approved disposable particulate respirators (filtering facepieces). Web site: http://www.cdc.gov/niosh/npptl/respirators/disp_part/particlist.html. Accessed October 8, 2003.
15. Carter BJ, Cammermeyer M. Emergence of real casualties during simulated chemical warfare training under high heat conditions. Mil Med 1985;150:657-63.
16. Carter BJ, Cammermeyer M. Biopsychological responses of medical unit personnel wearing chemical defense ensemble in a simulated chemical warfare environment. Mil Med 1985; 150:239-49.

17. Macintyre AG, Christopher GW, Eitzen E Jr, et al. Weapons of mass destruction events with contaminated casualties. JAMA 2000;283:242-9.

18. Sullivan J, Krieger G. Hazardous materials toxicology. Baltimore, MD: Williams and Wilkins; 1992.

19. Noll G, Hildebrand M, Yvorra J. Personal protective clothing and equipment. In: Daly P ed. Hazardous materials. Stillwater: Fire Protection Publications, Oklahoma State University, 1995; 285-322.

20. Cox R. Decontamination and management of hazardous materials exposure victims in the emergency department. Ann Emerg Med 1994;23:761-70.

21. Okumura T, Suzuki K, Fukuda A, et al. The Tokyo subway sarin attack: Disaster management. Part 1. Community emergency response. Acad Emerg Med 1998;5:613-7.

22. Okumura T, Suzuki K, Fukuda A, et al. The Tokyo subway sarin attack: Disaster management. Part 2. Hospital response. Acad Emerg Med 1998:5:618-24.

23. Occupational Safety and Health Administration. General description and discussion of the levels of protection and protective gear. Washington, DC: Occupational Safety and Health Administration; August 22, 1994. 29 CFR 1910.120 App B. Web site: http://www.osha.gov/pls/oshaweb/owadisp.show_document?p_table=STANDARDS&p_id=9767. Accessed October 6, 2003.

24. Hick JL, Hanfling D, Burstein HL, et al. Protective equipment for health care facility decontamination personnel: Regulations, risks, and recommendations. Ann Emerg Med 2003; 42:370-80.

25. OSHA Interpretation letter, September 5, 2002, from Richard E. Fairfax to Francis J. Roth. Washington, DC: U.S. Department of Labor, Occupational Safety, and Health, 2002. Web site: http://www.osha.gov/pls/oshaweb/owadisp.show_document?p_table=INTERPRETATIONS&p_id=24516. Accessed October 9, 2003.

26. Centers for Disease Control and Prevention. CDC recommendations for civilian communities near chemical weapons depots. 60 Federal Register 33307-33318, 1995.

27. Shapira Y, Bar Y, Berkenstadt H, et al. Outline of hospital organization for a chemical warfare attack. Isr J Med Sci 1991;27:616-22.

28. National Institute for Occupational Safety and Health. Letter to all respirator manufacturers. December 28, 2001. Web site: http://www.cdc.gov/niosh/npptl/respltr.html. Accessed October 22, 2003.

29. National Institute for Occupational Safety and Health. NIOSH issues first approval under program for certifying emergency responder respirators. June 3, 2002. Web site: http://www.cdc.gov/niosh/interspup.html. Accessed October 22, 2003.

30. National Institute for Occupational Safety and Health. Interim recommendations for the selection and use of protective clothing and respirators against biological agents. October 2001. 2002-109. Web site: http://www.cdc.gov/niosh/unp-intrecppe.htm. Accessed October 22, 2003.

29

All-Hazards Approach
To Decontamination

Richard N. Bradley

INTRODUCTION

A terrorist attack with chemical, biological, or radiological hazards may produce a number of contaminated victims. Many of these may arrive at the hospital within minutes of the event. In a multiple casualty situation, vehicles of opportunity, such as police cars, taxicabs, and private autos will transport the majority of casualties. Most of these will not be decontaminated prior to arrival (1). Despite this, most hospitals have not yet implemented adequate plans to decontaminate victims of a large-scale incident (2–7).

Since the dose of toxic substances influences the magnitude of the health effects, and since dose is a function of both concentration and time, hospital staff should act to decontaminate victims quickly. The decontamination process must not allow any contaminated individual into the hospital. That could lead to contamination of the building and exposure and possible harm to the hospital staff. Symptomatic staff would not be able to perform their duties and would add to the total number of victims needing treatment. Furthermore, a contaminated hospital may require extensive and costly decontamination.

Many different scenarios may result in contaminated patients arriving at the hospital. Rather than developing one plan for industrial chemicals, another for terrorist use of chemical weapons, another for a radiological incident, and yet another for biological warfare agents, hospitals should adopt an all-hazards approach to medical decontamination. This is important because the predictability, length of forewarning, onset, magnitude, scope, and duration will vary from one incident to the next. An all-hazards approach makes effective use of time, effort, money, and other resources. Furthermore, it helps avoid duplication of effort and gaps in disaster response (8).

As hospitals create an all-hazards plan for decontamination, they should keep three objectives in mind. First, they must not allow any contaminated patients to enter the interior of the hospital. Second, they should decontaminate patients as rapidly as possible. Third, they must plan to protect the hospital decontamination team from secondary exposure and injury.

PREPAREDNESS ESSENTIALS

All hospitals, regardless of size, should plan for providing medical decontamination. Given the widespread presence of hazardous substances and the unexpected nature of terrorist attacks, every hospital is at risk to receive contaminated patients. The ability to provide decontamination is required under national standards and federal law.

One such standard comes from the National Fire Protection Administration (NFPA). Because hospitals have such a vital role in the local response to incidents involving hazardous substances, the NFPA standards require medical facilities to have the ability to perform decontamination. These standards clarify the minimum level of competency required. Hospitals must have a decontamination area with proper ventilation, and plans for restricting access and containing runoff. These standards also require hospitals to provide trained, in-house personnel to decontaminate and care for affected patients. Personal protective clothing must be readily available (9).

Recent revisions to the Joint Commission for Accreditation of Healthcare Organizations (JCAHO) standards also address the need for an all-hazards approach to decontamination. JCAHO element of performance 21 from Standard EC.4.10 requires that each hospital's emergency management plan "identifies means for radioactive, biological, and chemical isolation and decontamination" (10).

Most importantly, the Occupational Safety and Health Administration (OSHA) Hazardous Waste and Emergency Response (HAZWOPER) standard requires hospitals to train workers to perform their anticipated job duties without endangering themselves or others. Federal law does not allow hospitals to deny emergency treatment to anyone who comes to the hospital (11). Thus, all hospitals must be able to care for any contaminated patient who arrives with an emergency medical condition. This requires them to have plans and a trained decontamination team available. It does not require them to train to the same level as hazardous materials teams. Rather, they are required to train decontamination staff to the "first responder operations level," with emphasis on the use of personal protective equipment (PPE) and decontamination procedures (12a). In addition to the personnel trained to the operations level, those employees who are likely to witness or discover a hazardous substance release or incident should be trained to the "awareness level". Additionally, "skilled support personnel" are defined as personnel who are not part of the decontamination or response team but have special skills that are emergently required in the contaminated area. Examples of these persons could be security personnel, specialty physician consultants, and respiratory therapists. Skilled support personnel do not require training in advance of an incident. They must be provided with a preentry briefing and be assisted with donning and doffing their PPE. An on-scene incident commander or decontamination team leader should be on site to coordinate the activities of casualty decontamination. This individual requires additional training beyond the operations level and does not need to be present for decontamination to begin (12b,12c).

ORGANIZE

Local Coordination

One of the key elements in organizing for medical decontamination is to ensure that the hospital is active in planning for the local response to terrorism and other disasters. Hospitals should be equal partners with local government, fire, police, and EMS providers. Communication plans must explicitly describe the process for two-way communication with the local government during the response to a terrorist attack. Rapid alerting after an incident and frequent status updates are vital to a successful operation.

An important forum for coordination of response plans is the Local Emergency Planning Committee (LEPC). Federal statutes require the designation of LEPCs. The U.S. Environmental Protection Agency's Chemical Emergency Preparedness and Prevention Office (CEPPO) coordinates them. Hospitals should play an active role in their LEPC. Plans and exercises should be coordinated through them to allow all parties to gain a mutual understanding of each other's capabilities and limitations (13).

Incident Command

The medical decontamination area will be organized and controlled as an extension of the Hospital Emergency Incident Command System (HEICS) (14). A medical Decontamination Group supervisor provides overall direction to the Decontamination Group; this individual is also termed the on-scene incident commander or decontamination team leader by OSHA (15). This individual appoints unit leaders to the various functions within the medical decontamination area. Following the principles of HEICS, each individual should have a job action sheet that gives simple instructions on how to carry out assigned responsibilities.

Set-up

Since patients may arrive with only a very brief warning, the Decontamination Group must be able to set up its work area quickly. This requires regular training. The team should establish the decontamination area near an entrance to the hospital. There should be some consideration for protecting patient privacy, such as screens or tents.

Initial Reception Area

Patients coming to the medical decontamination area will first encounter the initial reception area. The unit leader in this area is responsible to determine which individuals require decontamination, to set decontamination priorities, and to determine the mode of decontamination. This unit leader directs those who can walk independently to a supervised self-decontamination process. Others will require assisted decontamination. It is essential that medical personnel with training in the recognition of clinical toxidromes be located at the initial reception area. These trained providers along with the on-scene incident commander and hazmat personnel will determine what decontamination process will occur.

An immediate treatment area should be located in the initial reception area and may provide lifesaving treatment prior to decontamination. This may be limited to insertion of an oral airway, bag-valve-mask ventilation, control of severe bleeding, and immobilization of the cervical spine. In some cases, providers who have previously practiced the procedures in PPE may insert advanced airways. They may also administer chemical agent antidotes and anticonvulsant medication as needed. Reference charts for chemical agent symptom recognition and treatment may be helpful (16).

The initial reception area should have a plan for dealing with individuals who are armed. This may include victims who are law enforcement officers, civilians in lawful possession of a firearm, and criminals. There is also some risk that a perpetrator could come to the hospital with an improvised explosive device. The initial reception area should have a plan to deal with these contingencies. The plan must allow for a rapid request for assistance from local law enforcement authorities and evacuation of the decontamination area when necessary.

Clothing Removal

The first priority in decontamination is clothing removal. Removing the clothing will usually remove most of the contamination. When clothing is removed it should be placed inside of a plastic bag. The decontamination team will hold the bags until local authorities issue instructions on how to deal with them. Besides being a contamination hazard, the clothing may contain forensic evidence of interest to law enforcement officers. The staff will place patient valuables in another plastic bag. They must mark each bag with a name or number matching it with its owner. One solution is to use a multipart set of wristbands, such as those that nurseries use to match parents and newborn children. Each set of the three or four wristbands has the same number. The person assisting with disrobing places one band on the patient and attaches one to each bag of clothing or valuables. At some point, the decontamination staff may be able to decontaminate some objects, such as metal jewelry, keys and credit cards, and return them to their owners.

Dry Decontamination

In a chemical MCI the greatest number of victims affected may be those exposed to a vapor hazard only. The traditional

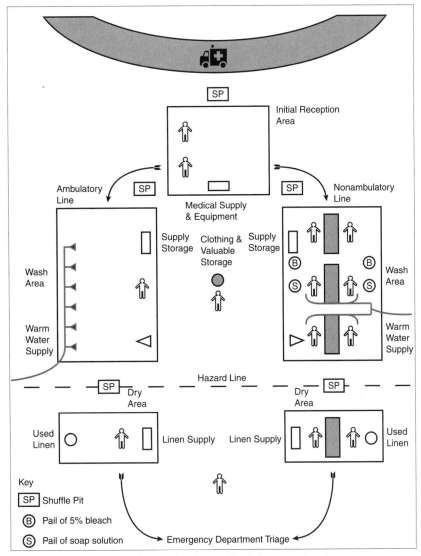

Figure 29–1. A possible layout for the medical decontamination area.

approach of washing patients down in showers may not be effective in the face of hundreds or thousands of casualties. The need for wet decontamination of all patients should be assessed in the initial reception area. Victims who have only been exposed to a vapor do not require decontamination beyond the removal of their clothing and replacement with suitable clean clothing. This "dry decontamination" effectively removes any vapor retained in the clothing. A number of commercial products available for dry decontamination allow for the clothing removal while maintaining the victim's privacy, and the victims can also be shielded and protocols followed to assure safety of their valuables while they are changing clothes. Another type of dry decontamination that may be seen in the literature is the adsorption and physical removal of chemical agents by the use of dry compounds such as diatomaceous earth or the military M291 kit. This process is not commonly used in the civilian setting.

Wash

The core of the wet decontamination process is washing with high volumes of water with a mild soap or detergent.

For nonambulatory patients, the attendants initially cover wounds with a water barrier while washing the rest of the casualty's body with detergent. They should use disposable soap bars or liquid detergent to reduce cross-contamination. They may use sponges, soft brushes, or washcloths for gently scrubbing the patients. They will subsequently flush wounds with sterile saline solution or potable water. Ambulatory casualties perform monitored self-decontamination in a similar fashion. Table 29-1 outlines the details of an example of the decontamination process.

Hazard Line

The decontamination process should follow the process of flow from the contaminated area (hot zone) to the clean area (cold zone). The area where the decontamination is occurring is often referred to as the contamination reduction corridor or the warm zone. The hazard line must be clearly identified as the line that marks the end of the contamination reduction corridor and separates the warm from cold zones. Decontamination team members in the warm zone should be in PPE whenever contamination may be present; those on the cold zone side do not require PPE. Decontamination team members in the contamination reduction corridor do not cross the hazard line after they have finished with a patient. Rather, they pass the patients across the line. They move nonambulatory patients to a clean stretcher and turn care over to team members in the dry area. They decontaminate the litter by washing with soap/detergent and water or wiping it with bleach and then return it to the initial reception area.

SECURITY

Hospital security personnel should be part of the medical decontamination team. At least some security personnel must be capable of functioning in PPE. Although their primary function may be to establish and enforce the perimeter, they must be able to respond to disruptive or violent patients in the medical decontamination area when necessary.

SAFETY

The medical decontamination team must have a safety officer assigned. This individual should have no other assigned responsibilities during the decontamination process. The safety officer must coordinate with the on-scene incident commander to ensure that decontamination staff members practice appropriate work/rest cycles based upon thermal stress (17).

RUNOFF

Many organizations that will plan for medical decontamination may be concerned about the possibility of environmental contamination from the wastewater. Since they may generate large volumes of wastewater during the decontamination process, some runoff, possibly containing hazardous substances, may enter the storm drains. Section 107 (d) (1) of the Comprehensive Environmental Response, Compensation, and Liability Act states, "No person shall be liable under this sub chapter for costs or damages as a result of actions taken or omitted in the course of rendering care, assistance, or advice in accordance with the National Contingency Plan or at the direction of an on-scene coordinator appointed under such plan, with respect to an incident creating a danger to public health or welfare or the environment as a result of any releases of a hazardous substance or the threat thereof."

While this Good Samaritan clause does provide some general protection for the hospital, it does not eliminate all potential liability, nor does it excuse gross negligence or intentional misconduct. Thus, it is prudent to have a plan for the management of wastewater. Ideally, it will be contained and held for disposal as a hazardous substance. The facility's plan should include steps it will take to contain the water, such as damming and diking drainage areas. In cases where the wastewater does enter a storm drain, the hospital incident commander should notify local or state governmental officials. In terrorism incidents involving hazardous substances, there will be a designated federal on-scene coordinator. It is important to coordinate activities with that individual to reduce potential liability (18).

SHUFFLE PITS

The medical decontamination team should attempt to prevent cross-contamination between the initial reception area and the wash area, and between the wash area and the dry area. The team can utilize shuffle pits to reduce this cross-contamination. These are large, low-sided boxes filled with an absorbent material. All individuals moving between areas should walk through the shuffle pits. Staff should wheel stretchers through the shuffle pits to reduce contamination on the wheels. This will reduce the risk of moving liquid contaminants. The absorbent in the shuffle boxes is a material such as Fuller's or diatomaceous earth. The military decontamination process utilizes shuffle pits, but many civilian decontamination systems do not.

STAFF TRAINING

Administration at each hospital must select staff members for training. Physicians, midlevel providers, nurses, technicians, aides, registration or business office personnel, housekeepers, security officers, and building engineers may all be members of the Decontamination Group and require training. At least two levels of training should be available for hospital personnel. Those individuals who will actually perform decontamination operations and wear PPE must be trained to the "hazardous materials first responder operations level" (19a). Other hospital staff that may be in the area but not directly exposed to contaminated patients should receive Hazardous Material Awareness Level training (12a).

Training should be a combination of didactic sessions with small-group activities. Exercises in simulated emergencies and hands-on training with PPE and decontamination equipment are also important. The instruction should focus on the dangers of secondary contamination; procedures for small- and large-scale decontamination; integration with the hospital's disaster plan; medical treatment for chemical, biological, radiological, nuclear, and explosive incidents; and the various roles within the decontamination team (12a). Training programs are available for hospital personnel that meet these requirements. (19b,19c,19d)

In preparation for an all-hazards approach to decontamination, training and knowledge of agents is essential. Certain chemical agents that exist as a vapor will be effectively decontaminated with only removal of clothing with trapped vapor (dry decontamination). With biological agents, the need for patient decontamination will have passed before the disease would present clinically. In an overt terrorist attack where there is a notification by the terrorists that a population has been exposed to a biologic agent (such as the anthrax letters), the exposed individuals would need to be decontaminated with detergent/soap and water. For patients needing wet decontamination, the process is very similar for those contaminated with biological warfare (BW) agents, chemical warfare agents, and radiological agents. Hypochlorite solution, which is utilized in military decontamination, is generally not utilized in civilian decontamination due to the availability of large volumes of water and questionable efficacy of the hypochlorite decontamination solution. It is important to note, however, that decontamination will not eliminate the infectious risk for individuals with BW diseases that show person-to-person transmission (20a).

PERSONAL PROTECTIVE EQUIPMENT

The on-scene incident commander must evaluate the situation and determine the level of PPE that the medical decontamination personnel will use. OSHA has clarified that Level C PPE may be acceptable when performing medical decontamination away from the site of the initial release (20b,20c). The on-scene incident commander must review all information available and determine if higher levels of PPE are required based upon the known and unknown factors (21).

Clearly, every hospital should provide at least Level C PPE to its responders. Some hospitals may choose to make available higher levels of PPE (along with the higher levels of training required) to their decontamination staff. In general, however, based on a review of both actual cases of contaminated patients and on limited laboratory studies, it is likely

---

| TABLE 29-1 | Patient Decontamination Procedure |

Initial Reception Area
1. Evaluate all arriving patients for life-threatening conditions. These patients are put into the immediate treatment area. Perform simple medical procedures such as placing an oral or nasal airway, bag-valve-mask ventilation on patients with inadequate respiration. More advanced airway measures may be utilized if resources allow. Exsanguinating hemorrhage must be controlled. Cervical spine protection and the administration of chemical agent antidotes can be delivered in the immediate treatment area prior to decontamination.
2. Determine each patient's needs for decontamination.
3. Patients who require dry decontamination only should be directed to the dry decontamination area. These patients will have their clothing removed and replaced with clean clothing.
4. Place nonambulatory patients on decontamination stretchers or backboards and move to the nonambulatory decontamination area. These patients will all be wet decontaminated.

Ambulatory Patients (dry decontamination)
1. Direct patient to the ambulatory dry decontamination area.
2. Patient removes all clothing. Valuables are placed in a small plastic bag, and clothing is placed into a larger bag. Label patient and bags with matching numbers, such as a three-part nursery identification bracelet.
3. Pass clothing and valuables to the attendant. Attendant passes bags to the clothing and valuable storage area.
4. Patient moves through the contamination reduction corridor to the cold zone.
5. Patient dries self and deposits towel in designated container.
6. Patient dons gown and proceeds to emergency department triage.

Nonambulatory Patients
1. The staff continues life-saving measures such as bag-valve-mask ventilation or bleeding control that started in the immediate treatment area.
2. Decontamination staff moves the patient to the wash area.
3. In the wash area, team members remove all clothing and valuables from the patients. They place clothing in a large plastic bag and valuables in a small plastic bag. They label the patient and the belongings with matching numbers, such as a three-part nursery identification bracelet.
4. Staff passes patient belongings to the clothing and valuable storage area. The staff decontaminates scissors and any other equipment used by dipping in 5% bleach (or washing with copious water and detergent).
5. Staff rinses the patient from head to toe.
6. They gently wash the patient with detergent and a soft brush, sponge, or wash cloth from head to toe for at least 5 minutes, giving careful attention to washing areas such as the ears, eyes, axilla, and groin.
7. They log-roll the patient to wash the posterior surfaces, protecting the cervical spine if necessary.
8. They rinse the patient for at least one minute.
9. They move the patient to the cold zone. Decontamination staff should not move across the hazard line between the wash area and the dry area. Instead, members on one side should pass the patient off to team members waiting on the other side. In the process, they move the patient to a clean backboard or stretcher. The wash area staff wipes the empty stretcher with bleach (or washes with copious water and detergent).
10. Staff dries the patient and covers the patient with a sheet.
11. They move the patient to the emergency department triage area.
12. Patient dons gown and proceeds to emergency department triage.

that air purifying respirators along with liquid-impermeable clothing will provide sufficient protection for hospital decontamination personnel (22).

Each hospital will tailor its selection of decontamination equipment for its own situation. Table 29-2 shows a sample listing of equipment. The equipment for medical decontamination should include items to certify the completion of decontamination. A chemical agent monitor such as the APD 2000 (23), while relatively expensive at approximately US$11,000 in 2004 (24), is an excellent device for screening patients on arrival to determine if decontamination is necessary and to certify decontamination. The use of inexpensive monitoring capabilities such as pancake radiation detectors and M8 or M9 chemical paper may also be acceptable, but they are not able to detect as broad array of agents.

PREPAREDNESS HISTORIC EVENTS AND CASE HISTORIES

Hospital preparedness for contaminated patients is essential in order to avoid secondary contamination. There have been many cases where secondary contamination has injured hospital personnel. The keys to avoiding injury to hospital staff are appropriate decontamination procedures, good communication with out-of-hospital personnel, and appropriate levels of PPE with adequate staff training in its use (25).

The most famous case of secondary contamination causing casualties was the 1995 terrorist attack with sarin in the Tokyo subways. The hospitals did not establish any decontamination operations, and contaminated patients entered the facilities. This caused significant secondary contamination. Thirteen of the fifteen physicians who worked in the emergency department developed symptoms from exposure to sarin on the victims they were treating. Most of these doctors had visual complaints and several had severe miosis. Others had rhinorrhea, shortness of breath, chest tightness, and cough. Six of the physicians received treatment with nerve agent antidote (26). It is likely that this contamination was secondary to the entrapped sarin vapor in the casualties' clothing. The secondary contamination may have been avoided by removing this contaminated clothing before allowing the patients to enter the hospitals (dry decontamination).

PREPAREDNESS CHECKLIST TABLES AND SUMMARY

Medical decontamination is not an excessively complicated task. Nevertheless, it can require a significant commitment of personnel, time, and effort. The hospital must ensure that it has all-risk decontamination plans in place. Decontamination teams must obtain equipment. They must participate in training, both initial and annual refresher, so that they may operate safely and effectively and comply with accreditation standards and the law (Tables 29-1 and 29-2).

| TABLE 29-2 | Decontamination Area Equipment and Supplies |

ITEM
Bandage scissors
Litter stands
M8 chemical agent paper
5% (household) bleach
12-quart pails
Sponge, cellulose
Plastic bags
Plastic sheet
Black pencils
Chemical protective clothing
Decontamination litters
Atropine
Pralidoxime chloride
Diazepam
IV needles
IV infusion sets
IV fluid
Oral airways
Advanced airways (laryngeal mask airways, combitubes, or endotracheal tubes with laryngoscopes)
Battery-operated suction units
Bag-valve-mask resuscitators
Personal protective equipment
Chemical agent detector, such as the APD 2000
Dressing and bandaging supplies
Sterile saline for irrigation
Tourniquets
Washcloths
Towels
Patient gowns
Blankets and bed sheets
Diapers
Sanitary napkins
Knife
Duct tape
Flashlights
Spare batteries

The expected number of patients as determined by local hazard vulnerability assessments should determine the amounts of equipment and supplies required.

RESOURCES

1. The Occupation Safety and Health Administration publishes a pamphlet entitled "Hospitals and Community Emergency Response—What You Need to Know." This informational booklet provides a generic overview of the federal regulations governing hospital emergency response to situations involving hazardous substances. It is available on-line at http://www.OSHA.gov (27).

2. The Chemical Emergency Preparedness and Prevention Office (CEPPO) maintains a web page that provides a

directory to find the contact information on LEPCs throughout the country. It is available at http://www.epa.gov/ceppo/lepclist.htm.

3. Joint Commission on Accreditation of Healthcare Organizations (JCAHO) has published several resources to assist hospitals in meeting accreditation standards. "The Guide to Emergency Management Planning in Health Care" contains sections that pertain to all-hazards decontamination planning (28).

4. The Agency for Toxic Substances and Disease Registry has published the Managing Hazardous Materials Incidents series. This helpful series provides emergency medical services personnel and hospital emergency departments with guidance to plan for and respond to incidents with hazardous substances. Volume 2 contains specific guidance on the decontamination process (29). It is available on the Internet at http://www.atsdr.cdc.gov/mhmi.html.

5. The U.S. Army Medical Research Institute of Chemical Defense, Chemical Casualty Care Division has extensive materials on decontamination and management of contaminated individuals. Their web site includes several full-text books that may be useful to a decontamination team. Their Internet resources are available at http://ccc.apgea.army.mil.

REFERENCES

1. Okumura T, Takasu N, Ishimatsu S, et al. Report on 640 victims of the Tokyo subway sarin attack. Ann Emerg Med 1996; 28(2):129-35.

2. Cone DC, Davidson SJ. Hazardous materials preparedness in the emergency department. Prehosp Emerg Care 1997;1(2): 85-90.

3. Case GG, West BM, McHugh CJ. Hospital preparedness for biological and chemical terrorism in central New Jersey. N J Med 2001;98(11):23-33.

4. Ghilarducci DP, Pirrallo RG, Hegmann KT. Hazardous materials readiness of United States level 1 trauma centers. J Occup Environ Med 2000;42(7):683-92.

5. Treat KN, Williams JM, Furbee PM, et al. Hospital preparedness for weapons of mass destruction incidents: An initial assessment. Ann Emerg Med 2001;38(5):562-5.

6. Wetter DC, Daniell WE, Treser CD. Hospital preparedness for victims of chemical or biological terrorism. Am J Public Health 2001;91(5):710-6.

7. Greenberg MI, Jurgens SM, Gracely EJ. Emergency department preparedness for the evaluation and treatment of victims of biological or chemical terrorist attack. J Emerg Med 2002; 22(3):273-8.

8. Kreps GA. Organizing for emergency management. In: Drabek TE, Hoetmer GJ, eds. Emergency management: principles and practice for local government. Washington, DC: International City Management Association; 1991. p. 39-40.

9. National Fire Protection Association. Standard for competencies for EMS personnel responding to hazardous materials incidents. Quincy, MA: National Fire Protection Association; 2002.

10. 2003 automated comprehensive accreditation manual for hospitals [CD-ROM]. Version Update 2. Oakbrook Terrace, IL: Joint Commission Resources; 2003.

11. Special responsibilities of Medicare hospitals in emergency cases. 2003. 42 CFR 489.24, pp. 938-48.

12a. Williams-Steiger occupational safety and health act of 1970. 29 CFR 1910.120, pp. 369-411.

12b. Joint Commission on Accreditation of Healthcare Organizations. The 2001 Joint Commission Accreditation Manual for Hospitals. EC 1.4 and 1.6 (rev). Oakbrook Terrace, IL: Joint Commission Resources; 2001.

12c. Healthcare Facility Emergency Incident Command System III—January, 1998. San Mateo County Emergency Medical Services Agency. Available from: www.emsa.cahwnet.gov/dms2/heics3.htm.

13. Fairfax RE. Application of HAZWOPER (1910.120) to terrorist and weapons of mass destruction incident responses [Online]. 2003. Available from: URL:http://www.osha.gov/pls/oshaweb/owadisp.show_document?p_table=INTERPRETATIONS&p_id=24731. Accessed March 18, 2004.

14. San Mateo County Department of Health Services. The hospital emergency incident command system. 3rd ed. Sacramento: California Emergency Medical Services Authority; 1998.

15. Hazardous Waste Operations and Emergency Response (HAZWOPER) 29 CFR 1910.120.

16. Bradley RN. Toxic chemical agents reference chart—symptoms and treatment. In: Rakel R, Bope E, eds. Conn's current therapy 2003. Philadelphia: Saunders; 2003. pp. 1320-1.

17. Thermal injury (AFP 48–151). Andrews AFB MD: Air Force Medical Operations Agency, 2002.

18. U.S. Environmental Protection Agency. First responders' environmental liability due to mass decontamination runoff. Washington, DC; 2000.

19a. Clark RA. Training requirements for hospital personnel involved in an emergency response of a hazardous substance [online]. Available from: URL:http://www.osha.gov/pls/oshaweb/owadisp.show_document?p_id=20911&p_table=INTERPRETATIONS. Accessed March 22, 2004.

19b. Advanced disaster life support. From National Disaster Life Support Publications, American Medical Association; 2004.

19c. Basic disaster life support. From National Disaster Life Support Publications, American Medical Association, 2004.

19d. Core disaster life support. From National Disaster Life Support Publications, American Medical Association, 2004.

20a. Kortepeter M, Christopher G, Cieslak T, et al., editors. Medical management of biological casualties. 4th ed. Fort Detrick: U.S. Army Medical Research Institute of Infectious Diseases; 2001.

20b. OSHA interpretation letter Sept. 5, 2002, from Richard E. Fairfax to Francis J. Roth. US Department of Labor, Occupational Safety, and Health, Washington, DC.

20c. OSHA interpretation letter Dec. 2, 2002, from Richard E. Fairfax to Kevin J. Hayden. US Department of Labor, Occupational Safety, and Health, Washington, DC

21. Fairfax RE. Training and PPE requirements for hospital staff that decontaminate victims/patients. [Online]. Available from: URL:http://www.osha.gov/pls/oshaweb/owadisp.show _document?p_table=INTERPRETATIONS&p_id=24523. Accessed March 19, 2004.

22. Hick JL, Hanfling D, Burstein JL, et al. Protective equipment for health care facility decontamination personnel: Regulations, risks, and recommendations. Ann Emerg Med 2003; 42(3):370-80.

23. Arrow-Tech. APD 2000. [Online]. Available from: URL:http://www.arrowtechinc.com/apd%202000_2.htm. Accessed March 26, 2004.

24. Fisher Scientific. Smiths Detection APD 2000 chemical warfare agent detector. [Online]. Available from: URL:https://www1.fishersci.com/Coupon?gid=177091&cid=1342. Accessed March 25, 2004.

25. Horton DK, Berkowitz Z, Kaye WE. Secondary contamination of ED personnel from hazardous materials events, 1995-2001. Am J Emerg Med 2003;21(3):199-204.

26. Nozaki H, Hori S, Shinozawa Y, et al. Secondary exposure of medical staff to sarin vapor in the emergency room. Intensive Care Med 1995;21(12):1032-5.

27. Occupational Safety & Health Administration. Hospitals and community emergency response—what you need to know. Washington, DC: Occupational Safety & Health Administration; 1997.

28. Joint Commission Resources. Guide to emergency management planning in health care. Oakbrook Terrace: Joint Commission Resources; 2002.

29. Agency for Toxic Substances and Disease Registry. Hospital emergency departments: a planning guide for the management of contaminated patients. 2000 ed. Atlanta: Agency for Toxic Substance and Disease Registry; 1992.

30

Detection, Prediction, and Surveillance

Warren L. Whitlock

INTRODUCTION

Surveillance is an all-encompassing activity that includes planned and unplanned information collection, statistical analysis, and the prediction reporting of possible future events. This definition encompasses the next generation of detection and surveillance systems on the horizon and provides the groundwork for both horizontal and vertical views of the requirements for successful surveillance systems. The Centers for Disease Control and Prevention (CDC) defines public health surveillance as "the ongoing, systematic collection, analysis, and interpretation of data (e.g., regarding agent/hazard, risk factor, exposure, health event) essential to the planning, implementation, and evaluation of public health practice, closely integrated with the timely dissemination of these data to those responsible for prevention and control" (1). Prediction of health trends depends on accurate detection data, dynamic data integration for surveillance, and Bayesian probability for sensitivity, specificity, and statistical accuracy. Identifying the requirements, components, and systems engineering for early detection of health states can provide a strategic decision capability concerning resources and disease prevention actions. However, surveillance systems can have severe shortcomings, based on the quality of the data collected and the detection methods used to provide surveillance. These are essential topics for a discussion of detection and surveillance capabilities and realities.

Although the CDC provides a reasonably clear general definition for health surveillance, it does not provide a specific definition of "detection," and the key to successful surveillance is early detection. Surveillance of specific detection information, when recognized, allows for early strategic intervention. Detection methodology is the historical foundation of epidemiology and surveillance and the primary key for effective actions to limit, control, and prevent potential disease outbreaks. Surveillance can be either accurate and valuable or inaccurate with little utility, based on its precision and accuracy for prediction of "true positive" public health outcomes.

One of the finest examples of detection and surveillance is Dr. John Snow's epidemiological research in 1854 in detecting cases of cholera and their location in London. Each cholera case detected and its location were painstakingly plotted by hand on a map of the city. The density of cholera cases in a concentric fashion based on their location made the association and conclusion obvious to anyone that it was the centrally located town well and its water that was contaminated with cholera. The mapping of each case detected provided for a surveillance system to understand the relationship between the disease and the source to form strategic decisions regarding resources and public health policy, which later formed the basis for modern epidemiology and public health activities. Snow's work constituted a case-controlled study demonstrating that people from low-risk areas outside of London who drank the cholera-contaminated water developed cholera. This confirmed his theory that cholera cases were associated with the well water before medical science had discovered it was a bacterial organism that caused the contamination and disease (2). It was the undeniable confirmation of Snow's surveillance prediction that caused a revolution in public health attitudes. Despite the profound effect of this methodology, it took almost 20 years to fully change the public behavior even after the causes and effects of cholera were known.

History teaches us that the ability to predict future health events from detection and effectively communicate this information to leaders can be devastating if not rooted in the daily management and administration of our government system. The Native Americans taught the early British and European settlers much important information, but perhaps no lesson from that period of history is as poignant as what was learned from the first recorded incidence of biological warfare use in North America. The French and Indian War was waged from 1754 to 1763. After seven years, a victory was still not foreseeable until a British commander approved a submitted plan to use blankets from a smallpox hospital to infect Native American tribes that had no natural resistance. William Trent, a commander of the local militia of the townspeople of Pittsburgh, notes in his journal on May 24, 1763, "[W]e gave them two Blankets and an Handkerchief out of the Small Pox Hospital. I hope it will have the desired effect" (3).

Without detection and surveillance capability, smallpox spread rapidly across the Native American tribes. After the initial cases, the true cause went unrecognized by Native

American leaders, and the morbidity and mortality resulted in devastation of the eastern Native American population, effectively ending the French and Indian War in less than a year. Native Americans continued to suffer from smallpox outbreaks for years afterward because they were not capable of understanding the public health strategic consequences.

Detection and surveillance requirements for protection of public health against weapons of mass destruction (WMD) will be no less an important requirement than the understanding of the contagion risk of smallpox might have been to Native Americans. The changes required in the United States to achieve effective detection and surveillance will be no less profound than what Snow faced in changing public health policy after discovering the relationship between cholera and water contamination. The understanding and transformational change in a global health detection and surveillance system required to prevent or limit the impact of a biological or chemical terrorism attack effectively could result in even more lives saved today than all the lives saved in history because of Snow's original discovery concerning cholera.

PREPAREDNESS ESSENTIALS

The possibility of the intentional spread of chemical, biological, radiological, nuclear, or explosive (CBRNE) agents by terrorists makes it essential that preparedness planning incorporate the use of advanced technology for medical surveillance. This must be done in support of a wide spectrum of professions to include first responders, public health officials, and military services (both active and reserve components) and by commercial companies that import products into the United States. Detection and surveillance for threat and risk reduction needs specifically to target CBRNE and, most recently, "cyber-terrorism attacks" (4). If surveillance is to be effective, it must be established within the federal standards for medical data but support the systematic processes of data collection, analysis, and dissemination among local, state, and federal agencies.

"All data concerning global disease incidence, including WHO data, should be treated as broadly indicative of trends rather than accurate measures of disease prevalence" (5). To further define the critical requirements for detection and surveillance, the real challenge is to distinguish among a *disease outbreak,* the *deliberate use of biological weapons,* and the *native fluctuations in the detection system* that *are not predictive of either one.* Early detection presupposes there is a system matrix for surveillance that can then predict future health events. Without the ability to discriminate between these incidents at an early point in time through detection, surveillance will only occur in a retrospective, asynchronous, postmortem fashion and result in "lessons learned" as a history archive footnote. Efforts under way on both the civilian and military community homeland security fronts and defense and preparations for potential bioterrorism agent deployment will have clear and measurable benefits to our current health surveillance systems used by the Department of Defense (DoD) and the CDC today.

In October 2000, the Defense Threat Reduction Agency's Advanced Systems and Concepts Office (ASCO) and the CDC cosponsored a workshop aimed at identifying the essential elements of a national health surveillance system. The National Health Surveillance Workshop described three types of surveillance systems: "data mining, rapid diagnostics, and syndromic systems" (6).

The data mining process is performed retrospectively and uses statistical methods to uncover relationships that otherwise would not be discovered or understood. Data mining evaluates existing data that is already archived, and it requires no effort to perform collection activities. But because it is retrospective, it is limited even in the most ideal of circumstances to providing information on "what happened in the past." Data mining cannot by itself provide the necessary prediction of trends needed for surveillance systems. The analogy would be to drive a car forward by only having the ability to look backward to see where you have been. Data mining also depends on the quality of legacy data recorded, which for most available surveillance systems is based in medical billing codes (ICD-9). In medical systems, this is the most prevalent methodology used for surveillance today. Other "legacy" data models are being explored, such as emergency department "chief complaint" or patient call-in information lines, but because of inconsistent definitions of the data and lack of systematic collection, they are all limited in meeting true surveillance requirements.

Because many of the CDC's identified high-risk bioagents have zoonotic or animal origins, surveillance systems must use more than just human insurance billing codes and incorporate standards in broad categories of agriculture, animal, and human data for aggregation. Future surveillance systems must include veterinary medicine, agricultural system data, and U.S. Trade and Immigration information, as well as medical health data.

Just as the CDC has classified bioterrorism agents/ diseases by category (7), the International Office for Epizootics (OIE) has classified animal diseases into categories based on their risk of negatively impacting international trade and global economy. The class A list is defined by "Transmissible diseases which have the potential for very serious and rapid spread, irrespective of national borders, which are of serious socio-economic or public health consequence and which are of major importance in the international trade of animals and animal products." The class B list is defined by "Transmissible diseases, which are considered to be of socio-economic, and/or public health importance within countries and which are significant in the international trade of animals and animal products" (8). Bioterrorism agents such as anthrax, Q fever, tularemia, brucellosis, and glanders are on both the CDC and the OIE lists.

The spectrum of detection systems to support surveillance must include environmental, agricultural, and occupational field detection evidenced by the growing number of stationary and mobile *rapid detection and diagnostic devices* (RD3) that provide immediate identification of biological, chemical, and radiation agents. RD3 can provide real-time detection with a high degree of sensitivity in multiple sites over long periods of time. However, the RD3s still need an integrating system for surveillance prediction of events using multiple disparate data sources that yield a high probability and accuracy. These types of systems are generally more expensive and more sensitive to environmental conditions and therefore of limited utility because they are subject to variable specificity in the detection thresholds. The validation of alarm thresholds and higher quality devices for proven field use is needed before deploying these systems as part of surveillance systems in real-world operations.

The importance of research and technology enhancement of medical surveillance is clear from the largest retrospective investigation injury and disability studies in DoD. This work took 9 years to complete by review of medical records and resulted in these five recommended steps for surveillance system development:

1. Surveillance: Determine problem to be investigated.
2. Research: Identify the specific data for cause and risk factor detection.
3. Research/intervention trials: Use for prevention and surveillance strategies.
4. Policy, behavioral changes, and equipment: Optimize the use of technology for implementation.
5. Ongoing surveillance and research: Evaluate effectiveness of future planning and forecasting capabilities (9).

The requirement for "Research" is listed in three of the five categories from this study compiled by military and civilian experts. The most notable conclusion concerning detection and surveillance is that current systems are not adequate to meet our national, state, or local agency requirements for early detection, accurate prediction, and valid decisions concerning resources by public health, federal, and state government officials.

The two categories of clinical surveillance are *direct* and *indirect* methodology. Indirect surveillance is analogous to taking a census based on current information systems and medical codes. This can provide general information concerning past or current events but by itself it cannot necessarily provide for early or accurate identification of future trends. The direct type of surveillance is more formal because of its specific data collection and examination to determine factors or conditions that predict health events in a given population, location, and time period. An example of indirect surveillance is when the recorded atmosphere and weather conditions monitored from satellite by NASA were combined with recorded outbreaks of the West Nile virus in Egypt. Matching of these historical trends showed an association of flooding of the Nile River during the summer season to epidemics of West Nile virus infection. Because mosquitoes are the carrier and vector of the West Nile virus, pooled water and warm seasons provide conditions necessary for West Nile epidemics. Public health actions to address these conditions were based on the understanding of this indirect surveillance and subsequently were proven to reduce the number of cases of West Nile virus infection (10). This type of surveillance of environmental conditions provided valid prediction of human and animal disease risk in large geographical areas and populations, which are used now in other areas of the world with West Nile virus infections. The ability to collect clinical information within our indirect medical information system must have the capability to use patient symptoms and signs, or what is known as "syndromic surveillance."

Serological surveillance in populations is a more specific measure, which can be conducted under both direct and indirect methods. Indirect surveillance is similar to the monitoring of HIV-positive rates routinely reported to public health and the CDC. Direct surveillance is illustrated by the specific and systematic monitoring for coronavirus (cause of the severe acute respiratory syndrome [SARS] epidemic), the seroconversion rate in both human and animal populations to predict background population exposure, predict risk for potential epidemic, and institute tighter infection control policies in high-risk countries (11). Because one of the critical predictors of epidemics is a population's native resistance to a disease, serological data can also have great value for epidemic probability and forecasting. Direct surveillance of serological conversion rates in a targeted population can provide evidence of subclinical disease exposure, risk of disease epidemic, and assist with prediction information for other areas and populations. If direct surveillance for serological conversion is used in a large target population, it can have very high costs and present implementation problems for training and education across many organizations. Both direct and indirect serological surveillance methods can provide predictions of prevalence and risk in geographical distributions for many human and veterinary diseases. Serological surveillance provides objective information concerning the frequency of specific findings in a population and is therefore more quantifiable than subjective billing code surveillance. For medical surveillance to be used effectively by health care providers and decision makers, it must be available in a near "real-time" capability for accurate probability prediction. This requirement provides an opportunity for technology and equipment to support a "next-generation" surveillance capability to deter and prevent potential terrorist attacks and deployment of bioterrorism agents. This chapter provides a glimpse of some near-term and long-term products that are in development for both civilians and military.

PREPAREDNESS HISTORIC EVENTS AND CASE HISTORIES

The concept of a modern biological warfare and research development program was developed after World War II when investigations showed evidence that Japan had conducted systematic and comprehensive research on potential biological agents for use during the war. Records show the testing of these agents on human prisoners, the modifying and weaponizing of the bioagents, and the development of delivery systems, such as aerosol delivery of anthrax spores (12). The U.S. research efforts on the atomic bomb ended the war with Japan before these biological research efforts could come to fruition and be used against the Allied forces.

The dropping of the atomic bomb at Hiroshima and Nagasaki ended not only the war but the deployment of Japan's considerable biological warfare capability. Planning the ideal future surveillance system might be based on determining the requirements to meet the worst case scenario.

Therefore the "ideal surveillance system" would provide enough sensitivity and specificity for early detection, accurate prediction, and effective preventive actions in preparedness against the "ideal CBRNE agent." The ideal syndromic surveillance system should be simple to use, supplied at no or low cost to end users, and be of great value in their job performance, but still provide for data collection at point of care in a wide range of settings (public health clinics, physicians' offices, emergency departments, pharmacies). It would also provide for alert thresholds and transmission (data synchronization) of information and alerts across jurisdictions, regions and states, and network domains. This type of system would be able to provide data query over time for valid predictions of trends that lie outside of historical trends and provide indications for in-depth ad hoc query and investigation.

Asynchronous data is analyzed retrospectively, whereas synchronous data enable the concept of real-time information analysis. Microsoft defines real-time data (RTD) as data that updates on its own schedule (for example, stock quotes, manufacturing statistics, Web server loads, and warehouse activity) (13). RTD for the perfect surveillance system would allow for "synchronous data" and RTD update, which is defined as a RTD architecture and RTD server. The next generation surveillance system must have RTD forecasting and analysis with thresholds (predefined "panic value"), duplicate data certification, and transmission logging of alarms, recommendations, and actions for appropriate agencies (i.e., telephone, pagers, e-mail lists, and data-synchronized client alarms). The ability to respond dynamically to specific detection information is an example of the capability to differentiate "signal" from "noise." This type of system will incrementally collect better information about high-risk populations and reduce the burden of time and effort by first responders and health care providers.

PREPAREDNESS SUMMARY

From news reports, federal, DoD, and state agency reports, there are hundreds of parallel health surveillance systems being developed. The National Association of County and City Health Officials is funding more than $400 million of separate public health surveillance and training programs (14).

Jerry Hauer, a senior advisor to the Secretary for the Department of Health and Human Services for national security and emergency management, said in the proceedings of the Department of Health and Human Services National Committee on Vital and Health Statistics meeting held in February 2002, "I think one of the greatest concerns we have is that as different systems have been developed, be it syndromic or data mining, there has not been a commonality of data that is required. We will wind up with a group of systems around the country that don't necessarily talk with one another" (15). Hauer is absolutely correct in saying that no surveillance system can be realized when confronted with our current medical detection coding methodology. Effective health and environmental standardized data detection information for data mining and syndromic surveillance function is not an option, it is a critical requirement.

A discussion of the Framingham Heart Study, one of the greatest modern research programs, illustrates this point clearly. Before 1950, it was believed coronary disease was

unavoidable and people could not change their risk because the risk factors for disease surveillance were not understood. To determine what constellation of factors from the biological, environmental, and living style spheres could predict risk for myocardial infarction was one-half of the researchers' objective. The other half was the novel concept that physicians and their patients take action and prevent what was thought to be inevitable. The detection of high blood pressure, serum cholesterol, age, dietary habits, and exercise habits were not incorporated into a surveillance program for heart disease until the results of this study changed risk behavior in the United States forever. However, the final results of this direct syndromic surveillance study took decades to make its predictions and be validated in subsequent trials. The value of standardized medical data to deliver medical care information more effectively and collect detection information without error will also provide the key to early identification of disease trends and the ability to make strategic decisions to protect the health of the population.

The U.S. military developed an innovative health care strategy called Force Health Protection (FHP), which uses preventive health techniques and emerging technologies in environmental surveillance and combat medicine to protect service members before, during, and after deployment. The overarching goal of FHP is casualty prevention, achieved through a physically and mentally fit force trained for modern combat. FHP prevention concentrates on environmental and health hazards and preventive strategies to reduce the largest number of military casualties caused by disease and nonbattle injury (DNBI) (16).

To reduce the DNBI threat, a system for conducting and maintaining continuous surveillance of the force health and the DNBI threat includes global medical intelligence to support the capability to implement countermeasures early. These may include immunizations, environmental, and public health or preventive measures. The Joint Force Medical Surveillance Program analyzes illness rates in two broad categories: "battle injury" and "disease nonbattle injury" (DNBI) (17). Battle injuries are caused by conventional small arms and fragmentation ordinance and explosive munitions including high-velocity weapons, land mines, rockets, bombs, artillery, as well as bayonets and other wounding devices used or employed by a single individual or a crew. However, the direct mortality from military conflict is not historically the reason that major campaigns are lost, and in one study it was found to contribute less than 1 percent of overall cause of death globally in the year 2000 (18).

The DoD DNBI surveillance program aggregates disease and injury into 16 categories that have established thresholds determined from historical military injury and disease rates during deployments. These categories are reported weekly by all deployed medical units for visibility of the threat to soldiers in a given environment or from endemic diseases. This is a type of syndromic surveillance based on aggregated symptoms and diagnoses and is used today by the U.S. Army's Center for Health Promotion and Preventive Medicine (CHPPM). The U.S. Army and other services have engaged large resources and considerable academic acumen from lessons learned within the U.S. Army War College and calls to "tailor the use of preventive medicine assets to enter the area of operations at each level of conflict" and to establish an "effective DNBI (surveillance) prevention program" (19). Military medical leaders understand the importance of conducting systematic health surveillance of soldiers to make decisions concerning resources that protect their soldiers. Thresholds for which a commander must not exceed are based on rate of occurrence 1/1,000 over a 7-day time period (17). Because the aggregation of the symptom and disease categories are at risk for variables, the time period of 7 days adjusts the sensitivity to avoid frequent false positives.

DoD is perhaps one of the greatest test beds to prove and establish these medical standards for use in clinical situations at the patient interface and for military leaders' command and control requirements to protect their soldiers under worldwide conditions. The DNBI data can be used by the medical staff to identify local- or theater-level trends in health status and target feasible means of reducing the incidence of preventable disease and injury. An example of how DNBI data is aggregated is in the infectious gastrointestinal category. This category contains "all diagnoses consistent with infection of the intestinal tract and includes any type of diarrhea, gastroenteritis, 'stomach flu,' nausea/vomiting, hepatitis, etc., but does NOT include noninfectious intestinal diagnoses such as hemorrhoids, ulcers, etc." (17).

This constellation of symptoms and diagnoses in military operations has a threshold level of 5/1,000/week. If the rate of gastrointestinal infectious category exceeds twice this threshold or the rate doubles from the prior week, commanders are advised to realign resources and conduct a complete investigation into the causes.

DoD GLOBAL EMERGING INFECTIOUS SURVEILLANCE

The DoD program for Global Emerging Infectious Surveillance (GEIS) supports global surveillance, training, research, and response to emerging infectious disease threats through military research laboratories around the world and within the United States. GEIS epidemiological capabilities serve U.S. interests through early warnings of new infectious diseases, enable preventive medicine to combat epidemics, and enhance military hospitals' capability to treat disease outbreaks. The DoD GEIS laboratories in Cairo, Egypt; Nairobi, Kenya; and Bangkok, Thailand work closely with the CDC to monitor emerging infections across the globe.

The U.S. Air Force (USAF) provides a medical data collection, assessment, and surveillance program called the Global Expeditionary Medical System (GEMS) inside its modular deployable hospitals. As former Air Force lieutenant general Paul Carlton said in his testimony to the House Armed Service Committee, "Technology is key with portable C2 (command and control)-linked test platforms that aid the field medic in determining the nature and cause of the biological hazard to facilitate mitigation" (20).

During the coalition exercise Bright Star in Egypt, September to October 2001, the Third Medical Command (3rd MEDCOM) evaluated a modified GEMS system to conduct deployed health surveillance. The GEMS was modified to use the Portable Data File (PDF-417) two-dimensional bar code on the military ID card for error-free identification of patient information to include name, rank, social security number, age, service, and blood type. The modified GEMS included updated patient symptoms in drop-down categories organized in a Subjective, Objective, Assessment, Plan (SOAP) format for intuitive navigation for health care providers. Although the exercise was shortened due to Operation Enduring Freedom (OEF), the medical surveillance portion called "Digital Force Health Protection" was a marked achievement in demonstrating advanced surveillance capabilities in deployed military populations using detection and surveillance technology tools. A single PDF-417 symbol carries up to 1.1 kilobytes of readable data in two-dimensional symbology. A major advantage not appreciated by many is that, unlike the one-D bar code, which is useless without a complete database application, the PDF-417 serves as its own mobile database in a standard that is now used for nonmedical purposes by both federal and state governments. It can provide a coded identification information system for medical and health surveillance purposes, and the information content meets federal, state, and Health Insurance Portability and Accountability Act (HIPAA) requirements for privacy.

The demonstration of the GEMS application provided the 3rd Medical Command in Egypt with force health strength surveillance, monitoring of the illness rates over all of the DNBI categories, and generation of maps with highlighted areas where the DNBI thresholds were exceeded. Exported data was exported into encrypted files and sent via Internet to the Southeast Regional Medical Command, where all surveillance information could be further analyzed in less than 24 hours after a soldier had been seen at a clinic in Egypt. Early detection of health threats and subsequent command decisions to protect the health of deployed soldiers can be accomplished using computerized technology. The use of computerized data detection capabilities, surveillance query, and archival transmission of data is an absolute requirement for military operations abroad and at home.

Digital Force Health Protection during Bright Star Exercise and the subsequent testing by Medical Research and Materiel Command at Fort Detrick, Maryland, resulted in the first demonstration of personnel using developed bar-code technology for medical surveillance systems (21). A second phase of this work involved a two-D handheld scanner that could automatically read the two-D matrix data (raster) in less than 2 seconds. All health care encounters begin with the identification of the patient and end with a medical outcome. The PDF-417 is a personnel file data standard for all U.S. military service identification cards to include active and reserve components as well as dependent family and retired service members. It is now used on the drivers' licenses of over 30 states for storage of identification information and organ donor status. It is being used most recently by commercial retail stores to check identification of purchases using check or credit cards, but it has tremendous potential for integration of data and information standards in disasters and emergency response for homeland security.

RESOURCES

The United States is a major hub of global travel, immigration, and commerce and supports a military presence overseas and has wide-ranging global economic interests. The greatest risk to national security and national economic interest is the disruption and degradation of U.S. security and economy in the worldwide market through some multipronged chemical and biological terrorist campaign. A global *integrated surveillance and response system* that includes the World Health Organization, International Emerging Infections Programs (IEIPs), CDC's National Center for Infectious Diseases (NCID), DoD's Global Emerging Infectious Surveillance System (GEIS), and the CDC's Emerging Infectious Surveillance program is the essential requirement. These surveillance systems must provide real-time and accurate ongoing systematic collection, analysis, and interpretation for evaluation of public health trends and forecasting from local, state, federal, and international organizations. The surveillance systems must be closely integrated with the distributed networked dissemination of information to public health personnel responsible for prevention and control. Table 30-1 lists all the functional areas for a global integrated surveillance system. Examples of government and commercial surveillance applications covering some of these areas are listed in Table 30-2 and Table 30-3.

A CDC initiative to promote the use of standardized data is the National Electronic Disease Surveillance System (NEDSS). It is anticipated that it could achieve the needs for an interoperable surveillance system for federal, DoD, state, and local public health and medical organizations. It encourages the use of automatic capture and analysis of data that are already available to include ICD-9 codes and electronic Health Level Seven (HL7) Reference Information Models (22). NEDSS system architecture is designed to integrate legacy surveillance system such as the National Electronic Telecommunications System for Surveillance (NETSS) and will ideally use other more robust coding systems such as the Systematized Nomenclature of Medicine-Clinical Terms (SNOMED-CT) and the PDF-417 bar codes in use across DoD and the majority of U.S. states for drivers' license identification. Currently NEDSS has a long way to go to provide data interoperability for systematic comprehensive electronic data architecture needed across the global

TABLE 30-2	DoD Surveillance Tools and Agencies in 2002

SURVEILLANCE TOOL	DEPLOYING AGENCY
LEADERS	USAF
ESSENCE	GEIS
SAMS	Navy/SPAWAR
MDSS	NHRC/SPAWAR
DMSS	AMSA
RDSS	NEHC
FMSS	NHRC
MSS/LERSM	TMIP-J
DHSS	CHPPM/SOCOM
GEMS	USAF
JMO-T	DUSD

medical system. The NEDSS standards for future development could provide standard operating procedures using current infrastructure for secure transmission, archival of sensitive or critical data, and federal-and state-secure Internet and gateway for the future CDC's Secure Data Network (SDN). Integration of legacy system architecture and defining the requirements for interchangeable data within the developing DoD, federal, state, and commercial standards remains the greatest challenge.

The Joint Service Installation Pilot Project (JSIPP) is a DoD program managed by the Defense Threat Reduction Agency to model DoD support systems for homeland security and defense around the requirements for response to weapons of mass destruction or natural disaster events. The sites will be provided with equipment and training to enhance protection, detection, and emergency response. The installations selected to be the first participants in the JSIPP are Camp Lejeune, NC; Fort Campbell, KY; Pope Air Force Base (AFB), NC; Barksdale AFB, LA; Fort Lewis, WA; Navy Region Southwest, San Diego, CA; Fort Gordon, GA; Robins AFB, GA; and Naval Surface Warfare Center, Dahlgren, VA. Chemical and biological detector data will be integrated with medical surveillance for testing and evaluation over both military and civilian computerized networks. Fort Gordon, Georgia, the U.S. Army Signal Center & School and the Southeast Regional Medical Command, is one of the nine installations of the JSIPP that is testing the latest chemical and information technologies for use as a "DoD backbone" for common capability at all military installations.

Improving the health detection and surveillance for a global system is therefore not just altruistic; it strengthens and stabilizes U.S. deployed military and foreign interests as well as prevents destabilizing epidemics that could negatively impact on U.S. interests and allies. Contributing to a global surveillance standard provides monitoring for mitigation planning and provides support by reducing risk through effective surveillance to foreign populations and economies. Detection and surveillance systems can reduce the risk of effective biological warfare and terrorism and reduce the threat to the U.S. national security and economy.

The International Organization for Standardization (ISO) and the International Electro-Technical Commission (IEC)

TABLE 30-1	Requirements for a Global Integrated Surveillance System

- Surveillance of U.S. population health
- Surveillance of all immigrations into the United States (people, cargo, information)
- Surveillance of U.S. military and coalition forces health
- Surveillance of allied countries' population health
- Surveillance of adversary countries' population health
- Surveillance of animal health
- Surveillance of agriculture
- Surveillance of wildlife and natural resources

TABLE 30-3	Selected Commercial Tools in 2002	
TOOL	**COMPANY**	**URL**
BASIICS	Health Hero Network, Inc.	http://www.healthhero.com/
RSVP	Sandia National Labs	http://www.sandia.gov/
SURVEIL	DSHI Systems, Inc.	http://www.dshisystems.com/?mt=2&st=3
RedBat	ICPA, Inc.	http://www.icpa.net/SoftwareProd.htm#redbat
LEADERS	IDAHO Technology, Inc.	http://www.armytechnology.com/contractors/nbc/idaho/

created a Joint Technical Committee on Information Technology (ISO/IEC JTC1) in 1998. The JTC1 Information Technology Sub-Committee 17 (SC17) has the responsibility for developing standards for identification cards and personal identification technology to include biometrics (23). Bar-code scanning as a medical standard for medication logistics and dispensing is being presented to the Food and Drug Administration (FDA) (24). It could assist with medical error reduction and provide a candidate technology for global data use and for NEDSS. If used in a matrix format such as the PDF-417, it could also provide portable database storage for patients.

Identification codes such as bar-code technology are currently a data standard under ISO and commonly used for global merchandise tracking. The Automatic Identification and Data Capture (AIDC) is a global trade association for commercial companies and providers of identification and data technology. Data standards that offer great promise are multidimensional bar-code matrix, data-rich technology-enabled cards (magnetic stripe, "smart" card, contactless card, optical card), embedded biometric, and the Radio Frequency Identification (RFID) wireless data collection capability (25).

The lead for DoD research and development is the Defense Advanced Research Projects Agency (DARPA). It is tasked with managing basic and applied research and development for the next generation war fighter. One of the DARPA projects is the Bio-Surveillance prototype systems capable of detecting a covert release of a biological pathogen through monitoring and automated reporting of current information technologies. The key to mitigating a biological attack is early detection so the technology of Bio-Surveillance could provide the capability to initiate preventive medications and reduce numbers of casualties (26).

This increase in monitoring of nontraditional data sources in animal health, behavioral indicators, and prediagnostic and diagnostic medical data will require sustained effort and long-term funding. The Bio-Surveillance could dramatically increase the ability to detect a clandestine biological warfare attack for early response (26).

The technical challenge is to correlate and integrate information derived from heterogeneous data sources (medical, environmental, veterinary, agricultural, and personnel identification) for development of autonomous detection algorithms while at the same time providing for privacy protection and patient confidentiality (26).

Other DARPA projects include the Tissue Based Biosensors and Activity Detection Technology to detect a wide range of threats such as genetically engineered bacteria and viruses or unknown emerging infectious agents. The capability to use technology sensors inside of living systems was pioneered in the field of invasive cardiology with pacemakers but may have a new role inside living cells to detect either nonspecific or specific agents in an environment. To address the preexposure detection, discrimination, and identification of the threat requirement, DARPA is developing detection systems as well as biological sensors that function at the molecular level. Some of these use technology similar to recently developed medical laboratory tests like the direct fluorescent antibody test for *Legionella pneumophila,* the organism that causes Legionnaires' disease. These technologies promise the capability for fluorescent reaction to chemical and biological agents that are highly sensitive and specific. At the molecular level of genes is another technology called Triangulation for Genetic Evaluation of Risks (TIGER) for the capability of detecting genetic differences or mutations in the environment. This novel approach to biodetection could yield benefits not only against the intentional development of drug-resistant or more virulent biological agents but could also have tremendous value in monitoring for normal biological changes in the genes of pathogens such as in hospitals with drug-resistant bacteria or for antigenic "shift" in influenza virus. Detection technology is a major direction with current DARPA research and will provide an important piece of the total surveillance picture (26).

With GEIS support, scientists at the Walter Reed Army Institute of Research started developing the Electronic Surveillance System for the Early Notification of Community-based Epidemics (ESSENCE) in 1999. ESSENCE is a clinically based application for syndromic surveillance of daily outpatient encounters from over 300 U.S. military treatment facilities (MTFs) around the world. It uses the clinic or facility location, date, and ICD-9 codes to provide a mapping system (27) similar to John Snow's original work in epidemiology.

Real-Time Outbreak and Disease Surveillance (RODS) is an open source public health surveillance project that resulted from the academic collaboration of hospitals, foundations, and public health industries. It is based on ICD-9 billing codes and intended to be used by health departments or urban regions for surveillance of common disease trends. It is written in Java hardware compatibility and downloadable for noncommercial use (28).

Most experts agree the legacy coding for medical billing is not nearly robust enough to support data spectrum for the symptom and early disease detection or monitoring necessary for an adequate surveillance system. The National Library of Medicine endorses the Unified Medical Language System (UMLS) for moving one medical coding system into a compiled and compatible version of another. The most robust of the medical coding systems that covers human and animal disease, etiology, pathology, laboratory, and treatment is the Systematized Nomenclature of Medicine (SNOMED-CT) (29). This multiaxial database of disease, etiology, associations, and conditions has now a robust concept and relationship architecture that links "symptoms," "physical findings," "environmental conditions," "geography," "preventions," and "diagnostic tests" to "diseases" and "potential treatments" (30). However, the more robust and comprehensive any data diction system for surveillance, the more likely the violation of patient privacy. The Health Insurance Portability and Accountability Act (HIPAA) sets new standards for electronic medical data and records. Recently efforts directed to integration of billing codes, clinical terminologies, and robust medical data structure like SNOMED-CT offer some of our best hopes for a functional NEDSS capability.

Because all pathology laboratories in accredited hospitals across the United States currently use SNOMED to report the incidence of diagnoses, a SNOMED-CT-enabled health care and information system could provide surveillance over symptom complexes, disease diagnoses, laboratory findings, vaccines, and treatments for virtually any location in the world. Research efforts to use SNOMED-CT to encode clinical information contained in electronic medical records and references to organize symptoms, physical findings, possible diagnoses, and medical planning as part of a military and DoD research program show that it can provide the necessary capability to identify and respond to bioterrorism events in a real-time modality (31).

Surveillance involves the detection of critical points: areas under direct threat of disease such as federal, DoD, state, and public areas; border crossings for personnel and shipping and receiving areas; agricultural areas to include food, soil, and watershed resources; and the monitoring for activity in other countries worldwide. Surveillance resource deployment should then be implemented and maintained at these critical points, with planned surveillance frequency to detect clinical/pathological signs, serology conversions, and identification of infectious causative agents under normal and heightened alarm conditions. The frequency of surveillance at these critical points must be determined by the risk at each point. Financial constraints and predeployment testing of surveillance systems will also be a major determinant of the capability, frequency, and effectiveness of such systems.

The Internet's communication technology uses routing computers (routers) to maintain a mapping of the fastest route for information packets to travel around the world in under several hundred milliseconds or less. Computer engineers design networks to avoid system fragility: "A common goal that designers of complex systems strive for is robustness. Robustness is the ability of a system to continue to operate correctly across a wide range of operational conditions, and to fail gracefully outside of that range" (32). This design of a robust complex that anticipates the scale of operations demanded to avoid failure is defined as "precognitive technology."

In reality, precognition, or the "knowing of what is going to happen" based on scientific facts confirming hypotheses, provides the basis for distinction between modern science and the magic and alchemy that abounded during the Middle Ages. Automated detection and archival systems using synchronous distributed database networks as the technical

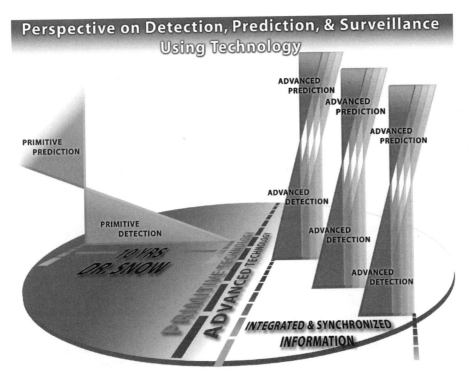

Figure 30–1. Detection and prediction are the two major components of a simple surveillance system. The difference between a primitive surveillance system used since the 19th century and an advanced technology enhanced surveillance system is the ability to enable integrated information networked using precognitive technology. Precognition in surveillance-predictive architecture depends on synchronous rather than asynchronous information technology. The advanced prediction synchronous technology achieves real-time analysis for current and future surveillance.

architecture achieves information access, precognition that supersedes current understanding of enhanced information systems (33). This relationship is shown in Fig. 30-1 and illustrates how the integrated technology supports precognitive surveillance. Not only does synchronous technology provide the architecture for real-time predictive models and the basis for proactive decisions and plans, it allows for early surveillance actions. This chapter has provided the essentials for detection, prediction, and surveillance understanding and a platform to assimilate the requirements for a technology architecture. The definition of surveillance must therefore include both a defined role for detection and prediction, using data standards and technology to achieve a robust precognitive surveillance across the global spectrum of operations.

Detection and prediction technology requirements for surveillance, with other requirements for implementation, characterize a road map for future investment and research to meet the public health challenge on a global scale. Incorporation of deployment and operations requirements, such as personnel training and logistical support of technology, are essential to achieve a final robust surveillance system. Recognizing the current deficits in our surveillance system and the essential components needed to achieve a fail-safe system using advanced information system technology and standards is a critical step. Achieving global surveillance will be a significant milestone in human history that if not achieved within this generation could result in detrimental change affecting the dominant species on this planet (Fig. 30-2).

REFERENCES

1. Centers for Disease Control and Prevention [no date]. Definition of public health surveillance. Web site: http://www.cdc.gov/epo/dphsi/phs/overview.htm. Accessed October 2003.
2. Snow J. On the mode of communication of cholera. London: John Churchill Publishers; 1855.
3. Harpster JW. Pen pictures of early western Pennsylvania. Journal of William Trent, 1763. Pittsburgh: University of Pittsburgh Press, 1938;99,103-4.
4. Garrison L, Grand M. Cyberterrorism: an evolving concept. In: National Infrastructure Protection Center highlights (Issue 06-01). Washington, DC: June 15, 2001. Web site: http://www.nipc.gov/publications/highlights/2001/highlight-01-06.htm. Accessed December 2003.
5. National Intelligence Council. [January 2000]. The global infectious disease threat and its implications for the United States (NIE 99-17D) Web site: http://www.cia.gov/nic/graphics/infectiousdiseases.pdf. Accessed October 2003.
6. Defense Threat Reduction Agency. National Health Surveillance System Workshop summary report. 2000. Web site: http://www.dtra.mil/about/organization/ab_health.html. Accessed October 2003.
7. Centers for Disease Control and Prevention. [November 2003]. Bioterrorism agents/diseases. Web site: http://www.bt.cdc.gov/agent/agentlist-category.asp. Accessed November 2003.
8. World Organization for Animal Health [February 2003]. Classification of animal diseases. Web site: http://www.oie.int/eng/maladies/en_classification.htm. Accessed November 2003.
9. Jones BH, Amoroso PJ, Canham ML, et al. Atlas of injuries in the U.S. armed forces: conclusions and recommendations of

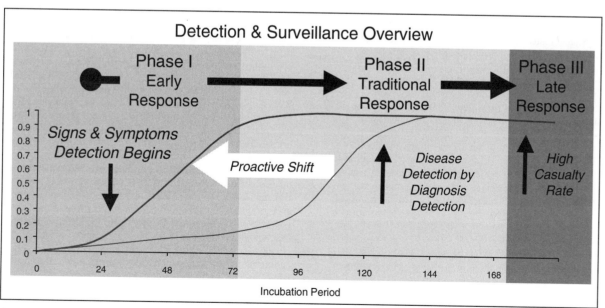

Figure 30–2. The graphic depiction of number of disease cases shows that early spread is usually not detected until the diagnosis is confirmed and large number of cases is affected in Phase II. Phase III outcomes are demonstrated by the SARS epidemic in China when in less than 60 days, the disease spread from Hong Kong to Beijing and the rest of the world before significant quarantine and preventive action was taken (34). For surveillance to be effective, the detection must be proactive and occur early in Phase I.

the DoD Injury Surveillance and Prevention Work Group. Mil Med Suppl 1999;164(8):1-633.

10. Campbell GL, Marfin AA, Lanciotti RS, et al. West Nile virus. Lancet Infect Dis 2002;2(9):519-29.

11. Paskin R. Food and Agriculture Organization of the United Nations [no date]. Manual on livestock disease surveillance and information systems. Web site: http://www.fao.org/WAICENT/FAOINFO/AGRICULT/AGA/AGAH/EMPRES/Info/other/surveill.htm. Accessed October 2003.

12. U.S. Army Medical Research Institute of Infectious Diseases. Medical management of biological casualties handbook. History of biological warfare and current threat. 4th ed. Fort Detrick, MD: 2001.

13. Getsch T, Cornell P. Microsoft Developer Network [July 2001]. Real-time data: frequently asked questions. Web site: http://msdn.microsoft.com/library/default.asp?url=/library/enus/dnexcl2k2/html/odc_xlrtdfaq.asp. Accessed November 2003.

14. Department of Health and Human Services Subcommittee on Labor, Health and Human Services and Education Committee on Appropriations [March 2001]. Statement of National Association of County and City Health Officials. Web site: http://www.naccho.org/advocacydoc298.cfm. Accessed November 2003.

15. Department of Health and Human Services. [February 2002]. National Committee on Vital and Health Statistics Proceedings. Web site: http://www.ncvhs.dhhs.gov/020226tr.htm. Accessed October 2003.

16. United States Department of Defense. Instruction, implementation and application of joint medical surveillance for deployments (DoD Instruction 6490.3). Washington, DC: 1997.

17. Department of Defense. Chairman, Joint Chiefs of Staff Memorandum (MCM 0006-02). Updated procedures for deployment health surveillance. Enclosure C: Weekly disease and non-battle injury report instructions. Washington, DC: 2002.

18. Murray CJL, King G, Lopez AD, et al. Armed conflict as a public health problem. BMJ 2002;324:346-9.

19. United States Army. Operational concept for combat health support (TRADOC Pamphlet 525-50). Fort Monroe, VA: United States Army Training and Doctrine Command, 1996.

20. United States House Armed Services Committee [January 2001]. Statement of: Lieutenant General Paul K. Carlton Air Force Surgeon General. Web site: http://www.house.gov/hasc/openingstatementsandpressreleases/107thcongress/01-07-13carlton.html. Accessed December 2003.

21. Whitlock WL. Using a PEM and a medical database in Operation Bright Star. Proceedings of the 7th Annual American Telemedicine Association; June 2-5, 2002, Los Angeles.

22. Centers for Disease Control and Prevention [no date]. An overview of the National Electronic Disease Surveillance System. Web site: http://www.cdc.gov/nedss/About/overview.html. Accessed October 2003.

23. Information Technology Standards [no date]. The International Organization for Standardization and the International Electrotechnical Commission. Web site: http://www.sc17.com. Accessed November 2003.

24. Department of Health and Human Services [March 2003]. US Food and Drug Administration FDA News: FDA proposes drug bar code regulation. Web site: http://www.fda.gov/oc/initiatives/barcode-sadr/fs-barcode.html. Accessed December 2003.

25. Association for Identification and Data Capture Technologies [no date]. Web site: http://www.aimi.org/technologies/. Accessed November 2003.

26. Department of Defense [April 2002]. Defense Advanced Research Projects Agency Fact File: A compendium of DARPA programs. Web site: http://www.darpa.mil/body/NewsItems/darpa_fact.html. Accessed November 2003.

27. Department of Defense Global Emerging Infections Systems. ESSENCE IV User Guide, 2003.

28. University of Pittsburgh Center for Biomedical Informatics: The Realtime Outbreak and Disease Surveillance Laboratory (RODS) Mission and Background [2003]. Web site: http://www.health.pitt.edu/rods/default.htm. Accessed October 2003.

29. National Library of Medicine [July 2003]. Unified medical language system. Web site: http://www.nlm.nih.gov/research/umls/Snomed/snomed_announcement.html. Accessed December 2003.

30. Systematized Nomenclature of Medicine [no date]. Clinical terms. Website: http://www.snomed.org. Accessed October 2003.

31. Whitlock W, Thompson GD, Bowman W. A medical knowledge coupler for deployed environments incorporating Systematized Nomenclature of Medicine Clinical Terms. September 14-16, 2003, San Diego.

32. Gribble, SD. Department of Computer Science and Engineering, The University of Washington [no date]. Robustness in complex systems Web site: http://www.cs.washington.edu/homes/gribble/papers/robust.pdf. Accessed December 2003.

33. Hopper M. Massachusetts Institute of Technology Comparative Media Studies [July 2001]. Wisdom from MIT's Athena: a paradigm for precognition. Web site: http://web.mit.edu/mehopper/www/listen.htm. Accessed December 2003.

34. Riley S, Fraser C, Donnelly CA, et al. [June 2003]. Transmission dynamics of the etiological agent of SARS in Hong Kong: impact of public health intervention. Science 1961-66;300 (5627). Web site: http://www.sciencemag.org/cgi/content/full/300/5627/1961.

SUGGESTED READINGS

1. Barthell EN, Cordell WH, Moorhead JC, et al. The frontlines of medicine project: a proposal for the standardized communication of emergency department data for public health uses including syndromic surveillance for biological and chemical terrorism. Ann Emerg Med 2002;39(4);422-9.

2. Bioterrorism preparedness and response: use of information technologies and decision support systems. Summary, Evidence Report/Technology Assessment 59, July 2002. Agency for Healthcare Research and Quality, Rockville, MD. Web site: http://www.ahrq.gov/clinic/epcsums/bioitsum.htm.

3. Centers for Disease Control and Prevention. Draft framework for evaluating syndromic surveillance systems for bioterrorism preparedness. Web site: http://www.cdc.gov/epo/dphsi/syndromic/framework.htm. Accessed October 2003.

4. Duchin JS. Epidemiological response to syndromic surveillance signals. J Urban Health 2003;80(3)Suppl 1:i115-6.

5. Emanuel PA, Calvin C, Kerr L, et al. Validating the performance of biological detection equipment: the role of the federal government. Biosecurity Bioterrorism: Biodefense Strategy, Practice, Sci 2003;1(2):131-7.

6. Hutwagner L, Thompson W, Seeman GM, et al. The bioterrorism preparedness and response early aberration reporting systems (EARS). J Urban Health 2003;80(3)Suppl 1:i89-i96.

7. Lober WB, Trigg LJ, Karras BT, et al. Syndromic surveillance using automated collection of computerized discharge diagnoses. J Urban Health 2003;80(3)Suppl 1:i97-i106.

8. Lombardo J, Burkom H, Elbert E, et al. A systems overview of the electronic surveillance system for the early notification of community-based epidemics (ESSENCE II). J Urban Health 2003;80(3)Suppl 1:i32-i42.

9. Morrissey J. A defining moment. Mod Healthcare 2003;30-2.
10. Pavlin JA. Investigation of disease outbreaks detected by "syndromic" surveillance systems. J Urban Health 2003;80(3)Suppl 1:i107-14.
11. Pavlin JA, Mostashari F, Kortpeter MG, et al. Innovative surveillance methods for rapid detection of disease outbreaks and bioterrorism: results of an interagency workshop of health indication surveillance. Am J Public Health 2003 9(8):1230-5.
12. Peters KI. Pattern recognition. Government Executive [serial online]. Web site: http://www.govexec.com/features/0903/0903s2.htm. Accessed November 2003.
13. Platt R, Bocchino C, Caldwell B, et al. Syndromic surveillance using the minimum transfer of identifiable data: the example of the national bioterrorism surveillance demonstration program. J Urban Health 2003; 80(3)Suppl 1:i25-i31.
14. Riengold A. If syndromic surveillance is the answer, what is the question? Biosecurity and Bioterrorism: Biodefense Strategy, Practice, Sci 2003;1(2):77-81.
15. Strang N, Cucherat M, Boissel JP. Which coding system for therapeutic information in evidence-based medicine. Comput Methods Programs Biomed 2002;68(1):73-85.
16. Tsui FC, Wagner MM, Dato V, et al. Value of ICD-9-coded chief complaints for detection of epidemics. J Am Med Inform Assoc 2002;9:41-7.

Communications Preparedness for Terrorism

31

Health Care Facilities and Interagency Communication During Terrorism

Raymond L. Fowler, Peter Moyer, Crawford Mechem, and Paul Moore

INTRODUCTION

A terrorist event threatening life and property is perhaps one of the most dreaded incidents that can befall a civilian population. Preparedness is vital to the protection of the citizens of a population to mitigate the potentially adverse consequences of such an action. This chapter of *The Medical Response to Terrorism* will set out the breadth of the need for interagency communication in preparation for and during terrorist events. By necessity, this discussion must be abbreviated, since a comprehensive discussion of all relevant areas of interagency communication would comprise several volumes of text. However, this chapter will lay a foundation in which a comprehensive plan can be constructed.

Communication allows people to work together on a common task. It is the process whereby individuals and organizations figure out their roles and how they interface with others to carry out the task at hand. Disasters place particular demands on interagency communication. In fact, communication is often sited as the major problem in multiple agency/multiple jurisdiction disaster response. Communication during a disaster provides for the assessment and determination of several key aspects vital to interagency management (Table 31-1).

No aspect of preparedness calls for greater attention to detail than the ability of the various agencies involved in the

management of terrorist events than to be able to communicate effectively. The reasons for effective communication are legion. Citizens must be able to call for help. Dispatch agencies must have the capability to immediately send appropriate responding personnel, vehicles, and equipment to areas of concern. Responding personnel need the ability to update the agency's dispatch center and leadership regarding the nature of the problem and the potential or actual need to expand the scope of the response. In addition, they must be able to convey their assessments of hazards that may represent terrorist activities and then to pass this on to other community response organizations, such as hospitals; public safety, public works, public health, and emergency management agencies; and the military. Public safety agencies, in turn, require a broad set of communications abilities to keep the scene as safe as possible for both responders and citizens.

PREPAREDNESS ESSENTIALS: BASIC FEATURES

To best assist community planners responsible for optimizing available community resources, this chapter will lay out the basic communication requirements for each agency called upon to respond to a terrorist event. The design, implementation, monitoring, and periodic redesign of equipment, policies, protocols, and personnel will flow from these basic requirements and provide emergency response

TABLE 31-1	Interagency Communication: Key Areas During a Disaster

- An ongoing assessment of what the disaster situation is, including an assessment of potential danger to responders
- An ongoing assessment of what resources are necessary to respond to the disaster, what resources are immediately available, and how and when others can be obtained
- A determination of the priority of needed resources
- A determination of what individuals and organizations will be responsible for and the different response measures

Source: Aufderheide, E. Disaster response principles of preparation and coordination. Mosby; 1989. Chapter 5, p. 3.

organizations with a foundation upon which to expand. The design of a communication plan for mitigation of a terrorist event must have a number of basic features (Table 31-2).

Any given terrorist event will place specific populations at risk in a given geographic area, the mitigation of which may require *multimethod functionality*, which is the response and cooperation of multiple agencies. Thus, multimethod functionality of any municipal communication system is vital. The communication system developed by a municipal area should be flexible, integrating the information pathways of many different agencies, though each may have its own communication network. Public safety matters must be dealt with. People may be injured, requiring field triage, management, and transport. Hospital facilities must be put on notice, including the communication of an accurate rapid assessment of their capabilities and current load factors to appropriate agencies. The local, state, and/or federal emergency management agencies may require notice. A need for public works (water, power, sewer, road maintenance, etc.) to be placed on alert may also arise. Thus, appropriate community planning for terrorist events must, of necessity, provide for communications media that blend on a moment-to-moment basis a poly-agency network of providers from all areas of community response.

Inclusion is a basic feature of interagency communication. It is vital that all appropriate agencies be included in the communications network. Community planners must enumerate the facilities available for response to events that could affect their areas. Such planning requires the collective imagination of the members of all planning groups responsible for emergency preparedness. Entities at risk, such

TABLE 31-2	Interagency Communication: Basic Features

- Response and cooperation of multiple agencies (multimethod functionality)
- Inclusion of all agencies involved in event mitigation
- Hardening
- Simplicity
- Continuous functionality

as public gathering areas, mass transit, and public works facilities, require identification and assessment of their unique vulnerabilities. Extrapolation of communication needs from potential hazards, merged with current and anticipated modes of information sharing that must take place during events, will reveal an appropriate functionality of community response to the planners.

Many jurisdictions have studied these areas extensively. The governor of Oregon in 1972, for example, established the Oregon Emergency Response System (OERS). It was designed to manage the resources of the state during various emergencies, including "natural and technological . . . and civil unrest." Its program includes a prospective, multijurisdictional series of agreements between local, regional, and state levels, as well as with the private sector. OERS established a "primary point of contact" through which any responding entity would provide the state appropriate contact information and an assessment of the emergency event, including requests that must be forwarded to the state or federal government (1). OERS allows for a constant "state of readiness" of the state communications network, including routine testing and monitoring of available equipment and systems. This is an excellent example of a state-led effort to examine the needs of the citizenry within that governmental limit and provide a network of communications through prospective planning. However, appropriate limitations are highlighted in the Oregon Quick Response Report #149, which found that only 39% of representatives of responding agencies would be notified of the establishment and activation of an Emergency Communications Center (2). Clearly this state plan, at the time of that publication, had more work to do in developing an adequate notification system that would notify the appropriate agencies of a potential event. An important take-home message to community, regional, and state planners is the need for continuous monitoring of the readiness of on-call personnel. Communications systems must be *hardened* to withstand the impact of terrorist events. It is within the realm of imagination that attempts to injure a population might target the various communications agencies serving that population. The 911 call-taking centers and dispatch facilities must be reasonably prepared to withstand adverse events, including possible physical attacks. Precedent exists for such efforts. For example, the San Ramon Valley Fire Protection District in California has provided for the site hardening of one of its stations and its administration building, which is equipped with food, water, and emergency power so that it may serve as a principle emergency operations center for the municipalities that it serves. Thus, it may be strongly suggested both by reason and by precedent that adequate community protection includes an awareness of potential damage or destruction of central call-taking and dispatching agencies and the prudent securing of these facilities. In addition to hardening of the central call-taking and dispatching areas, redundant systems must be available to assume some or all of these responsibilities, should the central facility be damaged.

One potential method for technologically hardening a municipality's central facility is to arrange for neighboring agencies to share communication responsibilities should the given municipality's system be damaged. Another hardening possibility is the utilization of the Radio Amateur Civil Emergency Service, or RACES, under a standing protocol from the fire chief or other authorized agent of the community. RACES could be used to contact a neighboring fire department or appropriate emergency management agency, to activate mutual aid, alert surrounding hospital facilities, and/or contact the vertical governmental structure, including notifying the state or federal governments for military assistance. Thus, limitations of community budgets need not place undue constraints on the capacity of an area or region to maintain hardened communications abilities, thus providing continual multiagency connection during the evolution of a hostile event against a community.

The value of *simplicity* in design and coordination of multiagency communication cannot be overemphasized. In the second section of this chapter, significant emphasis is placed on the potential for adverse outcomes when interagency communication is not part of community planning. Indeed, substantial information may be available to one agency that may affect the welfare of other responders, but without adequate planning for communication of that information, needless harm may fall to others responding to the event. Thus, it is stressed herein that barriers to interagency communication must be broken down at the drawing board. Egos must be sacrificed to the greater good of the citizens and the responders. The breadth of the commitment of public and private facilities appointed to plan for the common protection of citizens and responders must be a uniform agreement to bypass unnecessary interagency conflicts.

Emergency response systems have a common element, namely the requirement that these hardened systems have *continuous functionality*, defined as being available 24 hours a day, 7 days a week. EMS and fire agencies, as well as public safety entities, have maintained such accessibility to the public since their early days. This allows these groups to respond to emergencies with the appropriate resources in prompt order. Indeed, responders have arrived at the scene of explosions and bombings so rapidly that significant numbers of fatalities have occurred in the ranks of the responders themselves due to secondary explosive devices specifically targeted against them and timed to detonate just as they were staging or initiating patient triage.

These basic features are essential to interagency communications and can be demonstrated in many ways. Public health agencies must be included in the community planning for terrorist incidents such as biohazard releases. Public health agencies, for example, have significant control over the availability of vaccine supplies. If these supplies cannot be made available promptly to initiate widespread community immunization in accordance with community-wide plans, it could be reasonably predicted that the number of casualties might be greater; therefore, including public health agencies early in interagency planning is essential.

Interagency planning for community response to an epidemic of an especially deadly agent such as smallpox or perhaps the agent causing the Severe Acute Respiratory Syndrome (SARS) virus requires careful attention by community planners. For example, should the index case in the setting of a smallpox outbreak occur in an apartment complex, it may be necessary to exercise authority that limits the freedom of individuals, who either are already becoming ill or who have been exposed. The term "isolation" applies to the removal from public contact of those who are already ill, whereas the term "quarantine" applies to the removal from public contact of an individual who has been exposed, but is

not yet ill. Preparation for either of these restraints on personal freedom requires a broad community agreement and prior education of the citizens as to what actions must be taken by agency officials in the event of such an outbreak.

To provide sufficient powers to allow for the isolation or quarantine of appropriate individuals, the United States Code Section 264, which is found in Section 361 of the Public Health Service Act, provides the Secretary of Health and Human Services with the duty to stop "the introduction, transmission, and spread of communicable diseases from foreign countries into the United States and within the United States and its territories/possessions" (3). This law comes under the aegis of regulations found in the 42 CFR Parts 70 and 71. Under its delegated authority, "the CDC is empowered to detain, medically examine, or conditionally release individuals suspected of carrying a communicable disease." This regulation further states that "in the event a passenger infected with SARS were to arrive in the United States on board an international flight, the Executive Order provides HHS with clear legal authority to detain or isolate the non-compliant passenger and prevent the passenger from infecting others. This authority would only be used if someone posed a threat to public health and refused to cooperate with a voluntary request" (3). To provide such detainment, isolation, or quarantine in real time, a carefully thought-out community plan of cooperation between hospitals, public health officers, and public safety personnel is necessary. For example, if an index case were found to have exposed a significant number of persons at a sporting event, then the tracking and isolation of persons at risk of becoming ill, as well as exposing additional persons, would truly present a substantial problem for any community. Sufficient planning requires the collective cooperation and imaginations of community agencies. It is useful to comment at this point that the use of quarantine in the United States is a power that has been used rarely. Indeed, again from the CDC, "The last litigated case involving the involuntary quarantine of a passenger arriving into the United States occurred in 1963 and involved a suspect case of smallpox. On the other hand, CDC routinely temporarily detains incoming planes and interviews passengers for health reasons. For example, CDC temporarily detained an incoming plane and interviewed passengers in Seattle in December 2001 to verify that a report of smallpox aboard the flight was in fact a hoax" (3).

PREPAREDNESS ESSENTIALS: SYNDROMIC SURVEILLANCE

The medical response to terrorism involves gathering information from a wide variety of health care providers and facilities in a timely fashion. The earliest possible warning to a community at risk of a terrorist event is essential. Public service agencies in communities regularly receive vital data that, when submitted to analysis, can reveal patterns in the "background noise" of day-to-day life which might otherwise be undetected. In application to public health, this is referred to as *syndromic surveillance*, or the ability to detect diseases demonstrating a risk to the public health through patterns of illness recognition in a given area. Syndromic surveillance is not a new process. It has been used for generations by public health officers to determine if communities are at risk through incidences of disease cases being reported. It is possible to use automated computer-aided techniques to filter through incoming information to public service agencies, such as 911 dispatch centers. However, the practices of physicians and community support services is now amplified by using computers to analyze cases reported to many 911 agencies or presenting to many emergency departments across the United States, indeed providing automated syndromic surveillance of these reports. The reports produced by such enhancements to the information systems of these agencies can provide for immediate data linking to area epidemiologists on an automated basis, with this data automatically falling within federal information-sharing guidelines. Information that can be sent includes patient demographics, the type of clinical problem, and the findings from specific clinical data points, focused by the patients' postal codes. However, again according to the CDC, "syndromic surveillance will be affected by the selection of data sources, timeliness of information management, definition of syndrome categories, selection of statistical detection thresholds, availability of resources for follow-up, recent experience with false alarms, and criteria for initiating investigations" (4). Finally, recent work with computerized Emergency Medical Services (EMS) medical record creation has indicated that the field computers can instantly update the central data server regarding the chief complaints of patients presenting in the field. Thus, even the medical record data server can serve a useful role in the gathering of data useful in syndromic surveillance.

Community syndromic surveillance may also reveal unexpected results, such as Edwards, Stout, and Overton found when monitoring the 911 dispatch using electronic syndromic surveillance from the 911 Computer-Aided Dispatch during a recent marathon through Richmond. Many cases of "acute shortness of breath," were identified by the software, and the trend was noted exactly along the route of the race (5).

PREPAREDNESS ESSENTIALS

INTERPERSONAL COMMUNICATION

As important as the technologic challenges with communication are, the human factors of *interpersonal communication* may be more important. This section addresses the importance of the people aspects of communication, general areas that demonstrate problems in disaster-related communication, and suggested solutions (Table 31-3).

TABLE 31-3	Interpersonal Communication: Focus Areas

- Autonomous behavior
- Inadequate command and control authority delineation
- Inadequate fixed and mobile command and control structures
- Agency-specific jargon or radio transmission codes

Organizations that typically act on their own often fail to change their approach when multiple organizations are involved. Such organizations give priority to their internal information needs rather than the overall response effort. This *autonomous behavior* is exaggerated by interagency territorialism and rivalry.

Preincident planning is key to effective communication during a disaster. Individual organizational roles and how they "interdigitate" with other organizations' roles are spelled out in advance. These roles are formalized in statutes and charters. They are operationalized through standard operating procedures and are meshed under a jurisdiction's Comprehensive Emergency Management Plan (CEMP). A CEMP ensures that an appropriate agency is assigned responsibility for every important function in the plan and defines the roles and responsibilities of each agency under different scenarios.

Joint training across agencies and jurisdictions is necessary to understand organizations' respective roles and how they interface with one another. An example played out in many communities is the decontamination of chemically contaminated patients. Is there a role for EMS (such as triage and administration of antidotes) in the warm zone? Assuming that some, if not the majority of, patients will arrive at the hospital having bypassed the fire department and EMS in the field, how will decontamination be carried out at the hospital?

Plans and training are tested in multiagency, multijurisdictional exercises. On a local level, exercises test relationships between different agencies and neighboring jurisdictions. They must also look at the interface of local agencies with regional, state, and federal resources. Open, honest "after action evaluations" postdrills and actual disasters are often difficult for agencies to participate in but are absolutely necessary if plans are to adapt, change, and improve. At times such critiques may need the help of outside facilitation.

Formal organizational roles need buy-in and stewardship from agency leaders and secondary leaders as well as the rank and file. Local political leadership must understand the community's disaster response plan and play an active part in clarifying roles and resolving disputes.

Cross-agency planning, training, and drilling build awareness of others' roles, how they operate, and what their needs are. They build familiarity—both individual and organizational. They build trust in individual and organizational competences and reliability. Finally, they build mutual respect for other organizations' contributions.

In many communities, local emergency management plays the vital role of coordinating disaster response both in the preincident phase and during the disaster itself. A major part of that coordination is communication.

Inadequate command and control authority delineation is a common and serious limitation to effective communication and scene management. California fire services created the Incident Command System (ICS) in the 1960s to enable mutual-aid fire companies to work together more effectively after a series of urban/wildland interface fires in Los Angeles. ICS has since been adopted by public safety agencies and other organizations nationally. Under ICS, a lead agency is determined. Fire is the lead agency at fires, hazardous materials, and building collapses; public health is the lead agency during infectious disease outbreaks, law enforcement is the lead agency at crime scenes, and so on. The lead agency provides the incident commander (IC) who works collaboratively in a unified command structure consisting of senior representatives from each of the responding agencies.

Establishing and maintaining this collaboration is easier said than done. Organizational representatives have to join forces. The nature of an incident, as well as changes in that nature over time, creates questions as to who is in charge at what time. Additionally, how collaborative is the incident commander—is it really unified command?

Inadequate fixed and mobile command and control structures often leads to poor communication and a potentially negative impact on incident management. A fundamental requirement for interagency communication is proximity of different agencies' leadership to share information on an ongoing basis and together plan a response during disasters. At the incident, this is called the command post. Off-site this is termed the emergency operations center (EOC). The command post coordinates incident operations. The EOC looks at the larger picture, providing support for the incident while coordinating with other local assets and regional and federal resources. While part of the composition of command posts and EOCs is technologic, an equally important part is human. Agencies must agree to send senior, decision-making representatives to meet and work together.

Agency-specific jargon or radio transmission codes can be a limitation to effective incident management. Terminology and procedures used to communicate vary among different organizations. Many police, fire, and ambulance services use radio codes for communication. These codes may vary from agency to agency making interagency communication difficult. To enhance interagency communication, many agencies are abandoning codes in favor of plain English ("clear text" or "clear speech"). Agencies sharing radio frequencies must avoid "stepping" on one another and congesting radio traffic. Interagency command channels must be established. Incident frequencies must be agreed upon. Backup means of communication need to be in place. Alternative means of communicating such as mobile data terminals help reduce radio traffic during disasters.

HOSPITAL CONSIDERATIONS IN INTERAGENCY COMMUNICATION

The vital role that hospitals play in community emergency preparedness has been receiving increased attention in recent years (6). Experience gained from the Oklahoma City bombing, the Tokyo subway sarin attack, and the 2001 attack on the World Trade Center indicates that in the event of a large-scale terrorist incident, many, if not the majority, of casualties may arrive at local hospitals by means other than EMS. Because local fire, EMS, and law enforcement personnel may be too occupied with the incident to come to their aid, hospitals should be prepared to draw on their own resources to mount an effective response (7). Hospital personnel may have to decontaminate large numbers of patients if indicated, perform rapid triage and patient care, maintain adequate supplies of pharmaceuticals and equipment, track patients, preserve the confidentiality of patient information, address security issues, and interface with the media, while also handling the normal

patient load unrelated to the immediate incident. Despite this increased emphasis placed on hospital self-reliance, when faced with a local, regional, or national terrorist incident, hospitals will have to maintain effective lines of communication with other hospitals as well as local, state, and federal agencies (8). There are many reasons for this. If one hospital is being overwhelmed with patients, or if the hospital itself has been the target of a terrorist attack, it may be necessary to transfer patients, staff, or supplies from one hospital to another. For this to occur, a large number of ambulances or other means of transportation would be required. Both facilities would have to track patients and supplies carefully. Credentialing medical personnel sent to work in the other hospital would have to be addressed. Finally, how to pay for the operation must be determined. This process would be easier if such transfers were made between member hospitals of a larger health system. However, regardless of the scenario, a reliable communications system to maintain the flow of information would be critical. Rather than attempting to solve communications problems in the heat of the crisis, such issues must be addressed in advance through careful planning.

In the event of a terrorist incident, hospitals may need to communicate with the local agency leading the response to the crisis. This may be a fire or law enforcement agency or may be the municipal government. In many cases, a local or regional EOC may be activated and staffed by personnel from all responding agencies. If this is the case, hospitals must be able to communicate with the EOC to determine the status of the crisis and what may be expected of them.

Hospitals must be able to communicate with the local EMS system, relaying such important information as their availability of beds and other resources and how many patients of varying levels of acuity their inpatients services and emergency departments can handle, including both isolation and intensive care unit beds that may be available. This is also true of hospitals with specialized capabilities, such as burn centers, trauma centers, pediatric hospitals, or those with toxicology services. Such information will allow the EMS system to distribute the patients they are transporting in such a way that no one hospital receives an inordinate proportion of the patients and those patients with specialized needs are transferred to the most appropriate facility. In addition, medical command hospitals that provide online medical command to ambulance services must still be able to perform that function throughout the course of the incident. Depending on the nature of the incident, there may be an increased need to treat and release patients at the scene or to deviate in some way from the ambulance service's standard operating procedures. Input from medical command physicians may be crucial in these cases.

In communities where EMS and fire suppression are performed by separate agencies, hospitals may have to communicate with local fire personnel for actual fire suppression in the facility or for guidance with the management of patients exposed to potentially hazardous agents, such as nerve agents or vesicants. Such information may also be obtained from local or regional poison control centers.

Hospitals responding to terrorist incidents involving a biological agent would have very different communications needs. The time frame of the response would be over a matter of days or weeks, rather than minutes or hours. Hospitals would have to be able to communicate with local public health officials regarding appropriate patient care and the need for mass vaccination of employees or the public. At the same time, the hospitals could convey the numbers of patients their emergency departments are seeing as well as their presenting symptoms and presumptive diagnoses. This would help public health agencies to identify the sentinel case or cases and, through ongoing surveillance, monitor the progression of the disease outbreak (9,10). The development of a Web-based regional surveillance system would be one way to facilitate information transfer. For such a system to be effective, multiple hospitals would have to be involved. Issues of compliance with Health Insurance Portability and Accountability Act, the location of the data warehouse, who would analyze the data, and funding would have to be addressed. Designating the local public health department as the lead agency in such an endeavor may help to resolve some of these issues (11). While the likelihood of a systemic communication failure would be small in this scenario, an effective way to convey a large amount of clinical data from hospitals to public health officials in as close to real time as possible would have to be developed. The confidentiality of patient information must be guaranteed. Finally, the impact of this system on day-to-day hospital operations would have to be minimized.

In the course of the response to a terrorist incident, hospitals may rapidly deplete their available supplies, including pharmaceuticals. Rather than maintaining large inventories of pharmaceuticals and other needed material on-site, in recent years hospitals have moved to the practice of stocking smaller inventories that are replenished every few days from contracted companies. If these supplies are exhausted, hospitals would need a reliable means of communicating with local vendors to replenish their stock rapidly. If the traditional means of communication between hospital and vendor were disrupted, a backup system would have to be used to ensure that needed supplies are delivered.

An ongoing dialogue between hospitals and the media may be necessary during the course of the response to a terrorist incident. If casualties arrive at a hospital, the media would not be far behind with inquiries about the number of patients and their medical condition. Hospital administration must have a means of conveying a clear and consistent message to the media, and thereby to the public. This could also be a good time for medical personnel to educate the public on the nature of the threat and the steps that can be taken to mitigate the threat. Finally, any hospital, receiving patients from a terrorist incident should be prepared for ongoing interaction with local, state, or federal law enforcement agencies. The Federal Bureau of Investigation (FBI) is the law enforcement agency with the ultimate responsibility for responding to a terrorist incident. However, local and state law enforcement agencies would be invariably involved as well. In the event of disruption of the usual means of communications, hospitals must have alternative means of communicating with these agencies.

The need for hospitals to have reliable communications during a response to a terrorist incident is apparent. Hospitals have responded to this need in a variety of ways over the past few years. A recent survey of thirty emergency department directors and nurse managers reported that all of their facilities had developed communication systems based on

telephone lines or radios for use in disasters. All of these individuals, in addition, had call-out systems using telephone call lists or paging systems (12).

PREPAREDNESS HISTORIC EVENTS AND CASE HISTORIES

The September 11, 2001, terrorist attack on the World Trade Center uncovered major problems with the "people" aspect of interagency communication during disasters in New York City. Partly because of preincident planning, training and drilling, the Washington area's interagency communication during the response to the terrorist attack on the Pentagon was overall successful.

Minutes after the South Tower collapsed at the World Trade Center, police helicopters hovered near the remaining tower to check on its condition. "About 15 floors down from the top, it looks like it's glowing red," the pilot of one helicopter, Aviation 14, radioed at 10:07 A.M. "It's inevitable." Seconds later another pilot reported: "I don't think this has too much longer to go. I would evacuate all people within the area of that second building."

Those clear warnings, captured on police radio tapes, were transmitted 21 minutes before the building fell, and officials say they were relayed to police officers, most of whom managed to escape. Yet most firefighters never heard those warnings, or earlier warnings, to get out. Their radio systems failed frequently that morning. Even if the network had been reliable, it was not linked to the police system. The police and fire commanders guiding the rescue effort did not talk to one another during the crisis. Cut off from critical information, at least 121 firefighters, most in striking distance of safety, died when the North Tower fell (13).

Long-standing interagency turf battles between the New York City Police Department (NYPD) and the New York City Fire Department (FDNY) and between the commissioners heading NYPD and New York City's Office of Emergency Management (OEM—the local agency charged with coordinating disaster response) made the lack of communication seen at the World Trade Center predictable (14). In retrospect, New York City had held only one interagency disaster drill in the 18 months leading up to the September 11 attack, and that was a table top exercise, not a field one (14).

No common command post was established (15), and no senior NYPD representative was sent to the FDNY incident command post. The failure of the NYPD surveillance helicopter to warn FDNY of the North Tower's imminent collapse would have been avoided were the helicopter to have had on board an FDNY representative. On paper, that had been the formal agreement since 1993. No common radio frequency was shared between the agencies (15). OEM Commissioner Hauer had devised an 800-MHz radio system for interagency communication, but no agreement to use the system had been reached. On 9/11 the previously distributed radios sat idle.

The McKinsey after action report on the World Trade Center noted the following additional NYPD communication weaknesses: aviation units, intelligence, and detectives responded quickly but were not well coordinated; there was minimal intelligence sharing between local and federal agencies; there was a lack of incident reporting and documentation; no clearinghouse for distilling, correcting, and disseminating accurate information to responders was set up; regular briefings did not occur throughout the event; and there was little command or disaster response training for NYPD leaders after Captain school (16).

The McKinsey critique describes congestion on EMS radio frequencies and EMS dispatchers who were too overwhelmed to be able to synthesize information and disseminate it effectively. A message from a distraught caller on the 105 floor of the South tower said at 9:37 A.M. that the "90th something" floor had collapsed. Although the message got through to police, it never made it to fire before the South Tower collapsed at 9:59.15 A.M.

As events unfolded in New York City, another aircraft took aim at the Pentagon, located in Arlington County, Virginia. The Arlington County Fire Department witnessed the impact and notified the Arlington Emergency Communications Center (ECC). The ECC in turn invoked the Greater Metropolitan Washington Area Police and Fire/Rescue Services Mutual Aid Plan (COG Mutual Aid Plan) and the Northern Virginia Mutual Aid (NOVA) agreement and contacted surrounding jurisdictions to request mutual aid. More than 50 agencies responded (17).

Interoperability planning in Metropolitan Washington, D.C., began with the crash of Air Florida in January 1982 (18). This planning resulted in "interagency operational agreements that allowed responders from one jurisdiction to operate on the other area public safety radio systems" (18). By the mid-1990s, these agreements had been incorporated into the Northern Virginia Truncated Mutual Aid Agreement (NVTMA), which resulted in the majority of northern Virginia agencies using compatible 800 MHz trunking technologies" (18). Because of existing mutual-aid agreements, the majority of the first responders to the Pentagon had Arlington County's radio frequencies preprogrammed into their portable radio equipment. They were able to switch to the designated frequency and communicate directly with the Arlington County dispatchers and the on-scene incident commander (18).

The COG Mutual Aid Plan and the NOVA agreement addressed more than compatibility of radio frequencies. They also described procedures for requesting assistance and, via the ICS, accountability for issuing and obeying orders. COG and NOVA called for the elimination of signals and codes in favor of clear text messages (17). The NVTMA established talk groups, common standard operating procedures for radio operators, and protocols for directing out-of-jurisdiction units (17).

"Finally it is difficult to overstate the value of personal relationships formed and nurtured among key players long before the Pentagon attack. Chief Plaugher served in the Fairfax County Fire and Rescue Department for 24 years before moving to Arlington. Chief Tom Hawkins of Alexandria spent 15 years with Arlington County. Chief Brown of Loudin County is a Fairfax alumnus. One of Special Agent Combs' jobs with the FBI NCRS was to establish and maintain close working relationships with the regional fire and rescue departments. His relationship with Chief Schwartz was well established before September 11. The list of beneficial personal relationships extended throughout the ranks. Firefighters from neighboring jurisdictions had often worked and trained together, which built valuable trust and confidence" (19).

There were, of course, problems with the Pentagon response as well. As the number of state and federal agencies at the Pentagon increased, interoperability presented new challenges. No means of direct interoperability was available to those secondary responders (19). Ambient noise made it hard to talk on the radio. Earpieces might have diminished that noise. In the first few hours, cellular phones did not work well. Public Safety cellular priority service was not in place. Nextel telephones with two-way radio capability were somewhat more reliable. Bullhorns were used for evacuation instructions. At times foot messengers were the most reliable form of communication. Pagers seemed to be the most reliable means of personnel recall, but most firefighters didn't have pagers (19).

Many surviving victims reported to the Pentagon's DiLorenzo Tricare Health Clinic (DTHC), located away from the west side of the building, which is the side that had been struck. The DTHC did not transmit patient disposition information to the EMS Control. Triage, treatment, and transport activities at the DTHC were not coordinated with EMS Control (19). No designated clearinghouse hospital was identified. Thus, communication around patient treatment and disposition between EMS Control at the incident site and area hospitals was deficient (19). Arlington County EMS units are not equipped with mobile data terminals. This technology would have allowed better communication with EMS Control without congesting radio traffic (19).

Arlington County does not have a facility specifically designed and equipped to support the emergency management functions specified in the CEMP. The conference room currently used as the EOC does not have adequate space and is not configured or properly equipped for that role. The ACFD does not have a mobile command vehicle. During the Pentagon attack it had to rely on vehicles belonging to other agencies (19).

PREPAREDNESS CHECKLIST TABLE AND SUMMARY

The breadth of the advance of civilization is submitted significantly to review in outline format by the community services that define and support its citizens. Preparation for the mitigation of deadly events that may be plotted against the people mandates comprehensive research and the laying of groundwork, which can guarantee the most optimal outcome from whatever maladies may be cast upon the citizens and their property. Equal to any other aspect of planning is the need to define carefully the areas of interagency communication that will allow for the exchange of data and support, providing therein the assurance that all of the efforts of rescuers, public safety officers, medical providers, support services, and the rest of those who participate in community reinforcement can be measured to the mission as best as possible given the available community resources.

Thus, herein presented were found some of the successes and failures of communication from the efforts of diverse communities across the country during terrorist events that have befallen the country. Also, the framework requiring attention by those who plan communication techniques on the behalf of communities has been provided; this outline for action will hopefully allow the user to see a bit more clearly into the needs of the future.

Above all, it is vital that all players be brought to the deliberation table, with appropriate guidance and authorization being applied by clear-minded leaders who examine the experiences and information available to date, borne upon the beneficent stanchion of public and private funding. Only through the thoughtful inclusion of all community cast members whose duty it is to protect the public welfare can the necessary resources be brought to bear and most accurately applied during the tragic drama of distress.

RESOURCES

1. Medtronics "Medusa" EMS Medical Record Software, released 2004, provides for syndromic surveillance through a central data collection server which is maintained in real time. Web site: www.medtronics.com.

2. Einolf, D. HAZWOPER incident command: A manual for emergency responders. Government Institutes Publisher; 1998.

3. American Medical Association Advanced, Basic, and Core Disaster Life Support Courses.

4. Centers for Disease Control and Prevention, Emergency Preparedness and Response. Web site: http://www.bt.cdc.gov/.

5. Radio Amateur Civil Emergency Service (RACES). Web site: www.races.net.

REFERENCES

1. Oregon Emergency Management web site. Available at: http://www.osp.state.or.us/oem/index.html. Accessed on January 2002.
2. Parker R, et al. Oregon Emergency Management: evaluating interagency communication in the post-disaster environment. Quick Response Report #149. Eugene, Oregon: Community Service Center; 2002
3. The Centers for Disease Control web site. Severe acute respiratory syndrome: questions and answers on executive order and interim final rule. Accessed October 2003.
4. Buehler JW, Berkelman RL, Hartley DM, Peters CJ. Syndromic surveillance and bioterrorism-related epidemics. Available at: CDC web site section on Syndromic Surveillance.
5. Edwards DP, Stout T, Overton J. Using EMS CAD data, statistical methods & GIS mapping to create a bio-surveillance alert system for an urban U.S. population. National Association of EMS Physicians Annual Meeting Research Abstracts; 2003.
6. Waeckerle JF. Domestic preparedness for events involving weapons of mass destruction. JAMA 2000; 283: 252-4.
7. Bradley RN. Health care facility preparation for weapons of mass destruction. Prehosp Emerg Care 2000 Jul-Sep;4(3): 261–9.
8. Centers for Disease Control. Biological and chemical terrorism: strategic plan for preparedness and response. Recommendations of the CDC Strategic Planning Workgroup. MMWR Recomm Rep. 2000 Apr 21;49:1-14.
9. Flowers LK, Mothershead JL, Blackwell TH. Bioterrorism preparedness. II: the community and emergency medical services systems. Emerg Med Clin N Am 2002 May;20(2): 457-76.
10. Pavlin JA. Investigation of disease outbreaks detected by "syndromic" surveillance systems. J Urban Health 2003 Jun;80[2 Suppl 1]:i107-14.
11. Irvin CB, Nouhan PP, Rice K. Syndromic analysis of computerized emergency department patients' chief complaints: An opportunity for bioterrorism and influenza surveillance. Ann Emerg Med 2003; 41: 447-52.
12. Treat KN, Williams JM, Furbee PM, et al. Hospital preparedness for weapons of mass destruction incidents: an initial assessment. Ann Emerg Med 2001 Nov;38(5):562-5.
13. *New York Times,* Jul 7, 2002.
14. *New York Times,* Sep 9, 2002.
15. *New York Times,* Jul 7, 2002.
16. McKinsey and Company. Improving NYPD emergency preparedness and response. pp. 28, 29.
17. Lund, DA. Learning to talk, the lessons of non-interoperability in public safety systems. Justice Works, University of New Hampshire; April 2002. p.15.
18. Answering the call: communications lessons learned from the Pentagon attack. Public Safety Wireless Network; Jan 2002.
20. Arlington County after action report on the response to the September 11 terrorist attack on the Pentagon. p. A31.

32

Media and Communications Preparedness For Terrorist Events

Raymond L. Fowler, Paul E. Pepe, and Paul E. Moore

INTRODUCTION

The end of the Cold War and the breaking down of the Berlin Wall ushered into the last decade of the last millennium a brief sense of calm, creating a pervading feeling in many that, indeed, perhaps peace was a delicate organism that could indeed take root in the newly tilled spiritual soil of nations around the world. Yet, within a few short years, terrorist actions burst abundantly on a stunned world, from the initial attempts to destroy the New York World Trade Center in 1993, to the nerve gas attacks in Tokyo, to the destruction of the Murrah Building in Oklahoma City, to name but a few incidents.

These events have continued to escalate, as exemplified by the September 11, 2001, World Trade Center and Pentagon destructions, to multiple attacks against the seat of government of the United States with bioterrorist agents, to the horrible simultaneous destruction of four trains by ten devastating explosions in Madrid, killing hundreds and wounding almost 2,000 people. Indeed, suicide bombing appears to be one of the methods of choice by determined terrorists, rendering those who seek after and practice civil liberty at risk of life or limb at their hands.

A terrorist event set against a citizenry could pose potentially unforeseeable threats, and the availability of information about the event transmitted through various communication media can have a tremendous impact on the public. Proper community and agency preparation against such threats includes planning for security and availability of communications methods including the various elements of the media (1). This chapter provides reasons for communication in preparation for and during such events, examples of how these interfaces occur, and lays out a framework for planning for those organizations and individuals called on to prepare or manage such events.

PREPAREDNESS ESSENTIALS AND HISTORIC EVENTS

THE BASIC ELEMENTS OF COMMUNICATION IN RESPONSE TO TERRORIST EVENTS

The basic elements of communication in response to terrorist events must be understood. Four broad areas of great concern are identified for those organizations involved in the preparation for handling terrorist events or in the actual management of the event itself. Public service agencies that actualize situation containment, as well as initial victim management and mobilization, are important elements in effective communication during a terrorist event. Communications surrounding victim evaluation and care institutions are responsible for the health care needs of those affected by the incident. Well-defined protocols and responsibilities to communicate the request for outside support beyond local resources, such as military or other agencies, are vital. The release of information to the media is a key element in effective communication during and surrounding a terrorism incident (Table 32-1).

All responding providers have specific needs as well as related needs for the flow of information regarding these events. Related issues include obtaining resources for care of victims and supplies for various purposes such as provider protection, victim transportation, and containment of the event. Unique needs include staging of the event on scene, identifying the scope of the event, locating injured victims, bringing additional resources to bear, or communicating to the public for various reasons, including the prevention of further citizen exposure to the event. Some additional examples for prompt information flow include hospital notification

320

TABLE 32-1	Key Communication Areas During a Terrorism Event

1. Public service agencies
2. Health care workforce and facilities
3. Interagency response mobilization
4. Effective media management

and coordination, locating family members, dealing with the "worried well" and the "walking wounded" or for patients with routine needs, and providing supplemental resources. The list is, by necessity, incomplete.

The method(s) of communication during terrorist events employ the routine channels utilized in day-to-day life (2). The exceptions, of course, occur in the event of local resources being supplemented by federal agencies such as the FBI or the military, all outside the usual routine of municipalities. Such an event, though, may require a significant, even massive, upscaling of the level of information being transferred to various recipients. In the 9/11 bombing of the World Trade Center, for example, a vast increase in traffic within the member agencies responding to the event, to outside agencies in calls for assistance, and to the media and world at large flowed as a result of the event (3).

In the war on terrorism declared by President George W. Bush in 2001, an essential part of the endeavor is found in the increased requirements for communities to carefully examine and identify potential terrorism targets in their territories. Where possible, the potential for destruction of these targets—or the risk of harm to citizens utilizing them—may possibly be ameliorated by thoughtful planning.

Large sporting events, for example, such as those held in stadiums, present a huge potential as terrorist targets. Even minor explosives or gas releases could trigger both initial direct harm from the noxious agent as well as substantial victims through panic. Careful advance thought about crowd control methods that may help contain the spread of panic and mass fleeing from the event would be essential. However, it may be difficult to know what information is appropriate to convey to a frightened crowd should a release of a toxic agent occur, for example. It must be remembered that well-meaning building control officials in the bombing of the World Trade Centers announced over the public address system that evacuation was not necessary, leading many people to return to or remain within the (alleged) safety of the buildings that were soon to collapse. Thus thinking about the basics of communications concerning terrorist events naturally follows three basic paths: prevention, management, and amelioration.

PREVENTING TERRORIST EVENTS THROUGH COMMUNITY COMMUNICATIONS PREPARATION

The issue of the preservation of personal liberty in the context of providing the greatest good for the community has perhaps never been more vital than now. Community preparedness, however, requires a heightened level of awareness that begins with a framework of alertness and communication (4). This foundation is formed by municipal agents and involves citizens in a variety of ways. For example, especially during times of heightened alert from the Department of Homeland Security, increased screening of personal items—even the screening of the individuals themselves—entering into gathering areas, although onerous to some, plays an important role in protecting the greater good. This inspection is an element of the communication plan, requiring prompt notification of the appropriate public safety agencies in the event of positive identification of a hazard (5).

This requirement for communication methods for prevention must be extrapolated across the community landscape: from stadiums to churches to fire departments to EMS agencies. Key people in gatherings must be identified who can seamlessly interface with public safety, fire, and EMS. Methods of communication must be identified, and drills must be conducted.

Terrorist targets can either be anticipated or may not be obvious. The era of suicide bombers—a method of causing maximal effect with a minimal loss of life on behalf of the terrorist organization—makes a school bus full of children a target. Proper communication preparation for such an event might require a key point individual who is responsible for screening entrants to the vehicle. Clearly, though, preparation ultimately may have only a limited impact in terms of decreasing the scope of an incident.

An important example of such preparation is in changes that have been taken regarding parking around municipal buildings. The severity of the blast wave from the truck parked outside the Murrah Federal Building in Oklahoma City affected the framework of the structure, blasting floors upward, which then collapsed into rubble. Prevention of such destruction by vehicles has required substantial rethinking of parking plans for a host of structures. The prevention of destruction, in this case, requires municipal planning and agreement followed by communication to users of the parking areas in real time, plus the enforcement required to assure adherence to these plans.

The assassins who stalked the streets of Maryland, Virginia, and Washington, D.C., in 2002 proved very difficult to apprehend in spite of intense community awareness and media coverage. Yet comprehensive communications across multiple jurisdictions provided the final clues to the identity of the individuals and their vehicle. Media was employed as an active agent in the process of tracking and identification. Then it was left to an observant citizen at a late night hour in a roadside rest area to spot the snipers sleeping in their vehicle, bringing to a quiet end a nearly month-long terrorist event that had caused millions of people to be pierced with fear. Had not the alert Alabama officials' investigation of an apparently random liquor store robbery and murder a month prior produced vital evidence linking this event to subsequent investigative findings, it may only be speculated what the ultimate number of persons injured or killed may have been—and how long terror would have continued to grip the citizens of those states.

Prevention of terrorist events through communication programs is a comprehensive matrix that intermixes agency and public awareness through adept planning and identification of modes of technology, including media participation, sufficient to meet the challenge. No amount of preparation will be sufficient to prevent all determined malefactors from succeeding in at least a portion of the intended harm to a citizenry. However, clearly defined channels of communication established prospectively among agencies, citizen groups, and media sources can clearly help forestall, or at least ameliorate, the effects of a terrorist event (6).

MANAGING TERRORIST EVENTS THROUGH COMMUNITY COMMUNICATIONS PREPARATION

The spectrum of terror is vast. Broadly it may be said that terrorist events have two main elements: the actual physical impact on the target(s) and the emotional distress in the citizenry resulting from the event. Both elements are critical during the actual management of a terrorist event.

As an event unfolds, the facts of the issue gradually become evident, including any loss of life or injuries, physical damage to areas, and the requirements for bringing the situation under control. The intensity of the situation during such an occurrence veritably assures that great potential exists for a dramatically increased volume of utilization of typical communications media. Anxious family members commonly crowd the telephone lines with calls about loved ones. Well-meaning citizens contact public services such as police and fire departments to report what they have seen. Only a carefully prepared, thoughtful plan for protection of contact among involved member agencies can give significant assurance that information interchange can continue.

The intensity of communications among public service agencies may increase dramatically during a terrorist event, and channels of communication require careful design to allow proper function during an event. Unnecessary traffic must be suppressed. For example, prolonged patient presentations on radios by EMS providers must be restrained by protocol. Just as during a multicasualty incident, the initial physical examination process diminishes from the DOT primary survey to a "triage survey," such as the "red survey" found in the Advanced Disaster Life Support program; the patient presentation process to medical control should be abbreviated to only the information required to notify hospitals of patient destination and general basics concerning the patients' conditions.

Community all-hazards management plans include dealing with problems such as biohazard events (whether of a terrorist nature or otherwise) that require prompt activation to assure the best outcome. Thus activation of these plans through facility notification by public service agencies must be carried out early. Busy hospital emergency departments may have to discharge noncritical patients, empty out waiting rooms, place guards outside to prevent unnecessary traffic, establish and provide staffing for decontamination areas, set up hospital central communications centers, and contact additional physician, nursing, and support staff through callback procedures.

This example is on point for this discussion. Should an index case of smallpox present in an urban emergency room, the outpouring of agency notifications, emergency hazards plan activations, and media awareness will be nearly unimaginable. Intense efforts to identify the contacts of the individual, living quarters, recent travel, and otherwise determine how this case came to occur will be undertaken within an intense time frame. The Public Health Department will be activated. Citywide vaccination programs intended to encircle potentially infected persons will become operational. Many cities might initiate a prospectively designed plan to utilize fire department personnel and paramedics to become members of the vaccination team. Centers for vaccination will be established. The city—indeed the world—will be watching with bated breath.

In real time, the utilization of all appropriate communications programs, especially through careful contact with the media, will be essential to prevent community panic, to provide information for vaccination centers, to update the community on the disease progress (if any) in the community, and to optimize the resources available to prevent the spread of the infection while preserving community health (7). However, such an event may naturally be expected to have far-reaching consequences within that urban center, including the possibility of quarantine of the community, limiting of traffic flow in and out of the city until the infection appears to be controlled, and the provision of appropriate medical resources (perhaps such as a separate hospital for infected persons).

Much can be learned from the failure of communications programs to be used optimally during terrorist acts. The sarin nerve gas attacks by the Aum Shinriko against Tokyo in March 1995, resulted in hundreds of exposures of a greater or lesser degree. The number of deaths is somewhat disputed, but clearly in excess of 5,000 people were affected. Photographs of the event show people standing casually in the area of the release of the gas inside the subway. Thousands presented themselves to emergency rooms, over 600 to one facility alone. No decontamination or personal protective equipment was used initially by many of the hospital responders, and it was reported that over 23% of the hospital staff who treated victims sustained exposure themselves (8). Of the more than 1,300 EMS providers who responded to the scene, 10% of them were exposed and developed symptoms. Thus the medical infrastructure itself was threatened by failures in communication.

The reality that communication failures can kill and injure was demonstrated in the failure of police radio channels to interlink with fire and EMS channels in New York. This resulted, at least in part in over 100 fire rescue personnel being trapped and subsequently killed in the collapse of the North Tower of the World Trade Center, over 20 minutes after the pilot of the police helicopter flying above the building saw that the collapse of the building was imminent. Thus operationalizing system communications design, both in equipment and in protocol, is an essential element of limiting risk and exposure to both the citizenry being served and to the rescue/medical providers involved (9).

AMELIORATION OF TERRORIST EVENTS THROUGH COMMUNITY COMMUNICATIONS PREPARATION

The terrible disaster that was manifested in the 9/11 events riveted the attention of the world (10). For weeks, little programming on television strayed from the topics around the attacks against the United States, the destruction of property, and, most importantly, the evolving scope of the loss of life of both citizens and rescue providers. The horror of the death and devastation in Washington, New York, and in the aircraft involved presented a grisly scenario of such enormity that its scope challenged human ability to encompass the grief and shock of the event.

Media and communications played the simultaneous roles of linking rescue and recovery involving thousands of providers while presenting the unfolding drama and details to the watching world. This interplay of information supply served to coordinate the extinguishing of flames, rescue of the living, recovery of the slain, and the beginning of removal and rebuilding through bringing together local, state, and federal agencies. The continuous outpouring of television, radio, and the printed word provided a stream of messages to the public, both to assist concerned family and loved ones as well as to provide a steady flow of news to the hundreds of millions around the world watching in horror.

Thus the gradual relaying of the bits of news generated by hopeful discoveries or sorrowful results from the New York and Washington ground zero locations laid the foundation for both the construction of the reality of loss and the assembly of the framework for recovery. This steady coordination of responding resources and media elements through the common resources of coordinated communications simultaneously provided the guidance for the utilization of responder resources and for the easing of the malaise of a country suffering a terrible wound.

FURTHER PREPAREDNESS ESSENTIALS

HARDENING OF COMMUNICATIONS RESOURCES AGAINST TERRORIST EVENTS

All agencies that might be called on to provide response against a terrorist event in a given area must identify prospectively those methods of information transfer that should be hardened and will be reasonably expected to survive anticipated attacks. EMS dispatch agencies, for example, play a central role in sending appropriate rescue, treatment, and evacuation resources to scenarios that may occur. Such resources may be vulnerable to attack, and this vulnerability must be considered by the municipal planners responsible for implementing the design and construction of these facilities. Targeted attempts to enhance injury to a community may select certain power poles, for example, disrupting telephone services, radio stations, television stations, and dispatch agencies. It is essential, then, that scenario testing of potential losses of communication be conducted to allow a clear view of how municipalities could maintain all of their various communication needs should different modes of information transfer be momentarily disabled or even destroyed.

Reasonable caution should be taken to allow agencies to function as "communication free" as possible. For example, many municipalities require online medical control contact to authorize certain levels of advanced field medical care by EMS personnel. The EMS system medical director should provide presigned authorization of a certain set of skills that may be conducted in the absence of any direct communica-

tion with online medical control. An example of a suggested minimum set of skills that should be preauthorized by the medical director is provided at the end of this chapter. Such preparation may limit the real-time communications necessary for medical providers, perhaps during vital moments in a scenario when the ability to transfer information is extremely limited, decreasing the burden on the already stressed information transfer needs.

LIMITING COMMUNICATION TRAFFIC DURING TERRORIST EVENTS

Maintaining a strict policy toward limiting traffic during events such as terrorist actions is important to allow sufficient information bandwidth to be available. In incidents affecting many citizens and responders—whether it is a nerve gas strike on a subway or a bomb on a train—the information media, especially radio and cellular channels, are commonly overwhelmed. Should then, for example, only a single high-band radio channel be functioning during an attack on a football stadium, frequent brief reminders from the central radio agency—typically the dispatch agency—that "all users of that frequency should limit radio traffic" would be essential, especially should the channel become crowded. Communications should be strictly limited to essential information, including destination of patients being transported to care facilities and very brief scenarios of the problems that the ill or injured have experienced, allowing these care facilities to be as prepared as possible for incoming victims. Abbreviation of traffic is essential. Such abbreviation is not necessarily common practice, for example, in patient presentations via EMS traffic to online medical control, and thus reaching pre-event agreement on proper methods to limit communications traffic while optimizing information transfer should be part of planning and training. The shortening of information transfer requires prior preparation, instruction, and practice to be appropriately facilitated during an event.

CONTACT WITH THE EMA, THE MILITARY, PUBLIC HEALTH AGENCIES INCLUDING THE CDC, AND MUNICIPAL/GOVERNMENTAL AGENCIES

Medical care facilities and all public service agencies called on to provide response and care for a potential terrorist event must cooperate as part of acceptable civil community planning to set out those methods of initiating contact with the area and state emergency management agencies (EMAs), appropriate public health resources (such as the public health facilities in the area as well as the CDC), and any other appropriate municipal or governmental agencies whose participation might be anticipated or required.

In addition, all municipal and governmental agencies that might be called on to participate in response to a terrorist event must establish and maintain call and notification structures that allow for the timely dispatching of these resources in the event of a hostile action. These agencies include but are not limited to public safety, emergency dispatch, power companies, water management facilities, road repair, storm sewer management, vehicle maintenance, and telephone repair. These emergency notification lists must be tested periodically. The results must be submitted to appropriate quality control assessment for reliability.

A biological, chemical, or explosive event set against a citizenry may place extraordinary requirements on responding agencies to provide unusual supplies not commonly anticipated in communities. The National Pharmaceutical Stockpile, for example, provides large quantities of medications such as atropine and 2-PAM for use in the protection from or treatment of a nerve gas exposure, and this resource can be quickly mobilized to a geographical location. The receiving area, however, must have in place an appropriate plan for the receiving, opening, and distribution of the resources contained within the pushpack, should its delivery be required. Thus the actual communication notifying the federal agency of the need for activation of the stockpile must be part of a well worked-out process for the receiving and distribution of this resource.

Another example of such an issue would be found in the setting of an explosion at an emergency communications center in a metropolitan area that resulted in substantial damage to emergency communications systems in that area. A notification call might be required to the EMA, but immediately available communication resources might be damaged. The emergency response system should consider an alternative communication method as part of community planning. One such hardened response is the deployment of the Radio Amateur Civil Emergency Service (RACES). Under a preexisting agreement with the fire chief of the community, for example, a call would be needed to a neighboring fire department to then place a call for the EMA, for mutual aid, to notify surrounding hospital facilities, and perhaps even the military for assistance. A call to the RACES indeed could serve that function. Such a notification structure must be part of a prospective overall emergency communications plan.

PROTECTION OF RADIO AND CELLULAR TELEPHONE BANDWIDTH

A terrorist event would place severe demands on the limited information transfer methods available to communities. Public calls for help commonly come from land-line telephones, although the growing use of cellular telephones clearly indicates these devices are among the most common methods of notification and activation of emergency response agencies for all types of emergencies. Compelling evidence indicates that these personal communications devices (PCDs) are so ubiquitous that they have become the most common method of notification of emergencies. It would be prudent, then, as part of community municipal budgeting, that enhanced 911 systems be modified to allow for Wireless Enhanced 911 (WE911) ability, allowing for emergency communications centers to localize the site of the localization of callers in the setting of emergencies. Although such WE911 ability is important, it must be remembered that this ability only localizes the caller, not the site of the event. A PCD caller may indeed be quite far from the event, so the value of the WE911 localization must be considered a part of the total information being received, and its total value in localizing an event must be weighed in the balance.

Also given the wide use of cellular telephones and the common dependence of municipal agencies for the use of these devices as well, it is clear that restrictions must be placed, in advance, on cellular telephone channels for the purpose of suppressing unnecessary use of these channels and to provide access to municipal agencies for these channels. In a similar vein, emergency radio channels must be strictly protected for the use of those agencies that might respond to a terrorist event to allow for the needs of those agencies.

Also, planning agencies should consider making available direct satellite telecommunication devices, microwave linkups, and Internet channels for use during terrorist events (11). Such equipment can be quickly set into operation in the event of a disaster, provided the equipment truly meets the operational needs of the agency. A useful uplink is the establishment of direct Internet communication for victim tracking, resource allocation, and information provision. Indeed, municipal trials with such satellite uplinks have been conducted and have shown great promise, mirroring similar devices in use by the military, such as the instant availability worldwide of medical records of members of the armed services who may become ill or injured during military operations.

COMMUNICATIONS CENTERS DURING TERRORIST EVENTS

Planning for amelioration of and recovery from terrorist events must include the provision for centers for emergency communications (ECCs) (12). The ECC must be established in areas designated to provide coordinated communication among responding agencies. These centers provide a free flow of required information for the function of the facility in which the ECC is designated during such a catastrophe.

A hospital-based ECC should be established in a convenient, central, restricted, and hardened location in that facility. Access to the ECC should be restricted to authorized personnel, and security personnel should be posted at the entrance to the facility during the event and for some period during the aftermath. The ECC for a hospital must provide contacts to all appropriate agencies, including the fire department, EMS, public safety, public health, pharmacy, administration, central supply, surgery, intensive care, security, and maintenance on a real-time basis. The ECC must have adequate backup communications methods in case of electrical and/or telephone failure.

The municipal-based ECC should be located in a hardened facility to which access is restricted. Officers of the municipality, such as mayors and city council persons, should not necessarily receive routine access to the center except as permitted under local ordinance. This municipal ECC must preserve real-time connections with fire, EMS, dispatch, public safety, public health agencies, EMA, water/sewer authorities, power companies, media, and appropriate maintenance agencies during a terrorist event. Media connections within the ECC are essential, including real-time telephone and Internet availability. Logs of all communications activity must be maintained by ECC staff, including the investigations of past and ongoing threats that may be reported.

An ECC could be reasonably anticipated to be a target for terrorists. Any attack that could disrupt communications among assigned agencies could be expected to increase the potential for an increased number of victims, cause the committing of valuable community resources to areas inconsistent with optimal amelioration of the event, and create an increased potential for panic. The planning for the restriction of access to and the hardening of emergency communication centers, therefore, should pay careful consideration to the physical location of this center, its redundancy of communication methods, and its protection by security and public safety agencies. An important center to emulate in design and positioning is the ECC for Houston, Texas, whose location is well back from the road, whose ECC operations are housed in protected hardened locations, and whose access is strictly limited.

THE RADIO AMATEUR CIVIL EMERGENCY SERVICE

As discussed briefly earlier, private radio operators (known as ham radio operators) have created an organization known as the Radio Amateur Civil Emergency Service (or RACES). This organization is made up of licensed amateur radio operators who volunteer their time and equipment to provide supplemental communication to local, county, or state agencies during times of crisis or disaster. RACES is governed by regulations of the Federal Communications Commission (FCC) found in part 97, subpart E, of the FCC regulations.

The RACES Internet web site states that "as far as participation, by FCC regulations only RACES-affiliated stations may participate in RACES nets, including training drills. Furthermore, participation in SKYWARN nets are limited to those RACES station members who have attended a SKYWARN training class in the last two years." Through these training programs, a heightened degree of awareness is maintained by these individuals. They maintain a higher level of alert and preparation in the event that they might be contacted by their municipalities to render service in the event of terrorist or natural disasters.

Community planning should include the identification of these local communications resources. These individuals present a truly worldwide resource, making available to municipalities their equipment and time to provide secondary communications support in the event of primary communications failures.

A useful web site for reference to this organization is found at the URL http://www.eham.net/links/. The user may enter the selection "Emergency and Special Services" (without quotes) into the Search box.

FACILITATED COMMUNICATION THROUGH INTERNET-BASED SYSTEMS AND OTHER COMPUTER RESOURCES

The global revolution in information distribution through the Internet is unprecedented in its potential scope for the support of those who would supply resources against terrorist actions. Internet-based information is of such common availability and depth that virtually any information necessary to manage an emergency of any sort can be located on the Web

through either an "insecure" or a "secure" computer resource. Written resources such as textbooks may take years to produce, but a page on the Web can be written quickly and maintained in a current, dynamic, up-to-the-minute, even self-refreshing electronic state by the web site manager. Therefore a catalog of available web sites for anticipated information needs should be maintained by any municipal planner, providing the ECC with adequate computer resources, including bandwidth, so the ECC staff can get the information they need. Indeed, a municipal manager with access to appropriate web pages can be a very useful asset to those providing emergency response (13).

The Internet is a real-time, dynamic network. It may, therefore, serve a vital role for many purposes in the support of those responding to a terrorist action. Constant Web uplinks to assigned web sites can be utilized to inform responders regarding numbers and names of victims, causes of acute conditions of victims, and location of victim mobilization for care. Moreover, this uplink, established in a dynamic format, can provide hospitals with the numbers of victims, how they are being treated and have responded to treatment, and estimated times of arrival. Also, those utilizing the uplink in the field may also receive in virtually real time the status of area receiving facilities, including their current capabilities and resource alerts. The Dallas, Texas, central facility communication through the EMSystem project, managed jointly by the BioTel network and Parkland Hospital as well as the Dallas-Fort Worth Hospital Council, maintains just such a dynamic presence on the Internet in real time, connecting all area hospitals to prehospital providers through this information resource (14).

Mobile data terminals in emergency vehicles play an important role in many urban centers by sending data to various facilities from dispatch agencies to hospitals to public safety communications. Syndromic surveillance by fire/EMS dispatch software plays a vital role in detecting the appearance of multiple cases of symptoms that might be associated with terrorist events (15). Personal digital assistants (PDAs) may also play a role during the management of a terrorist event. For example, PDA software is now of such sophistication that comprehensive patient treatment algorithms, pharmacology texts, and toxicology references can quite literally be available in the palm of the hand of a responding provider or hospital facility medical staff member. Such resources can be extremely useful in the proper setting, especially in the event of a biological or chemical terrorist action that perhaps involves unfamiliar disease organisms or chemicals.

PRIVACY OF PATIENT INFORMATION DURING A TERRORIST EVENT

All citizens have rights to privacy regarding their bodies as well as certain information about themselves. Congress has come down strongly in favor of the protection of citizens' rights to control their medical information. The Health Insurance Portability and Accountability Act of 1996 (HIPAA) has provided strict regulations regarding how patient medical information must be managed (16). Any person providing medical care to anyone must closely adhere to these laws.

These rules apply to all health care organizations, including all health care providers, physician offices, health plans, employers, public health authorities, life insurers, clearinghouses, billing agencies, information systems vendors, service organizations, and universities. HIPAA calls for severe civil and criminal penalties for noncompliance with these regulations, including fines of up to $25,000 for multiple violations of the same standard in a calendar year as well as fines of up to $250,000 and/or imprisonment up to 10 years for the knowing misuse of health information that may be identifiable to an individual patient.

Because the risks associated with misusing patient medical information are so severe, it is clearly of the utmost importance that municipal agencies prospectively examine the use of any patient information in regard to those persons who might be provided any kind of medical service during a terrorist action. These regulations affect agencies broadly and deeply. For example, the required compliance responses are not standard throughout the industry because the various provider organizations are not standardized, complicating the application of any blanket rules. Just as an example, a particular organization that routinely maintains a computer network that might receive patient care information will be required to set in place appropriate security access mechanisms that can provide the required access control. Thus this matter, in terms of municipal disaster planning, must be addressed well in advance by a municipality, with appropriate legal reference and guidance obtained well in advance.

Generally speaking, any information items that might identify a patient, with the exception of age and sex, should not be broadcast in any medium at any time without clear, written patient consent. Obviously obtaining such consent during a crisis situation will be problematic. Thus it is prudent that municipal response agencies and hospitals resist releasing any patient identifiers by any medium at any time without the clear, prospective, and timely guidance of legal counsel.

THE ROLE OF THE MEDIA IN AMELIORATING TERRORIST EVENTS

The media can be a valuable asset during a terrorist action in two broad ways. First, the public health may require protection. A nerve gas attack against a subway might cause a substantial risk to public health both in the release of the toxin as well as in the disruption of the public transportation system. The citizenry might then be called on to avoid the use of public transportation and indeed to avoid approaching any of certain transportation centers within a given proximity. The local, state, or national media, because of the breadth of their broadcast coverage, could quickly and accurately inform the populace of the affected area regarding appropriate safety precautions via radio, television, Internet, and newsprint including both immediate and delayed public hazards (17). These hazards might include the need for evacuation, for alternative routes of travel, or for the potential of an event producing delayed hazards that might affect the public health. For example, smoke from a large explosion might cause such particulate contamination of the atmosphere in

the affected area that those at risk for bronchospastic conditions might need to take precautions. Such was the case in the New York downtown area following the 9/11 attacks. The information communicated by the media contained important warnings, including the use of masks where appropriate, how to obtain them, and when to wear them.

Medical advice and other information resources available through the media are essential to the proper management of a potential terrorist action in which the public health may be at risk. An attack against an airliner that then crashed into a community might, indeed, place hundreds (or, in large cities, thousands) of citizens at risk. Evacuation centers might be established, and the media, through the use of appropriate broadcast methods, might advise appropriate evacuation instructions, the location of available centers, and even contact information for those who may require municipal services to receive appropriate transportation and/or care.

The media can likewise serve a support role in a terrorist action. The broadcasting of a need for clothing, blankets, water, and other supplies to help emergency rescuers is commonly made through the media and has become an invaluable resource in such settings. For example, the outpouring from the goodness of a national population has been evidenced many times in such horrific events as the 9/11 attacks when calls for additional support supplies were made. Within hours, thousands of bottles of water and other materials were made available by a grateful public to lend assistance to those providing rescue and recovery operations.

The media can play an invaluable role in the dissemination of information regarding events that have occurred (18). The public has a right to know what is occurring that is newsworthy and of general public interest. A given population is a community, and the sense of participation in that community is measured in significant part by information distributed that is of public interest. Indeed, coincident with the World Trade Center bombings, an intense public interest was served by the media, sharing likewise information on the specifics of the management of the disaster as well as the airing of the communal grief of a nation and the world (19). The sharing of this outpouring of grief throughout the communications media served to inform, educate, support, and sharpen the determination of tens of millions toward the rescue of the wounded, the recovery of the dead, the removal of the debris, and the resolve for the future.

Important items that might be shared through the media include critical information for families of victims, especially whom to contact for information and where to gather for support or waiting. Thus in this manner the media becomes a public service agency in the broadest sense, bringing necessary vital assistance to those who need that service, at whatever distance the needy might be from the actual event.

Previous work has set out many essential elements in the management of media relations (20). These critical points are vital during the planning and training for how media elements will be utilized during a terrorist action. The important core elements for the management of media issues are found in Table 32-2.

TABLE 32-2	Ten Essential Elements for Effective Media Communication

1. The public must receive a single, clear message.
2. A redundancy of persons authorized to talk to the media must be created, preferably within a thoughtful protocol prepared well in advance of any MCI.
3. A cadre of close-working experts must be identified.
4. Persons involved in any portion of the MCI must be responsive and helpful to the media.
5. During communication, the nature of the content released must be carefully controlled. The individual communicating with the media must always tell the truth but should resist giving every detail.
6. The face shown to the media must be one of concern. To quote Pepe, the individual authorized to speak to the media should "be a human being, and act like one."
7. The communicator should try to avoid giving out factoid sound bites that sound good but have no ultimate consequences.
8. The authorized individual communicating with the media must remember not to panic, especially under media pressure.
9. When communicating with the media, those involved with the MCI and the populace at large should learn lessons from the past but consider future possibilities/threats, recalling that "when facts are scarce, words soon take their place."
10. Those caring for the MCI should also help care for the members of the media, appreciating how important they are to the management of the operation.

PREPAREDNESS SUMMARY

Municipal planners are compelled to take what action is possible to prevent, manage, and ameliorate the effects of a terrorist action against their communities. It may be stated broadly that a determined terrorist utilizing concealed means and shielded by the element of surprise can inflict damage of some measure, perhaps even terrible damage. However, equally determined emergency resource administrators can create a wall of detection, deflection, and direction that can either prevent or at least diminish the destructive intent applied against a population.

Only through a carefully designed program of coordinated communication resources that are current, active, and durable can these administrators most accurately manage the needs of the populations they serve and provide the protection that the coming years will demand.

RESOURCES

EMS ADVANCED LIFE SUPPORT SKILLS THAT MAY BE AUTHORIZED UNDER MEDICAL CONTROL STANDING ORDER IN THE EVENT OF COMMUNICATION FAILURE (21)

1. Endotracheal intubation
2. IV fluid replacement
3. Use of albuterol and ipratropium for bronchospasm
4. Use of nitroglycerin for chest pain suspicious for cardiac events
5. Advanced cardiac life support algorithms for the management of sudden death, including defibrillation, use of epinephrine, and the use of amiodarone
6. Use of antiarrhythmics as appropriate in the setting of myocardial infarction
7. Possibly field termination of cardiac arrest management in multiple casualty situations, requiring the concurrence of two team EMS advanced life support leaders and possibly the coroner or medical examiner, if these individuals are on scene
8. 12-lead EKG interpretation for signs of ischemia or injury
9. Needle decompression of tension pneumothorax
10. Needle cricothyrotomy
11. Pain management, including authorized narcotic medications such as incremental dosages of morphine sulphate

Note: All skills listed must only be conducted by trained, certified, and routinely quality-controlled individuals who have demonstrated competency in these areas.

REFERENCES

1. Centers for Disease Control, Atlanta. Imported plague—New York City, 2002. MMWR Morb Mortal Wkly Rep 2003; 52(31):725-8.
2. Kahan E, Fogelman Y, Kitai E, et al. Patient and family physician preferences for care and communication in the eventuality of anthrax terrorism. Fam Pract 2003;20(4):441-2.
3. Bradt DA. Site management of health issues in the 2001 World Trade Center disaster. Acad Emerg Med 2003;10(6):650-60.
4. Pavlin JA, Mostashari F, Kortepeter MG, et al. Innovative surveillance methods for rapid detection of disease outbreaks and bioterrorism: results on an interagency workshop on health indicator surveillance. Am J Public Health 2003;93(8):1230-5.
5. Ott WE. Emergency messaging and contingency communications. JEMS 2003;28(6):108, 110.
6. Palmer DJ, Stephens D, Fisher DA, et al. The Bali bombing: the Royal Darwin Hospital response. Med J Aust 2003; 179(7):358-61.
7. Pavlin JA, Mostashari F, Kortepeter MG, et al. Innovative surveillance methods for rapid detection of disease outbreaks and

bioterrorism: results on an interagency workshop on health indicator surveillance. Am J Public Health 2003;93(8):1230-5.

8. Okumura T, Suzuki K, Fukuda A, et al. The Tokyo subway sarin attack: disaster management. Part 2. Hospital response. Acad Emerg Med 1998;5(6):618-24.

9. Noji EK. Creating a health care agenda for the Department of Homeland Security. Managed Care. 2003;12(11 Suppl):7-12.

10. Marshall RD, Galea S. Science for the community: assessing mental health after 9/11. J Clin Psychiatry 2004;65(Suppl 1): 37-42.

11. Yellowlees P, MacKenzie J. Telehealth responses to bio-terrorism and emerging infections. J Telemed Telecare 2003; 9(Suppl 2):S80-2.

12. Kendra JM, Wachtendorf T. Elements of resilience after the World Trade Center disaster: reconstituting New York City's Emergency Operations Centre. Disasters 2003;27(1):37-53.

13. Ferguson NE, Steele L, Crawford CY, et al. Bioterrorism web site resources for infectious disease clinicians and epidemiologists. Clin Infect Dis 2003;36(11):1458-73. Epub May 22, 2003.

14. Dallas Area BioTel System. Parkland Memorial Hospital, Dallas, TX.

15. Greenko J, Mostashari F, Fine A, et al. Clinical evaluation of the Emergency Medical Services (EMS) ambulance dispatch-based syndromic surveillance system, New York City. J Urban Health 2003;80(2 Suppl 1):i50-6.

16. Bruce J. Bioterrorism meets privacy: an analysis of the Model State Emergency Health Powers Act and the HIPAA privacy rule. Ann Health Law 2003;12(1):75-120.

17. Pollard WE. Public perceptions of information sources concerning bioterrorism before and after anthrax attacks: an analysis of national survey data. J Health Commun 2003; (8 Suppl) 1:93-103; discussion 148-51.

18. Prue CE, Lackey C, Swenarski L, et al. Communication monitoring: shaping CDC's emergency risk communication efforts. J Health Commun 2003;8 (Suppl 1):35-49; discussion 148-51.

19. Klitzman S, Freudenberg N. Implications of the World Trade Center attack for the public health and health care infrastructures. Am J Public Health 2003;93(3):400-6.

20. Pepe P, Fowler R. Media and communications during disasters. Advanced Disaster Life Support 2003; 80-1.

21. The Dallas Area BioTel System, Dallas, Texas. Web site: www.biotel.ws.

Training Preparedness for Terrorism

33

Exercises and Educational Courses in Terrorism Preparedness

Myra M. Socher and Edwin K. Leap

INTRODUCTION

Very few emergency care workers have ever cared for the casualties of weapons of mass destruction. Terrorism, which is an enormous concern for all health care providers and emergency responders, is still relatively rare when held up against the background of our normal practices and concerns. That is, it is rare so far. But the world is a dangerous place, and the war on terror is in its infancy.

If we want to be prepared, we have roughly three options. We can turn away from all of the bad news and pretend, if we try hard enough, that it will never happen to us. Statistically, we may be right. The majority of persons in industrialized nations currently do not live in areas that are considered high risks for terrorist use of weapons of mass destruction (WMD). This approach has some undeniable practicality. A physician or paramedic may spend 30 years in practice and never see a case of weaponized plague, or care for a patient with radiation sickness. But then again, we could make the same argument for many of the problems we encounter in caring for the health needs of the public. We could say, for instance, that physicians in the rural South do not need to know about HIV if it is rare where they work. We could say that paramedics in ski areas need not learn to deliver babies because what are the odds? But this is a risky

way to play the numbers, and the results can be disastrous if our assessment of the risks turns out to be wrong. A little preparation, a little knowledge, just enough to recognize a problem and call for help, might save one life or thousands. So, ignoring the risk of terrorism may not be the best plan.

As a second alternative, we could go to the opposite extreme and seek to be exposed to terrorist events and mass casualty episodes. We could, if we have not already, join the military and travel to combat zones, just to get a feel for the danger, the heightened alertness, the sound of gunfire, and the look of exploded vehicles. There we would learn firsthand how to care for victims of bombs or bullets and learn, through our own wish to survive, how to be vigilant for signs of chemical, biological, and radiological illnesses. Or perhaps, we could work at a large urban emergency department.

If ignoring the problem is unacceptable, and if seeking it out is impractical, then we must obtain the knowledge and training by attending educational courses and exercises in terrorism preparedness.

Most emergency care workers have at least a little experience with preparedness exercises. Some of our more "seasoned" colleagues still remember the days of "duck and cover," when an entire nation practiced, to greater or lesser extents, what they would do in the case of nuclear war. In those days, the Civil Defense initiative existed because the world moved through its days and nights with the very real fear that nuclear weapons would fall like rain one day.

It was a fear with legitimate foundations, based on the very real existence of intercontinental ballistic missles (ICBMs) in silos and submarines around the world, possessed by the two most powerful military forces in the world, which were run by governments with philosophies diametrically opposed to one another. Whether anyone believed it would matter or not, they practiced the old duck-and-cover drill because doing something was better than doing nothing. The Cold War, which was covert and conducted mostly by spies and diplomats, was considered by some as the equivalent of World War III. If this is correct, then the advent of the recent major terrorist attacks is the equivalent of a fourth world war.

Most emergency workers have also had some experience with disaster drills. Medical schools and hospitals have traditionally held annual exercises that involve situations like tornadoes, earthquakes, plane crashes, and industrial accidents. These exercises are often attended by emergency department staff, EMS workers, residents, and students. Other hospital personnel, including administrators and health practitioners from nonemergency settings, often elect not to participate in these exercises.

It may be argued that the modern era has brought us a reality even more terrifying than the ICBMs, which dominated our attention in the Cold War. Nuclear missiles, for all of their potential apocalyptic power, were possessed by nations whose leaders and citizens generally wanted to see their grandchildren. And they were generally secured and maintained by large disciplined military forces. The modern threat of terror and weapons of mass destruction is quite different from those days. In terrorism, hatred combines with technology, and suicidal fervor combines with tremendous lethality. The result is that even the most jaded and cynical emergency care provider recognizes that "it could happen here." And since it could, preparation is essential.

Because of a number of widely publicized terrorist events in the 1990s, emergency care providers in the United States have made an enormous effort to prepare for the prospect of terrorism on American soil. This effort, like all great efforts, has been a combined labor. It involves all levels of health care, federal government, as well as the emergency providers in the field. We begin this chapter by describing the Domestic Preparedness (DP) training program, as a very positive example of how training has been taken to the population centers of the United States. Federal legislation that used resources and information from diverse and capable organizations in the government and private sectors was enacted, and then all of those assets were pooled into this program, which was disseminated to municipalities across the country.

If the essence of the program could be summarized, it would be in the phrase "NBC Delta," which is the concept at the heart of this training system. It means that, although the nation is well prepared for many emergency contingencies, there is a gap between existing preparation and the preparation needed for response to nuclear, biological, and chemical agents or weapons of mass destruction. The delta, or difference, was the critical gap that the Domestic Preparedness program sought to fill.

The program began in 1996, one year after the attack on Oklahoma City, and five years before the attack on the Twin Towers and the Pentagon. It might be said that the DP program was both reactionary and visionary. Those who con-

ceived and implemented it sensed a growing danger to the United States and acted on their intuition. Although most of those involved in running the DP program did not foresee the use of an airliner as a weapon of mass destruction, the DP program had already laid the initial framework that allowed the country to augment its response faster, and more effectively, in the weeks, months, and years since 9/11. The original program targeted the largest 120 cities and used a "train-the-trainer" format. It was thought that by preparing instructors across the nation, the effect of terrorism preparedness education would be multiplied. This program continues, now under the direction of the Office for Domestic Preparedness, within the Department of Homeland Security. It has evolved into a program with multiple course topics and multiple levels of training. It continues to provide an outstanding level of preparedness training for a nation that remains under the constant threat of terrorism.

However, preparedness training did not stop there. Humans are very creative creatures, and so we always try to reinvent, always try to improve. Some of the improvements in preparedness training we now see include self-assessments for organizations and individuals to take before training and open table-top exercises that are less intimidating and more entertaining than traditional didactics. Furthermore, because emergency responders and health care providers are not always able to travel long distances to receive training, the training is being taken to them. The Internet is a growing source of distance education in WMD preparedness issues; it also contains an enormous amount of accessible information that can be useful in real time, or as some have described it, "just in time," by those faced with possible WMD events, whether suspicious infectious outbreaks or dramatic chemical exposures.

This chapter is included in the text so that readers can have some perspective on preparedness exercises and education in weapons of mass destruction, as well as some insight into the new directions that preparedness training is taking. It is useful to review the progress that such training has taken. As we look at how training was conducted in the past, we can respond to current threats more easily. And as we assess what has been successful, we can make future courses and exercises more effective. It is the least we can do for the emergency responders and health care workers who will use them as they prepare to safeguard our nation against the terrifying, unthinkable, but all too real threat of terrorist use of weapons of mass destruction.

PREPAREDNESS ESSENTIALS

Preparedness is a continuum, with no real endpoint. We are better prepared today than we were yesterday, and tomorrow we will be even more prepared. If we try to define preparedness we can say that "it is a proactive effort by an institution to shift rapidly from a normal and routine state to a heightened state of alert and an increased level of operations in response to a disaster or a multiple casualty incident" (1). Although we can never be totally prepared for every eventuality, through education, planning, and exercises, we can progress to more advanced levels of preparedness.

Perhaps the most important element of preparedness is awareness. When students are aware of existing and potential threats, they will be better motivated and better able to deal with an act of terrorism. In light of their awareness, they can learn how to evaluate their current response systems and existing policies and procedures. Using their newly acquired knowledge, they will be able to "harden" their institution's ability to respond to an incident.

Preparedness is the result of planning, but even a good plan is only useful if it is exercised and the results of the exercise are used to improve its structure. Many valuable planning templates, from hospitals to Metropolitan Medical Response Systems, are available at the micro and macro levels. Geographically, efforts extend from local and regional efforts to programs conducted by federal agencies (e.g., CDC's Pandemic Influenza Plan) (2). Medical planners are encouraged to take advantage of these.

Emergency operations plans (EOPs) provide the roadmap to a response effort. They provide detailed instructions on how to navigate the obstacles that arise, how to manage the sudden influx of patients into the health care system, how to provide for their physical and mental well-being, and how to recover from an incident and return to normal day-to-day operations as quickly and efficiently as possible. Training is needed to incorporate these EOPs properly into the response plan (3).

Education follows planning. There are many different programs that use diverse media in both the public and private sectors, and educators must choose wisely when selecting the programs that are best suited to their particular audiences.

There is a trend to move away from the more traditional didactic courses to facilitated workshops, table-top exercises, and larger field exercises. Case-based teaching has increased in popularity in many so-called merit badge courses such as Advanced Cardiac Life Support (ACLS), and this trend is being translated to WMD training.

Exercises constitute an important component of any training program. "Experience and data show that exercises are a practical and efficient way to prepare for crises. They test critical resistance, identify procedural difficulties, and provide a plan for corrective actions" (4).

After any exercises or other case-based educational program, a session is typically conducted between the course moderators and the regional and local leaders, and a summary of the major suggestions and comments is prepared for distribution to all participants. This *after action report* provides an opportunity to receive input for improving the course content and to discuss application to the specific environment where the program was conducted. Major exercises in the United States deserve special discussion. The first of these was called TOPOFF (Top Officials) 2000, conducted in May of that year. It was a congressionally mandated, no-notice exercise that was staged at three locations and that simulated radiological, chemical, and biological attacks. After action reports provided valuable feedback, and the lessons learned were incorporated into the design of TOPOFF II.

TOPOFF II, also congressionally-mandated, was preceded by a series of WMD seminars and table-top exercises designed to educate the participants prior to the actual exercise. An "open exercise design" was used, where stakeholder participants worked in concert with exercise design experts to develop the program. The organizers considered the use of this technique a success. They cited enhanced learning by the participants due to their direct participation in the development of the exercise (5). It was also described as having allowed regional planners to "develop and strengthen relationships in the national response community."

Of significance to the medical community was the simulated public health emergency in Illinois, one of the largest mass casualty exercises to date, which examined the coordination between the medical and public health communities, and their ability to respond to and intervene in the spread of the epidemic. A significant finding, in keeping with the results of most, if not all, exercises was the lack of an effective communications system. Additionally, they described casualties among health care providers, a well-known factor in areas where terrorist bombings often involve a second device targeting responders.

More recently, a secret cabinet-level table-top exercise called Scarlet Cloud (anthrax), "showed that we are a lot better off today than we were two years ago before 9/11," according to a senior administration official. "It also showed that there has definitely been a fast learning curve on bioterrorism" (5)

Exercises provide an excellent tool to identify, analyze, and quantify the strengths and gaps in our response systems and our degree of understanding of WMD and its accompanying threats. So, we should use exercises of varying degrees of sophistication, duration, and intensity as an integral part of any education process.

PREPAREDNESS HISTORIC EVENTS AND CASE HISTORIES

In the early- to mid-1990s, several notable terrorist events had a great impact on planning for potential threats in the United States. The bombing of the World Trade Center in 1993, the terrorist chemical attack on the Tokyo subway system in 1995, the bombing of the Alfred P. Murrah Federal Building in Oklahoma City in 1995, and the Centennial Park bombing in Atlanta in 1996 led to the passing of legislation to better equip our nation's first responders (6). The Nunn-Lugar-Domenici (NLD) Defense against Weapons of Mass Destruction Act of 1996 (Public Law 104-201) mandated training for the 120 most populous cities in the United States (Fig. 33-1) (7).

The resultant Domestic Preparedness (DP) program provided the initial benchmark training for the medical response to terrorism for federal, state, and local agencies and is considered the prototype on which many other courses were built. This training was designed for federal, state, and local emergency responders to prepare for possible terrorist incidents involving Nuclear, Biological and Chemical (NBC) agents (8).

In February 1997 the Department of Defense's U.S. Army Chemical and Biological Defense Command (CBDCOM), now the Soldier and Biological Chemical Command (SBCCOM), took the lead with the support of five other federal agencies (Department of Energy, Federal Bureau of Investigation, Federal Emergency Management Agency, U.S. Public Health Service, and the Environmental Protection

1. New York, N.Y.	31. Kansas City, Mo.	61. Arlington, Tex.	91. Garland, Tex.
2. Los Angeles, Calif.	32. Long Beach, Calif.	62. Norfolk, Va.	92. Glendale, Calif.
3. Chicago, Il.	33. Tucson, Ariz.	63. Las Vegas, Nev.	93. Columbus, Ga.
4. Houston, Tex.	34. St. Louis, Mo.	64. Corpus Christi, Tex.	94. Spokane, Wash.
5. Philadelphia, Pa.	35. Charlotte, N.C.	65. St. Petersburg, Fla.	95. Tacoma, Wash.
6. San Diego, Calif.	36. Atlanta, Ga.	66. Rochester, N.Y.	96. Little Rock, Ark.
7. Detroit, Mich.	37. Virginia Beach, Va.	67. Jersey City, N.J.	97. Bakersfield, Calif.
8. Dallas, Tex.	38. Albuquerque, N. Mex.	68. Riverside, Calif.	98. Fremont, Calif.
9. Phoenix, Ariz.	39. Oakland, Calif.	69. Anchorage, Alaska	99. Fort Wayne, Ind.
10. San Antonio, Tex.	40. Pittsburgh, Pa.	70. Lexington, Ky.[a]	100. Newport News, Va.[a]
11. San Jose, Calif.	41. Sacramento, Calif.	71. Akron, Ohio	101. Arlington, Va.
12. Baltimore, Md.	42. Minneapolis, Minn.	72. Aurora, Col.	102. Worcester, Mass.
13. Indianapolis, Ind.	43. Tulsa, Okla.	73. Baton Rouge, La.	103. Knoxville, Tenn.
14. San Francisco, Calif.	44. Honolulu, Hawaii	74. Raleigh, N.C.	104. Modesto, Calif.
15. Jacksonville, Fla.	45. Cincinnati, Ohio	75. Stockton, Calif.	105. Orlando, Fla.
16. Columbus, Ohio	46. Miami, Fla.	76. Richmond, Va.	106. San Bernardino, Calif.
17. Milwaukee, Wis.	47. Fresno, Calif.	77. Shreveport, La.	107. Syracuse, N.Y.
18. Memphis, Tenn.	48. Omaha, Nebr.	78. Jackson, Miss.	108. Providence, R.I.
19. Washington, D.C.	49. Toledo, Ohio	79. Mobile, Ala.	109. Salt Lake City, Utah
20. Boston, Mass.	50. Buffalo, N.Y.	80. Des Moines, Iowa	110. Huntsville, Ala.
21. Seattle, Wash.	51. Wichita, Kans.	81. Lincoln, Nebr.	111. Amarillo, Tex.
22. El Paso, Tex.	52. Santa Ana, Calif.	82. Madison, Wis.	112. Springfield, Mass.
23. Cleveland, Ohio	53. Mesa, Ariz.	83. Grand Rapids, Mich.	113. Cleveland, Ohio
24. New Orleans, La.	54. Colorado Springs, Co.	84. Yonkers, N.Y.	114. Irving, Tex.
25. Nashville, Tenn.	55. Tampa, Fla.	85. Hialeah, Fla.	115. Chesapeake, Va.
26. Denver, Colo.	56. Newark, N.J.	86. Montgomery, Ala.	116. Kansas City, Kansas
27. Austin, Tex.	57. St. Paul, Minn.	87. Lubbock, Tex.	117. Metarie, La.[a]
28. Fort Worth, Tex.	58. Louisville, Ky.	88. Greensboro, N.C.	118. Ft. Lauderdale, Fla.
29. Oklahoma City, Okla.	59. Anaheim, Calif.	89. Dayton, Ohio	119. Glendale, Ariz.
30. Portland, Oreg.	60. Birmingham, Ala.	90. Huntington Beach, Calif.	120. Warren, Mich.

Figure 33–1. Cities selected for Domestic Preparedness program (in order of population). [a]Not a city government. (Source: US Army Chemical and Biological Defense command.)

Agency) to develop the DP program. They conducted four focus group meetings with first responders to determine core competencies and to develop comprehensive training performance objectives. Firefighters, hazardous materials (hazmat) specialists, on-scene incident commanders, emergency medical services, physicians, law enforcement officers, and 911 operators and call takers, as well as the appropriate federal agencies participated in this effort. The findings and recommendations of these focus groups formed the basis for a comprehensive set of 26 training performance objectives, details of which may be found in the matrix in Table 33-1 (9).

The performance objectives considered existing emergency response guidelines and standards prescribed by the Occupational Safety and Health Administration (OSHA), National Fire Protection Association (NFPA), and the Joint Commission for Accreditation of Healthcare Organizations (JCAHO). They were structured according to four competency levels (Awareness, Operations, Technician/Specialist [nonmedical and medical response], and Incident Command) with three separate levels of training (Basic, Advanced, and Specialized). These competencies reflected the levels identified in OSHA's 29 code of federal regulation (CFR) to ensure that the necessary competencies would be consistent from city to city while still permitting the cities the flexibility to determine those levels in which they needed more training (10).

It was decided that, where possible, existing courses within the Department of Defense and other federal agencies, like the Chemical Stockpile Emergency Preparedness program, would be modified to provide the basis of the initial programs of instruction. By using civilian medical personnel to rescript these courses, the military teaching materials would be tailored to meet the needs of the first response community. The train-the-trainer approach was adopted to increase the size of the audience reached and to foster the development of networks of instructors at the local level to provide ongoing education for their personnel using existing internal education structures. Leave-behind materials that could be reproduced included copies of the instructor and student manuals, video presentations, 35 mm PowerPoint slides, CD-ROMs, and training aids. A toll-free NBC Domestic Preparedness Helpline and a web site were provided to allow for technical assistance and as a resource to research additional questions that were raised during the course of training (11).

Prior to the program being taken to each city, the local governments were provided with a self-assessment tool to help determine the training requirements and needs of each municipality. Initially learning was primarily didactic in structure with few "show-and-tell" and "hands-on" sessions, although these did increase as the program evolved. The Technician–Emergency Medical Services (EMS) course was unique in that it concluded with a triage exercise with

TABLE 33-1   Performance Objectives Matrix

Performance Requirements

Legend for requirements: O - basic level ● - advanced level ◆ - specialized

AREAS OF COMPETENCY	REF.	AWARENESS — EMPLOYEES (FACILITY WORKERS, HOSPITAL SUPPORT PERSONNEL, JANITORS, SECURITY GUARDS)	AWARENESS — RESPONDERS (INITIAL FIREFIGHTERS, POLICE OFFICERS, 911 OPERATORS/DISPATCHERS)	OPERATIONS (INCIDENT RESPONSE TEAMS, EMS BASIC HAZMAT PERSONNEL ON SCENE)	TECHNICIAN/SPECIALIST (INCIDENT RESPONSE TEAM SPECIALIST, TECHNICIANS, EMS ADVANCED, AND MEDICAL SPECIALIST)	INCIDENT COMMAND (INCIDENT COMMANDERS)
1. Know the potential for terrorist use of NBC weapons:	C, F, M, m, G					
• know what the NBC weapons substances are		O	●	●	●	●
• know their hazards and the risks associated with them		O	●	●	◆	●
• know likely locations for their use		O	●	●	●	●
• know the potential outcomes of their use by terrorists		O	●	●	●	●
• know indicators of possible criminal or terrorist activity involving such agents			●	●	●	●
• know behavior of NBC agents			●	●	◆	●
2. Know the indicators, signs, and symptoms for exposure to NBC agents, and identify the agents from signs and symptoms, if possible.	C, F, M, m	O	●	●	◆	●
2a. Know questions to ask caller to elicit critical information regarding an NBC incident.	G, m		● (911 only)			
2b. Recognize unusual trends that may indicate an NBC incident.	G, m	O	●	●	◆	●
3. Understand relevant NBC response plans and SOPs and your role in them.	C, F, M, m	O	●	●	●	●
4. Recognize and communicate the need for additional resources during a NBC incident.	C, m, G	O	●	●	●	●

(continued)

TABLE 33-1 *(continued)*

Performance Requirements

Legend for requirements: O - basic level ● - advanced level ◆ - specialized

AREAS OF COMPETENCY	COMPETENCY LEVEL		AWARENESS		OPERATIONS	TECHNICIAN/ SPECIALIST	INCIDENT COMMAND
	EXAMPLES	REF.	EMPLOYEES — FACILITY WORKERS, HOSPITAL SUPPORT PERSONNEL, JANITORS, SECURITY GUARDS	RESPONDERS — INITIAL FIREFIGHTERS, POLICE OFFICERS, 911 OPERATORS/ DISPATCHERS	INCIDENT RESPONSE TEAMS, EMS BASIC HAZMAT PERSONNEL ON SCENE	INCIDENT RESPONSE TEAM SPECIALIST, TECHNICIANS, EMS ADVANCED, AND MEDICAL SPECIALIST	INCIDENT COMMANDERS
5. Make proper notification and communicate the NBC hazard.		C, F, M, m	O	●	●	●	●
6. Understand: • NBC agent terms • NBC toxicology terms		C, F, m	O	●	● ● (EMS-8 only)	● ●	● ●
7. Use individual protection at a NBC incident • Self-protection measures • Assigned NBC protective equipment		C, F, M, m	O	●	● ●	◆ ◆	● ●
8. Know protective measures and how to initiate actions to protect others and safeguard property in an NBC incident. • Selection and use of PPE		F, M	O	●	● ●	◆ ●	● ●
8a. Know measures of evacuation of personnel in a downwind hazard area for an NBC incident.		M, G		●	●	●	●
9. Know CB decontamination procedures for self, victims, site, equipment, and mass casualties: • Understand and implement • Determine		C, F, M, m	O self	●	● ● ●	◆ ◆ ●	● ● ●
10. Know crime scene and evidence preservation at an NBC incident.		F, M, m	O	● (except 911)	●	●	●

	Description	Codes	Col 1	Col 2	Col 3	Col 4
10a.	Know procedures and safety precautions for collecting legal evidence at an NBC incident.	F, G, m	●	◆	●	●
11.	Know federal and other support infrastructure and how to access in an NBC incident.	C, F, M, m	◆	●	○	○ (911 only)
12.	Understand the risks of operating in protective clothing when used at an NBC incident.	C, F, m	●	●	●	○
13.	Understand emergency and first aid procedures for exposure to NBC agents, and principles of triage.	F, M	○	◆	●	○
14.	Know how to perform hazard and risk assessment for NBC agents.	C, F, M, m	●	◆	●	
15.	Understand termination/all clear procedures for an NBC incident.	C, F, m	●	●	●	
16.	Incident Command System/ Incident Management System • Function within role in NBC incident • Implement for NBC incident	C, F, M	◆	●	●	
17.	Know how to perform NBC contamination control and containment operations, including for fatalities.	C, F, M, m	◆ ●	◆	●	
17a.	Understand procedures and equipment for safe transport of contaminated items.	G, m	●	◆	●	
18.	Know the classification, detection, identification, and verification of NBC materials using field survey instruments and equipment, and methods for collection of solid, liquid, and gas samples.	C, F, M, m	●	◆	○	
19.	Know safe patient extraction and NBC antidote administration.	F, m	○	◆ (medical only)	● (medical only)	
20.	Know patient assessment and emergency medical treatment in NBC incident.	M, m, G		◆ (medical only)	● (medical only)	

(continued)

TABLE 33-1 (continued)

Performance Requirements

Legend for requirements: O - basic level ● - advanced level ◆ - specialized

		AWARENESS		OPERATIONS	TECHNICIAN/SPECIALIST	INCIDENT COMMAND
		EMPLOYEES	RESPONDERS			
AREAS OF COMPETENCY	REF.	FACILITY WORKERS, HOSPITAL SUPPORT PERSONNEL, JANITORS, SECURITY GUARDS	INITIAL FIREFIGHTERS, POLICE OFFICERS, 911 OPERATORS/ DISPATCHERS	INCIDENT RESPONSE TEAMS, EMS BASIC HAZMAT PERSONNEL ON SCENE	INCIDENT RESPONSE TEAM SPECIALIST, TECHNICIANS, EMS ADVANCED, AND MEDICAL SPECIALIST	INCIDENT COMMANDERS
21. Be familiar with NBC, related public health and local EMS issues.	G			●	●	O
22. Know procedures for patient transport following NBC incident.	F, G			● (medical only)	● (medical only)	O
23. Execute NBC triage and primary care.	G			● (medical only)	◆ (medical only)	
24. Know laboratory identification and diagnosis for biological agents.	G			(medical only)	◆ (medical only)	
25. Have the ability to develop a site safety plan and control plan for an NBC incident.	C, F				◆ (medical only)	◆
26. Have ability to develop NBC response plan and conduct exercise of response.	G, m					●

Legend for references: C, 29 CFR 1910.120 (OSHA Hazardous Waste Operations and Emergency response); M, Macro objectives developed by a training subgroup of the Senior Interagency Coordinating Group); m, Micro objectives developed by U.S. Army Chemical & Biological Defence Command; G, Focus Group workshop; F, NFPA Standard 472 (Professional Competence of Responders to Hazardous Materials Incidents) and/or NFPA Standard 473 (Competencies for EMS Personnel Responding to Hazardous Materials Incidents).

moulaged victims; most students found it to be the highlight of the training session.

It is interesting to note that an ongoing quality improvement process, using feedback from the student evaluations and city officials, resulted in the program creating eight updated versions by the time it transitioned from its original sponsor, the SBCCOM to the Department of Justice (DOJ) in October 2000. During the Department of Defense's tenure, 28,500 responders (medical and nonmedical) in 1,700 classes were trained in 105 cities.

One of the authors of this chapter was the primary developer of the first DP program medical module, which began as a component of the first responder program of instruction used in Denver, Colorado. This module was later replaced by two distinct medical courses—one for prehospital providers and one for hospital providers.

The DP program visited each city for one week, during which time six courses were offered. The courses were Responder Awareness, Responder Operations, Technician–EMS, Technician–HazMat, Technician–Hospital Provider, and Incident Command System. The final day was set aside for a table-top exercise, which was intended to reinforce the lessons learned earlier in the week while providing the opportunity for participants of different disciplines to interact with one another, sometimes for the first time. The first city to receive the complete DP program was Philadelphia.

Once the train-the-trainer program was completed, subsequent return visits to the cities were used to conduct broader table-top exercises integrating local and state participants, with the endpoint of the learning process being a wide-scale field exercise. The exercises were also intended to reinforce the training, to evaluate its efficacy, and to provide feedback to the participants in the form of after action reports.

The DP program Awareness level training (the basic, introductory course) incorporated a paradigm described with the acronym "RAIN"—*recognize, avoid, isolate, and notify*. These are great umbrella concepts for any medical response to terrorism and serve to heighten awareness by early *recognition* and suspicion, which are even more relevant in today's times of "heightened vigilance" recommended by the Department of Homeland Security. *Avoiding* contact with victims and/or toxic substances protects the responder and reduces any possible spread of contamination as does *isolation. Notification* alerts the appropriate authorities and opens the lines of communication for requesting additional resources from state and federal agencies.

Two unique teaching methods were utilized. One was teaming an emergency responder with a subject matter expert to combine the skills and expertise of the nation's nuclear, biological, and chemical experts with the skills and expertise of experienced emergency responders (12). The other was the emphasis on what was coined the NBC Delta—the "difference between the standard HazMat incident and one involving the use of nuclear, biological or chemical, materials often referred to as Weapons of Mass Destruction (WMD)" (13). It is interesting to note that these terms have been used interchangeably, and, as knowledge has become more sophisticated and different organizations have tried to personalize their training efforts, many new acronyms have emerged. Examples include B-NICE (Biological, Nuclear, Incendiary, Chemical and Explosive agents) and CBRNE (Chemical, Biological, Radiological, Nuclear and high-yield Explosive) which is the current acronym of choice for the Department of Defense (DOD).

The NBC Delta can be graphically illustrated (Fig. 33-2) (14) as a triangle with the broader base representing

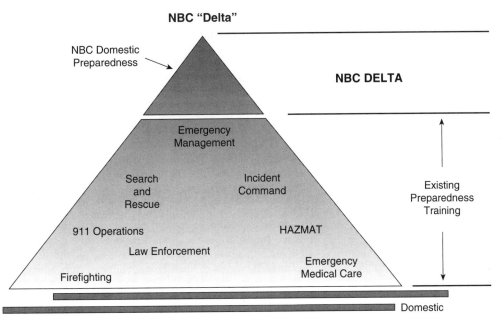

Figure 33–2. NBC Delta.

existing emergency response training and the narrower apex the additional NBC information provided in the DP program. Using a "building block approach" (15) existing training is supplemented with terrorism and NBC training (Fig. 33-2).

Many similarities exist between a hazmat incident and an NBC attack (16). Terrorist events will likely result in many individuals presenting with medically unexplained physical symptoms (the "worried well"), which could rapidly overwhelm the health care system and necessitate the use of novel triage methods to isolate actual from potential victims (17). Hospitals currently operate at maximum bed capacity and use just-in-time supplies. In order to cope with the sudden increased needs resulting from a terrorist attack, the ability to increase surge capacity must be developed ahead of time. One of the goals of the DP program was to help enhance the surge capacity, while also making it practical and applicable to normal disasters, epidemics, and other times of increased use of health care and emergency response resources.

One of the major advantages of the DP program was the integration of local, state, and federal agencies at the regional level. This merger has set the precedent for more recent planning and educational efforts including those now funded by the Centers for Disease Control and Prevention (CDC) and the Health Resources Service Administration (HRSA), both of which call for regionalization of planning efforts.

A serious disadvantage was the decision to select cities based on population size, without considering either their possible vulnerability or proximity to one another. As a result, some large geographical regions of the country were bypassed. It was also thought that by directly interacting with the city administrations, DOD may not have taken advantage of existing training structures and emergency management already in place in the states (18).

The DP program laid a solid groundwork for future WMD training. But it is important to note that the program did not operate in a vacuum. During the same period, the U.S. Army Medical Research Institute of Chemical Defense (USAMRICD) and the U.S. Army Medical Research Institute of Infectious Diseases (USAMRIID) were providing courses both at their facilities in Maryland

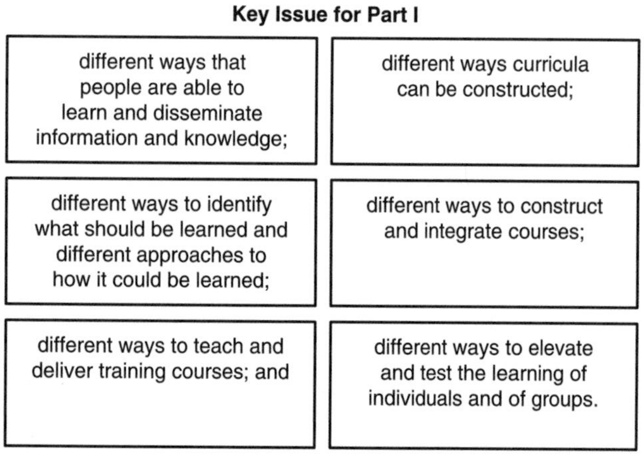

and, starting in 1998, via satellite broadcast. Both organizations developed for the military handbooks that became widely used by first responders and were distributed to the students who participated in the medical modules of the DP program (19). These handbooks, together with the *Textbook of Military Medicine* (see the Resources section at the end of this chapter), are available both on CD-ROM and on the Internet for download to a PDA.

The Department of Justice's Office of Justice Programs (OJP), which was responsible for the DP program after its transition from DOD, developed the National Domestic Preparedness Consortium, whose five members, Louisiana State University, Texas A&M University, the New Mexico Institute of Mining and Technology, the Department of Energy's Nevada test site, and OJP's Center for Domestic Preparedness at Fort McClellan, Alabama, received funding to develop and implement specialized training for first responders.

The General Accounting Office's report "Combating Terrorism: Observations on the Nunn-Lugar-Domenici Domestic Preparedness Program" describes an effort to coordinate multiple training efforts (20). This task fell to the Department of Justice, which uses several different mechanisms to unify a fragmented system and to ensure that trainers and educators are provided with a compendium of courses from which to select those most suited to their purposes. The Office for Domestic Preparedness (ODP) training catalog (21) gives the educator detailed descriptions of courses offered. Local organizations apply to their state's training point of contact who, once this has been approved, works with the ODP training partner to schedule the course either at a location within the requesting jurisdiction or at the training partner's site.

A task force convened for the purpose of identifying objectives and competencies for training in NBC preparedness concluded that there is a lack of NBC response training in U.S. medical and nursing schools (22). There is only limited training in NBC preparedness in emergency medicine residency training programs.

The OJP ODP, formerly the Office for State and Local Domestic Preparedness Support (OSLDPS), developed a training strategy for first responders regarding who should be trained and what tasks they should be trained to perform. They describe how to select delivery methods and training sites for optimum results, evaluation methods, and how to determining the gaps in the existing training (23,24). This is summarized in the six key issues that are basic to teaching efforts relating to NBC terrorism as documented in Fig. 33-3 (25). The ODP model process for WMD training is illustrated in Fig. 33-4 (26).

The resultant ODP Training Strategy and ODP Emergency Responder Guidelines give detailed discussions on the skills, knowledge, capabilities, and recommendations needed for an effective response and provide an excellent tool for educators to use to ensure that all the different pieces of the response can be coordinated into a cohesive unit (i.e., interoperability). (See the Resources section at the end of the chapter.) In the electronic version of the responder guidelines, each response element is linked to the appropriate training courses for easy access.

Key Issue for Part I

different ways that people are able to learn and disseminate information and knowledge;	different ways curricula can be constructed;
different ways to identify what should be learned and different approaches to how it could be learned;	different ways to construct and integrate courses;
different ways to teach and deliver training courses; and	different ways to elevate and test the learning of individuals and of groups.

Figure 33–3. Key issues for part one.

Model Process for WMD Training

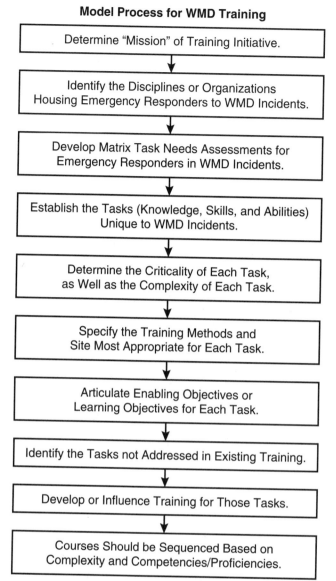

Figure 33–4. Model process for WMD training.

EVOLUTION OF INNOVATIVE EDUCATION

Since the attacks on the World Trade Center and the Pentagon on September 11, 2001, and the anthrax attacks of October 2001 many innovative training programs have been developed. The urgency of improving the preparedness status of the first response community and that of the hospitals—"first receivers"—combined with additional funding from the Department of Homeland Security, CDC, and HRSA, have provided incentives to find better methods to reach larger audiences as quickly as possible. For example, following the anthrax attacks of 2001 and the discovery of SARS, many just-in-time Internet-based learning tools were provided to the medical community to teach the pathophysiology of these diseases, how to protect oneself, recognition of signs and

symptoms, decontamination, isolation, treatment, etc. Another example of such adaptation is a program entitled "Terrorism Response and Emergency Care" (TREC) that was developed in the southwestern United States. It uses a 4-hour teaching module delivered twice-daily at various sites and electronic audience participation systems. The goal of such a course is to provide teaching to busy health care providers to whom such information is essential, in a concise, efficient format. (14, personal communication).

It is becoming clear that some flexibility needs to exist in training formats and techniques. Based on this premise, ODP is now pursuing a blended learning approach to provide modular training content in a variety of mediums. The ODP is advocating the application of technological advances with more traditional training methods. Two examples of the blended learning approach are Navy Medicine's Disaster Preparedness, Vulnerability Analysis, Training and Exercise (DVATEX) program and Dartmouth's Virtual Terrorism-Response Academy (VTRA). Next-generation methods are being used to better prepare our nation's medical providers and to improve their ability to respond to an act of terrorism.

The U.S. Navy Medicine Office of Homeland Security developed the DVATEX program to help Navy hospitals and clinics worldwide strengthen their level of emergency preparedness to meet new threats in the environment. This program uses two new self-assessment tools. The first of these is described as the "Hospital Emergency Analysis Tool" or HEAT, which assesses the presence of over 250 factors contributing to effective hospital emergency response. The second is the Analysis Tool for Ambulatory Care (ATAC). After the self-assessment process is complete, a multidisciplinary team of emergency preparedness experts visits each Navy hospital and clinic and conducts CBRNE training for hospital staff, performs a vulnerability analysis, and stages an infectious disease table-top exercise to validate the facility's emergency management plan. The DVATEX program endeavors to identify vulnerabilities and provides recommendations for remedies, while helping develop long-term plans to improve preparedness levels. Table-top exercises, which are simulated NBC attacks, have been conducted both in the continental United States and at U.S. Navy facilities overseas.

The VTRA model is being developed by Dartmouth's Program on Counterterrorism Preparedness and Training (PCPT) (27,28). This program focuses on developing multimedia and Web-based education and sometimes uses advanced video gaming software techniques in a novel way to engage students in terrorism preparedness. Students are being taught how to recognize terrorist attacks, respond to incidents properly, and protect themselves and members of their communities.

This chapter provides an introduction to various methods either currently available or in development to educate health care providers on how best to respond to acts of terrorism. The discussion includes an introduction to the DP program and other training programs, an evaluation of the value of realistic exercises, and a review of some Internet and technology-based courses, as well as an assessment of the importance of curriculum design.

RESOURCES

1. "Emergency Preparedness and Response Competencies for Hospital Workers," "Bioterrorism and Emergency Readiness for All Public Health Workers," and "International Nursing Coalition for Mass Casualty Education—Educational Competencies for Registered Nurses Responding Mass Casualty Incidents." Available from: http://www.nursing.hs.columbia.edu/institute-centers/chphsr/index.html.

2. *Textbook of Military Medicine—TMM8 Medical Aspects of Chemical and Biological Warfare,* Office of the Surgeon General, Dept. of the Army.

3. *Medical Management of Chemical Casualties Handbook.* Available at http://www.gmha.org/bioterrorism/usamricd/Yellow_Book_2000.pdf.

4. *Medical Management of Biological Casualties Handbook.* Available from: http://www.nbc-med.org/SiteContent/HomePage/WhatsNew/MedManual/Feb01/handbook.htm.

5. *Medical Management of Radiological Casualties,* 2nd edition., Bethesda, MD: Armed Forces Radiobiology Research Institute; April 2003. Available from: http://www.afrri.usuhs.mil/www/outreach/pdf/2edmmrchandbook.pdf; Site visited on April 18, 2004.

6. Office for Domestic Preparedness, *Approach for Blended Learning.* Available from: http://www.ojp.usdoj.gov/odp/blendedlearning/pdfs/bls.pdf.

7. Office for Domestic Preparedness Weapons of Mass Destruction Training Program: Enhancing State and Local Capabilities to Respond to Incidents of Terrorism. Available from: http://www.ojp.usdoj.gov/odp/docs/coursecatalog.pdf.

8. *Jane's Mass Casualty Handbook: Hospital Emergency Preparedness and Response.*

9. *Jane's Mass Casualty Handbook: Pre-hospital Emergency Preparedness and Response.*

10. Centers for Disease Control and Prevention. Useful information on education, including announcements of satellite broadcasts and Web-based training courses are also available to the reader on the CDC's web site: www.cdc.gov.

11. University web sites provide another excellent resource as do those of local and state government.

12. Texas Terrorism Response and Emergency Care course, 2002–2003, University of Texas Southwestern Medical Center, Dallas, Texas, and the Texas Department of Health. D. C. Keyes, personal communication.

13. Colombia University School of Nursing, Clinical Competencies for Different Health Care Providers and Public Health Workers. Available from: http://www.nursing.hs.columbia.edu/institute-centers/chphsr/index.html.

14. Office for Domestic Preparedness, ODP Approach for Blended Learning. Available from: http://www.ojp.usdoj.gov/odp/blendedlearning/pdfs/bls.pdf.

REFERENCES

1. Booz Allen Hamilton. Understanding needs for health system preparedness and capacity for bioterrorist attacks [report]. Maryland: Agency for Healthcare Research and Quality; 2002.

2. National Vaccine Program Office. Pandemic influenza: a planning guide for state and local officials (Draft 2.1) [planning guide]. Atlanta: Centers for Disease Control and Prevention; 2000.

3. Barbera JA, Macintyre AG. Jane's mass casualty handbook: hospital emergency preparedness and response, first edition. Surrey, UK: Jane's Information Group; 2003.

4. Office for Domestic Preparedness. Exercise development and support. [online]. Available from: URL: http://www.ojp.usdoj.gov/odp/exercises/state.htm#nep. Accessed on January 11, 2004.

5. Miller J. U.S. has new concerns about anthrax readiness. *New York Times,* Dec 28, 2003.

6. Domestic Preparedness Program. Training overview DPT 8.0 [CD-ROM]. Maryland: U.S. Army Soldier and Biological Chemical Command; 1999.

7. Report to Congressional Requesters. Combating terrorism: opportunities to improve domestic preparedness program focus and efficiency [report]. Washington, DC: General Accounting Office; 1999.

8. Domestic Preparedness Program. Training overview DPT 8.0 [CD-ROM]. Maryland: U.S. Army Soldier and Biological Chemical Command; 1999.

9. U.S. Department of Defense. Report to Congress annex A, volume I, domestic preparedness program in the defense against weapons of mass destruction: performance objectives matrix [online]. Available from: http://www.defenselink.mil/pubs/domestic/annexa/html. Accessed January 11, 2004.

10. Friel G. Congressional testimony for hearing on federal response to domestic terrorism involving weapons of mass destruction status or Department of Defense support program [online]. Available from: http://www.fas.org/spp/starwars/congress/1998_h/3-21-98friel.htm. Accessed on January 11, 2004.

11. Domestic Preparedness Program. Training overview DPT 8.0 [CD-ROM]. Maryland: U.S. Army Soldier and Biological Chemical Command; 1999.

12. Friel G. Congressional Testimony for hearing on Federal response to domestic terrorism involving weapons of mass destruction status or Department of Defense support program [online]. Available from URL: http://www.fas.org/spp/starwars/congress/1998_h/3-21-98friel.htm. Accessed on January 11, 2004.

13. Socher MM. NBC Delta: special training beyond HAZMAT in the USA. Resuscitation 1999;42:151-3.

14. Domestic Preparedness Program. Training overview DPT 8.0 [CD-ROM]. Maryland: U.S. Army Soldier and Biological Chemical Command; 1999.

15. Socher MM. NBC Delta: special training beyond HAZMAT in the USA. Resuscitation 1999;42:151-3.

16. Domestic Preparedness Program. Training overview DPT 8.0 [CD-ROM]. Maryland: U.S. Army Soldier and Biological Chemical Command; 1999.

17. Weedn VW, McDonald MD, Locke SE, et al. Crisis health risk self-assessment tools for personal biodefense and health infrastructure protection. Eng Med Biol In press.

18. Report to Congressional Requesters. Combating terrorism: opportunities to improve domestic preparedness program focus and efficiency [report]. Washington, DC: General Accounting Office; 1999.

19. USAMRICD. Medical management of chemical casualties handbook. Maryland; 1999. USAMRIID. Medical management of biological casualties handbook. Maryland; 1998.

20. Testimony before subcommittee on national security et al. Combating terrorism: observations on the Nunn-Lugar-Domenici

domestic preparedness program [testimony]. Washington, DC: General Accounting Office; 1999.

21. Office for Domestic Preparedness. Weapons of mass destruction training program: enhancing state and local capabilities to respond to incidents of terrorism [online]. Available from: URL: http://www.ojp.usdoj.gov/odp/docs/coursecatalog.pdf. Accessed January 11, 2004.

22. Waeckerle JF, Seamans S, Whiteside M, et al. Task force of health care and emergency services professionals on preparedness for nuclear, biological, and chemical incidents. Ann Emerg Med 2001;37(6):587-601.

23. Pelfrey WV, Kelley WD, May JW. Executive summary: the Office for Domestic Preparedness Training Strategy. Washington, DC: Office of Justice Programs, Department of Justice; 2002.

24. Pelfrey WV, Kelley WD, May JW. Executive summary: the Office for Domestic Preparedness Training Strategy. Washington, DC: Office of Justice Programs, Department of Justice; 2002.

25. Pelfrey WV, Kelley WD, May JW. Executive summary: the Office for Domestic Preparedness Training Strategy. Washington, DC: Office of Justice Programs, Department of Justice; 2002.

26. Pelfrey WV, Kelley WD, May JW. Executive summary: the Office for Domestic Preparedness Training Strategy. Washington, DC: Office of Justice Programs, Department of Justice; 2002.

27. Interactive Media Laboratory Dartmouth College. Program on counter-terrorism preparedness & training virtual terrorism-response academy [online]. Available from: http://www.ists.dartmouth.edu/IML/projects.htm.

28. Columbia University School of Nursing. Clinical competencies for different health care providers and public health workers. Available at: http://www.nursing.hs.columbia.edu/institute-centers/chphsr/index.html. Accessed on April 18, 2004.

34

Technology Applications in Preparedness Training

Timothy D. Peterson

INTRODUCTION

Preparedness education, training, and learning opportunities are absolutely essential for an efficient and effective medical response system to terrorism. The classrooms of today have a multiform appearance, with no standard single setting or method of teaching. The traditional classroom setting with students and teacher in the same room at the same time doing the same thing is often evolving into a virtual classroom where students are able to access instructional material and complete the course objectives at a time and place of their convenience. Education and training in health sciences have traditionally taken place both in the classroom and at the patient bedside to enable cognitive and psychomotor skills to be integrated in real time. Current demands for terrorism training are exceeding the means available by traditional settings alone.

The recent technological development of distance learning and simulators with the capability of physiological response monitoring associated with changing scenarios and hands-on intervention enables a larger number of students to participate in initial training and refresher experiences. It is becoming apparent that today's challenges of terrorism training will be increasingly addressed by emerging opportunities provided by new applications of technology, which are creating new paradigms for education. As participants in this new technology wave, both teachers and students have increasing access to rich learning environments.

In order to develop and implement a successful medical response to the terrorism training process, it is important to understand not only the fundamentals of the learning process but also to be aware of recent advances in technology and their potential applications. This chapter provides an overview of learning theory and process and then focuses on the technology available and the related challenges integrating technology into the health sciences for terrorism training. Because this is a relatively new challenge to educators and variables are unique to each setting, principles that apply for integrating new

technology into education and training are only recently beginning to emerge. As new applications develop, outcomes related to retention of skills and knowledge for terrorism training need to be monitored and published in peer-reviewed journals in order to provide further guidance as to what technology is cost effective in various settings. The information here can be used as a resource for planning in conjunction with needs assessments within individual geographical settings and jurisdictions. Because technical aspects are developing rapidly, there are likely some that have not been covered in this chapter and new ones that will have emerged at the time of this publication.

PREPAREDNESS ESSENTIALS

LEARNING BASICS

Learning refers to the acquisition of skills, knowledge, ability, and attitudes. *Education* refers to the core content and curriculum objectives designed to achieve the desired learning. *Training* refers to the specific process by which learning of the specific core content and curriculum objectives is achieved. Achieving and sustaining a level of learning with the desired impact on skills, knowledge, ability, and attitudes depend on the effectiveness of the training process to impart the core content and curriculum objectives to the student.

Individual students learn in a variety of ways. Three learning theories are briefly examined for consideration. These involve the *behavioral approach*, the *cognitive approach*, and *social learning*. Any one of a combination of these theories may or may not be relevant to a given technological application to learning. An understanding of how individuals learn may be useful when considering a specific technological application.

The *behavioral approach* (power of rewards) involves the repeated pairing of a stimulus and response that yields a reward. Pavlov's (1) groundbreaking work with dogs demonstrated that pairing the ringing of a bell with a meal several times eventually caused the dog to salivate with the ringing of the bell alone. Positive reinforcement of a stimulus was shown to produce a desired (conditioned) behavioral response. Training in a new work process must therefore involve positive reinforcement of a stimulus when the desired outcome is achieved. Likewise, negative stimulus should be reserved for an undesired outcome.

The *cognitive approach* uses the internal mental process and involves various cues in the environment to form a mental map. In early cognitive experiments, for example, rats learned to run through a maze to reach a goal of food (2). Repeated trials caused the rats to develop and strengthen cognitive connections that identified the correct path to the goal. People can also develop cognitive maps that show the path to a specific goal. Repeated use of an algorithm for assessment and treatment builds the association with an internal map and the desired outcome. Training in a new work process should therefore result in a new cognitive map of job performance. With increasing application, the individual should develop and sustain new links between the tasks that comprise the job and optimal ways of linking and performing them. Advances in technology provide a great opportunity for automated training. Such systems must use cues inherent in the situation to help learners develop cognitive maps around specific tasks.

People can also learn by modeling or imitating behaviors, as described in *social learning* theory (3). This theory integrates the behavioral and cognitive approaches and involves the following steps:

1. Learners watch others, who act as models.
2. Learners develop a mental picture of the behavior and its consequences.
3. Learners try the behavior themselves.
4. Learners repeat the behavior if positive consequences result. Learners do not repeat the behavior if negative consequences occur.

Studies analyzing the impact of social learning indicate an average gain of 17% in performance (4). Different types of reinforcement produce different outcomes. For example, performance feedback had a greater impact than monetary reinforcement in manufacturing organizations, whereas the reverse was true in service organizations (3).

Modeling and imitating behaviors as a way of learning can apply to both on-the-job and off-the-job training. Trainers present models of good performance, and the trainees see the relationship between these desirable behaviors and the consequences. Trainees then rehearse the behaviors and consequences, building cognitive maps that intensify the links and set the stage for future behavior. The learning impact occurs when the subject tries the behavior and experiences a favorable result. The learner develops a cognitive image of the situation, which provides a way of thinking about the steps in acquiring new skills, knowledge, ability, or attitudes (5).

The bottom-line question becomes "How can learning be encouraged?" The answer, fundamentally, is as follows: It must involve energetic presentations, provide information in an easily accessible manner, and provide some enjoyment or positive stimulus. Successful learning has been shown to involve the appropriate conditions, reinforcement of the desired learning behaviors, environmental cues that encourage learning, and a modeling strategy (6).

PERFORMANCE-BASED LEARNING

Education and training within the health sciences is increasingly using a performance-based or competency-based theory of design. In the computer science field, for example, Cisco System's RIO (Reusable Information Objects) project is explicitly performance based. Based on work from Ruth Clark (7) embracing contemporary learning theory, RIO views all training as a means to enable a worker to complete a task successfully (8). This process follows three steps:

1. Identify the job task.
2. Identify the skills and knowledge necessary to complete the task.
3. Develop training in modular chunks that are organized to support the task.

Using the RIO model, learning is based on outcome rather than content. It focuses on what people need to do, rather than on what there is to know.

Suppose, for example, a medical equipment company produced a new device. The content approach to training would list the product's features, develop instruction on these features, and then quiz for recall of the features. In contrast, an outcome approach would begin by assessing the patient's indications for use of the device and then match the patient's needs to the device's capabilities. The quiz would be performance based and involve the ability to use the device correctly in appropriate patient scenarios.

As technology applications are woven into the learning process, it becomes clear that suitable tools and resources depend on the overall core content and objectives of learning and how to achieve a successful performance-based outcome.

DISTANCE LEARNING

Within the context of rapid technological change and shifting market conditions, the American education system is challenged with providing increased learning opportunities, often with decreased budgets. Many educational institutions are answering this challenge by developing distance learning. The United States Distance Learning Association (USDLA) defines distance learning as "the acquisition of knowledge and skills through mediated information and instruction, encompassing all technologies and other forms of learning at a distance" (9). At its most basic level, distance learning takes place when a teacher and student(s) are separated by physical distance and technology (i.e., voice, video, data, and print), often in concert with face-to-face communication, is used to bridge the instructional gap (10). Distance learning therefore encompasses all technologies and supports the pursuit of lifelong learning for all (11).

Distance learning has the distinct advantage of providing students with limited time, distance, or physical disability the opportunity to update their knowledge at the place of their employment or even at home. The scheduling of courses for distance learning often takes into consideration that most of the students are working professionals who participate in continuing education programming in addition to their full-time job responsibilities. Therefore, a distinct advantage of distance learning is the ability to schedule at the learner's discretion regarding time and location.

Providing access across a wide geographical area involving not only the urban setting but also rural, remote, and wilderness areas makes the application of distance learning methodologies essential. Regardless of the classroom setting, a wide range of instructional methodologies is available to facilitate interaction on site or through distance learning. The decision regarding which methodology will be applied is often driven by cost, flexibility for the faculty and students, objectives, content, and outcomes supported by available technology.

Research comparing distance education to the traditional classroom setting indicates that teaching and studying at a distance can be as effective as traditional instruction when methods and technologies used are appropriate to the instructional tasks, there is student-to-student interaction, and there is timely teacher-to-student feedback (12,13). According to the USDLA, research studies have found consistently that distance learning classrooms can be as effective as traditional instruction methods. In addition, research studies often point out that student attitudes about distance learning are generally positive (14).

Distance learning has become increasingly common. Most students who enroll in distance education courses are over 25 years old, employed, and have previous college experience. More than half are women. As a group, distance learners are highly motivated (15). Therefore, the successful distance learner is, by definition, a committed student who will establish a schedule and adhere to it. A wide range of employers are finding it difficult to release employees for on-campus study and discovering it is a good investment to bring the classroom to their work sites. According to a survey conducted by the International Foundation of Employee Benefits Plans, employees rank continuing education as more important than child care, flextime, and family leave (15). Faced with retraining 50 million American workers, corporate America is using distance learning, both internally and externally, for all aspects of training (14).

A wide variety of technological options is available for distance learning. The four major categories of delivery, based on the University of Idaho College of Engineering Outreach overview (16), are as follows:

1. Voice: Instructional audio tools include the interactive technologies of telephone, audio conferencing, and short-wave radio. Passive (one-way) tools include tapes and radio.

2. Video: Instructional video tools include still images such as PowerPoint presentations, preproduced moving images (e.g., film, videotape), CD/DVD-based presentation with live and synchronized online component, and live and archived webcasting or utilization of learning platforms such as WebCT or Blackboard.

3. Data: Computers send and receive information electronically. For this reason, the term "data" is used to describe

this broad category of instructional tools. Computer applications for distance education are varied and include the following:

- Computer-assisted instruction (CAI): Uses the computer as a self-contained teaching machine to present individual lessons.
- Computer-managed instruction (CMI): Uses the computer to organize instruction and track student records and progress. The instruction itself need not be delivered via a computer, although CAI is often combined with CMI.
- Computer-mediated education (CME): Describes computer applications that facilitate the delivery of instruction. Examples include electronic mail, fax, real-time computer.

4. Print: Forms the foundation of all education programs and is the basis of all the other delivery systems. Various print formats include textbooks, study guides, workbooks, course syllabi, and case studies.

The four categories just listed form a basic model, but technology is rapidly leading to new applications as the World Wide Web related software and hardware expands with opportunities, speed, and access. Web-based instruction (WBI) is a hypermedia-based instructional method that utilizes the attributes and resources of the Web to create a meaningful learning environment where learning is fostered and supported. Kahn (17) reports that WBI should include many resources, support collaboration, implement web-based activities as part of the learning framework, and support both novices and experts in the context of the Web's potential in relation to instructional design principles. E-mail in a WBI instructional program can provide asynchronous communication among students and instructor. Likewise, e-mail, listserves, newsgroups, and conferencing tools can jointly contribute to the creation of a virtual community on the Web.

Although technology plays a key role in the delivery of distance learning, educators must remain focused on instructional outcomes, not the technology of delivery. The key to effective distance learning is focusing on the needs of the learners, the requirements of the content, and the constraints faced by the instructor before choosing a delivery system. Effective distance learning programs develop with careful planning and evolve with hard work and dedicated efforts of many individuals, including the integrated efforts of students, faculty, facilitators, support staff, and administrators. Meeting the instructional needs of the students to master the education content is the litmus test by which the effectiveness of distance learning programs must be judged.

Distance learning has the promise of being more efficient from a time and cost per student perspective. The USDLA reports that major corporations save millions of dollars each year using distance learning to train employees more effectively and more efficiently than with conventional methods (14). Effectiveness of achieving cognitive skills has been validated (12–14), but effectiveness related to psychomotor skills is not yet widely reported. Until recently, applications of distance learning in health sciences have been most suited to cognitive aspects of learning and are now widely reported in the literature (18–25). With the development of fiber-optic and satellite communication systems involving simultaneous audio and visual capabilities has come the possibilities of patient consultation, instruction, and oversight of diagnostic and surgical techniques and patient follow-up connecting the rural/remote/wilderness physicians and their patients with tertiary referral centers and their specialists. Medical literature is now beginning to report success stories regarding the psychomotor aspects of distance learning (26–39). The concept of a virtual medical campus is now breaking the barriers of time and space, a revolution that has great capacity to influence every aspect of medicine, the advent of which may prove crucial to meet current needs for disaster medicine training.

TELEMEDICINE

The first telemedicine standard to be developed, documented, and adopted widely was the radiology standard, which includes technical and image transmission standards as well as requirements and qualifications needed for teleradiology practice (37). Subsequently, many other subspecialties are engaging in telemedicine, finding the need and use of special skills and knowledge. For example, a surgeon faced with the need to provide an acute intervention can benefit from real-time operative assistance from colleagues in another state or country. When faced with implementing a new lifesaving procedure for the first time, in lieu of sending an unstable patient many miles away where the procedure is done routinely, telemedicine technology provides immediate access and can save considerable time and expense. The telepresence surgery system permits the surgeon to operate on a patient across a distance, achieved through real-time 3D video vision, stereo audio, and remote instrument control with haptic feedback (31). Surgical applications are reported for virtual reality simulator training in arthroscopy (28), endoscopic (38), laproscopic (26,39), and cardiac procedures (32) in a real-time learning environment where a series of tasks can be evaluated to determine when competence is achieved. Although virtual reality surgery exists, a number of challenges remain to improve realistic models of the human body: creating interface tools to view, hear, touch, feel, and manipulate these human body models, and integrating virtual reality systems into medical education and treatment (36).

Cruise ship medicine facilities are adding telemedicine consultation capabilities to benefit passengers with diagnostic and treatment challenges when at sea. Similarly, national and international networks of health service providers that offer telemedicine and teleconsultation services to remote, isolated places and to ship vessels for both routine and emergency situations are covering a gap not fulfilled by current bureaucratic and telematic procedures (35). Consultation and follow-up of primary care cases for dermatology, neurology, cardiology, otolaryngology, and many other specialties are finding telemedicine a useful adjunct for immediate feedback versus sending the patient miles away and awaiting the written report from the consultant by mail (25,27,29,30,34). Radiologists have the capability to read x-rays and scans on patients without needing to be at the facility, enabling timely interpretation for rural/remote/wilderness areas that are faced with treatment and transfer decisions dependent on the radiologist's report (37).

These and many other emerging applications hold promise to utilize telemedicine and other technical advances increasingly within not only the cognitive but also the psychomotor and decision-making processes of clinical medicine. Indeed, the practice of medicine has entered a virtual reality where we transmit more details about the patient directly to our medical colleagues with direct feedback instead of sending the patient, often in poor health, a long distance for evaluation and treatment, which is often further delayed by scheduling issues.

Telemedicine's potential to transform medical practice has become a reality, but many legal and ethical concerns have yet to be resolved. Silverman (40) reports four main areas of concern: the doctor-patient relationship, malpractice and cross-border licensure, standards, and reimbursement. Gaining widespread support from providers, patients, and regulatory bodies as an acceptable means of health service delivery will require consensus on standards of law and ethics. Additionally, the implications of confidentiality related to the practice of telemedicine are becoming more apparent with time and use. Recording, transfer, and storage of patient information are increasingly regulated to protect patient confidentiality, and failure to comply with requirements of the federal Health Insurance Portability and Accountability Act of 1996 (HIPAA) can place the clinician at risk for fines and licensure sanctions. A complete discussion of this is beyond the scope of this chapter, and additional detail may be found on the HIPAA web site at http://cms.hhs.gov/hipaa/. Health care providers must be aware of compliance issues and are encouraged to seek guidance specific to their clinical setting from their individual employers.

CAUTION AREAS FOR DISTANCE LEARNING

Recently there has been an explosion of distance learning programs at academic centers and on the Internet. Important red flags to watch for when considering distance learning programs, based on the work of Thomas (41), are as follows:

1. Have you looked deeper than the web site or catalog? Questionable organizations can produce spectacular web sites and call themselves bona fide educational institutions. It is time for the buyer to beware of bogus degree mills that can be mistaken for legitimate institutions by the uninformed.

2. Is the provider accredited by a recognized authority? Accreditation is the number-one verifier of the quality of a distance learning provider. All accreditation providers are not equal or recognized. The U.S. Department of Education (www.ed.gov) has a list of verified accreditors as does the Council for Higher Education Accreditation (www.chea.org). The Distance Education Training Council (www.detc.og) also can help verify accreditors. Check to see that the institution is properly licensed and approved in the state where it is located.

3. Will the certificate or credit apply and be recognized in your professional field? Especially for medical sciences that require medical licensure or certification within the state of practice, it is critical to know if the distance learning courses will meet state-established requirements for the particular professional field. Transferring credit is just as important. You must know ahead of time if the course will be credited at future institutions.

4. Does the provider have a track record of success? With distance learning evolving so quickly, it is often hard to judge quality based on longevity. Some very good programs are just getting started. At a minimum it is wise to ask if the course has been taught before or is part of a pilot. If there is no prior information about the course or program, investigate the track record of the organization itself.

5. Are the admissions policies too easy? Watch out for programs that admit students with few restrictions. Also, credit for past experience without close evaluation is unacceptable.

6. Is the class too big for adequate feedback from and interaction with the faculty? Without having to provide physical seating, the temptation for providers is to overfill a class with paying students. The more students per faculty member, the less apt students are to get the attention they need. Distance teaching and learning is often more difficult in that the contact between teacher and student can be more demanding, necessary, and time consuming to allow for adequate evaluation and feedback.

7. What is the course content and how is the material presented? In the rush to attract the growing number of students interested in distance learning, some institutions focus on high-demand fields without much regard for whether they possess the expertise. Seek information from professional societies and accrediting bodies about the history and performance of a provider as a way to access quality.

8. Are the faculty qualified? There is a big difference between instructing a room full of students and interacting with virtual students. To really teach, instructors can't simply tape their lectures and send them off. Because many courses are designed for working professionals, a combination of educational credentials, teaching experience, and real-world experience is important to look for in instructors.

9. What is the level of interaction between students and faculty members? Interaction is vital to the success of the student who sits alone instead of interacting in a classroom. Instructors must be open to questions and comments at all times, and e-mail makes this readily possible. Other options are by fax and phone.

10. What is the institution's response to your specific questions? If you send an e-mail about taking a course and do not receive a prompt response, this is a legitimate concern. Responses must be timely and complete.

11. What do current and past students who have completed the course(s) say about the program? Comments about courses and feedback from students should be available for prospective students. It can't hurt to observe or evaluate comments of peers about their distance learning experience.

PREPAREDNESS HISTORICAL EVENTS AND CASE HISTORIES

Applications of technology for domestic preparedness and disaster medicine are beginning to emerge from recent military experience (42–44). Disaster response application to telemedicine was well demonstrated in the aftermath of the tragic earthquake in Soviet Armenia in 1988. Using distanced learning to deliver first aid training in 1998 was reported successful in Alberta, Canada (45). The Alberta pilot study found that self-paced learning of the didactic component for first aid training worked well; however, hands-on evaluation of skills was mandatory to certification. Therefore, mass training where certification is needed requires a mixture of distance learning and hands-on testing. As virtual reality simulation teaching devices improve with advances in technology, evaluators may be able to participate in the certification or credentialing process from a distance. The examples described and references cited in the recent surgical literature just referenced demonstrate that confirming psychomotor aspects of learning can be done effectively from a distance.

TECHNOLOGY APPLICATIONS

Applications of technology for domestic preparedness and disaster medicine can now be envisioned. Required at this time is a series of well-structured and ongoing planning, implementation, and evaluation activities to determine what applications are cost effective in terms of skills and knowledge retention. The total financial requirements and how to support the costs associated with widespread implementation and evaluation are not fully understood, and the political intrigue of who gets what, where, when, and how has yet to be played out. These are some common complexities of the landscape that new technology faces among developers, marketers, suppliers, and consumers. How this will evolve and be paid for in the context of doing the most public good are beyond the scope of this chapter.

Nevertheless, live simulated patient encounters on management of urgent clinical problems that arose during management of the mannequin simulator in a highly realistic clinical setting have been reported as a successful learning model (46). Scenario preparation for disaster preparedness training using "smart mannequins" with the capability of physiological response monitoring associated with changing scenarios and hands-on intervention has recently been developed as part of the American Medical Association's (AMA) national training program, the Advanced Disaster Life Support (ADLS) course (47). Participants involve students interacting as coworkers of a clinical treatment team evaluating a series of patient scenarios involving any type of nuclear, biological, chemical, or environmental exposure event. The instructor and technical assistants change the physiological parameters of the mannequin based on the treatment team's assessment and interventions. For example, pupils dilate or constrict depending on type of chemical exposure and treatments given. Lung sounds diminish as a result of injury and increase after chest tube insertion. The quality and rate of pulses change in response to treatment or lack of appropriate treatment.

In relation to a battlefield or disaster situation, a virtual system can provide the environment to perfect skills and rehearse procedures before entering a hostile or chaotic live situation (48). Virtual environments involving tabletop scenarios using interactive computer-based technology have recently been developed to allow a team of responders (public safety, fire, EMS, etc.) to evaluate a given scenario, implement activities, watch the scenario evolve as a result of their decisions, and work as a team through a series of events until the exercise is completed. The intensity of the scenario can be adjusted to add a higher level of challenge for the team, such as an increased number of victims, more severe weather, and public interference at the scene. The scenario may require a sequential set of steps that the team must perform successfully in order for the conditions of the scene to mitigate and resolve.

CHALLENGES

A set of objectives for the training of emergency physicians, emergency nurses, and EMTs to care for casualties resulting from nuclear, biological, and chemical incidents was published in April 2001 by the U.S. Department of Health and Human Services Office of Emergency Preparedness and the American College of Emergency Physicians joint task force on disaster medicine training (49). Implementation of the core content and determining competencies for the nation's health care workforce in the out-of-hospital and hospital settings in order to assure timely and appropriate care along a seamless continuum will be a monumental challenge. In the United States today, there are approximately 700,000 EMTs. A significant number are volunteers, of whom approximately one-half are employed by private companies and the other half are working with local fire departments or local government agencies. There are approximately 90,000 emergency nurses and 32,000 emergency physicians working in approximately 5,000 emergency departments. Almost no course work specific to disaster medical response is currently included in the requirements for training and certification/licensure of any of these health care providers (49). The AMA has taken action to meet this national educational and training need. In collaboration with several founding academic institutions and a consortium of prominent health care provider and workforce organizations, agencies, and academic institutions, the AMA has developed the National Disaster Life Support (NDLS) program. This program is a national initiative involving a series of standardized courses that establish a uniform foundation in all-hazards disaster training for the comprehensive target audience of the health care workforce (50). The need for both initial and ongoing training of the nation's first-line health care providers is staggering and almost certainly cannot be met alone by traditional classroom instructional methods. Advances in technology described in this chapter unquestionably play a significant role in meeting the short-term training needs and long-term update training of these groups. Expansion of the virtual classroom into the remote and wilderness areas will provide an opportunity for volunteer EMS providers to continue to learn and lessen the hardships involved if they were required to leave their communities and jobs to complete additional training requirements. Nurses and physicians likewise will have more ready access and flexibility to complete learning objectives necessary to keep local hospitals and health care systems up to standard.

The October 2002 Report of the Terrorism Response Task Force by the American College of Emergency Physicians, "Positioning America's Emergency Health Care System to Respond to Acts of Terrorism," calls for the development of a technology-based, self-study program covering the awareness objectives as a short-term strategy (51). Coupled with the performance training and testing based on virtual reality described in this chapter, it will be possible to achieve mass training of the health care community in both the cognitive and psychomotor aspects of disaster medicine within the next few years. A number of federal grants now provide funds to further develop and implement the curriculum and the associated much needed training process (52,53).

PREPAREDNESS CHECKLIST

New advances in technology are being developed and marketed on an ongoing basis. The following is a checklist when considering applying existing and new technology to terrorism training:

1. Core content and curriculum objectives are designed to achieve the desired learning.

2. Accreditation of the provider by a recognized authority is present.

3. Faculty are qualified by educational credentials, teaching experience, and real-world experience.

4. Technology applications are suitable tools and resources to enable training through a process that assures the acquisition of the desired skills, knowledge, ability, and attitudes.

5. Educators focus on instructional outcomes, not the delivery of technology.

6. Learning results in a successful performance-based outcome involving appropriate patient scenarios.

7. Meeting the instructional needs of the students to master the education content is achieved.

PREPAREDNESS SUMMARY

Current and evolving technology advances have much to offer disaster medicine training. Over the next few years these advances will no doubt be tested in real time throughout the country. The result will be a more clearly defined methodology and effectiveness for the health sciences. The key to effectiveness is focusing on the needs of the learners, the requirements of the content, and the constraints faced by the instructor prior to choosing a delivery system. The evolution of the virtual classroom, computer-driven tabletop exercise simulation, and "smart mannequins" greatly enhance the capacity to meet current needs for disaster medicine training. Educators must remain focused on instructional outcomes, not the delivery of technology. Meeting the instructional needs of students to master the education content is the litmus test by which the effectiveness of technology applications must be judged.

RESOURCES

TELEMEDICINE AND TELEHEALTH JOURNALS

1. IEEE Transactions on Information Technology in Biomedicine, Guttenburg Information Technology Center, Room 5200, New Jersey Institute of Technology, 323 Martin Luther King Boulevard, Newark, NJ 07102, (201) 228-7068.

2. Journal of Telemedicine and Telecare, Royal Society of Medicine Press, Ltd., 1 Wimpole St., London W1M 8AE, United Kingdom.

3. Telemedicine Journal and e-Health, 2 Madison Avenue, Larchmont, NY 10538, (914) 824-3100.

4. Telehealth Practice Report, Civic Research Institute, P.O. Box 585, Kingston, NJ 08528, (609) 583-4450.

REFERENCES

1. Pavlov I. Conditioned reflexes: an investigation of the physiological activity of the cerebral cortex. London: Oxford University Press, 1927.
2. Tolman EC. Purposive behavior in animals and men. New York: Appleton-Century-Crofts, 1932.
3. Luthans F, Stajkovic AD. Reinforce for performance: the need to go beyond pay and even rewards. Academy of Management Executive 1999;13(2):49-57.
4. Stajkovic AD, Luthans F. A meta-analysis of the effects of organizational behavior modification on task performance. Academy of Management Journal 1997;40:1122-49.
5. Perception, attribution, and learning. In: Gordon JR ed. Organizational behavior—a diagnostic approach. 7th ed. Upper Saddle River, NJ: Prentice Hall; 2002;45-69.
6. Lewis NJ, Orton P. The five attributes of innovative e-learning. Training & Development 2000;54(6):45-51.
7. Clark RC. Recycling knowledge with learning objects. Training & Development 1998;60-1.
8. Reusable learning objects authoring guidelines: how to build modules, lessons, and topics-Cisco Systems White Paper 2003. Web site: http://business.cisco.com/prod/tree.taf%3Fasset_id=104120&ID=44748&public_view=true&kbns=1.html. Accessed September 8, 2003.
9. Distance learning glossary. Web site: http://www.usdla.org/html/resources/dictionary.htm. Accessed August 24, 2003.
10. Distance education: an overview. Web site: http://uidaho.edu/eo. Accessed June 18, 2003.
11. United States Distance Learning Association. [Homepage of the United States Distance Learning Association].Web site: http://www.usdla.org. Accessed September 8, 2003.
12. Moore MF, Thompson MM, Quigley AB, et al. The effects of distance learning: a summary of the literature. Research monograph. University Park, PA: Pennsylvania State University, American Center for the Study of Distance Education, 1990. Report No. ED 330 321.
13. Verduin JR, Clark TA. Distance education: the foundations of effective practice. San Francisco: Jossey-Bass, 1991.
14. Distance learning: research information and statistics. Web site: http://www.usdla.org/html/aboutUs/researchInfo.htm. Accessed August 19, 2003.
15. Who is learning at a distance? Web site: http://www.petersons.com/distancelearning/code/articles/who/asp. Accessed June 29, 2003.
16. College of Engineering Outreach. Distance education at a glance, guide 1. Moscow, ID: University of Idaho College of Engineering, 1995.
17. Kahn BH. Discussion of resources and attributes of the Web for the creation of meaningful learning environments [abstract]. Cyberpsychol Behav 2000;3(1):17-23. Available from Telemedicine Research Center: TIE ID 9312.
18. Ramsay DL, Benimoff A. The ability of primary care physicians to recognize the common dermatoses [abstract]. Arch Dermatol 1981;117:620-2. Available from Telemedicine Research Center: TIE ID 1266.
19. Blonde L, Spens R, Osheroff JA. American College of Physicians (ACP) medical informatics and telemedicine review [abstract]. J Med Sys 1995;2:131-7. Available from Telemedicine Research Center: TIE ID 1662.
20. Crandall LA, Coggan JM. Impact of new information technologies on training and continuing education for rural health professionals [abstract]. Rural Health 1994;10(3):208-15. Available from Telemedicine Research Center: TIE ID 1692.
21. Hou SM. Impact of medical informatics on medical education [abstract]. J Formosan Med Assoc 1999;11:764-6. Available from Telemedicine Research Center: TIE ID 8191.
22. Chen HS, Guo, FR, Lee FG, et al. Recent advances in telemedicine [abstract]. J Formosan Med Assoc 1999;11:767-72. Available from Telemedicine Research Center: TIE ID 7874.
23. Morris DG. Using telemedicine to facilitate training in cardiotocography interpretation [abstract]. J Telemed Telecare 2000;6(Suppl 1):53-5. Available from Telemedicine Research Center: TIE ID 7911.
24. France FHR. WHO views perspectives in health informatics [abstract]. Int J Med Informatics 2000;1:11-9. Available from Telemedicine Research Center: TIE ID 9241.
25. Coleman J, Nduka CC, Darzi A. Virtual reality and laparoscopic surgery [abstract]. Br J Surg 1994;81(12):1709-11. Available from Telemedicine Research Center: TIE ID 446.

26. Ota D, Loftin B, Saito R, et al. Virtual reality in surgical education [abstract]. Comput Biol Med 1995;25(2):127-37. Available from Telemedicine Research Center: TIE ID 1863.

27. Menn ER. Teledermatology in a changing health care environment [abstract]. Telemed J 1995;1(4):303-8. Available from Telemedicine Research Center: TIE ID 2462.

28. Ziegler R, Fischer F, Muller W, et al. Virtual reality arthroscopy training simulator [abstract]. Comput Biol Med 1995;25(2):193. Available from Telemedicine Research Center: TIE ID 1952.

29. Burgess LP, Holtel MR, Syms MJ, et al. Overview of telemedicine applications for otolaryngology [abstract]. Laryngoscope 1999;109(9):1433-7. Available from Telemedicine Research Center: TIE ID 7750.

30. Tooley MA, Forrest FC, Mantrip DR. MultiMed: remote interactive medical stimulation [abstract]. J Telemed Telecare 1999;5(Suppl 1):119-21. Available from Telemedicine Research Center: TIE ID 6644.

31. Kaufmann C, Rhee P, Burris D. Telepresence surgery system enhances medical student surgery training [abstract]. Stud Health Technol Informatics 1999;62:174-8. Available from Telemedicine Research Center: TIE ID 7711.

32. Rinisland H. ARTEMIS: a telemanipulator for cardiac surgery [abstract]. Eur J Cardiothorac Surg 1999;16(Suppl 2):106-11. Available from Telemedicine Research Center: TIE ID 7676.

33. Ross MD, Twombly A, Lee AW, et al. New approaches to virtual environment surgery [abstract]. Stud Health Technol Informatics 1999:62:297-301. Available from Telemedicine Research Center: TIE ID 7706.

34. Stat TY. Bringing health care and education within reach: distance learning, telepathology transform laboratory medicine [abstract]. Lab Med 2000;31(4):198-205. Available from Telemedicine Research Center: TIE ID 8497.

35. Samiotakis Y, Anagnostopoulou S, Alexakis A. A regulated telemedicine system for day to day application in remote areas [abstract]. Stud Health Technol Informatics 2000; 57-91-8. Available from Telemedicine Research Center: TIE ID 9284.

36. Lange T, Indelicato DJ, Rosen JM. Virtual reality in surgical training [abstract]. Surg Clin North Am 2000;9(1):61-79. Available from Telemedicine Research Center: TIE ID 8074.

37. Picot J. Meeting the need for educational standards in the practice of telemedicine and telehealth [abstract]. J Telemed Telecare 2000;6(Suppl 2):59-62. Available from Telemedicine Research Center: TIE ID 8980.

38. Tasto JL, Bauer JJ, Verstreken K, et al. Training simulator for endoscopic procedures [abstract]. Telemed J 2000;6(1):171. Available from Telemedicine Research Center: TIE ID 8452.

39. Sawyer MA, Lim RB, Wong SY, et al. Telementored laparoscopic cholecystectomy: a pilot study [abstract]. Stud Health Technol Informatics 2000;70:302-8. Available from Telemedicine Research Center: TIE ID 9273.

40. Silverman RD. Current legal and ethical concerns in telemedicine and e-medicine [abstract]. J Telemed Telecare 2003;9 (Suppl 1):67-9. Available from the Royal Society of Medicine Press: DIO 10.1258/135763303322196402.

41. Thomas C. Red flags to watch for when choosing distance education programs. Web site: http://www.petersons.com/distancelearning/code/articles/distancelearnquality5.asp. Accessed September 8, 2003.

42. Llewellyn CH. The role of telemedicine in disaster medicine [abstract]. J Med Sys 1995;19(1):29-34. Available from Telemedicine Research Center: TIE ID 1030.

43. Raymann RB. Telemedicine: Military applications [abstract]. Aviat Space Environ Med 1992; 63(2):135-7. Available from Telemedicine Research Center: TIE ID 1280.

44. Marchessault R, Benson P, Bigott T, et al. Digital training tools for the U.S. Army Medical Department (AMEDD) teledermatology project [abstract]. Telemed J 2000;6(1):181. Available from Telemedicine Research Center: TIE ID 8471.

45. Reichle CW, Cearns M. Using distance training to deliver first aid training [abstract]. J Telemed Telecare 2000;6(Suppl 2): 63-4. Available from Telemedicine Research Center: TIE ID 8981.

46. Cooper JB, Baron D, Blum R, et al. Video teleconferencing with realistic simulation for medical education [abstract]. J Clin Anesth 2000;12(3):256-61. Available from Telemedicine Research Center: TIE ID 8890.

47. Coule PL, Schwartz RB, Swienton RE eds. Advanced Disaster Life Support ADLS Provider Manual. Chicago: American Medical Association, 2003.

48. Stansfield S. Medisim: casualty care on the virtual battlefield. Mil Med Technol 1997-98;23.

49. American College of Emergency Physicians and the U.S. Department of Health and Human Services, Office of Preparedness. Developing objectives, content, and competencies for the training of emergency medical technicians, emergency physicians, and emergency nurses to care for casualties resulting from nuclear, biological, or chemical (NBC) incidents—final report. Dallas: American College of Emergency Physicians, 2001.

50. Report 1 of the Council on Scientific Affairs (I-03): AMA National Disaster Life Support Program. Web site; http://www.ama-assn.org/ama/pub/article/2036-8173.html. Accessed August 16, 2004.

51. American College of Emergency Physicians. Positioning America's emergency health care system to respond to acts of terrorism. Dallas: American College of Emergency Physicians; 2002.

52. U.S. Department of Health and Human Services Health Resources and Services Administration Maternal and Child Health Bureau. National bioterrorism hospital preparedness program—cooperative agreement guidance. Washington, DC: HRSA, 2003.

53. U.S. Department of Health and Human Services Health Resources and Services Administration Maternal and Child Health Bureau. Terrorism training program grant guidance. Washington, DC: HRSA, 2003.

The author would like to acknowledge Tanya Uden-Holman, PhD, Associate professor with the Department of Health Management and Policy at the University of Iowa College of Public Health and Janet McMahill, PhD, Interim Dean, School of Education, Drake University for their assistance with the preparation of this chapter.

Operational Medical Preparedness for Terrorism

35

Strategic Response to Explosive and Traumatic Terrorism

Brian A. Krakover

INTRODUCTION

Although the United States has been spared the frequent terrorist attacks experienced by Israel, the United Kingdom, Malaysia, and other countries, the 2001 World Trade Center attack and the Murrah Federal Building bombing in Oklahoma City adequately demonstrated that the United States is not immune (1). This chapter reviews trends in terrorist bombing tactics and a system of preparing and dealing with explosive terrorism in accordance with the all-hazards approach to established disaster management. After reading this chapter, the reader should feel comfortable planning for and responding to bomb detonations, major explosive calamities, and the resulting mass casualty situations.

PREPAREDNESS ESSENTIALS

The major medical challenge posed by explosive terrorist acts is that they frequently generate a multiple-casualty situation. Even though nuclear, biological, and/ or chemi-

cal weapons have received a great deal of attention over the last decade, conventional explosives have been, by far, the most common type of weapon employed in terrorist attacks in modern history (2). In the past, this usually occurred during wars or other military operations. More recently however, more ambitious terrorists have brought more critically injured patients to the civilian medical setting. The civilian medical establishment in most countries is not geared toward managing multiple casualties on a daily basis. Moreover, responders are often not acquainted with the different guidelines that should be followed in this type of situation. The problem is to identify the number of casualties who are in critical but salvageable condition in the field and upon arrival to the hospital. Such individuals are usually mixed in with a large number of minimal casualties presenting to all available medical facilities and creating a significant triage and management problem (3).

TARGETS OF TERRORISM

Public places with little or no security presence are easy targets. Examples are religious sites, dance clubs, shops or markets, and public transport, especially during the rush hour. Between 2000 and 2003 there have been scores of bombings in Israeli markets, night clubs, and restaurants. Strictly ethnic or religious targets are also common. The August 2003 bombing of the Imam Ali Mosque in Najaf, Iraq, killed scores including a major religious leader (4). Earlier in April 2002 the oldest synagogue in North Africa was attacked by suicide bombing, killing 19 people (5). Figure 35-1 presents a breakdown of terrorist attacks in 2001. Note the disproportionate number of bombings and armed assaults compared to all other tactics (6).

BOMB BASICS

Blast injuries are usually caused by explosive devices such as bombs, mines, or missiles. They function by the burning of certain fuels. The combustion process happens so rapidly that the gases produced by the combustion are pushed outward at tremendous speed and in such a violent manner so as to produce a shock wave. This shock wave propagates at the speed of sound in all directions (7). The combination of this shock wave as well as the thermal products of the explosion in conjunction with their effects on

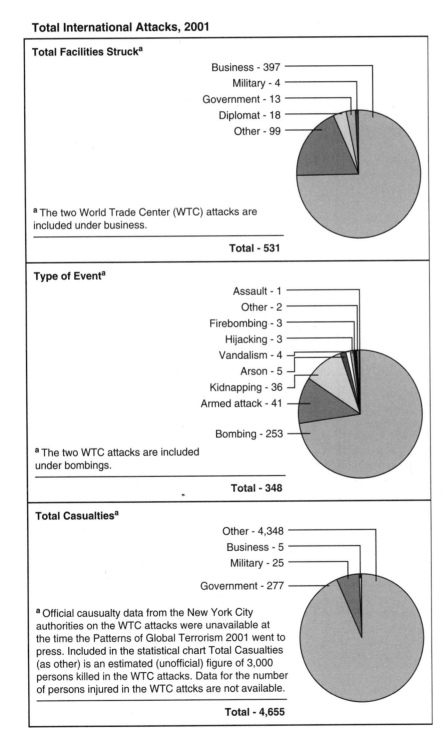

Total International Attacks, 2001

Total Facilities Struck[a]

Business - 397
Military - 4
Government - 13
Diplomat - 18
Other - 99

[a] The two World Trade Center (WTC) attacks are included under business.

Total - 531

Type of Event[a]

Assault - 1
Other - 2
Firebombing - 3
Hijacking - 3
Vandalism - 4
Arson - 5
Kidnapping - 36
Armed attack - 41

Bombing - 253

[a] The two WTC attacks are included under bombings.

Total - 348

Total Casualties[a]

Other - 4,348
Business - 5
Military - 25
Government - 277

[a] Official causalty data from the New York City authorities on the WTC attacks were unavailable at the time the Patterns of Global Terrorism 2001 went to press. Included in the statistical chart Total Casualties (as other) is an estimated (unofficial) figure of 3,000 persons killed in the WTC attacks. Data for the number of persons injured in the WTC attcks are not available.

Total - 4,655

FIGURE 35–1. Total International attacks 2001. Source: U.S. State Department, Washington, DC. *2001 patterns of global terrorism.* 2001.

TABLE 35-1 Composite High Explosives

NAME	COMPOSITION	FORMULA
AMATOL	80/20 Ammonium nitrate/TNT	$C_{0.62}H_{4.44}N_{2.26}O_{3.53}$
ANFO	94/6 Ammonium nitrate/#2 diesel oil	$C_{0.365}H_{4.713}N_{2.000}O_{3.000}$
COMP A-3	91/9 RDX/WAX	$C_{1.87}H_{3.74}N_{2.46}O_{2.46}$
COMP B-3	64/36 RDX/TNT	$C_{6.851}H_{8.750}N_{7.650}O_{9.300}$
COMP C-4	91/5.3/2.1/1.6 RDX/Di(2-ethylhexyl) sebacate/oolyisobutylene/motor oil	$C_{1.82}H_{3.54}N_{2.46}O_{2.51}$
DYNAMITE	75/15/10 RDX/TNT/plasticizers	

Source: United Nations Office on Drugs and Crime. Conventional terrorist weapons. Available at: http://www.unodc.org/unodc/terrorism_weapons_conventional.html.

structures and personnel makes explosions ideal terror weapons.

Military explosives are divided into two general classes, high explosives and low explosives, according to their rate of decomposition.

HIGH EXPLOSIVES

A high explosive is characterized by the extreme rapidity with which its decomposition occurs; this action is known as detonation. When initiated by a blow or shock, it will decompose almost instantaneously in a manner similar to an extremely rapid combustion or with rupture and re-arrangement of the molecules themselves. In either case, gaseous and solid products of reaction are produced and generate an overpressurization wave. High explosives are usually nitration products of organic substances, such as toluene, phenol, pentaerythritol, arnines, glycerin, and starch, and may be nitrogen-containing inorganic substances or mixtures of both. TNT is an example of a high explosive (Table 35-1).

LOW EXPLOSIVES

Low explosives are mostly solid combustible materials that decompose rapidly but do not normally detonate or produce significant overpressures. This action is known as deflagration. Upon ignition and decomposition, low explosives develop a large volume of gases that produce enough pressure to propel a projectile in a definite direction. The rate of burning is an important characteristic that depends upon such factors as combustion gas pressure, grain size and form, and composition. Under certain conditions, low explosives may be made to detonate in the same manner as high explosives.

CHARACTERISTICS OF EXPLOSIVES

The closer the victim or structure is to the site of an explosion, the stronger the shock wave. The term "blast overpressure" is used to describe the power of a shock wave. Commercial explosives can produce tremendous peak overpressures on the order of thousands of pounds per square inch, but this lasts

only milliseconds and dissipates rapidly over distance. Water extends the lethal radius of explosives due to its increased density compared to air (7). Several other factors influence the effects of an explosive reaction (Table 35-2).

Velocity

An explosive reaction differs from ordinary combustion in the velocity of the reaction. The velocity of combustion of explosives may vary within rather wide limits, depending upon the kind of explosive substance and upon its physical state. For high explosives, the velocity, or time of reaction, is high (usually in feet per second), as opposed to low explosives, where the velocity is low (usually in seconds per foot).

Heat

An explosive reaction of a high explosive and a low explosive is always accompanied by the rapid liberation of heat. The amount of heat represents the energy of the explosive and its potential for doing work.

Gases

The principal gaseous products of the more common explosives are carbon dioxide, carbon monoxide, water vapor, nitrogen, nitrogen oxides, hydrogen, methane, and hydrogen cyanide. Some of these gases are suffocating, some are actively poisonous, and some are combustible. For example, the flame at the muzzle of a gun when it is fired results from the burning of these gases in air.

TABLE 35-2 Relationship Between Explosive Mass and Lethal Radius

MASS OF EXPLOSIVE	LETHAL RADIUS
30 kg	5.5 m
200 kg	9.6 m
400 kg	11.4 m
700 kg	18 m
1,200 kg	20 m
2,000 kg	24 m

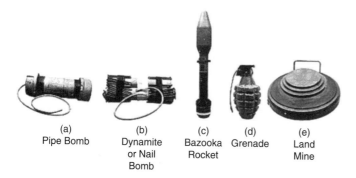

(a) Pipe Bomb   (b) Dynamite or Nail Bomb   (c) Bazooka Rocket   (d) Grenade   (e) Land Mine

Figure 35–2. Various explosive devices. Source: Emergency Response and Research Institute. http://www.emergency.com/ explosives-misc.htm. Courtesy of Bureau of Alcohol, Tobacco, and Firearms.

Pressure

The high pressure accompanying an explosive reaction is due to the formation of gases that are expanded by the heat liberated in the reaction. The work that the reaction is capable of performing depends upon the volume of the gases and the amount of heat liberated. The maximum pressure developed and the way in which the energy of the explosion is applied depends further upon the velocity of the reaction. The rapidity with which an explosive develops its maximum pressure is a measure of the quality known as brisance. A brisant explosive is one in which the maximum pressure is attained so rapidly that a shock wave is formed, and the net effect is to shatter material surrounding or in contact with it. Thus brisance is a measure of the shattering ability of an explosive.

Stability

The stability of an explosive is important in determining the length of time it can be kept under normal stowage conditions without deterioration and its adaptability to various military uses. A good, general explosive should withstand a reasonable exposure to such extremes as high humidity in a hot climate or cold temperatures of arctic conditions (8).

The number of potential materials available to the committed terrorist is impressive. Materials ranging from stolen military-grade explosives to gasoline drums to household fertilizer can be incorporated into an explosive device capable of devastating any modern structure. Most military-style munitions such as bombs and missiles are too cumbersome to be employed as a single unit. The exception to this generalization is the mine—both the anti-personnel and antitank mine. Mines can be adapted without much difficulty with average engineering experience. Some 300 different types of mines are buried under the soil, killing tens of thousands every year.

Most bombs assembled by terrorists are improvised. The raw material required for explosives is either stolen or misappropriated from military or commercial blasting supplies or made from fertilizer and other readily available household ingredients. Such assembled bombs are known as Improvised Explosive Devices (IEDs) (9).

COMPONENTS

The purpose of most IEDs is to kill or maim. Some IEDs, known as incendiaries, are intended to cause damage or destruction by fire. IEDs have a main charge, which is attached to a fuse, which is attached to a trigger. In some types of IEDs, these three components are integrated into a single unit. The trigger activates the fuse. The fuse ignites the charge, causing the explosion. The effects of the IED are sometimes worsened by the addition of material, such as scrap iron or ball bearings. Sometimes the trigger is not the only component that activates the fuse; there can also be an antihandling device that triggers the fuse when the IED is handled or moved (Fig. 35-2).

EXAMPLES OF IEDs

Pipe Bomb

The pipe bomb is the most common type of terrorist bomb and usually consists of low-velocity explosives inside a tightly capped piece of pipe. Pipe bombs are very easily made using gunpowder, iron, steel, aluminum, or copper pipes. They are sometimes wrapped with nails to cause even more harm.

Molotov Cocktail

This improvised weapon (first used by the Russian resistance against German tanks in the Second World War) is used by terrorists worldwide. Molotov cocktails are extremely simple to make and can cause considerable damage. They are usually made from materials like gasoline, diesel fuel, kerosene, ethyl or methyl alcohol, lighter fluid, and turpentine, all of which are easily obtained. The explosive material is placed in a glass bottle, which breaks upon impact. A piece of cotton serves as a fuse, which is ignited before the bottle is thrown at the target.

Fertilizer Truck Bomb

Fertilizer truck bombs consist of ammonium nitrate. Hundreds of kilograms may be required to cause major damage. The Irish Republican Army, Tamil Tigers, and some Middle Eastern groups use the ammonium nitrate bomb. This was also the type of bomb employed in the Oklahoma City bombing.

Letter and Parcel Bombs

Letter and parcel bombs can be constructed of many different explosives and detonators based on the parcel size and method of opening. Most parcel and letter bombs target an individual and not a large population.

Remotely Controlled Bombs

A bomb can be set off by remote control. This system uses radio waves to complete a circuit, causing an electric detonator to be connected to a voltage source at the desired moment. In practice, terrorist groups use this system for large quantities of explosives, which they hide in light vehicles, cars, or trucks (the normality of the means of transport helps the approach to the target; the explosive charge is thus camouflaged by an everyday vehicle) (10).

Barometric Bomb

The barometric bomb is one of the more advanced weapons in the terrorist's arsenal and is utilized primarily to attack aircraft or tall buildings. This IED utilizes an altitude meter detonator that can be placed in an aircraft or elevator. The detonator is set to go off when a certain altitude is reached. Ted Kaczynski, the Unabomber, fashioned a crude barometric bomb that he sent through the mail system. The bomb was placed in the cargo hold of American Airlines flight 444 from Chicago to Washington, D.C. When the plane reached 35,000 feet, the bomb detonated a crude explosive device filling the cabin with smoke. The pilot was able to land the aircraft and the only injury to passengers and crew was mild smoke inhalation (11).

The Effects of a Bomb

Explosives are devices used to convert chemical into kinetic and/or thermal energy. This is accomplished in three ways depending on the speed of propagation of the chemical reaction.

The environment can have a decisive influence on the type and amount of damage produced by a bomb. The effect of the shock wave varies in particular with the pressure and temperature of the ambient surroundings. The climatic or meteorological conditions can, in turn, have major consequences for the propagation of the shock wave, as can the wind. Physical structures such as walls or vehicles play a major role as well. Walls or alleys can reflect or focus a single or multiple blast waves, magnifying their impact significantly. The amount of damage sustained is also influenced by the distance from the explosion (see Table 35-3).

Building collapse is a major hazard for both victims as well as rescue workers. In practice, even though construction methods can mitigate the damage from a blast, ordinary buildings are vulnerable. The bomb attack on the American Embassy in the center of Nairobi on August 7, 1998, caused the collapse of a neighboring Gateway House building on to several dozen offices and a secretarial school (213 dead and more than 5,000 injured). Tragically, the horrific collapse of the two towers of the World Trade Center attack transformed a mass casualty situation into a mass fatality situation. Some constructional elements (e.g., lightweight dividing walls made of brick, coverings of various types, and glass) are more susceptible to blast. Many investigators attribute the World Trade Center collapse to structural failure caused by the intense fires after the initial aircraft collision.

RESPONSE ESSENTIALS

Known or suspected explosives, of any type, should be handled only by qualified explosives ordinance disposal (EOD) or bomb squad personnel. In the event you discover any of the devices pictured in Fig. 35-2,

1. Evacuate the area.
2. Do not touch or remove the device.
3. Immediately contact the nearest police agency and notify them that you believe you have found an explosive device.
4. Request assistance (11).

Responding to a traumatic explosive event requires planning and training utilizing the all-hazards approach to prevent unnecessary morbidity and mortality to victims. The response to blast events can be organized into three phases: the preparatory phase, the response phase, and the recovery phase.

Preparatory Phase

Successfully defeating the goals of the terrorist requires saving lives and preventing panic, fear, and disorder. The first step is to think like a potential terrorist. Emergency planners must identify critical targets within their jurisdiction.

TABLE 35-3 Characteristics of Explosives

PROCESS	CHARACTERISTICS	SPEED OF TRANSFORMATION	EFFECTS
Combustion	Reaction depends on thermal conduction	Moderate (cm/sec)	Thermal burns
Deflagration	Combustion accelerated by increases in pressure and temperature	Rapid (100s m/sec)	Shrapnel, blast trauma, thermal burns
Detonation	Creation of shock wave—near complete conversion to kinetic energy	Very rapid (km/sec)	Large blast effect, aftershock, shattering effects

Municipal buildings, sports arenas, critical infrastructure, and commercial targets should all be considered for attacks taking place any time of day, year, and climate.

Once the list of possible targets has been established, a plan must be developed for each target to include establishment of casualty collection points, the prevention of further damage to surrounding structures or environmental assets, the formation of routes of ingress and egress, and the creation of scene security both for the protection of first responders as well as the collection of forensic evidence (this is also a crime scene). Other things to consider include daily traffic patterns, weather or seasonal effects, resupply factors, and communications. Furthermore, it is vital that media outlets be involved from the very beginning. During the World Trade Center attack, mobile phone networks were quickly overloaded and communications became difficult. Providing media outlets with preprinted reports and instructions in the event of an explosive attack may save vital time and keep communications resources free.

Evacuation and Route Analysis.

Evacuation and Route Analysis. An important item to consider is that recently first responders have become targets of terrorists. In both the September 11 attacks as well as at a summer 2003 concert in Moscow, secondary devices (the second tower attack for the former and a second bomber in the latter) were used to attack first responders effectively. This trend must provoke careful thought for emergency planners. In addition to determining the most direct route to nearby health care facilities or casualty collection points, the routes must be secured. This can be done on the scene by law enforcement personnel or, more importantly, by prior route analysis. That is to say, planners can look at potential routes and clear them of structures such as mailboxes, news stands, traffic signal control boxes, or other structures or objects that could hide a secondary device or provide tactical advantage to a would-be terrorist. It is always easier to plan in peacetime than to make rapid decisions during a time of crisis. An additional component should be considering alternate routes for contingencies such as construction, inclement weather, secondary attack, or rush hour traffic.

Crime Scene.

Crime Scene. As mentioned earlier, blast events are frequently crime scenes as well as mass casualty events. Proper care must be taken to preserve evidence where possible, and law enforcement authorities should be an integral component of disaster plan preparation. In addition, several organizations at the federal level should be integrated into major event planning to include disaster medical assistance teams (DMATs) and urban search and rescue (USAR) teams. Furthermore, appropriate engineering resources for rescue, evacuation, and recovery should be procured in advance for aid in preventing structural collapse and assisting with scene safety.

Logistics.

Logistics. A crucial component to any disaster plan is logistics. Explosive events happen in an instant but can produce cataclysmic amounts of damage requiring large amounts of material, personnel, and financial resources. All of these elements must be coordinated in advance of an event to allow for seamless resupply operations and rotations of personnel who may easily become exhausted or injured during rescue operations, as well as for ensuring that involved organizations are paid in a timely manner for their goods and services.

Rehearsals and Drills.

Rehearsals and Drills. The most essential element of any good plan is rehearsal and drills. The disaster plan for a blast event should be integrated into existing disaster planning and should involve as realistic an approach as is feasible. Multiple event scenarios such as radiological, biological, and chemical as well as secondary devices should be included in a rehearsal event. These exercises should be utilized to identify areas that can be changed to improve the response to the event.

Evaluation.

Evaluation. In any plan, there is always room for improvement. All involved personnel must be prepared to evaluate and critique their component of the response plan and make necessary changes when, not if, indicated.

Response Phase

A unified algorithm called the D.I.S.A.S.T.E.R. Paradigm is utilized in the American Medical Association's disaster response training courses. This paradigm provides an organized approach for the management of disasters.

D—Detect

I—Incident Command

S—Scene Safety and Security

A—Assess Hazards

S—Support Required

T—Triage and Treatment

E—Evacuation

R—Recovery

D—Detect.

D—Detect. One advantage of dealing with an explosive event is the fact that it is loud, conspicuous, and instantly affects a great deal of people. Therefore, notification and detection are not as difficult as a chemical or biological attack might be, although an explosive device may be used to detonate or disperse nuclear, radiological, chemical, or biological materials, so be sure to involve hazmat or weapons of mass destruction teams early.

I—Incident Command.

I—Incident Command. The incident command system needs to be activated to achieve several components of an effective response: (a) unity of command, (b) accountability, and (c) a single voice for the media, general public, employees, and law enforcement.

S—Scene Security and Safety.

S—Scene Security and Safety. Secure the scene in order to prevent subsequent attacks and further injury to victims, to preserve the crime scene, and to prevent building collapse or spread of contamination in the event of a chemical, biological, or radiological attack. This is also the time to secure preplanned evacuation routes to prevent secondary device explosions. It is essential to have a coordinated response with Emergency Medical Services, law enforcement, hazmat, and other agencies to ensure the safety and security of the incident site.

A—Assessment of Hazard. As stated previously, building collapse, and nuclear, biological, and chemical threats should be assessed, as should environmental hazards such as fire, toxic smoke and fumes, and structural integrity of the building if one is involved. With the high likelihood of unstable structures, well-meaning medical responders may enter in an attempt to assist and lose their own lives due to structural collapse. The risk benefit of entry into structures in this setting must be carefully weighed and expert advice utilized to minimize the risk to responders. Additionally, consideration of secondary devices must be a high priority. Vigilance and awareness of the threat will be key in identification of these hazards and their mitigation.

S—Support. Once the nature of the threat is determined and the ICS is notified, the various elements of the chain of command need to maneuver resources and materials to the site of the disaster as well as provide accurate and timely information to the public, victims, and law enforcement in the most secure manner available. This will need to be a coordinated response and decisions must be made early in the course of the event to determine if local resources will be adequate to respond or if state or federal resources will be required. Requests for this support will come from the incident command system to the appropriate local, state, and federal agency. Early reports to the hospitals through the ICS and Medical Control pathways should be provided. These reports should include the estimated numbers of casualties and estimated times of arrival, along with specific requirements such as decontamination.

T—Triage and Treatment. Standard triage principles should be used to evacuate the most critically wounded who would be amenable to available treatment resources. The use of a standardized system such as MASS Triage will allow better coordination and information flow between the incident site and the hospitals (13–15). Specific areas of treatment that will need to be addressed and are covered in other areas of this book include primary, secondary, and tertiary blast injury; crush syndrome; and compartment syndrome. Medical responders must be familiar with the management of these conditions. However, they should also be aware that because these events are often crime scenes that the preservation of forensic evidence is very important.

E—Evacuation. Utilizing preplanned evacuation routes, evacuation of critical patients should proceed as quickly as possible. Given the potentially large number of patients requiring evacuation, traffic coordination and logistical support is critical (16).

R—Recovery. A number of steps are involved with the recovery process. For the medical community, the treatment of patients and the return of the hospital to it's preevent sta-

tus is a high priority. This recovery may be complicated if contaminated casualties were allowed into the facility without appropriate decontamination and highlights the importance of preplanning. Additionally, the psychological impact of these events may last for years and have a considerable impact on the required assets to provide this care. For law enforcement, bringing the perpetrators to justice is a high priority. For the community at large, the process of rebuilding infrastructure and trust will take time and may be shortened by the community's assurance that appropriate steps had been taken prior to the event. This highlights the idea that recovery must begin before the event occurs through planning, training, and exercises.

Review

The vast majority of modern terrorist attacks have been with conventional weapons in the form of firearms and explosives—most notably improvised explosive devices. Optimal response to explosive terrorism requires thorough prior planning and an all-hazards approach to terrorism management.

RESOURCES

1. Counterterrorism/Weapons of Mass Destruction Training Links. Web site: http://www.fbi.gov/hq/td/academy/ctwork12.htm
2. Preparing for Terrorism: An Emergency Services Guide. Pamphlet written by G. Buck and published in October 1997.
3. Federation of American Scientists. Web site: http://www.fas.org
4. Patterns of Global Terrorism. Pamphlet produced yearly by U.S. State Department. Web site: http://www.state.gov.
5. Emergency Response and Research Institute. Web site: http://www.emergency.net.

REFERENCES

1. Wightman JM, Gladish SL. Explosions and blast injuries. Ann Emerg Med 2001 Jun;37:664-78.
2. Stein M, Hirshberg A. Medical consequences of terrorism. Surg Clin N Amer 1999 Dec; 79(6).
3. Terror Attack Database (International Policy Institute for Counter-Terrorism Web site). Available at: http://www.ict.org.il. Accessed August 18, 2004.
4. CBS News/ Associated Press. Mosque Blast: 19 Al Qaeda nabbed [online]. Available at: http://www.cbsnews.com/stories/2003/08/31/iraq/printable570944.shtml. Accessed August 30, 2003.
5. Hooper J, Tremlett G. Tunisian synagogue bomb tied to al-Qaida. The Guardian April 23, 2002. Available at: //www.guardian.co.uk/print/0,3858,4399571-103681,00.html. Accessed August 18, 2004.
6. U.S. Department of State. Manchester, UK: Guardian Newspapers, LTD: Patterns of global terrorism. 2001.

7. DeLorenzo RA, Porter RS. Care of Blast and Burn Casualties. Tactical Emergency Care. Prentice-Hall 1999.
8. Integrated Publishing. High and low explosives [online]. Available at: http://www.tpub.com/gunners/2.htm. Accessed August 18, 2004.
9. Explosive devices [online]. Available at: http://library.think quest.org/CR0212088/terweapex.htm. Accessed August 18, 2004.
10. Emergency Response and Research Institute. http://www.emergency.com/explosives-misc.htm
11. United Nations Office on Drugs and Crime. Conventional terrorist weapons [online]. Available at: http://www.unodc.org/unodc/terrorism_weapons_conventional.html. Accessed August 18, 2004.
12. Miscellaneous Explosives Used as Improvised Explosive Devices (IED's) American Medical Association, Chicago, IL. Advanced disaster life support. National Disaster Life Support Publications; 2004.
13. American Medical Association, Chicago, IL. Basic disaster life support. National Disaster Life Support Publications; 2004.
14. American Medical Association, Chicago, IL. Core disaster life support. National Disaster Life Support Publications; 2004.
15. Emergency Response and Research Institute. Available at: http://www.emergency.com/explosives-misc.htm. Accessed August 18, 2004.
16 Peleg K, Aharonson-Daniel, et al. Patterns of injury in hospitalized terrorist victims. Am J Emerg Med 2003 Jul;21(4): 258–62.
17. U.S. Navy Surface Warfare Officer School. Chemical explosives: introduction to naval engineering course syllabus. Rev. Jan 20, 1998.

36

The Forensic Evaluation of Gunshot Wounds Associated With a Terrorist Event

William S. Smock

The United States has been forever changed by the domestic and international terrorist events on our soil over the last 10 years. In the aftermath of a terrorist incident involving U.S. citizens, its assets, or an assassination attempt on American leaders, either in this country or abroad, a forensic investigation will be swift and obligatory. Wound evaluations and evidence collection will be integral components of the law enforcement response. All patients, surviving and deceased, who are victims of blunt, blast, thermal, chemical, biological, radiological, or penetrating trauma will require a forensic evaluation to determine the nature of the injury and to document, collect, and preserve evidence.

Victims of gunshot wounding have unique forensic issues. The determination must be made as to whether a wound is an entrance or an exit wound. If possible, the projectile must be recovered, and a determination must be made as to the range of fire. Medical providers, from the tactical medic to the emergency physician, should understand the basic forensic principles associated with the assessment of gunshot wounds. The forensic lessons learned from the assassination of President Kennedy: from the treatment at Parkland Hospital, to the fallacious interpretation of wounds based on size, to the failure to have an autopsy performed by a forensic pathologist in Dallas, to the failure to document adequately the wounds photographically have all contributed to an example of how well-meaning medical providers can confound a criminal investigation of a gunshot wound. Failure of medical providers to identify, document, and analyze entrance and exit wounds, preserve short-lived evidence, and collect clothing and projectiles correctly could jeopardize future criminal and civil proceedings against both domestic and international terrorists (1–11).

FORENSIC EVALUATION OF HANDGUN WOUNDS

The life of the patient and the medical care required to guard it obviously take precedence over the need for forensic evaluations and evidence collection. Yet it is possible for treating EMTs, paramedics, nurses, emergency physicians, and trauma surgeons to perform a forensic evaluation while providing lifesaving care (3,11). At a minimum, every gunshot wound should have its anatomical location accurately documented, its physical characteristics described, and associated short-lived evidence preserved (11,12).

Nonforensic medical providers should always avoid describing a wound as "entrance" or "exit." Unfortunately, many practitioners enter forensic opinions into the medical records regarding wound type based solely on the size of the wound, assuming the large hole is the exit and the small hole is the entrance (10,13–15). Exit wounds, from handguns, are *not* consistently larger than their corresponding entrance wounds (11,15–18). The size of any wound, entrance or exit, is determined by multiple factors: the size, shape, configuration, and velocity of the projectile as it contacts or leaves the tissue and the physical characteristics of the tissue itself (17,18).

ENTRANCE WOUNDS

Gunshot wounds of entrance can be divided into four categories: distant or indeterminate range, intermediate range, close range, and contact. Each entrance wound category is based on the distance of the gun muzzle to the target and is called the "range of fire." Each range-of-fire category is associated with specific wound characteristics: distant-range wounds have only an abrasion collar, intermediate-range wounds have an abrasion collar and tattooing, close-range wounds have an abrasion collar and soot, and contact wounds have seared skin, soot, and triangular-shaped tears of the skin (Table 36-1).

The size of the entrance wound bears no relationship to the caliber of the bullet, and physicians should never render opinions on caliber based on the size of the entrance wound (17,18). Depending on the elasticity of the epithelial tissue, entrance wounds may contract around or expand beyond the tissue defect caused by the bullet.

| | | | CONTACT RANGE | |
DISTANT RANGE	INTERMEDIATE RANGE	CLOSE RANGE	LOOSE CONTACT	TIGHT CONTACT
Abrasion collar (Figs. 36-1, 36-2).	Abrasion collar with tattooing (Figs. 36-4, 36-5, 36-6).	Abrasion collar with soot (Figs. 36-7, 36-8).	Soot-covered abrasion collar. Contusion and triangle-shaped tears may be present (Fig. 36-9).	Seared skin, soot, contusion, triangle-shaped tears. Muzzle contusion may be present (Figs. 36-10, 36-11, 36-12, 36-14, 36-15, 36-16).

TABLE 36-1 Wound Characteristics of Entrance Wounds Based on the Range of Fire

DISTANT WOUNDS

In a distant- or indeterminate-range entrance wound, only the bullet makes contact with the skin. As the bullet penetrates the skin, the friction between the projectile and the epithelial tissue creates an "abrasion collar" (Fig. 36-1). Abrasion collars vary in appearance depending on the angle of penetration (Fig. 36-2). All entrance wounds have an abrasion collar with the exception of those on the palms of the hands and the soles of the feet, where the epithelium is highly keratinized (17). Entrance wounds in these locations appear slitlike and lack the abrasion collar (Fig. 36-3). Other terms, which may be used interchangeably with "abrasion collar," include "abrasion margin," "abrasion rim," and "abrasion ring." Abrasion collars are a pure friction phenomenon and not the result of a so-called hot bullet.

INTERMEDIATE RANGE

The intermediate-range wound is characterized by the presence of punctate abrasions, "tattooing" or "stippling" on the skin in the area of the abrasion collar (Figs. 36-4, 36-5). The tattooing is caused by unburned or partially burned pieces of gunpowder impacting the skin. Intermediate objects like clothing, furniture, or hair block the grains of gunpowder from making contact with the skin. Tattooing on the skin may be visualized from distances as close as 1/2 inch or as far away as 4 feet. The density and pattern of the punctate abrasions depend on the muzzle-to-skin distance, the length of the gun barrel, the presence of intermediate objects, the amount of gunpowder within a particular cartridge, and the physical shape of the gunpowder. Tattooing abrasions are visible for several days (Fig. 36-6). Unburned gunpowder can also be deposited and leave punctate nitrate residues on clothing. .

CLOSE RANGE

Close range is defined as the range at which the carbonatous residue of combustion or "soot" is visible around the wound or on clothing (Fig. 36-7). Close range is generally within a range of 6 inches but soot can be seen as far away as 12 inches in magnum loads. The type of gunpowder, the gun barrel length, and intermediate objects influence the concentration and pattern of soot. As in all entrance wounds, an abrasion collar or microtears are present, but with close-range

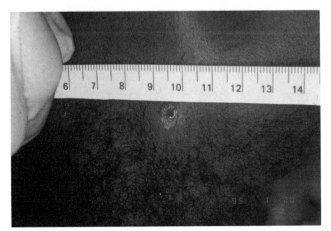

Figure 36–1. An abrasion collar is the result of friction between a projectile and the skin. Other appropriate forensic terms include "abrasion rim" or "abrasion ring."

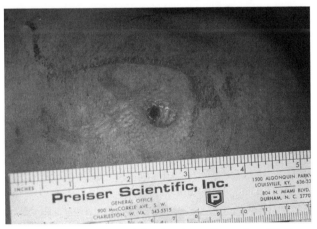

Figure 36–2. The width of the abrasion collar varies with the angle of the projectile's impact. The trajectory of the projectile here is from right to left.

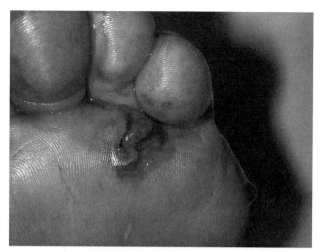

Figure 36–3. Entrance wounds on the palms of the hands and the sole of the feet lack an abrasion collar due to the highly keratinized nature of the skin.

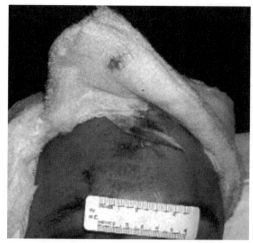

Figure 36–6. The punctate abrasions may be present for days. This patient's tattooing is easily visible 4 days postinjury.

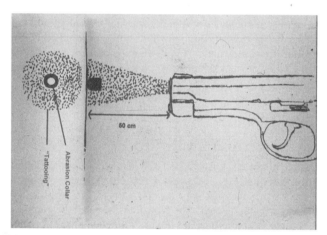

Figure 36–4. "Tattooing" is the result of partially or unburned gunpowder striking the skin. The "tattoos" are punctate abrasions.

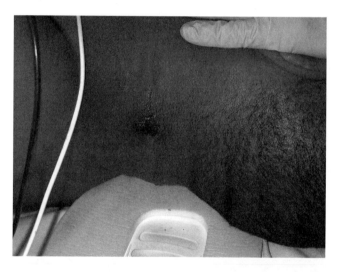

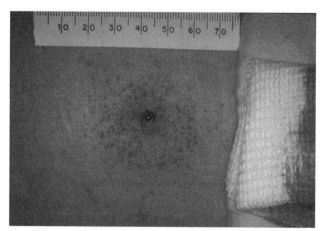

Figure 36–5. Tattooing is associated with the intermediate range of fire. This patient was shot in the back at a distance of 12 inches by a 9mm Smith & Wesson, model 6906.

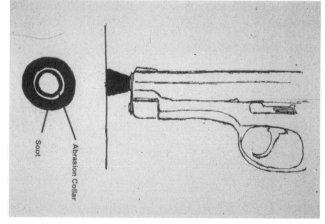

Figure 36–7 A, B: The deposition of soot surrounding this wound to the posterior neck is associated with a close range of fire, generally 6 inches or less.

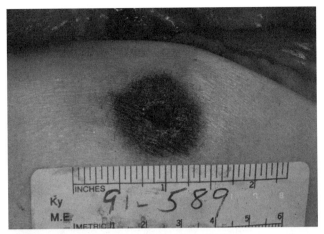

Figure 36–8. The presence of soot in a close-range wound may obscure the presence of an abrasion collar. This victim was shot at a distance of 1 inch with a .38 caliber revolver.

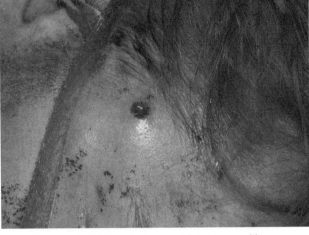

Figure 36–10. A tight-contact wound from a .22 caliber revolver. The wound displays soot, seared skin, and small triangular-shaped tears with surrounding contusion.

wounds it will be covered or obscured by the deposition of soot (Fig. 36-8). Soot is short-lived evidence and can be easily washed away in the rendering of patient care or surgical debridement of the wound. Do not describe soot as "powder burns." This is an outdated term used to describe epithelial thermal injuries associated with the use of black powder that initiated a thermal event on the clothing of a victim. Black powder, as opposed to the smokeless powder of commercial ammunition, is found in muzzle-loader rifles, antique weapons, and in the blanks used in starter pistols.

CONTACT WOUNDS

In a contact wound, the barrel is in contact with the victim's clothing or skin. Contact wounds can be subdivided into "tight contact," when the barrel is pushed hard against the skin or clothing, or "loose contact," when the barrel is not in full contact with the skin and may be angled (Fig. 36-9). Wounds sustained in tight-contact woundings vary in ap-

pearance depending on the elasticity of the skin and the volume of gas injected. For example, a contact wound to the temple from a .22 caliber short cartridge appears as a small hole with seared blackened edges and only tiny triangle-shaped tears (Fig. 36-10). Compare the .22 caliber wound (Fig. 36-10) to a contact wound to the forehead from a .357 caliber magnum load (Fig. 36-11). The large volume of gas from a magnum load injected into scalp tissue results in a large, gaping stellate wound from a ripping and tearing of the skin. It is these large wounds that are frequently misinterpreted as exit wounds based solely on their size (13–15). Close examination of the wound margins of all contact wounds will reveal the presence of soot and seared skin from the discharge of hot gases and an actual flame (Fig. 36-12). In addition to the projectile and gases, soot and unburned gunpowder are also driven into the wound and can be recovered from the underlying tissue.

Wound elasticity plays a significant role in the appearance of a contact wound. When tissue is very elastic (e.g., the anterior abdominal wall), injected gases will not expand

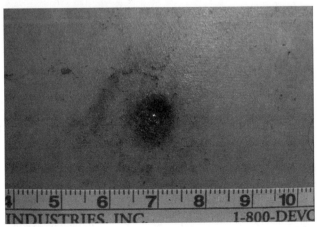

Figure 36–9. A loose-contact wound from a .25 caliber semiautomatic pistol. Soot and a surrounding contusion are visible.

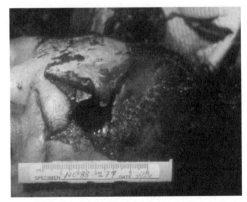

Figure 36–11. A tight-contact wound from a .357 caliber revolver. The wound displays large triangular-shaped tears with soot and seared wound margins. The large wound size is the result of large quantities of gas being injected into the scalp tissue.

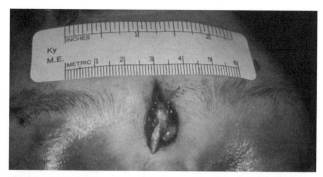

Figure 36–12. Seared wound margins and a triangular-shaped laceration at the 12 o'clock position from a tight-contact wound from a .38 caliber revolver. Soot was also visible within the wound.

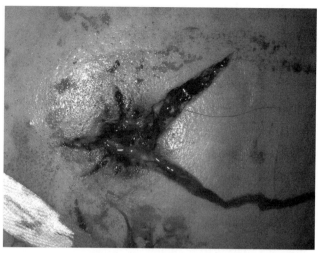

Figure 36–14. A muzzle contusion from a revolver is visible surrounding this tight-contact wound.

the tissue beyond the point at which it will tear. The same .357 caliber magnum load to the abdominal wall will only result in the deposition of soot at the wound margin and seared skin without triangle-shaped tears (Fig. 36-13).

With the injection of gases, the rapidly expanding skin may be pushed against the barrel or muzzle of the handgun with sufficient force to impart to the skin a contusion that mirrors the pattern of the barrel. This contusion is called a "muzzle contusion" or "muzzle abrasion" and may provide forensic investigators with critical information on the characteristics of the weapon's barrel, revolver versus semiautomatic handgun, used in the assault (Figs. 36-14, 36-15).

The loose-contact wound, from an angled pistol, exhibits an angled soot pattern (Fig. 36-9). The degree of tearing, if any, is dictated by the quantity of gases injected into the tissue. Incomplete muzzle contusions are possible if only a portion of the wound is pushed back against the weapon's barrel (Fig. 36-16).

A contact wound through clothing imparts a mixed picture depending on the number of layers of clothing and the

quantity of gases injected. Some of the gases will be injected into the tissues and may impart a blurred or muted muzzle contusion (Fig. 36-17). The gases can also dissect between the layers of clothing and the skin, resulting in a diffuse soot pattern overlying the muted muzzle contusion (Fig. 36-17).

EXIT WOUNDS

The size, shape, and configuration of an exit wound is dictated by the following variables: the projectile's velocity or energy as it exits the skin, the size and shape of the projectile, and the presence and nature of underlying tissue (17,18). When tissues, most commonly bone, are pushed out of the wound by the exiting bullet, the tissue will enlarge the wound itself. Exit wounds from handguns are not consistently larger than their associated entrance wounds

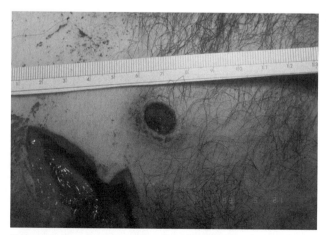

Figure 36–13. A contact wound to the abdomen from a .357 caliber magnum. The wound margins are seared, but triangular-shaped lacerations are not present due to the elasticity of the anterior abdominal wall.

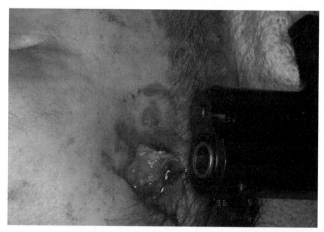

Figure 36–15. A muzzle contusion from a 9mm semiautomatic pistol. The contusion results from the forceful expansion of the skin against the barrel of the gun.

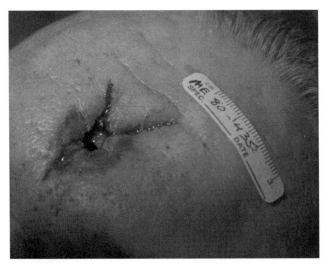

Figure 36–16. An incomplete muzzle contusion is present from the 3 o'clock to the 9 o'clock position on the forehead from a .38 caliber revolver.

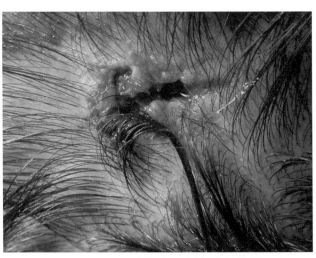

Figure 36–18. An exit wound generally has irregular borders and will lack the abrasion collar, soot, and tattooing of entrance wounds.

(11–18). The margins of exit wounds are generally irregular and lack the presence of abrasion collars, soot, and tattooing but may be slitlike if the projectile has only minimal energy as it exits the skin (Figs. 36-18, 36-19). Exit wounds may have a triangular shape that are very similar to contact wounds, but these wounds will not have any associated soot and seared skin (Fig. 36-20). A close inspection of the wound for soot is warranted if the practitioner is in doubt.

A "shored-exit" wound may exhibit what is termed a "false abrasion collar" (12,16,17). If the skin of the exit wound is pressed against a firm surface, the expanding skin may be forcibly compressed against the surface of an object (e.g., wall, door, or wallet) by the exiting projectile. This forcible contact can result in a visible abrasion that could easily be confused with an abrasion collar of an entrance wound (Figs. 36-21, 36-22).

FORENSIC EVALUATION OF CENTER-FIRE RIFLE WOUNDS

Projectiles discharged from center-fire rifles have the potential to inflict massive tissue damage (Fig. 36-23). Any bullet's wounding potential is based on the kinetic energy it possesses. The calibers of center-fire bullets, .223 to .308, are similar in diameter to handgun ammunition, but their wounding potential is greatly enhanced by the velocity of the round. The higher the velocity of a projectile, the greater the potential to inflict tissue damage based on the formula kinetic energy = mass × velocity^2/G. Injuries result from the transference of energy from the projectile to organs and bony structures. With high-velocity rounds, velocities greater than 2,000 feet/second, a temporary cavity is formed

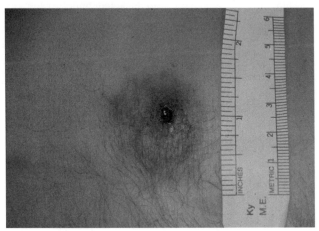

Figure 36–17. A contact wound through clothing will give a diffuse soot pattern overlying a muted muzzle contusion. Soot can be deposited between the layers of clothing.

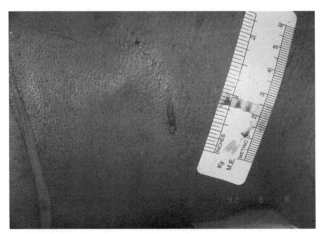

Figure 36–19. A slitlike exit wound from a 9mm projectile. Exit wounds are not consistently larger than their corresponding entrance wound.

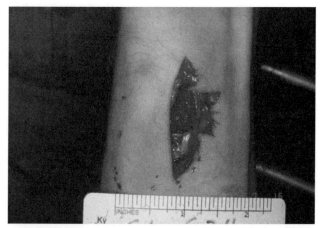

Figure 36–20. Exit wounds may exhibit triangular-shaped lacerations similar to contact entrance wounds but without the associated soot and seared skin.

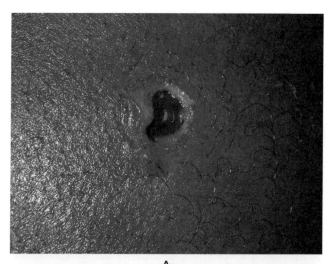

A

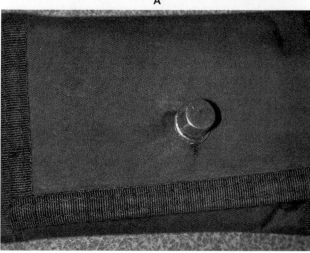

B

Figure 36–22. A, B: A "shored-exit" wound from a .40 caliber projectile that exited the lateral thigh and impacted the victim's wallet.

along the wound tract. The temporary cavity may approach 11 to 12 times the diameter of the bullet and can result in tissue damage away from the physical tract taken by the projectile itself (19). Temporary cavitation, in combination with the direct tissue disruption and energy transfer from a fragmenting or yawing (turning sideways) projectile, is what determines the size of the internal injury and that of the exit wound. Due to the amount of energy possessed and transferred to underlying tissue, exit wounds associated with center-fire rifles are, in contrast to those associated with handguns, generally larger than their corresponding entrance wounds (Fig. 36-24).

Entrance wounds associated with high-velocity center-fire projectiles do not significantly differ from those of handguns. Entrance wounds generally exhibit abrasion collars or microtears on the skin surface (Fig. 36-25). Wounds also have associated soot deposition and tattooing, but due to a number of variables (e.g., muzzle length, amount of power in a given cartridge, muzzle configuration, and type of gunpowder—ball vs. cylindrical), the range of fire in rifle wounds is not as clearly defined as in handgun wounds. The

determination of an exact range of fire for rifles and shotguns is best established through controlled testing performed by a firearms examiner at a crime laboratory.

High-velocity lead core and jacketed bullets generally break up into hundreds of fragments, called a "lead snowstorm," upon entering tissues, creating significant damage (Fig. 36-26). If the tissue is deep, the bullet fragments may fail to exit and be embedded within the victim. Thus it is possible to sustain an injury with a high-velocity round and not exhibit an exit wound. High-velocity rounds with steel cores almost uniformly exit intact and continue downrange. Both of these facts can confound the forensic investigator's efforts to find an adequate projectile sample to submit to the firearms examiner as evidence for ballistic analysis.

EVIDENCE COLLECTION

In a terrorist event involving firearms, law enforcement agencies, specifically the FBI, will attempt to collect forensic evidence from the victims. It is incumbent on the treating

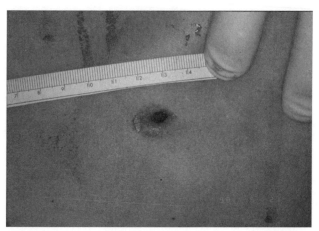

Figure 36–21. A "shored-exit" wound exhibits a "false" abrasion collar and occurs when the skin is supported or shored by a firm object as the projectile exits.

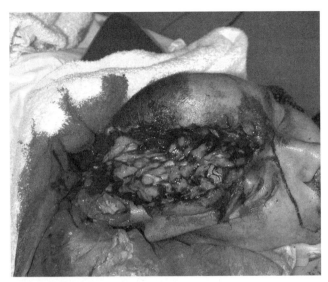

Figure 36–23. Massive head trauma from a .223 caliber high-velocity round fired at close range. Soot is present on the bridge of the victim's nose.

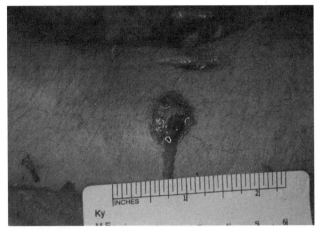

Figure 36–25. An abrasion collar associated with a high-velocity entrance wound.

medical providers to recognize, preserve, and collect short-lived evidence and not destroy valuable forensic evidence by omission or commission. Surgeon General Richard Carmona reported that trauma physicians "usually have little or no training in the forensic aspects of trauma care and therefore necessary evidence may often be overlooked, lost, inadvertently discarded or its admissibility denied because of improper handling or documentation" (20).

The practitioner's first step in evidence collection must be to describe the wound properly, including its precise anatomical location and the presence or absence of: an abrasion collar, soot, or tattooing. Ideally, this description would be supplemented with photographic documentation (21). Second, the practitioner must preserve articles of clothing so a range of fire can be determined from the presence or absence of soot, lead residue, or nitrate residues deposited on the surface of the victim's clothing (Fig. 36-27). Third, the health care provider must collect any projectiles or projectile frag-

ments that may be present in or around the victim. A "chain of custody," a written record of who has been in possession of the evidence, must be clearly documented in the medical record. Lastly, the investigating law enforcement agency may request assistance from the provider for additional assistance in collecting evidence (e.g., gunshot or explosive residue testing and radiographs of retained projectiles). At institutions where evidence collection protocols have been implemented, wounds are documented in a forensic fashion and evidence is collected in concert with medical treatment without compromising patient care (2,3).

DOCUMENTATION

An accurate description, using appropriate forensic terminology, with the anatomical location, wound characteristics, and size, is what the practitioner should strive to achieve. Wound characteristics will change, punctate abrasions will heal, and trace evidence will be lost with exploration,

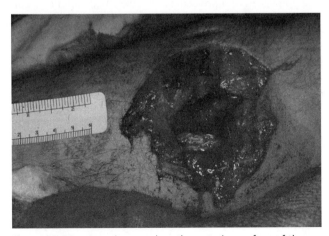

Figure 36–24. An exit wound on the anterior surface of the victim's leg from a .30 06 caliber high-velocity round. The wound is large due to the energy transferred to the underlying bone as it was extruded from the wound.

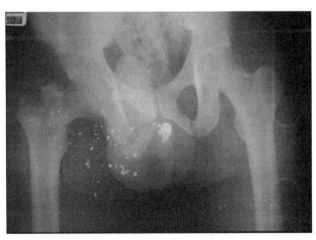

Figure 36–26. "Lead snowstorm" from a high-velocity round. Lead core and jacketed high-velocity rounds have a tendency to fragment into hundreds of pieces.

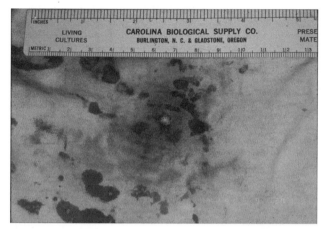

Figure 36–27. Soot deposition on a victim's shirt associated with a close-range gunshot wound. Each article of a victim's clothing should be packaged individually to avoid cross contamination.

cleansing, debridement, and the passage of time. The supplementation of an accurate wound description with a forensic photograph is ideal (21). A forensic photograph, by definition, must represent an accurate and objective depiction of its subject to be accepted as evidence in a court of law (22). To ensure a photograph's admissibility and withstand any legal challenges to its authenticity or integrity, the medical practitioner should be able to articulate the following (16):

- Exactly when and where the photograph was taken
- What the photograph depicts
- The precise anatomical location of the wound
- The size and shape of the injury
- The camera (digital or film) and type of film used
- Whether the photograph was obtained by court order versus informed or implied consent
- Where the film was developed/downloaded and if this process is standard protocol
- Whether the image has been altered and if so how (filters, computer-aided image enhancement)
- Whether the photograph "fairly and accurately" depicts what the medical provider observed

A photograph taken for forensic purposes and for admission in a court should be able to withstand any legal challenge. If the purpose of the photograph is to document the size of the gunshot wound, a scale must be placed next to the wound and the photograph must be taken at 90 degrees to the wound (Fig. 36-28). If the photograph is not taken at

90 degrees to the wound, the scale will not be accurate because perspective distortion is introduced (21). At a minimum, an orientation photograph, showing the general anatomical location of the wound as well as a close-up photo, should be obtained. This will permit investigators and a potential juror to not only visualize and understand the medical provider's forensic description and evidence associated with the wound but also its location on the victim.

The physician is required by law to obtain consent from the victim prior to the taking of the photograph (21). If the patient is unconscious, incapacitated, or unable to give consent, the photograph may be taken using implied consent. The use of implied consent is based on the assumption that the victim of a crime or terrorist event would want short-lived forensic evidence collected to assist in the investigation of the assault. If a patient, victim, or suspect is under arrest, presents with a court order for photographic documentation, or is dead, he or she has given up the right of refusal.

CLOTHING

Clothing can be an extremely valuable piece of forensic evidence in determining entrance from exit wounds and the range of fire. Visible and invisible residues from nitrates and lead can be deposited on the clothing. The pattern and concentration of these residues can be evaluated and reconstructed at the crime laboratory (Fig. 36-29). Each piece of the victim's clothing should be preserved in separate paper bags (23). Separate bagging also prevents the cross contamination of the residues to nonaffected articles of clothing. The use of paper bags permits any moisture present on the clothing to evaporate and minimizes the possibility of molding. Examination of the clothing fibers may also help in the determination of entrance versus exit wound because the fibers will deform in the direction of the passing projectile (Fig. 36-30). "Bullet wipe," a deposition of lead or lubricants, may also be present on clothing overlying a distant entrance wound (Fig. 36-31).

PROJECTILES

The propulsion of a projectile down the rifled barrel of a gun imparts multiple unique microscopic marks, "rifling impressions," on the side of the bullet (Fig. 36-32A). These microscopic marks, or "fingerprints," can be examined with a comparison microscope by the firearms examiner to determine if the projectile was fired from a specific gun (Fig. 36-32B). The medical practitioner should make every effort not to destroy or compromise these marks when removing or collecting the bullet from a patient. These bullets should be handled without any metal-to-metal contact (i.e., dropping the projectile into a metal pan or removing it from tissue with hemostats). Hemostats or pickups can be covered with gauze to prevent the destruction of the microscopic "fingerprints" (Fig. 36-33).

Projectiles, like other evidence collected from a shooting victim, must be collected in a breathable container such as an envelope or paper box (Fig. 36-34A). Bullets placed in an airtight container, such as a specimen container or film canister, will result in contamination and degradation of the evidence from moisture and proliferation of bacteria (Fig. 36-34B).

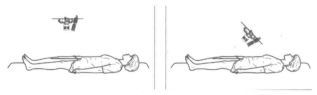

Figure 36–28. A forensic photograph for documentation of wound size must contain a scale and be taken at 90 degrees to the subject. If the lens is less than 90 degrees to the subject, perspective distortion is introduced.

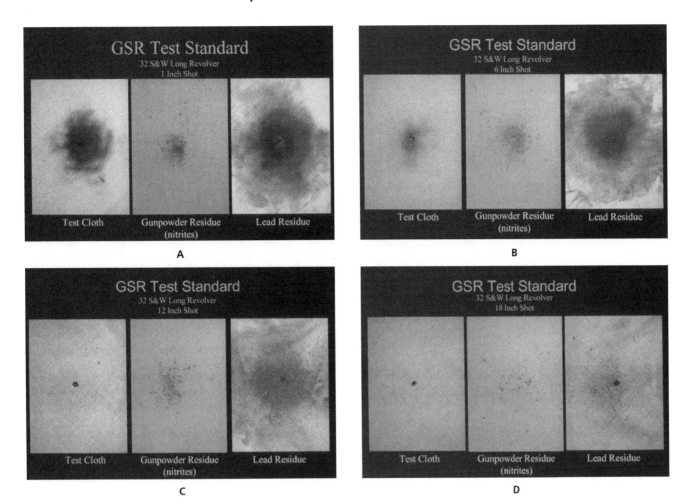

Figure 36–29 A–D: Testing of a victim's clothing for the presence of gunshot residues is an important component in determining a range of fire. Soot, nitrate, and lead residue deposition will vary with the muzzle to target distance. Lead and nitrate residues, invisible to the naked eye, are demonstrated at the 18-inch range in Figure 36–29D. Test firing under controlled conditions at the crime laboratory can be used to determine an accurate range of fire.

Radiographs, taken in the normal course of providing medical treatment, may also hold valuable forensic evidence on the number of projectiles, a projectile's characteristics, and the direction of fire. However, the medical provider should never estimate a bullet caliber on the basis of a routine x ray.

Traditional diagnostic radiography will induce projectile magnification unless the x-ray source is exactly 72 inches from the bullet. Radiographs will also assist the physician in determining when a high-velocity projectile was used by visualizing the "lead snowstorm" pattern (Fig. 36-26).

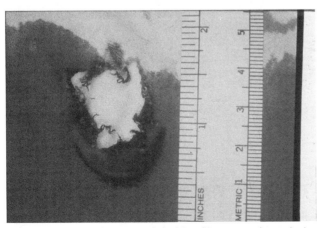

Figure 36–30. Examination of clothing fibers may also assist in the differentiation of entrance from exit.

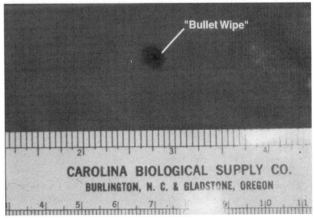

Figure 36–31. "Bullet wipe" is the deposition of lead residues and lubricants on clothing as the projectile penetrates.

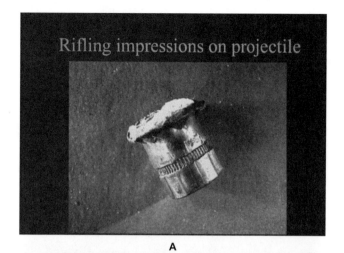

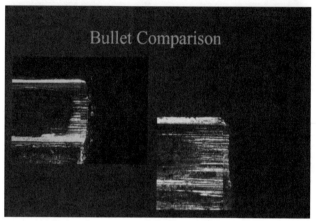

Figure 36–32 A, B: Microscopic rifling impressions are a unique fingerprint of a gun's barrel. The firearms examiner utilizes a comparison microscope to compare a projectile from a victim from one test fired from a suspected weapon. The split screen on the comparison microscope permits the examiner to rotate the projectiles to look for a match.

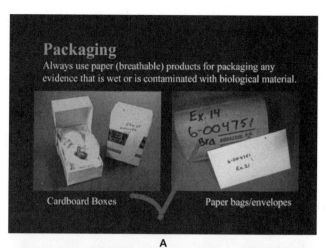

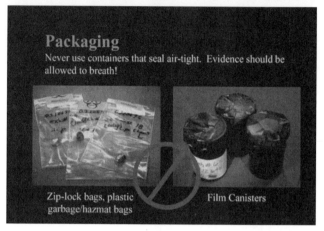

Figure 36–34. A, B: Projectiles recovered from victims must be collected in breathable containers (i.e., paper envelopes or boxes). Placement of bullets with blood or tissue in an airtight container will result in degradation of the projectile from the presence of moisture and the proliferation of mold.

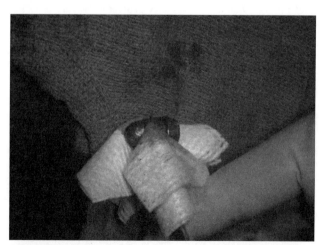

Figure 36–33. Medical providers must avoid metal-to-metal contact in the retrieval of projectiles to prevent destruction of critical evidence. Placement of gauze over the end of the hemostat or pickups will prevent the destruction of a bullet's microscopic impressions.

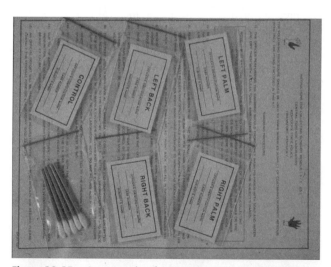

Figure 36–35. An example of a FART (Firearms Residue Test) or GSR (Gunshot Residue Test). This test involves the wiping of the front and back of a suspect's hands with a 5% nitric acid solution looking for the presence of primer and gunshot residues.

SUMMARY

The forensic evaluation of gunshot wounds and the collection of their associated evidence—whether at the crime scene, in the emergency department, or in the autopsy suite—will be critical components of the investigation and reconstruction of a terrorist incident. Questions still linger in the JFK assassination on the number and type of wounds present on his head and neck. Wouldn't the forensic world loved to have known what the president's neck wound looked liked, in proper forensic terms, prior to surgical intervention? The medical response to a terrorist event must include trained physicians, nurses, and prehospital responders who have not only expert medical skills but also possess the knowledge to evaluate and document gunshot wounds from a forensic perspective. This information, coupled with an evidence collection component, will permit law enforcement to prosecute successfully those responsible. Medical providers should strive to provide outstanding medical care in terrorist incidents without compromising the forensic elements of the criminal investigations that will follow.

RESIDUE TESTING

The investigating law enforcement agency may request that a gunshot residue test, or GSR, be performed on a victim or suspect (Fig. 36–35). This test, which looks for the presence of barium nitrate, antimony sulfide, or lead peroxide residues from the primer of the cartridge, only indicates the victim has been in an area where a weapon has been discharged (23–32). A positive GSR does not indicate, within reasonable scientific certainty, that the individual fired the weapon, only that he or she has been in an area where a weapon was discharged. A false-positive test can result from the transfer of residues from the shooter's hands to the hands of another individual (e.g., a police officer discharges a weapon and handcuffs a suspect) (32). Residues can fall to a tabletop and be picked up by someone other than the shooter, who inadvertently places a hand on the tabletop and has a so-called positive test.

REFERENCES

1. Smialek JE. Forensic medicine in the emergency department. Emerg Med Clin North Am 1983;1(3):693-704.
2. Smock WS, Nichols GR, Fuller PM. Development and implementation of the first clinical forensic medicine training program. J Forensic Sci 1993;38(4):835.
3. Smock WS. Development of a clinical forensic medicine curriculum for emergency physicians in the USA. J Clin Forensic Med 1994;1(1):27.
4. Smock WS, Ross CS, Hamilton FN. Clinical forensic medicine: how ED physicians can help with the sleuthing. Emerg Legal Briefings 1994;5(1):1.
5. Eckert WG, Bell JS, Stein RJ, et al. Clinical forensic medicine. Am J Forensic Med Pathol 1096;(3):182.
6. Mittleman RE, Goldberg HS, Waksman DM. Preserving evidence in the emergency department. Am J Nurs 1983;83(12):1652-6.
7. Godley DR, Smith TK. Some medicolegal aspects of gunshot wounds. J Trauma 1977;17(11):866-71.
8. Ryan MT. Clinical forensic medicine. Ann Emerg Med 2000;36(3):271-3.
9. Goldsmith MF. US forensic pathologists on a new case: examination of living patients. JAMA 1986;256(13):1685.
10. Fackler ML, Riddick L. Clinicians' inadequate descriptions of gunshot wounds obstruct justice: clinical journals refuse to expose the problem. Proc Am Acad Forensic Sci II:150. Colorado Springs: McCormick-Armstrong, 1996.
11. Smock WS. Forensic emergency medicine. In: Marx JA, Hockberger RS, Walls RM, et al. eds. Rosen's emergency medicine: concepts and clinical practice. 5th ed. St. Louis: Mosby, 2002;828-41.
12. Dana SE, DiMaio VJM. Gunshot trauma in forensic medicine: clinical and pathological aspects. In: Payne-James J, Busuttil A, Smock W eds. Greenwich Medical Media (GMM), 2003; 149-68.
13. Collins KA, Lantz PE. Interpretation of fatal, multiple, and exiting gunshot wounds by trauma specialists. J Forensic Sci 1994;39(1):94-9.
14. Marlow AL, Smock WS. The forensic evaluation of gunshot wounds by prehospital personnel. Proc Am Acad Forensic Sci II:149. Colorado Springs: McCormick-Armstrong, 1996.
15. Randall T. Clinicians' forensic interpretations of fatal gunshot wounds often miss the mark. JAMA 1993;269(16): 2058-61.
16. Smock WS. Forensic emergency medicine. In: Olshaker JS, Jackson MC, Smock WS eds. Philadelphia: Lippincott Williams & Wilkins: 63-83.
17. DiMaio VJM. Gunshot wounds: practical aspects of firearms, ballistics, and forensic techniques. 2nd ed. In: Geberth VJ, series ed. Boca Raton, FL: CRC Press, 1999.
18. Spitz WU. Spitz and Fisher's medicolegal investigation of death: guidelines for the application of pathology to crime investigation. In: Spitz WU ed. 3rd ed. Springfield, IL: Charles C. Thomas, 1993.
19. Sellier KG, Kneubuehl BP. Wound ballistics and the scientific background. Amsterdam: Elsevier Science, 1994.
20. Carmona R, Prince K. Trauma and forensic medicine. J Trauma 1989;29(9):1222-5.
21. Smock WS. Forensic photography. In: Stack LB, Storrow AB, Morris MA, et al. eds. Handbook of medical photography. Hanley and Belfus, 2001;397-408.
22. Osborne TL. Demonstrative evidence. In: Osborne TL, ed. Trial handbook for Kentucky lawyers. 2nd ed. Rochester, NY: Lawyers Cooperative Publishing, 1992.
23. Lee HC, Palmbach T, Miller MT. Henry Lee's crime scene handbook. San Diego: Academic Press, 2001.
24. Andrasko J, Maehly AC. Detection of gunshot residues on hands by scanning electron microscopy. J Forensic Sci 1977; 22(2):279-87.
25. Matricardi VR, Kilty JW. Detection of gunshot particles from the hands of a shooter by SEM. J Forensic Sci 1977;22(4):725.
26. Wolten GM, et al. Particle analysis for the detection of gunshot residue. I. Scanning electron microscopy/energy dispersive x-ray characterization of hand deposits from firing. J Forensic Sci 1979;24(2):409.
27. Wolten GM, et al. Particle analysis for the detection of gunshot residue. II. Occupational and environmental particles. J Forensic Sci 1979;24(2):423.
28. Wolten GM, et al. Particle analysis for the detection of gunshot residue. III. The case record. J Forensic Sci 1979;24(4):864.

29. Tillman J. Automated gunshot residue particle search and characterization. J Forensic Sci 1987;32(1):62.

30. Kee TG, Beck C. Casework assessment of an automated scanning electron microscope/microanalysis system for the detection of firearms discharge particles. J Forensic Sci Soc 1987;27(5):321.

31. Zeichner A, Levin N. Casework experience of GSR detection in Israel, on samples from hands, hair, and clothing using ok? An autosearch SEM/EDX system. J Forensic Sci 1995;40(6): 1082.

32. Gialamas DM, et al. Officers, their weapons and their hands: an empirical study of GSR on the hands of non-shooting police officers. J Forensic Sci 1995;40(6):1086.

37

Homeland Security

F. Marion Cain III

INTRODUCTION

With the exception of the Revolutionary War over two hundred years ago, the vast majority of Americans have never felt threatened inside the borders of the continental United States. America is surrounded on both sides by large oceans making physical attacks against U.S. territory all but impossible. This situation began to change during the Cold War. With the advent of ballistic missile technology and large-scale atomic and nuclear weapons, the homeland was now vulnerable to direct physical attack.

The federal government attempted to deal with this relatively new threat by establishing the Civil Defense program and by increasing expenditures in strategic weapons such as bombers, submarines, and missiles. A medical system was created to handle the large number of mass casualties that would be created by a thermonuclear attack on the United States.

When the Cold War ended in 1989, Americans began to feel safe from direct attack, and many Civil Defense programs, such as fallout shelters, were discontinued altogether. Many federal agencies played a role in the Civil Defense program, the Federal Emergency Management Agency (FEMA), began to focus more on preparation and response to natural disasters such as floods, fires, and hurricanes. The medical system created to handle mass casualties of a nuclear holocaust began to atrophy.

1995—THE YEAR TERRORISM STRIKES: TOKYO SUBWAY AND THE MURRAH FEDERAL BUILDING

On March 20, 1995, an event that was truly unique in the annals of terrorism took place (1). An obscure religious sect calling themselves Aum Shinrikyo unleashed an attack on the Tokyo subway system using the deadly nerve agent sarin. The immediate effects of the attack were staggering as 12 people died and over 5,000 reported to local hospitals with suspected signs and symptoms of nerve agent poisoning.

Also, over 10% of the responders who rushed into the subway became casualties (1).

Unbeknownst to the Japanese government, the group had been experimenting with weapons of mass destruction (WMD) agents for some time. Following a failed attempt to gain political power through elections in 1990, the group decided to develop unconventional weapons as a path to power and influence. Originally, Aum Shinrikyo tried to develop biological weapons. Fortunately the group's attempts were unsuccessful, and after investing millions of dollars in failed attempts to develop botulinum toxin, Ebola virus, anthrax, the venom of poisonous snakes, and mushrooms, Aum Shinrikyo shifted its development effort to chemical weapons (1).

Beginning in 1993, the group spent over $30 million to develop a chemical weapons arsenal. At various times Aum Shinrikyo produced at least limited quantities of VX, tabum, mustard gas, hydrogen cyanide, and phosgene. However, beginning in 1993, the group began to focus almost exclusively on the manufacture and production of sarin. On the night of June 27, 1994, the group was ready for its first dress rehearsal. In an attack on the mountain city of Matsumoto, the sect used a truck mounted with sprayers to disperse the deadly agent. The resulting attack left 7 dead and 58 hospitalized. Another 253 sought medical treatment on an outpatient basis (1).

Finally, on March 20, 1995, Aum Shinrikyo was ready. Using five assault teams consisting of two men each, the sect members planned an attack on the crowded Tokyo subway system at the height of Monday morning rush hour. Each team boarded a different train carrying two brown paper bags containing a plastic container of sarin. Between 7:46 A.M. and 8:01 A.M., cult members punctured the bags with an umbrella and stepped off the trains. As the trains continued down the track to the next station, toxic fumes began seeping from the bags. The effects were rapid. Passengers began displaying signs of coughing, vomiting, and convulsing within a few stops (1).

The first fire and emergency medical units began to respond shortly after eight o'clock and were quickly overwhelmed by the number of casualties flooding the train stations and pouring out onto the streets. Initial responders were not equipped with personal protective equipment (PPE). Consequently, many of them became casualties as they descended into the stations. Patients were not decontaminated at the incident scene before being transported to hospitals. In addition to almost 700 casualties transported to hospitals by ambulances, hospitals were quickly overwhelmed by over 4,000 victims self-referring to hospital emergency rooms. Of the 5,510 patients eventually treated, 85% were psychogenic, displaying no real chemical injuries. Tokyo police took over 2 hours to identify the agent as sarin. Meanwhile, hospitals had only limited stocks of 2-PAM and atropine sulfate to administer to the most seriously ill patients. Failure to decontaminate patients at the incident scene before transporting resulted in about 10% of the emergency medical technicians (EMTs) displaying symptoms of nerve agent poisoning, probably from off-gassing. The emergency room (ER) staff was also susceptible to off-gassing with approximately 16% of some ER staffs becoming casualties themselves (1).

Aum Shinrikyo's attack was significant because it represented the first chemical weapons attack by a nonstate group on a civilian population. This was a major turning point in the history of terrorism. After March 20, 1995, no one ever looked at terrorism quite the same.

Within less than a month following Aum Shinrikyo's deadly attack on the Tokyo subway, another terrorist attack would occur in the heartland of the United States and would shake America to its very core. At 9:02 A.M. on April 19, 1995, Timothy McVeigh exploded a rented truck containing a mixture of 4,800 pounds of ammonium nitrate (common fertilizer) and nitromethane (racing fuel) in front of the Alfred P. Murrah Federal Building in Oklahoma City, Oklahoma. The explosion destroyed several concrete columns at the front of the building causing a structural collapse of a major portion of the building's nine floors. The blast killed 168 people—19 of them children who attended a day care center located on the building's ground floor. Over 600 people were injured, and 25 surrounding buildings were severely damaged or destroyed. Prior to the attacks of September 11, 2001, the terrorist attack on the Murrah Federal Building was the largest domestic terrorist attack in the history of the United States (3).

AMERICA RESPONDS: PRESIDENTIAL DECISION DIRECTIVE 39 AND NUNN-LUGAR-DOMENICI ACT OF 1996

The Aum Shinrikyo nerve agent attack on the Tokyo subway and the bombing of the Murrah Federal Building in Oklahoma City clearly demonstrate that the nature of the terrorist threat has changed significantly over the last few years. Twenty years ago the purpose of the majority of terrorist attacks was to gain publicity for the terrorist group. To get their name and particular cause broadcast across the world was usually their primary objective. Invariably these terrorist attacks would result in relatively few casualties. The economic impact of these attacks was also very limited. The terrorist attacks of 1995 showed that the very nature of terrorism had changed fundamentally. Now, publicity and notoriety were no longer the primary objectives. The purpose of the new attacks was to create human casualties and to effect as many economic and social consequences as possible. These objectives could only be achieved by use of WMD.

Following these attacks, the federal government took several steps to better prepare the nation's responders to deal with this new threat posed by WMD. On June 21, 1995, President Clinton signed Presidential Decision Directive-39 (PDD-39), U.S. Policy on Counterterrorism. This classified document laid out the national policy and assigned specific missions to designated federal departments and agencies. PDD-39 reaffirmed existing Department of Justice (DOJ) and Federal Bureau of Investigation (FBI) responsibilities for counterterrorism and the threats or acts of terrorism within the United States. The directive further clarified the role of FEMA as the primary federal agency responsible for managing the on-scene response to an act of terrorism in the United States. PDD-39 also established U.S. policy for combating terrorism. It recognized that terrorism is a threat to national security as well as a criminal act. Therefore, the policy of the United States was to use all appropriate means to deter, defeat, and respond to all terrorist attacks on U.S. territory and resources, both with people and facilities, wherever they occur (4).

To ensure that the United States was better prepared to combat terrorism in all of its forms, a number of measures were directed. These included reducing vulnerabilities to terrorism, deterring and responding to terrorist attacks, and having capabilities to prevent and manage the consequences of terrorist use of WMD. To reduce vulnerabilities to terrorism, both at home and abroad, all departmental/agency heads were directed to ensure that their personnel and facilities were fully protected against terrorism. The Domestic Emergency Support Team (DEST) was created to respond to domestic incidents of terrorism. DEST membership was limited to those agencies required to respond to the specific incident. These teams included elements capable of responding to specific types of threats such as nuclear, chemical, and biological. The development of effective capabilities for preventing and managing use of WMD materials or weapons was given the highest priority. Senior officials were very concerned about the possibility of terrorists acquiring WMD, and preventing the acquisition of such materials/weapons or removing the capability from terrorist groups was given the highest priority (4).

Concerned that WMDs were becoming increasingly available to terrorists, Congress passed the Defense Against Weapons of Mass Destruction Act of 1996, commonly known as the Nunn-Lugar-Domenici Act (Public Law 104-201, September 23, 1996). The act designated the Department of Defense (DOD) as the lead agency to enhance domestic preparedness for responding to the use of WMD. Under the act, DOD was tasked to provide training, exercise, and expert advice to emergency response personnel and lend equipment to local jurisdictions.

The DOD identified the nation's 120 largest cities for receipt of training, exercises, and equipment to enhance their capacity to respond to WMD incidents. On April 6, 2000, President Clinton transferred this program to the Department of Justice (DOJ). Prior to the program's transfer, DOD trained over 28,000 first responders, delivered all three program elements to 68 of the 120 cities, and delivered the training components to an additional 37 cities. The program was again transferred on March 1, 2003, to the Department of Homeland Security (DHS) for completion of training for the remaining cities (5).

REFINING THE PROCESS: PRESIDENTIAL DECISION DIRECTIVES 62 AND 63

In an attempt to clarify several aspects of PDD-39, and to strengthen the nation's defenses against emerging unconventional threats, President Clinton issued Presidential Decision Directives 62 and 63 in May 1998. PDD-62 focused on terrorist acts and the use of WMD, while PDD-63 focused on unconventional assaults on the United States' critical infrastructures and cyber-attacks.

Combating Terrorism Directive, PDD-62, highlighted the growing threat of unconventional attacks against the United States. It detailed a new and more systematic approach to fighting terrorism by bringing a program management approach to U.S. counterterrorism efforts. The directive also established the Office of National Coordinator for Security, Infrastructure Protection and Counter-Terrorism to oversee a broad variety of relevant policies and programs, including areas such as counterterrorism, protection of critical infrastructure, and preparedness and consequence management for WMD. It reinforced the mission of the many federal agencies charged with defeating terrorism and codified and clarified their activities in a wide range of counterterrorism programs (5).

The Presidential Decision Directive 63 (PDD-63) specifically addressed critical infrastructure protection and called for a national effort to ensure the security of the vulnerable and interconnected infrastructures of the United States. These infrastructures included telecommunications, banking and finance, energy, transportation, and essential government services. The directive required immediate federal government action, including risk assessment and planning to reduce exposure of the critical components of America's economy. It stressed the importance of cooperation between the government and the private sector by linking designated agencies with private sector representatives (6).

PDD-63 built upon the recommendations of the President's Commission on Critical Infrastructure protection. In October 1997, the commission issued its report calling for a national effort to ensure the security of the United States' increasingly vulnerable and interconnected infrastructures. PDD-63 was the culmination of an intense, interagency effort to evaluate those recommendations and produce a workable and innovative framework for critical infrastructure protection. The president's policy set a goal of achieving a reliable, interconnected, and secure information system infrastructure by the year 2003 and significantly increased security to government systems by establishing a national center to warn of and respond to attacks. The directive also addressed the cyber and physical infrastructure vulnerabilities of the federal government by requiring each department and agency to work to reduce its exposure to these new threats (6).

PDD-63 was unique in that it was one of the first documents to seek the voluntary participation of private industry to meet common goals for protecting critical systems through public-private partnerships. PDD-63 set up a new structure to deal with this important challenge by establishing the National Infrastructure Protection Center (NIPC) to combine representatives from FBI, DOD, U.S. Secret Service, Energy, Transportation, the intelligence community, and the private sector in an unprecedented attempt at information sharing among agencies. The NIPC also provided the principal means of facilitating and coordinating the federal government's response to an incident, mitigating attacks, investigating threats, and monitoring reconstitution efforts (6).

9/11 AND THE CHANGES TO HOMELAND SECURITY

Following the unprecedented terrorist attacks against the World Trade Center and the Pentagon on September 11, 2001, the president and congress took several steps to enhance homeland security against terrorist attacks. On October 17, 2002, the National Security Counsel published the National Security Strategy of the United States of America. The purpose of this document was to establish a new national security strategy focused on homeland security by deterring attacks abroad and protecting against attacks at home (7).

To further emphasize the importance of homeland security, the National Security Counsel also published the first National Strategy for Homeland Security on July 16, 2002. This document was written with the expressed purpose to "mobilize and prepare The United States to secure the U.S. homeland from terrorist attacks." The strategy provided a national framework for homeland security by setting direction for federal departments and agencies that have a role in homeland security. It suggested steps that state and local governments, private companies, organizations, and individual Americans could take to improve their security. The document stated three strategic objectives: (a) prevent terrorist attacks within the United States; (b) reduce America's vulnerability to terrorism; and (c) minimize the damage and recover from attacks that do occur. Additionally, the strategy identified several major initiatives to help the nation better prepare for homeland security: (a) integration of several separate federal response plans into a single all-discipline incident management plan, (b) creation of a national incident management system, (c) preparation of health care providers for catastrophic terrorism, (d) augmentation of America's pharmaceutical and vaccine stockpiles, and (e) introduction of several initiatives to strengthen the capability of the nation's first responders to respond to a terrorist attack (8).

Published in December 2002, the National Domestic Preparedness Strategy was developed to help deal with various homeland security issues. This document articulates a national strategy specifically focused on combating WMD. The strategy recognized that the threat of a WMD attack represents one of the greatest security challenges facing the United States and conveys a comprehensive strategy to counter this threat. The document clearly states that the United States ". . . will not permit the world's most dangerous regimes and terrorists to threaten us with the world's most destructive weapons." The strategy outlines three principal pillars for combating WMD. The first is counterproliferation. The United States will use interdiction, deterrence, defense, and mitigation to counter the threat of WMD. Second, the United States will pursue an active nonproliferation strategy through the use of diplomacy, threat reduction cooperation, controls of nuclear materials, export controls, and sanctions. Finally, the strategy recognizes that all levels of government must be prepared to respond to the effects of a WMD attack (9).

One of the most important documents published by the White House following the terrorist attacks of September 11, 2001, was Homeland Security Presidential Directive 5 (HSPD-5). Published in February of 2003, this document further clarified roles of federal agencies in homeland security and mandated several important policy issues that would have a far-reaching impact on state and local response to acts of terrorism. First, HSPD-5 established the Secretary of Homeland Security as the principal federal official for management of domestic incidents. The secretary is responsible for coordinating the federal response within the United States and to prepare for, respond to, and recover from terrorist attacks, major disasters, or other emergencies. Previously, the director of FEMA had been responsible for these functions. (10).

HSPD-5 also called for the establishment of a single, comprehensive approach to incident management. Previously, incident management was not standardized, and many state and local jurisdictions developed their own unique approach. While the individual incident management systems worked well for small, localized events, such as fire or other local emergencies, response to a larger event involving multiple organizations from many different jurisdictions would require a more standardized approach. Therefore, the Secretary of Homeland Security was directed to develop a National Incident Management System (NIMS). The system would provide a consistent nationwide approach for federal, state, and local governments to work effectively together to plan for and respond to domestic incidents regardless of size or complexity. NIMS would provide for interoperability and compatibility among federal, state, and local levels of government by establishing a common set of concepts, principles, and terminology. All federal, state, and local agencies are required to adopt NIMS by fiscal year 2005 (10).

Furthermore, HSPD-5 established a National Response Plan (NRP). Although FEMA had long been responsible for a Federal Response Plan for natural disasters, response planning was not standardized across the federal, state, and local levels. Previously, many government agencies developed specific response plans that often dealt with just one threat or emergency and were not integrated with other agencies or response requirements. The NRP would be an integrated document focusing on an all-hazards approach to planning. The NRP would provide structure for a national-level response to include protocols for operating under different threats or threat levels, a consistent approach to reporting incidents, and a standard method of providing assessments. HSDP-5 also recognized that the initial responsibility for managing domestic incidents would fall on state and local authorities and called upon these entities to develop their own all-hazards plans and capabilities (10).

THE HOMELAND SECURITY ACT OF 2002 AND PUBLIC LAW 107-296

Perhaps the most important action taken by the federal government following the September 11, 2001, terrorist attacks was passage of the Homeland Security Act of 2002. Signed into law as Public Law 107-296 by President Bush on November 25, 2002, this important law established the Department of Homeland Security (DHS). The bill specifies the mission, functions, organization, and authorities of the new department. Congress' intent is the primary mission of the new department, including preventing terrorist attacks within the United States, reducing the vulnerability of the United States to terrorism at home, and minimizing the damage and assisting in the recovery from any attacks that may occur. The department's primary responsibilities correspond to the five major functions established by the bill: (a) information analysis and infrastructure protection; (b) chemical, biological, radiological, nuclear, and related countermeasures; (c) border and transportation security; (d) emergency preparedness and response; and (e) coordination with other parts of the federal government; state and local governments; and the private sector. The bill also established a secretary of Homeland Security and under secretaries for each of the major divisions within the department. In addition to specifying the major departments within Homeland Security, Congress also specified the 22 existing federal agencies to be transferred into the new department (11).

THE DEPARTMENT OF HOMELAND SECURITY—ORGANIZATION AND FUNCTIONS

The creation of the Department of Homeland Security is the most significant reorganization within the U.S. government since 1947 when President Truman merged the various branches of the U.S. armed forces into the Department of Defense. On March 1, 2003, over 170,000 federal employees were transferred to the new organization.

The Department of Homeland Security's first priority is to protect the nation against further terrorist attacks. To accomplish this mission successfully, the DHS is organized into four major directorates: (a) Border and Transportation Security, (b) Emergency Preparedness and Response, (c) Science and Technology, and (d) Information Analysis and Infrastructure Protection. The following is a description of each of the agencies transferred into the DHS:

The Border and Transportation Security directorate is responsible for: (a) preventing the entry of terrorists and the instruments of terrorism into the United States; (b) securing the borders, territorial waters, ports, terminals, waterways, air, land, and sea transportation systems; (c) administering the immigration and naturalization laws; (d) administering the customs laws; and (e) ensuring the speedy, orderly, and efficient flow of lawful traffic and commerce in carrying out these responsibilities (11). The agencies listed in Table 37-1 were transferred to this directorate (12).

The mission of the Border and Transportation Security directorate is staggering given that 730 million people travel on commercial aircraft and that there are more than 700 million pieces of baggage being screened for explosives each year. Additionally, there are 11.2 million trucks and 2.2 million rail cars that cross into the United States each year. Also, 7,500 foreign flagships make 51,000 calls in U.S. ports annually. DHS is responsible for protecting the movement of international trade across the nation's borders, max-

TABLE 37-1 Agencies Transferred to DHS, Directorate of Border and Transportation Security

AGENCY	TRANSFERRED FROM
U.S. Customs Service	Department of Treasury
Immigration and Naturalization Service (part)	Department of Justice
Federal Protective Service	General Services Administration
Transportation and Security Administration	Department of Transportation
Federal Law Enforcement Training Center	Department of Treasury
Animal and Plant Health Inspection Service (part)	Department of Agriculture

imizing the security of the international supply chain, and engaging foreign governments and trading partners in programs designed to identify and eliminate security threats before they arrive at U. S. ports and borders (12).

To better perform this mission, DHS combined the Animal and Plant Inspection Service, the Immigration and Naturalization Service, the Border Patrol, and the U.S. Customs Service to form the Customs and Border Protection Agency (CBP). CBP secures the nation's borders by providing border and ports of entry security, interdicting the passage of illegal goods, and working overseas to prevent illegal smuggling and immigration. Also, the responsibility for providing immigration-related services and benefits such as naturalization and work authorization was transferred from the Immigration and Naturalization Service (INS) to the Bureau of Citizenship and Immigration Services (BCIS) (12).

Transferred from the Department of Treasury, the Federal Law Enforcement Training Center (FLETC) trains the majority of federal officers and agents. It not only services 76 federal agencies but also provides training to state, local, and international police in selected advanced programs. Its headquarters are located on a 1,500-acre campus at Glynco, near Brunswick, Georgia, but FLETC also operates satellite federal training facilities at Artesia, New Mexico, and Cheltenham, Maryland. FLETC oversees the operations of the International Law Enforcement Academy at Gabarone, Botswana, and supports training for the U.S. Border Patrol at Charleston, South Carolina (13).

In the event of a terrorist attack, natural disaster, or other large-scale emergency, the DHS will assume primary responsibility for coordinating and directing the federal response. The DHS directorate, Emergency Preparedness and Re-

sponse, is responsible for overseeing domestic disaster preparedness training and coordinating the U.S. government response to a major event. Functions transferred to this directorate include (a) helping to ensure the preparedness of emergency response providers for major disasters and other emergencies; (b) establishing standards, conducting exercises, and training and evaluating performances; (c) coordinating the federal government's response to terrorist attacks and major disasters; (d) aiding the recovery from terrorist attacks and major disasters; (e) working with other federal and nonfederal agencies to build a comprehensive national incident management system; (f) consolidating existing federal government emergency response plans into a single, coordinated national response plan; and (g) developing comprehensive programs for interoperative communications technology and ensuring that emergency response providers acquire such technology. This directorate is also responsible for several specific functions: (a) coordinating the overall response; (b) directing the Domestic Emergency Support Team, the Strategic National Stockpile, the National Disaster Medical System, and the Nuclear Incident Response Team; (c) overseeing the Metropolitan Medical Response System; and (d) coordinating other federal response resources (11). The agencies listed in Table 37-2 were transferred to this directorate (12).

In connection with an actual or threatened terrorist attack, major disaster, or other emergency, the Secretary of Homeland Security is authorized to call certain elements of the Department of Energy (DOE) and the Environmental Protection Agency (EPA) into service as an organizational unit of DHS. These organizations provide expert personnel and specialized equipment to deal with the various nuclear emergencies, accidents, and terrorism. These teams include expertise in such

TABLE 37-2 Agencies Transferred to DHS, Directorate of Emergency Preparedness and Response

AGENCY	TRANSFERRED FROM
Federal Emergency Management Agency	FEMA
Strategic Pharmaceutical National Stockpile	Department of Health and Human Services
National Disaster Medical System	Department of Health and Human Services
Nuclear Incident Response Team	Department of Energy
Domestic Emergency Response Team	Department of Justice
National Domestic Preparedness Office	FBI
Office of Emergency Preparedness	Department of Health and Human Services
Metropolitan Medical Response System	Department of Health and Human Services

areas as device assessment and disablement, intelligence analysis, credibility assessment, and health physics (12).

Urban search and rescue (USAR) is another important aspect of the Emergency Preparedness and Response directorate. USAR involves the location, rescue, and initial medical stabilization of victims trapped in confined spaces. Structural collapse is most often the cause of victims being trapped, but victims may also be trapped in transportation accidents, mines, and collapsed trenches. USAR is considered a "multihazard" discipline, as it may be needed for a variety of emergencies or disasters, including earthquakes, hurricanes, typhoons, storms and tornadoes, floods, dam failures, technological accidents, terrorist activities, and hazardous material releases. Each USAR task force is composed of 62 positions. The task forces often include more than 130 highly trained members and are formed as a partnership between local fire departments, law enforcement agencies, federal and local governmental agencies, and private companies. A task force is totally self-sufficient for the first 72 hours of a deployment. The entire team and its equipment can be deployed in a U.S. Air Force C-141 or two C-130 aircraft. Team training requirements are very intense. In addition to being an EMT, each task force member must complete hundreds of hours of specialty training such as K-9, search and rescue, and rigging. Each task force is capable of (a) conducting physical search and rescue in collapsed buildings, (b) providing emergency medical care to trapped victims, (c) using search and rescue dogs, (d) assessing and controlling of gas, electric service, and hazardous materials, and (e) evaluating and stabilizing damaged structures (14).

DHS is also responsible for overseeing several public health-related response activities. The National Disaster Medical System (NDMS) is a cooperative asset-sharing program among federal government agencies, state and local governments, private businesses, and volunteers to ensure that resources are available to provide medical services following a disaster that overwhelms the local health care resources. NDMS is a federally coordinated system that augments the nation's emergency medical response capability. The overall purpose of the NDMS is to establish a single, integrated national medical response capability for assisting state and local authorities in dealing with the medical and health effects of major peacetime disasters and providing support to the military and veterans health administration medical systems in caring for casualties evacuated back to the United States from overseas (15).

NDMS also promotes the development of Disaster Medical Assistance Teams (DMATs). A DMAT is a group of professional and paraprofessional medical personnel (supported by a cadre of logistical and administrative staff) designed to provide emergency medical care during a disaster or other event. Each team has a sponsoring organization, such as a major medical center, a public health or safety agency, or a nonprofit, public, or private organization. The DMAT sponsor organizes the team and recruits members, arranges training, and coordinates the dispatch of the team. In addition to the standard DMATs, there are highly specialized DMATs that deal with specific medical conditions such as crush injury, burn, and mental health emergencies. Other specialty teams include Disaster Mortuary Operational Response Teams (DMORTs) that provide mortuary services, Veterinary Medical Assistance Teams (VMATs) that provide veterinary services, and National Medical Response Teams (NMRTs) that are equipped and trained to provide medical care for victims of weapons of mass destruction (15).

DMATs are required to deploy to disaster sites with sufficient supplies and equipment to sustain themselves for a period of 72 hours while providing medical care at a fixed or temporary medical care site. In mass casualty incidents, their responsibilities include triaging patients, providing austere medical care, and preparing patients for evacuation. In other types of situations, DMATs may provide primary health care and/or serve to augment overloaded local health care staffs. DMATs may also be activated to support patient reception and disposition of patients to hospitals. DMAT members are required to maintain appropriate certifications and licensure within their discipline. When members are activated as federal employees, licensure and certification is recognized by all states (15).

NDMS also provides victim identification and mortuary services. These responsibilities include temporary morgue facilities, victim identification, forensic dental pathology, forensic anthropology methods, processing, preparation, and disposition of remains. To accomplish this mission, NDMS entered into a Memorandum of Agreement with the National Association for Search and Rescue (NASAR), a nonprofit organization, to develop DMORTs. These mortuary affairs teams are composed of private citizens, each with a particular field of expertise, who are activated in the event of a disaster. DMORT members are required to maintain appropriate certifications and licensure within their discipline. When members are called to duty, licensure and certification is recognized by all states, and the team members are compensated for their duty by the federal government. During an emergency response, DMORTs works under the guidance of local authorities by providing technical assistance and personnel to recover, identify, and process deceased victims. Teams are composed of funeral directors, medical examiners, coroners, pathologists, forensic anthropologists, medical records technicians and transcribers, fingerprint specialists, forensic odontologists, dental assistants, x-ray technicians, mental health specialists, computer professionals, administrative support staff, and security and investigative personnel. The Office of Emergency Preparedness maintains a Disaster Portable Morgue Unit (DPMU) as a depository of equipment and supplies for deployment to a disaster site. It contains a complete morgue with designated workstations for each processing element and prepackaged equipment and supplies (15).

The NRP tasks the NDMS to provide assistance in assessing the extent of disruption and need for veterinary services following major disasters or emergencies. These responsibilities include assessing medical needs of animals, medical treatment and stabilization of animals, animal disease surveillance, zoonotic disease surveillance and public health assessments, technical assistance to ensure food and water quality, hazard mitigation, animal decontamination, and biological and chemical terrorism surveillance. To accomplish this mission, NDMS entered into a Memorandum of Agreement with the American Veterinary Medical Association (AVMA), a nonprofit organization, to develop VMATs.

TABLE 37-3	Agencies Transferred to DHS, Directorate of Science and Technology	
AGENCY		**TRANSFERRED FROM**
CBRN Countermeasures Programs		Department of Energy
Environmental Measurements Laboratory		Department of Energy
National BW Defense Analysis Center		Department of Defense
Plum Island Animal Disease Center		Department of Agriculture

These special veterinary teams are composed of private citizens who are activated in the event of a disaster. VMAT members are required to maintain appropriate certifications and licensure within their discipline. When members are activated, all states recognize licensure and certification. Teams are composed of clinical veterinarians, veterinary pathologists, animal health technicians (veterinary technicians), microbiologist/virologists, epidemiologists, toxicologists, and various other scientific and support personnel (15).

The Science and Technology directorate focuses on the use of technology to assist in homeland security. DHS operates under one roof with the capability to anticipate, preempt, and deter threats to the homeland whenever possible and the ability to respond quickly when such threats do materialize. Also, DHS is responsible for assessing the vulnerabilities of the nation's critical infrastructure and cyber security threats. The department will evaluate any potential threat and coordinate with federal, state, local, and private entities to ensure the most effective response. DHS's Science and Technology directorate is tasked with researching and organizing the scientific, engineering, and technological resources of the United States and leveraging these existing resources into technological tools to help protect the homeland. Universities, the private sector, and the federal laboratories are also an important part in this endeavor (11). Table 37-3 lists the major assets that were transferred to this directorate (12).

The department's research and technology efforts focus on developing capabilities to detect and deter attacks on information systems and critical infrastructures. The Science and Technology directorate oversees a national research program to support homeland defense. This research and development effort is driven by a constant examination of the nation's vulnerabilities, repeated testing of security systems, and a thorough evaluation of the strengths and weaknesses in the system. Advanced research and development of software and technology that will protect information is an important part of this program. DHS's Science and Technology directorate

conducts the research efforts to meet emerging and predicted needs and works closely with universities, the private sector, and national and federal laboratories (12).

The new department's Information Analysis and Infrastructure Protection directorate analyzes intelligence and information from other agencies, to include the Central Intelligence Agency, FBI, Defense Intelligence Agency, and National Security Agency, involving threats to homeland security. Functions transferred to this directorate include (a) receiving and analyzing law enforcement information, intelligence, and other information in order to understand the nature and scope of the terrorist threat and to detect and identify potential threats of terrorism within the United States; (b) comprehensively assessing the vulnerabilities of key resources and critical infrastructures; (c) integrating relevant information, intelligence analysis, and vulnerability assessments to identify protective priorities and support protective measures; (d) developing a comprehensive national plan for securing key resources and critical infrastructures; (e) taking or seeking to effect necessary measures to protect those key resources and infrastructures; (f) administering the Homeland Security Advisory System, exercising primary responsibility for public threat advisories, and providing specific warning information to state and local governments and the private sector, as well as advice about appropriate protective actions and countermeasures; and (g) reviewing, analyzing, and making recommendations for improvements in the policies and procedures governing the sharing of law enforcement, intelligence, and other information relating to homeland security within the federal government and between the federal, state, and local governments (11). Table 37-4 lists the federal agencies that were transferred to the Information Analysis and Infrastructure Protection Directorate (12).

Over the past several years, the range of computer crimes has increased from simple hacking by juveniles to sophisticated intrusions that may be sponsored by foreign powers. As

TABLE 37-4	Agencies Transferred to DHS, Directorate of Information Analysis and Infrastructure Protection	
AGENCY		**TRANSFERRED FROM**
Critical Infrastructure Assurance Office		Department of Commerce
Federal Computer Incident Response Center		General Services Administration
National Communications System		Department of Defense
National Infrastructure Protection Center		FBI
Energy Security and Assurance Program		Department of Energy

the threat and number of cyber crimes continue to increase, the Information Analysis and Infrastructure Protection directorate will continue to play an ever-increasing and vital role in homeland security. The directorate is responsible for detecting, warning, responding to, and investigating computer intrusions and unlawful acts that threaten or target critical infrastructures of the United States. Furthermore, the directorate not only provides a reactive response to an attack that has already occurred but also actively seeks to discover planned attacks and issue warnings before they occur. This large and difficult task requires the information to be collected and analyzed from all available sources, including, but not limited to, law enforcement, intelligence sources, data provided by industry and open sources, and the dissemination of warnings of possible attacks to potential victims (16).

The directorate includes representatives from 22 other government agencies, the private sector, state and local law enforcement, and international partners. This directorate is also responsible for computer intrusion investigations and for providing subject matter, equipment, and technical support to cyber investigators in federal, state, and local government agencies involved in critical infrastructure protection. It also provides a cyber emergency response capability to help resolve a cyber incident, as well as analytical support during computer intrusion investigations and long-term analysis of vulnerability and threat trends. Through its 24/7 watch and warning capability, it distributes tactical warnings to all the relevant partners, informing them of potential vulnerabilities and threats and long-term trends. It also reviews numerous government and private sector databases, media, and other sources daily to gather information that may be relevant to any aspect of its mission, including a possible attack (16).

Additionally, the Department of Homeland Security includes the U.S. Secret Service. This agency was transferred from the Department of Treasury and now reports directly to the secretary. Although transferred to DHS, its mission remains relatively unchanged. It continues to be responsible for (a) protection of the president and vice president, their families, heads of state, and other designated individuals; (b) investigation of threats against these protectees; (c) protection of the White House, vice president's residence, foreign missions, and other buildings within Washington, D.C.; and (d) planning and implementing security designs for designated national special security events. The Secret Service also investigates violations of certain laws relating to counterfeiting of obligations and securities of the United States; financial crimes such as identity theft, access device, and financial institution and computer fraud; and computer-based attacks on financial, banking, and telecommunications infrastructures (17).

The U.S. Coast Guard was also transferred to the new department from the Department of Transportation. The Coast Guard's traditional missions of maritime safety and security remain unchanged, and the service reports directly to the secretary of Homeland Security.

While FEMA is charged with planning and coordinating the federal response and mitigation of a terrorist attack, the Office of State and Local Coordination and the Office of Domestic Preparedness (ODP) have the primary responsibility of preparing the nation's responders for acts of terrorism. These offices provide training, funds for purchase of equipment, support for planning and execution of exercises, and

technical assistance for first responders and the medical community to help them prevent, plan for, and respond to acts of terrorism. ODP achieves its mission by providing grants to states and local jurisdictions, providing hands-on training through its residential training facility, the Center for Domestic Preparedness as well as in-service training at the local level, funding and working with state and local jurisdictions to plan and execute exercises, and on-site technical assistance to state and local jurisdictions (18).

ODP was established in 1998 in response to congressional concerns regarding the real potential of catastrophic effects of a chemical or biological act of terrorism. Congress realized that while the federal government plays an important role in preventing and responding to terrorist attacks, state and local public safety personnel are typically first to respond to the scene when such incidents occur. As a result, congress authorized the attorney general to assist state and local public safety personnel in acquiring the specialized training and equipment necessary to safely respond to and manage terrorist incidents involving WMD (18).

Training and exercises play an important role in preparing for acts of terrorism. In May 2000, at the direction of the congress, ODP conducted the TOPOFF (Top Officials) exercise, the largest federal, state, and local exercise of its kind, involving three separate locations and a multitude of federal, state, and local agencies. TOPOFF simulated chemical, biological, and radiological attacks around the country and provided valuable lessons for the nation's communities. In May 2003, ODP sponsored TOPOFF 2 exercise to build upon the success of the May 2000 TOPOFF. TOPOFF 2 was the most comprehensive terrorism response exercise ever undertaken by the U.S. government with more than 100 federal, state, and local agencies participating (18).

Development of state strategies has been another important ODP program. Beginning in 1999 and updated in 2003, each state was asked to provide an assessment of their training and equipment requirements to respond to acts of terrorism. These state strategies formed the basis for structuring grant and training programs to better meet state and local needs. Beginning with an allocation of $12 million in 1998, ODP's grant program has grown to over $4 billion in fiscal year 2004. Training for state and local responders is provided through grants and ODP's training center, the Center for Domestic Preparedness (CDP) located in Anniston, Alabama. Established in 1998, CDP utilizes facilities vacated by the closure of the U.S. Army's Chemical School to train state and local responders in advanced hands-on techniques to handle a terrorist attack. One of the more unique aspects of CDP's training program is the use of the chemical nerve agents sarin and VX in a controlled environment to simulate an actual terrorist attack. This training is provided at no cost to state and local responders (18).

STATE AND LOCAL RESPONSE EFFORTS

Americans tend to view security as a federal issue. However, in the new war against terrorism, security is now very much a state and local responsibility. In response to the massive commitment to homeland security by the federal government, states and many major metropolitan areas have also begun to organize themselves to better prepare for and respond to acts of terrorism. All state governments now have an office devoted specifically to homeland defense. However, actions to better prepare for terrorist attacks vary significantly from state to state. Some states have placed the National Guard in charge of all aspects of homeland security. Others have assigned this function to the Department of Public Safety or State Emergency Management Office, while a few states have followed the federal government's example by creating a new department to deal with this emerging threat. Many major metropolitan jurisdictions have also established new offices devoted entirely to homeland security issues. With the assistance of federal grants and other programs, state and local first responders, as well as medical personnel, have begun to receive specialized equipment and training to help them respond to such an attack.

CONCLUSION

The terrorist attacks of September 11, 2001, represent a clear fault line in the history of the United States. The United States is now engaged in a long, and most probably, protracted struggle against terrorism. The threat of catastrophic casualties caused by a terrorist attack using WMD is very real. The medical aspects of combating terrorism are both complex and daunting. Preparing to respond to such an attack requires new skills and procedures.

A unique aspect of homeland security is that although the federal government is the best prepared to respond to a terrorist attack, federal assets may not be immediately available at the scene of an attack. In fact, federal assets may take several hours if not days to reach the scene. Therefore, state and local health care providers must be able to formulate their own response with assets immediately available to them. America is now faced with a new enemy who strikes from the shadows and cannot be held at bay by the two gigantic oceans that have protected America for almost three centuries. Homeland security will play an important role in this struggle.

Establishment of an entire department of the federal government devoted to homeland security is without precedence in the history of the United States. As the Department of Homeland Security continues to mature, it will undoubtedly continue to evolve and change to meet future demands of securing the homeland against terrorist attacks. Preparing the nation to respond to the terrorist threat will take considerable time and effort; however, the journey is now well underway.

REFERENCES

1. Kaplan DE, Marshall A. The cult at the end of the world: the incredible story of Aum Shinrikyo. London: Hutchinson; 1996.
2. First annual report of the advisory panel to assess domestic response capabilities for terrorism involving weapons of mass destruction, submitted to the President and the Congress on 15 December 1999. Santa Monica, CA: RAND; 1999. pp. 40-51.
3. Alfred P. Murrah Federal Building bombing April 19, 1995 final report. Stillwater, OK: Oklahoma State University; 1996. p. 9-10.
4. Presidential Decision Directive 39. 1996; (3). Available at: http://www.ojp.usdoj.gov/odp/docs/pdd39.htm. Accessed on September 1, 2003.
5. Presidential Decision Directive 62, fact sheet. 1998; (2). Available at: http//:www.fas.org/irp/offdocs/pdd-62.htm. Accessed on September 18, 2003.
6. Presidential Decision Directive 63. 1998; (13). Available at http//:www.fas.org/irp/offdocs/pdd/pdd-63.htm. Accessed on September 18, 2003.
7. The national security strategy of the United States. 2002. Available at: http://www.whitehouse.gov/nsc/nss.pdf. Accessed on September 18, 2003.
8. The national strategy for homeland security. 2002; (90). Available at: http://www.whitehouse.gov/homeland/book/nat_strat_hls.pdf. Accessed on September 27, 2003.
9. National strategy to combat weapons of mass destruction. 2002; (9). Available at: http://www.whitehouse.gov/news/releases/2002/12/WMDStrategy.pdf. Accessed on September 27, 2003.
10. Homeland security directive 5. 2003; (6). Available at: http://www.whitehouse.gov/news/releases/2003/02/20030228-9.html. Accessed on March 3, 2003.
11. Homeland Security Act of 2002, Public Law 107-296. 2002; (485). Available at: http://www.whitehouse.gov/deptofhomeland/bill/hsl-bill.pdf. Accessed on August 2, 2003.
12. DHS Organization, DHS Agencies. 2003. Available at: http://www.dhs.gov/dhspublic/display?theme=13. Accessed on September 27, 2003.
13. The Federal Law Enforcement Training Center, DHS; Available at: http://www.fletc.gov/. Accessed on September 27, 2003.
14. US&R, National urban search and rescue system. Available at: http://www.fema.gov/usr/. Accessed on September 28, 2003.
15. National disaster medical system. (6). Available at: http://ndms.dhhs.gov/NDMS/ndms.html. Accessed on September 28, 2003.
16. Threats and protection, synthesizing and disseminating information. (10). Available at: http://www.dhs.gov/dhspublic/theme_home6.jsp. Accessed on September 29, 2003.
17. U.S. Secret Service homepage. (35). Available at: http://www.secretservice.gov/index.shtml. Accessed on September 29, 2003.
18. Office of Domestic Preparedness homepage. (11). Available at: http://www.ojp.usdoj.gov/odp/welcome.html. Accessed on October 1, 2003.

38

The Role of Military Medicine in Civilian Disaster Response

Brian A. Krakover

INTRODUCTION

Military medical units have played an important role in recent natural disasters and may be called on in the future to assist civilian agencies with medical response to future terrorist attacks (Fig. 38-1). Emergency response to future terrorist events will likely require federal assistance, and there is a plan in place, aptly named the Initial National Response Plan, which addresses many of the mechanics associated with that aid. This plan replaces the Federal Response Plan and will be replaced with a final National Response Plan at a future date. However, there are over 85,000 local jurisdictions for the military to support, and the doctrine that governs how the military will support civil authorities in disaster response is still under development (1).

PREPAREDNESS ESSENTIALS

In response to the events of September 11, the president of the United States and Congress established the Department of Homeland Security (DHS) to consolidate homeland security and civil support under a single organization, and the Department of Defense (DoD) established Northern Command (NORTHCOM) to consolidate homeland defense and civil support under a single command. Critical homeland security plans, policies, and procedures are still being debated and have not been finalized by national and state decision makers. The interaction of the DHS, the assistant secretary of defense for HLS, and NORTHCOM is still developing (1).

RULES REGARDING THE USE OF FEDERAL TROOPS

The policy that governs most limitations placed on the military's actions in domestic conflict is the well-known but less well understood Posse Comitatus Act of 1878 (2). The act was initially intended "to end the use of federal troops to police state elections in former Confederate states" (2). However, this Reconstruction era law is used today to keep the military from participating in domestic law enforcement. This restriction was one of the principal issues in the investigation of the military's involvement in the Branch Davidian assault, and it continues as a source of controversy for DoD domestic counternarcotic and counterterrorist operations (3). Many questions remain regarding the military's role in domestic terror incidents (3). As long as the federal bureaucracy defines terrorism as a law enforcement issue rather than a national security issue, the DoD faces considerable legal limits on its ability to act to counter domestic terrorism. However, Posse Comitatus is not the absolute prohibition that many consider it to be (4). A rather significant loophole is written directly into the law:

> Whoever, *except in cases and under circumstances expressly authorized by the Constitution or Act of Congress,* willfully uses any part of the Army or the Air Force (later to include Navy and United States Marine Corps as well) as a Posse Comitatus or otherwise to execute the laws shall be fined not more than $10,000 or imprisoned not more than two years, or both (5).

Thus it appears that the president or Congress may authorize the use of federal military forces for domestic use if they deem an indication exists (3). Significant recent exceptions to the act have included disaster relief operations under the Stafford Act, the "drug exception" authorized by Congress to fight the "war on drugs," border patrol operations along the Mexican border, and the military assistance provided to state and local governments under the Domestic Preparedness Program (3).

CHAIN OF COMMAND

At Oklahoma City, New York City, and the Pentagon, the incident commander in each case was a civilian fire chief,

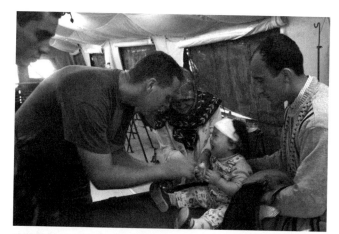

Figure 38–1. Lieutenant Jeff Bledsoe provides medical attention to a Turkish girl in a U.S. Navy medical tent in Izmit, Turkey, on August 25, 1999. DoD (Photo courtesy of Petty Officer 1st Class Robert Benson, U.S. Navy).

and the military was in support of that fire chief. That will most likely be the model for the future. Although a standardized incident command system is a step in the right direction, more still needs to be done in order to mitigate efficiently the damages that come from a terrorist attack. Under these circumstances, it is often not possible to evacuate all those who would benefit, and the ability to move surgical beds and health care providers into the area of operations may become important. To affect mortality significantly, however, trauma surgery must be available within minutes or hours, and overall surgical needs after an earthquake fall off sharply after the initial 72 hours (6). Although causing severe damage to health care facility structures, recent hurricanes in the United States have not resulted in large numbers of deaths and serious injuries, but they provide an appropriate analogy for a response to future terrorist attack. Military medical units offer an attractive way to augment patient care capabilities rapidly in a civilian disaster situation (6). In order to activate military medical forces for civilian disaster assistance, the state or local authorities, usually the governor, must make a request to the assistant secretary of defense for special operations and low-intensity conflict (SOLIC) for additional resources. The ASD-SOLIC is authorized by the DoD to designate the U.S. Army as the lead agency in cases of suspected domestic terrorism.

NATIONAL DISASTER MEDICAL SYSTEM

The National Disaster Medical System is a federally coordinated network of health care facilities that augments the nation's emergency response capability in case of disaster. The NDMS has the main responsibility for assisting state and local authorities in responding to major peacetime domestic disasters as well as augmenting the VA and DoD Contingency Hospital System for receiving casualties in times of war. DoD military hospitals, also known as MTFs (medical treatment facilities), make a significant contribution to the NDMS in civilian disasters by serving as Federal Coordinating Centers, or FCCs. The FCC, according to the Federal Response Plan, is a facility located in a U.S. metropolitan area responsible for daily coordination of planning and operations in an assigned NDMS region or Patient Reception Area (PRA) (7) (Table 38-1).

HISTORICAL EVENTS

MILITARY MEDICINE IN SUPPORT OF RECENT NATURAL DISASTERS

The U.S. armed forces have been involved in domestic disaster response activities since the end of the Civil War, and the reasons for using the military during these operations, including the ability to provide resources and organizational capabilities quickly, have not changed greatly since those early years (6). The medical literature describes two major deployments of military medical units to help with civilian disaster response.

On the evening of September 15, 1995, Hurricane Marilyn struck the island of St. Thomas in the U.S. Virgin Islands (USVI). The U.S. Army's 28th Combat Support Hospital was alerted for deployment on day 3. The territorial governor requested federal assistance because the island's only hospital was severely damaged by the storm. The CSH was able to provide medical and surgical beds, a neonatal ward, labor and delivery rooms, an eight-bed emergency room, and two 12-bed intensive care units (ICUs) based out of tents. They were also able to provide hospital laundry, pharmacy, radiology, and maintenance capabilities. Despite legal, financial,

TABLE 38-1	U.S. Contingency Bed Hospital Capacity (16)	
FACILITY TYPE	**NUMBER OF FACILITIES**	**BEDS AVAILABLE WITHIN 30 DAYS**
Department of Defense Military Treatment Facilities	45	7,603
Department of Veterans Affairs Facilities	64	6,904
NDMS-Affiliated Acute-Care Civilian Medical Centers	1,700	91,638
Total		106,145

and political concerns, the unit was able to care for a desperate patient population in need and to provide sustained capabilities while local health care facilities were rebuilt.

In June 2001, 87 airmen from the Air Force's 59th Expeditionary Medical Squadron, based at Wilford Hall Air Force Medical Center in San Antonio, Texas, deployed to Houston after rains from tropical storm Allison flooded the city. Five of the city's major hospitals were flooded and closed, bringing Houston's emergency room capabilities down to 75% of normal. In 12 days, they treated more than 1,000 patients (8). According to Major (Dr.) Andy C. Chiou, a staff surgeon with the 59th Medical Wing based in San Antonio, the field hospital enhanced Houston's emergency room capabilities by seeing over 100 patients a day and operated at roughly the equivalent of any major Air Force installation hospital with about one-tenth the staff (8).

In the case of Hurricane Marilyn, the critical contribution of the military was far-forward surgical and stabilization services for critically ill trauma patients (6). This capability is one of the main factors influencing the steady improvement in the survival of combat casualties since the Civil War, and it will play an important role in reducing morbidity and mortality of future terrorist attacks (9).

Local and regional resources may be rapidly used and cost effective and are vital for the immediate care of disaster victims. Most important to trauma patients will be an operational surgical capacity. These resources could be developed in the civilian sector within either the emergency management agency or the local trauma system. National Guard units could also support assets, and these could be located regionally with state National Guard compact (mutual-aid) agreements to provide for their shared use. Other local assets, such as local capacity for engineering assessment and health facility planning, could be developed within National Guard units or contracted in advance with civilian professionals. Inclusion of these personnel in predisaster mitigation projects would familiarize them with the health facilities they would be responsible for assessing during the response phase (6).

MILITARY RESPONSE CAPABILITIES

U.S. ARMY, U.S. NAVY, U.S. MARINE CORPS, AND U.S. AIR FORCE

The U.S. Army has organized Special Medical Augmentation Response Teams (SMART) to deliver a small number of highly skilled specialists within hours to evaluate a situation, provide advice to local authorities, and organize military resources to support response to a disaster or terrorist act. These teams, located at the Regional Medical Commands and subordinate commands throughout the country, have critical expertise in nuclear, biological, and chemical casualties; evacuation; trauma and critical care; burn treatment; preventive medicine; medical command, control, communications, and telemedicine systems; health facilities support; veterinary support; stress management; and pastoral care. These teams are organized, equipped, trained, and ready to deploy within 12 hours of notice. Their capabilities were most recently demonstrated when seven members from Tripler Army Medical Center deployed from Hawaii to the Pacific island of Chuuk to assist

residents injured during a typhoon. Since last fall, patient decontamination equipment has been fielded to 23 medical treatment facilities with emergency rooms, and personnel have been trained in its use. With this equipment, up to 20 ambulatory patients an hour can be decontaminated (10).

The U.S. Army Medical Research Institute of Infectious Diseases (USAMRIID) at Fort Detrick, Maryland, is a formidable national resource of expertise in dealing with dangerous diseases, whether natural outbreaks or the result of biological warfare. When anthrax-laced letters were sent in the mail in late 2001, USAMRIID geared up for a phenomenal effort to analyze thousands of samples collected from possibly exposed sites, looking for the deadly bacterium (10).

The army has also provided new patient care products to civilian law enforcement and trauma environments such as a rapid coagulant powder and a natural fiber bandage that rapidly treats life-threatening hemorrhage. Both were developed for soldiers but are now being made available to the civilian sector (11).

A major component of the army's deployment to the hurricanes mentioned previously is a system known as Deployable Medical Systems, or DEPMEDS. The DEPMEDS system is a modular, container-based system of bringing a tailor-made field medical system as far forward as possible. The DEPMEDS units are the size of a shipping container but assemble with a small crew of individuals. They come in a variety of packages ranging from operating suites, med/surg wards, intensive care units, pharmacy, laboratory, and radiology units (6). They are readily deployable by ship, rail, or ground transportation and provide rapid expansion of patient care facilities in the event of a mass casualty situation or replacement of existing facilities if local resources are damaged by natural or human-made forces.

The U.S. Army and U.S. Marine Corps have collaborated in the development of a compact, rapidly deployable surgical facility called the Advanced Surgical Suite for Trauma Casualties (ASSTC). The ASSTC is designed for trauma management and resuscitative surgery. It is contained in a single $5 \times 5 \times 10$ foot transit package and can be carried by aircraft or ship or towed behind a truck or light tactical vehicle. It can be air delivered by parachute where no runways exist, and it can be made operational within 18 to 30 minutes of arrival.

The U.S. Air Force has expeditionary medical support (EMEDS) teams consisting of numerous modular teams ranging in size from two personnel with equipment in backpacks to components of the modular Air Force theater hospitals (AFTH). Specifically, the two-person preventive medicine/aerospace medicine (PAM) team can provide initial medical assessment of disasters, public health/preventive medicine, and emergency/flight/primary-care medicine. Ground critical-care teams (GCCT), three-person intensive-care units based on critical-care air-transport teams (CCATT), have performed critical care and patient transport in hundreds of real-world missions. The five-person mobile field surgical team (MFST) provides emergency general and orthopedic surgery to 10 patients. Together, these teams—PAM, GCCT, and MFST—make up the 10-person small portable expeditionary aeromedical rapid-response (SPEARR) team, a disaster-response "force package" that travels with backpacks only (no pallet space) or with a small trailer (one pallet equivalent) that can be loaded by a sling. It does not require a forklift, and it can be pulled with a standard pickup truck or airlifted by helicopter. The team provides a broad scope of care and has intrinsic communication capability for aeromedical coordination, consultation, or resupply (12).

The U.S. Navy has already contributed to the war on terror. The Comfort was used to support operations during the World Trade Center attack. It docked near the WTC site and provided medical care and quarters to the disaster relief workers at ground zero. The Mercy and the Comfort are large-capacity hospital ships that could provide surge capacity for civilians when the ships are not deployed (13).

NATIONAL GUARD

The National Guard has traditionally been the key military element in both homeland defense and homeland security. Their rich and proud tradition going back to the 17th century has always stressed protecting U.S. citizens (14). Currently, the Air National Guard is in the process of reconfiguring its 89 medical squadrons into building blocks to provide EMEDS capabilities in each of the 10 FEMA regions (14).

The National Guard also maintains a host of specialized disaster response teams. Over 30 states have Civil Support Teams for Weapons of Mass Destruction (CST-WMD). These teams provide complementary capabilities to meet the needs of the first responder. In addition, the NGB (National Guard Bureau) maintains RAID, Rapid Assessment and Initial Detection Teams. The National Guard has equipped and certified nine Weapons of Mass Destruction Civil Support Teams (WMD-CST) whose mission is to assist local first responders in determining the nature of a terrorist attack, provide medical and technical advice, and pave the way for identification and arrival of follow-on assets. Congress has authorized 32 teams, including 17 teams added in fiscal year (FY) 2000 and 5 added in FY 2001. The first 10 teams were

funded as part of the National Defense Appropriations Act for FY 1999. As of September 2001, nine of these were certified by the secretary of defense as deployable (15,16).

Overseeing the WMD-CST teams is the Joint Task Force–Civil Support (JTF-CS), which was created as DoD's command and control center for military support to civilian authorities. JTF-CS will respond to requests for assistance from FEMA for the purposes of domestic WMD response. The Joint Task Force for Civil Support (JTF-CS) has no standing military personnel. The JTF-CS is commanded by a flag officer (general or admiral) and supported by full-time civilian personnel trained to organize and integrate first responders, federal law enforcement agencies, and emergency management personnel. The JTF-CS coordinates Department of Defense support to FEMA for WMD events in the United States, drawing on the DoD's logistical and medical assets and capabilities in detection and decontamination of toxic agents.

ADDITIONAL RESOURCE UNITS

The Armed Forces Institute of Pathology, a DoD agency, is internationally known for its expertise in consultative pathology and medical research. Within the Institute, the Office of the Armed Forces Medical Examiner and the National Museum of Health and Medicine employ forensic anthropologists specializing in mass disaster victim identification. The Office of the Armed Forces Medical Examiner (OAFME) is responsible for investigating all military fatalities as well as civilian deaths under federal jurisdiction. When called for emergency assistance, OAFME sends a team comprised of pathologists, dentists, anthropologists, and forensic scientists. OAFME has a close relationship with a number of federal investigative agencies (16) (Table 38-2).

TABLE 38-2 Anthropological Skills in Mass Disasters

SKILL	EXAMPLES
Devise grid systems for search and recovery	U.S. Air 427 Oklahoma City bombing
Devise search criteria based on size and scope of disaster	Hardin cemetery flood Oklahoma City bombing
Identifying and reassociating fragmentary remains	U.S. Air 427 American Eagle 4184 Valujet 592 TWA 800
Forensic anthropological analyses (age, sex, stature, etc.)	All cases
Radiographic comparisons of skeletal structures	Oklahoma City bombing
Positive identification based on biological criteria	All cases
Reconstructing injury and fragmentation patterns	Operation Desert Storm U.S. Air 427 Oklahoma City bombing
Determine reburial criteria based on remains recovered	Hardin Cemetery

From Sledzik. Federal Resources in Mass Disaster Response. CRM No. 10—1996.

The Armed Forces DNA Identification Laboratory (AFD-NAIL) is responsible for the DNA identifications of military fatalities, including those from the Vietnam and Korean wars. The staff of the AFDNAIL have also been involved in the identification of victims from several recent mass disasters. In addition, both OAFME and the National Museum of Health and Medicine offer courses in forensic pathology, forensic dentistry, forensic anthropology, and DNA identification methods (16).

The Office of the Armed Forces Medical Examiner and the National Museum of Health and Medicine have supported local resources in several recent mass disasters, including U.S. Air 427, American Eagle 4184, the Oklahoma City bombing, and TWA 800. Under a mandate to investigate all federal and military crashes and deaths, OAFME staff have identified remains from the crash of Department of Agriculture Secretary Ron Brown's plane in Bosnia in 1996 and the downing of two U.S. Army Blackhawk helicopters over Iraq in 1994. National Museum of Health and Medicine staff also provided technical guidance for cemetery floods in the towns of Hardin, Missouri (1993) and Albany, Georgia (1994) (16).

PREPAREDNESS SUMMARY

In light of the recent creation of the Department of Homeland Security and the new Northern Command, the role of the military in civilian disaster response is evolving to deal with emerging threats of terrorism as well as natural and environmental disasters. Future terrorism incidents may result in mass casualty, mass fatality, or mass damage to critical infrastructure that far exceeds the capabilities of civil authorities. One source of assistance may come from the U.S. military. In addition to clinical resources, the military can provide specialized analytical and detection capability for possible WMD scenarios as well as technical expertise for recovery and investigative operations. The military also brings to the table one of the largest and most robust logistical support capability anywhere in the world.

PREPAREDNESS CHECKLIST

- Future terrorist attacks may overwhelm civilian resources. The military may help.
- The Initial National Response Plan contains important information regarding the use of military resources.
- NORTHCOM is the military unified command with responsibility for homeland security.
- Use of federal troops for domestic response is addressed by Posse Comitatus, which may be amended by the president or Congress.
- Activation of military assets is controlled by the assistant secretary of defense for special operations and low-intensity conflict.

- Military treatment facilities can function as Federal Coordinating Centers as components of the NDMS.
- All branches of the active component military have deployable medical units that can help with surge capacity, logistical support, and technical support.
- The National Guard has several specialized units for detection and response to WMD incidents as well as humanitarian and disaster relief.

RESOURCE

U.S. Air Force Counterproliferation Center. Web site: http://c21.maxwell.af.mil/frstresp.htm.

REFERENCES

1. Williams TJ. Strategic leader readiness and competencies for asymmetric warfare. Parameters 2003;33(2):19-36.
2. Larson EV, Peters JE. Preparing the U.S. Army for homeland security: concepts, issues, and options. Appendix D. Overview of the Posse Comitatus Act. RAND MR-1251/A. Santa Monica, CA: RAND, 2001;243.
3. Quillen C. Posse Comitatus and nuclear terrorism. Parameters 2002;32(1):60-74.
4. Lujan TR. Legal aspects of domestic employment of the army. Parameters 1997;27:90.
5. U.S. Code, Title 18, sec. 1385.
6. Weddle M, Prado-Monje H. The use of deployable military hospitals after hurricanes: lessons from the Hurricane Marilyn response. Mil Med 2000;165:411-8.
7. Department of Veterans Affairs. VISN 11 preparedness activities: Mideast military conflict. Web site: http://www1.va.gov/emshg/docs/PRT-Briefing.ppt.
8. Elliot L. AF hospital leaves Houstonians grateful, points to Guard medical future. Texas National Guard Public Affairs Office, July 5, 2001.
9. Coupland RM. Epidemiological approach to surgical management of the casualties of war. BMJ 1994;308:1693-7.
10. Peake J. Training to respond to terrorism. Reprinted from U.S. Medicine, January 2003. Web site: www.armymedicine.army.mil.
11. Schwanke J. Military medicine: how far can we go? U.S. troops armed with the latest lifesaving medical breakthroughs. WebMD Medical News, Friday, April 4, 2003. Web site: http://content.health.msn.com/content/article/63/71927.htm.
12. Carlton PK. New millennium, new mind-set: the Air Force Medical Service in the air expeditionary era. Aerospace Power J, December 6, 2001;15(4).
13. Carmona RH. "The Role of Military Medicine in Civilian Emergency Response" http://surgeongeneral.gov/news/speeches/mercy.07262003.htm.
14. Reimer DJ. Statement to institute for the prevention of terrorism before the Subcommittee on National Security, Emergency Threats and International Relations April 29, 2003.
15. Clark E. Weapons of mass destruction civil support teams. Web site: http://www.cdi.org/terrorism/wmdcst.cfm.
16. Web site: http://www.defenselink. mil/news/Jan2000/b01132000_bt017-00.html.

39

Law Enforcement-Related Agencies

William Fabbri and Nelson Tang

INTRODUCTION

The response to terrorism-related events by law enforcement agencies necessitates coordinated medical support. Emergency physicians familiar with the special requirements of law enforcement are integral to this coordination.

Until recently, medical support of police operations was limited largely to nonemergent occupational medicine matters. Similarly, emergency medical services (EMS), like their fire service colleagues, planned, trained, and responded to contingencies without preplanned coordination with law enforcement, frequently gaining access to the scene only after termination of active police activity (1).

This past arrangement was acceptable in a time when body armor, tactical prowess. and superior numbers were generally sufficient for the police to safely contain and terminate a potentially violent confrontation. It is not applicable to the current threat of coordinated, near-simultaneous terrorist attacks with significant potential for the use of weapons of mass destruction (WMD). To accomplish their expanding missions, law enforcement agencies must now coordinate their activities with EMS, fire/rescue services, and specialists in other disciplines including hazardous materials (hazmat) operations, industrial plant and power generation operations, and public utilities.

Special Weapons and Tactics (SWAT) and evidence recovery operations conducted by the police in the context of WMD and hazmat also require personal protective equipment (PPE) and procedures previously unfamiliar to most law enforcement officers.

In addition, the containment and safe conclusion of a suspected WMD incident involving potential biological agents require cooperative efforts between law enforcement and elements of the medical community not traditionally associated with police, EMS, or fire/rescue services, such as public health investigators.

The threat of large-scale terrorist attacks involving WMD demands that law enforcement officers adopt new methodologies in response to nontraditional threats against themselves and the public. Medical support of police counterterrorist response and of law enforcement investigations conducted in proximity to chemical, biological, or radiological contamination requires communities to develop interoperability between law enforcement, emergency medical, fire/rescue, and special technical agencies. These relationships require the support and sponsorship of physicians and other health professionals familiar with the law enforcement mission.

PREPAREDNESS ESSENTIALS

THE ROLE OF EMERGENCY PHYSICIANS IN CONTINGENCY PLANNING

Prospective planning requires that emergency medical personnel, both EMS and hospital based, be familiar with the basic principles of personal and operational security utilized by police organizations and develop and exercise interoperative procedures for providing emergency care in the context of a law enforcement contingency.

TACTICAL EMERGENCY MEDICAL SUPPORT

The direct involvement of physicians in tactical law enforcement operations is a relatively new phenomenon. As recently as 1996, a survey of large metropolitan SWAT teams in North America demonstrated that 23% did not utilize a protocol for support by EMS, and 78% did not utilize a physician for medical planning (1).

The need for specialized medical support of law enforcement has recently been recognized by officers responsible

Disclaimer: The views expressed in this article are those of the authors and do not necessarily represent the views of the Federal Bureau of Investigation, The United States Secret Service, or the United States.

for tactical (SWAT) operations (2). Some law enforcement agencies combine tactical with search and rescue or technical rescue capabilities, and therefore have tactical officers trained and equipped for EMS operations within their special operations teams. Many other communities and jurisdictions provide technical rescue capability as part of a broader fire/rescue service, with variable degrees of interaction between EMS and law enforcement (3). Additional law enforcement specialty teams, such as negotiation units, may also benefit from medical support intrinsic to law enforcement (4). Evidence teams must develop protocols and procedures for evidence collection in the context of a suspected or actual release of biohazardous materials.

APPLYING EXISTING WMD PROCEDURES TO LAW ENFORCEMENT

Some aspects of the law enforcement counterterrorism mission have required direct interaction with the medical community, both to ensure the safety of officers working to contain and control hazards during actual terrorist attacks and to assist law enforcement investigators tasked to collect evidence and other information necessary to protect the public from future attack. Existing procedures used by medical and other non-law enforcement public safety agencies are applicable to WMD counterterrorist contingency response and investigation (5).

Current public safety doctrine dictates that any counterterrorism contingency response assumes the potential for involvement of WMD. Police tactical teams must be capable of containing and potentially engaging terrorists in a setting of suspected or actual biohazard contamination. More frequently, investigators must conduct evidence collection in the context of potential or confirmed contamination. These incidents may involve preplanned evidence collection, as in the investigation of violations of laws governing hazardous waste disposal or in response to a terrorist act, as demonstrated in the criminal deployment of anthrax bacillus in Florida, New York, and Washington, D.C., in 2001. Associated requirements for PPE and plans for the management of potential exposure of officers due to breach of PPE require those law enforcement agencies without EMS or field medical capability to develop appropriate medical support plans.

The Federal Bureau of Investigation (FBI) has adapted the training, equipment, and procedures proven in fire service and industrial hazmat operations to the problem of evidence collection in a potential or actual contaminated crime scene. Requirements for medical monitoring (6), work-rest cycles, and emergency response within the contaminated zone are addressed by law enforcement in a manner consistent with existing hazmat regulations (7) and procedures applied in the fire service and civilian industry. Integration into and collaboration with the existing local public safety infrastructure is an important part of these operations, which have served as a model for similar activities at various levels of government, both domestically and internationally.

The introduction of hazmat PPE and procedures to SWAT operations was initially necessitated in police operations involving clandestine drug laboratories. As a result of this institutional experience, the presence of materials representing hazards of fire, explosion, and toxic emissions at a police raid is not entirely new to current tactical law enforcement officers. With the addition of the counterterrorism scenario to SWAT doctrine, a need for medical consultation and support similar to that of conventional hazmat teams (8) is increasingly present in law enforcement nationally.

THE ROLE OF EMERGENCY PHYSICIANS IN LAW ENFORCEMENT

Emergency medicine physicians experienced in the support of EMS operations, particularly those of specialized hazmat teams, are particularly well suited to advise law enforcement special operations officers and evidence response investigators on appropriate PPE and medical support. As is the case in consultation with the fire/rescue community, those physicians serving in an advisory or medical oversight capacity must be familiar with the unique aspects of these operations when applied in a law enforcement context.

PHYSICIAN LIABILITY PROTECTION AND COMPENSATION

Issues related to compensation and liability protection for physicians supporting SWAT operations have been addressed in various ways (9). Even though relatively few physicians are employed directly by law enforcement agencies, as is the case at the FBI, the participation of the emergency medicine and trauma surgery staff of hospitals and trauma centers may support law enforcement and provide medical oversight by means of a contract or memorandum of understanding (MOU) between the medical institution and the law enforcement agency. This arrangement offers unique training and practice opportunities for hospital-based medical personnel, while providing for the specialized needs of law enforcement (10).

SECURITY PRECAUTIONS

Operational and individual security measures are integral to law enforcement operations, including SWAT and evidence response. Physicians and other medical professionals must maintain a clear awareness of those aspects of police operations deemed "law enforcement sensitive." Such matters involve tactical and investigative information, techniques, procedures, and other operational details that must remain confidential to retain their effectiveness and to ensure the safety of the officers and the public. Physician awareness courses serving as an introduction to law enforcement tactical operations are available (11).

Recent recognition of the potential for cyber intrusion and attack against critical national infrastructures has identified potential vulnerabilities in emergency services (12), such as computer-based public safety dispatch, emergency response, and interagency contingency planning. Appropriate security of information technology supporting the planning and implementation of community emergency response must extend to both the prehospital- and hospital-based components of EMS. Systems access, software architecture, and hardcopy documents related to EMS information systems should be reviewed for security in coordination with the law enforcement and fire/rescue components of public service response.

EVIDENCE COLLECTION PROCEDURES

Certain field procedures, including medical activities, may require modification to ensure the integrity of the evidentiary process. While the safety of patients and the effectiveness of medical interventions are of primary importance, treatment transport and personal protective procedures may require modification for compatibility with legal documentation and evidence collection techniques. These changes conducted at a contaminated crime scene are analogous to the modified medical procedures used for physical evidence collection during medical treatment of crime victims in the emergency department and operating suite.

The involvement of emergency physicians familiar with law enforcement operations is crucial in effective counterterrorist operational planning, within both the law enforcement and the medical communities. These physicians contribute to prospective planning of police response to WMD events, ensuring that a medical annex to tactical operations provides for an uninterrupted continuum of care for all injured personnel from the site of injury to a definitive care facility (13,14). They also serve as liaison to hospital staff and administration, as well as the public health community, to ensure effective coordination of effort in the event of a WMD terrorism contingency.

Recognition of the effectiveness of partnerships between law enforcement and medical agencies across the spectrum of local, state, and federal levels is increasing as a result of the application of multiagency activities such as real-time telephone conferences. The triage of responses to the large numbers of citizen calls regarding suspicious packages, powders, and other substances following the 2001 anthrax releases in the United States proved effective in relieving the burden placed upon responding public service and public health agencies (15).

THE INCIDENT COMMAND SYSTEM

The incident command system, initially utilized by the fire service (16,17) with more recent application to contingencies involving multiple agencies, is increasingly employed by law enforcement (18). Emergency physician participants in counterterrorism contingency planning must seek the opportunity to include other nontraditional participants in jurisdictional incident command planning. The inclusion of law enforcement and public health investigators, representing local, state, and federal levels is required if WMD discovered at a crime scene are to be met with a prompt and effective response (20).

SUMMARY

The complexity and potential lethality of law enforcement contingencies in the 21st century demand a coordinated response by law enforcement; fire/rescue, and both field and hospital-based emergency medical services. Leadership by emergency physicians familiar with the special requirements of law enforcement, other public safety agencies, and hospital and public health authorities is critical to the effective management of these incidents, to the safety of the public, and to the continued security of the United States.

RESOURCES

1. The National Academies of Science. Institute of Medicine. Public Health and Prevention. Available from: http://www.iom.edu/topic.asp?ID=3735

2. The White House. National Strategy for Homeland Security. Available from: http://www.whitehouse.gov/homeland/book/

3. U.S. Department of Defense. National Guard Bureau. Weapons of Mass Destruction Civil Support Teams. Available from: http://www.ngb.army.mil/downloads/fact_sheets/wmd.asp

4. U.S. Department of Defense. U.S. Army Medical Research Institute for Infectious Diseases. Available from: http://www.usamriid.army.mil/education/

5. U.S. Department of Energy. Emergency Response. Available from: http://www.energy.gov/engine/content.do?BT_CODE=NS_SS5

6. U.S. Food and Drug Administration. Counterterrorism Topics. Available from: http://www.fda.gov/oc/opacom/hottopics/bioterrorism.html

7. U.S. Department of Health and Human Services-Centers for Disease Control and Prevention. Available from URL: http://www.bt.cdc.gov

8. U.S. Department of Homeland Security—Federal Emergency Management Agency. Compendium of Federal Terrorism Training for State and Local Audiences. Available from: http:/www./fema.gov/compendium/index.jsp

9. U.S. Department of Homeland Security—U.S. Secret Service. National Security Special Events. Available from: http://www.secretservice.gov/nsse.shtml

10. U.S. Department of Justice. Counter-Terrorism Training and Coordination Working Group. Available from URL: http://www.counterterrorismtraining.gov/

11. U.S. Department of Justice—Federal Bureau of Investigation. Counterterrorism Programs. Available from: http://www.fbi.gov/terrorinfo/counterrorism/waronterrorhome.htm

12. U.S. Department of State. Counterterrorism Office. Available from: http://www.state.gov/s/ct/

REFERENCES

1. Jones JS, Reese K, Kenepp G, Krohmer J. Into the fray: Integration of emergency medical services and special weapons and tactics (SWAT) teams. Prehosp Disaster Med 1996;11(3): 202-6.
2. Heiskell LE, Carmona RH. Tactical emergency medical services: An emerging subspecialty of emergency medicine. Ann Emerg Med 1994;23(4):778-85.
3. Carmona RH. The history and evolution of tactical emergency medical support and its impact on public safety. Top Emerg Med 2003;25(4):277-81.
4. Greenstone JL. The role of tactical emergency medical support in hostage and crisis negotiations. Prehosp Disaster Med 1998; 12(2-4):55-7.
5. United States Government. Criminal and epidemiological investigation handbook. Washington DC: US Department of Justice—US Army Soldier Biological Chemical Command; 2003.
6. National Fire Protection Association. Chapter 10, Medical-monitoring. NFPA Document 471. National Fire Protection Association; 2002
7. Occupational Safety and Health Administration. Hazardous waste operations and emergency response. 29 CFR 1910.120. Occupational Safety and Health Administration; 1998.
8. National Fire Protection Association. NFPA Document 472. National Fire Protection Association; 2002.
9. Vayer JS, Schwartz RB. Developing a tactical emergency medical support program. Top Emerg Med 2003;25(4):282-98.
10. Lavery RF, Adis MD, Doran JV, et al. Taking care of the "good guys": a trauma center based model of medical support for tactical law enforcement. J Trauma 2000;48(1):125-9.
11. Boseman WP, Eastman ER. Tactical EMS: an emerging opportunity in graduate medical education. Prehosp Emerg Car 2002;6(3):322-4.
12. US Department of Homeland Security. May 1998. White Paper, Critical Infrastructure Protection: Presidential Decision Directive 63. [Online]. Available from: http://www.ciao.gov/publicaffairs/pdd63.html. Accessed February 2004.
13. Tang N, Fabbri W. Medical direction and integration with existing EMS infrastructure. Top Emerg Med 2003;25(4): 326-32.
14. Rinnert KJ, Hall WL 2nd. Tactical emergency medical support. Emerg Med Clin North Am 2002;20(4):929-52.
15. Tengelsen L, Hudson R, Barnes S, Hahn C. Coordinated response to reports of possible anthrax contamination, Idaho, 2001. Emerg Infect Dis 2002;8(10):1093-5.
16. Londorf, D. Hospital application of the incident management system. Prehosp Disaster Med 1995;10(3):184-8.
17. "Incident Command" in Emergency Response to Terrorism, US Fire Academy Administration, June 999. p. 41.
18. Eckstein M, Cowen AR. Scene safety in the face of automatic weapons fire: a new dilemma for EMS? Prehosp Emerg Car 1998;2(2):117-22.
19. Crupi RS, Asnis DS, Lee CC, et al. Meeting the challenge of bioterrorism: lessons learned from West Nile virus and anthrax. Am J Emerg Med 2003;21(1):77-9.

Special Considerations for Terrorist Events

40

Psychological Impact of Terrorism

Gregory Luke Larkin and Jay Woody

INTRODUCTION

By fostering insecurity both within and across geopolitical boundaries, terrorism represents a significant challenge to the health and safety of the global populace. Although the risks of physical annihilation at the macro level may be overstated, no person or earthly society is immune from the psychological trauma of terrorism (1). Teleologically, terrorism is a direct assault on the emotional health and mettle of society, having as its specific aim the mass dispersion of panic, fear, and anxiety among the public at large (2,3). Conventional, chemical, biological, and nuclear terrorism can kill or maim, but the most profound burden of all such human-made disasters to date has been psychological. Indeed, terrorists seek to shape future events through intimidation or coercion of civilians and government. Their recent success at holding society hostage through the threat of violence and physical harm to individuals and communities has lead to a crescendo in terrorist activity worldwide (4). It is therefore increasingly important for emergency department clinicians, as well as other treatment providers, to recognize the psychiatric manifestations of traumatic stress among the terrorized and respond in a medically appropriate manner.

Terrorism can cause severe short-term and long-lasting psychological effects related to perceived threats to life and liberty (5). The emotional fallout from events occurring in the United States in the autumn of 2001 highlight this point. Many months and even years after the coordinated terrorist attacks in Manhattan and Washington, D.C., the most powerful nation on earth continues to find itself enmeshed in a web of insecurity. Today, a shroud of uncertainty remains, stifling many aspects of Western life via cognitive and emotional (rather than physical) mechanisms. Similarly, the biological attack utilizing anthrax (*bacillus anthracis*) in the immediate aftermath of 9/11 resulted in few deaths, but the concern of additional anthrax release haunts the American psyche to this day. By its very nature, *terrorism depends more on its use of human psychology than on its access to weapons of mass effect for either its success or its failure.* For even in the complete absence of physical bloodshed, terrorism affects all aspects of life including one's ego strength, independence, autonomy, perceived safety, perceived freedom of movement, leisure time, daily activities, religious practices, economic decisions, risk behaviors, and lifestyle. In short, terrorism targets mental hygiene. Thus it is mental hygiene that holds the greatest promise of vaccinating a population against the emotional trauma of terror, and thereby constitutes the central subject of this chapter.

PREPAREDNESS ESSENTIALS AT THE MICRO LEVEL

VICTIM ISSUES

Psychological trauma is defined as psychological injury caused by extreme emotional and/or physical assault. Key elements of psychological trauma include a sense of abject powerlessness in the face of the terroristic experience and a related disruption of normal routine for some time thereafter (6). For most survivors of terrorism, however, there is hope; fully two thirds of survivors of a terroristic experience display only minimal, normal-range symptomatology that remits within days to weeks of the initial trauma (7,8).

A variety of acute psychobiological response patterns are regarded as "normal" during and immediately after traumatic experience, including (a) cognitive problems such as confusion, poor concentration, memory lapses, diminished attentional focus; (b) physical problems such as fatigue, insomnia, gastrointestinal problems, muscle tension, heightened autonomic activity; (c) emotional problems including anxiety, depression, guilt, anger, and denial; and (d) behavioral problems including social withdrawal, listlessness, substance abuse, aggressive behaviors. Among those individuals terrorized most severely, a host of trauma-induced syndromes may manifest either singly or in combination in the weeks after the event.

The most widely researched emotional aftershock is *posttraumatic stress disorder (PTSD)* and its subclinical forms involving *traumatic stress-related (TSR) symptoms*. Terrorist attacks clearly meet the definition of a "traumatic event," a core requirement for the development of PTSD (9). This syndrome involves a specific cluster of psychophysiological responses to the experience, frequently characterized by moments of apparent reexperiencing or intrusive memories/nightmares of the event coupled with attempts to avoid stimuli that might elicit these unbidden memories or dreams for weeks and perhaps even months and years after the critical incident. In full-blown PTSD, these clinical phenomena co-occur with evidence of sympathetic nervous system hyperarousal such as insomnia, elevated startle, hypervigilance, restlessness, irritability, and concentration difficulties (9).

Based on a review done by Gidron, the prevalence of PTSD after terrorist attacks worldwide is estimated to be 28%. The general public appears to have a considerably higher prevalence rate than trained security and emergency response professionals (10). Based on experience from the September 11, 2001, terrorist attacks, both the social distance to the traumatized victim and the temporal distance to a traumatic event were key determinants of who developed PTSD (11). Among direct survivors of the Oklahoma City bombing, 41% reported seeking professional mental health treatment within 6 months (12), whereas only 8.5% of the general Oklahoma City population sought help within 3 months.

Similarly, in the months following September 11, those with exposure to daily images of the World Trade Center developed more than double the usual baseline prevalence of PTSD and major depressive disorder (5), and the prevalence of PTSD in the New York City metropolitan area where the attacks took place was substantially higher than elsewhere in the country (13). At 6 months after 9/11, over 5% of New York City residents had continued PTSD symptoms and impaired functioning (14). Other longitudinal studies suggest that 33% to 50% of individuals affected initially go on to develop chronic stress symptoms (7,8), and subclinical levels of hostility, anxiety, depression, paranoid ideation, hypochondria, and phobias may continue for years after an encounter with terrorism (15).

Beyond PTSD, individuals directly exposed to a traumatic event are also at increased risk for developing other psychiatric disorders, somatic symptoms, and physical illness. *Trauma-induced depression* is a second, albeit poorly-understood, syndrome that is even more widely endorsed than PTSD symptoms after traumatic experience. Clinicians have observed that depressive syndromes brought on by experiences of terror and horror often develop into major depressive disorder, even among victims with previous lifetime mood stability, and it may take years to remit or treat successfully.

Finally, panic attacks, panic disorder, increased alcohol or substance abuse, and/or trauma-induced grief are often part of the posttrauma sequelae. *Posttrauma panic symptoms* are frequently associated with agoraphobia and involve cognitions related to a loss of a sense of safety. The symptoms may or may not be a manifestation of trauma-induced depression but frequently require psychotherapeutic intervention as well as psychopharmacology to treat successfully. *Trauma-induced grief* processes are inevitably a complicated bereavement and may involve survivor's guilt, outrage and horror, and difficulties in working through the grief issues because of the presence of hyperarousal, the risk of inducing flashbacks, and other painful memories and related symptomatology.

COURSE OF ILLNESS AND RISK FACTORS

The impact of traumatic experience, including exposure to terrorism, is most severe immediately postevent for both direct and vicarious victims, and, in general, it decreases with time (5,16). Both demographic and event-exposure factors are associated with adverse psychological outcomes after terrorism (7,17,18). The mental health of the New York City community improved with time after the terrorist attacks of 2001, with the initial 59% of general residents having four or more emotional symptoms dropping to 17% at 5 months. Those in their 40s and 50s seemed to have had relatively higher emotional distress than both younger and older groups (11). Analyses done on survey responses by lower Manhattan residents 30 days after the September 11 bombing of the World Trade Center indicated that those exposed to two or more lifetime traumas and those who were female were three times as likely as males to have been newly medicated after the attack (14). In addition, those who experienced a panic attack within hours of the incident were most likely to have sought psychiatric help within 30 days of the trauma. Related studies have confirmed higher levels of postevent PTSD and major depressive disorder

TABLE 40-1	Incidence of Traumatic Stress Response Symptoms by Type of Trauma Exposure			
STUDY	N	TRAUMA TYPE	TRAUMA-ASSESSMENT INTERVAL	PTSD/TSR SYMPTOM %
Feinstein (1989)	14	Ambushed soldiers	2–24 days	100%
Patterson et al. (1990)	54	Burn	<1 month	30%
Green et al. (1993)	24	Motor vehicle accident (MVA)	1 month	8%
Rothbaum et al. (1992)	95	Rape	<1 month	94%
North et al. (1994)	136	Mass shooting	1 month	Men = 20% Women = 36%
Riggs et al. (1995)	130	Assault	<1 month	Women = 71% Men = 50%
Delahanty et al. (1997)	130	MVA	14–21 days	Responsible for MVA = 19% Not responsible for MVA = 29%

Source: Bryant R. Acute stress disorder. 2000. Reprinted by permission.

(MDD) for females, those with less education, those who are single or unmarried, those who have a prior history of mental health problems or psychological trauma (19), and those who use alcohol and cigarettes as coping mechanisms (20) (Table 40-1).

Converging evidence suggests that more than acute trauma exposure, early anxiety reactions may also serve as important predictors of subsequent maladjustment (14,21,22). Peritrauma dissociation, defined as disruption in the usually integrated functions of consciousness, memory, identity or perception of the environment, may also be predictive of subsequent psychiatric difficulties. Dissociative defenses highlight this risk and may include numbing (i.e., detachment from expected emotional reactions), reduced awareness of surroundings, memory impairment, depersonalization (i.e., a sense that one is seeing oneself from another's perspective), and derealization (i.e., perception that one's environment is unreal, dreamlike, or occurring in a distorted time frame).

Beyond time and space, the protective factors that insulate exposed individuals from later symptom development are not well understood. In an Israeli study in which the survey respondents appeared to be functioning unusually well given the scope of terrorism they endured, the most prevalent coping mechanisms were active information search about loved ones and social support (20). Among families of kidnapped victims held for ransom in Colombia, the quality of family system was positively correlated with outcome. Individuals from cohesive family systems who showed interest in each other's concerns and let members share feelings presented less PTSD and psychological distress after kidnapping. In addition, certain patterns of adapting to terrorism appear to be more constructive than others. Avoiding avoidance, for example, may be healthy for some individuals because, according to Horowitz (1992), "avoidance blocks the assimilation of the traumatic experience leaving it encapsulated in a traumatic memory that may cause PTSD or other symptoms" at a later time.

ASSESSING AND TREATING THE PSYCHOLOGICAL IMPACT OF TERRORISM IN THE EMERGENCY DEPARTMENT

Researchers and clinicians alike now recognize that it is normal for people to experience psychophysiological changes following terrorism. However, certain emergency department (ED) protocols may still be warranted to treat the acute manifestations of terror (Table 40-2).

Questioning the Victim about the Event

Recent findings have raised serious questions about the advisability of detailed peritraumatic questioning about the traumatic experience. Patients are often in a state of heightened arousal, and verbalizations and elaboration of a traumatic experience at this point can exacerbate distress; severe peritraumatic distress has been associated with long-term psychopathology. Some experts go on to speculate that arousal-inducing peritraumatic questioning may actually result in pathological consolidation of long-term memories into neural patterns leading to long-term adverse effects.

In response to these concerns, the Academy of Cognitive Therapy released a position paper after the September 11 tragedy recommending that, in the initial weeks after a trauma, those people who seek acute care for psychological harm be offered *only* "psychological first aid":

> The goal of psychological first aid is facilitation of normal emotional processing of the traumatic event(s). Helpers are advised not to include psychological techniques at this early phase but instead to (1) assess and provide for immediate physical needs (e.g., injury treatment, food and water), (2) ensure the person's physical safety (e.g., arrange safe shelter if necessary), (3) offer practical help (e.g., arrange childcare alternatives for a parent who is overwhelmed, protect from media intrusions, etc.), (4) make sure the traumatized

TABLE 40-2	Treatment of Emergency Manifestations of Psychiatric Symptoms Commonly Associated with Traumatic Victimization

SYNDROME	EMERGENCY MANIFESTATION	TREATMENT ISSUES
Posttraumatic stress disorder	Panic, terror, suicidal ideation, flashbacks	Reassurance; encouragement of return to responsibilities; avoid hospitalization if possible to prevent chronic invalidism; monitor suicidal ideation
Trauma-induced depression	Suicidal ideation or attempts; self-neglect; substance abuse	Assessment of danger to self; hospitalization if necessary; nonpsychiatric causes of depression must be evaluated individually
Trauma-induced panic	Panic, terror; acute onset	Must differentiate from other anxiety-producing disorders, both medical and psychiatric; ECG to rule out mitral valve prolapse; propranolol (10 to 30 mg); alprazolam (0.25 to 2.0 mg); long-term management may include an antidepressant
Bereavement	Guilt feelings, irritability; insomnia; somatic complaints	Must be differentiated from major depressive disorder; antidepressants not indicated; benzodiazepines for sleep; encouragement of ventilation
Brief psychotic reactions	Emotional turmoil, extreme lability; acutely impaired reality testing after obvious psychosocial stress	Hospitalization often necessary; low dosage of antipsychotics may be necessary but often resolves spontaneously
Insomnia	Depression and irritability; early morning agitation, frightening dreams; fatigue	Hypnotics only in short term; (e.g., triazolam [Halcion], 0.25 to 0.5 mg, at bedtime); treat any underlying mental disorder; rules of sleep hygiene
Increased alcohol and substance abuse	Intoxication at the time of presentation for services	Referrals as warranted; education about the need to develop alternative coping techniques

From Kaplan and Sadock, Synopsis of psychiatry, Copyright 2000, Lippincott & Williams. With permission.

person makes contact with the people who might be a normal source of comfort in his or her life (e.g., family, friends, spiritual community), (5) facilitate contact with loved ones (nearby and far away), (6) educate patients about the normality of a variety of peri-trauma responses, (7) support real life task decisions (what can you continue to do? what needs to be delayed? Help the individual prioritize life tasks that need attention).

Any discussion of the trauma in the initial weeks should include only what the individual wants to talk about [23] and are advised not to encourage the person to retell the trauma story again and again in the belief that this will help prevent PTSD. In fact, such retelling . . . in the early weeks following a trauma may encourage unhelpful rumination, linked to risk for persistent PTSD. Also [24], should be careful not to overwhelm the person with information.

SUMMARY OF MENTAL HEALTH ISSUES FOR VICTIMS

In general, patients who experience a natural recovery from trauma are likely to appraise their peritraumatic responses as normal reactions to an abnormal event and to believe they are strong enough to cope (25). Recovery is hastened with resumption of normal routine and deliberate efforts not to avoid reminders of the trauma. In contrast, some patients who go on to experience persistent PTSD view their trauma symptoms as evidence of permanent, negative emotional damage that will not be overcome. Many experts believe persistent PTSD is maintained by excessive avoidance (of trauma reminders), rumination (viewing images over and over and cannibalizing all news media), and excessive safety-seeking behaviors (staying home, hypervigilance to danger). However, one size does not fit all. In the wake of a terrorist experience, it is not always possible to normalize daily routine and generalize emotional responses. Thus the physician treating these victims must be versatile and ready to respond with situation-specific, person-specific interventions that are compassionate and appropriate to the circumstance.

PREPAREDNESS ESSENTIALS AT THE MESO LEVEL

PROVIDER ISSUES

Health care workers and emergency response personnel may become both direct and collateral casualties in large-scale disasters or mass casualty events. These events are sometimes called *critical incidents* and include the examples found in Table 40-3.

TABLE 40-3 Examples of Critical Incidents

- Hostage or siege situations
- Direct exposure situations
- Aggravated assaults
- Robbery
- Sudden or unexpected death
  - Murder, suicide, or attempted suicide
  - Vehicle accidents
  - Serious injuries or fatality
- Discharge of firearms
- Death of a peer or coworker
- Death of a child
- Events involving mass casualties
- Disasters with prolonged intense media coverage

Exposure of emergency health care workers (EHCWs) to extraordinary collateral trauma evokes what is known as *critical incident stress (CIS)*. Others have referred to CIS as traumatic stress, combat fatigue, and rapid-onset burnout, to name a few. For EHCWs, CIS can be operationalized as *an unusually strong emotional, behavioral, psychological, or physiological reaction of an emergency worker who is confronted with an acute traumatic event outside the usual human experience.* Emergency personnel are susceptible to CIS when exposed to unexpected mission failure, excessive human suffering, unusual sights, smells, and sounds, or personal threats to life and limb. Such stress can interfere with the worker's ability to cope and function on scene or later, both at work and at home.

Several factors make trigger stressors more psychologically troubling to health care workers than others, including young victim age, overidentification with the bereft, longer exposure, enhanced perception of gravity, and the intensity of the exposure. In addition to disasters that are natural or humanmade, critical incidents such as homicide or suicide that involve one's own family, friends, or coworkers are particularly high risk. High-publicity crimes and disasters that are magnified via the ubiquitous media can also amplify the likelihood of an event causing critical stress. Colleagues who are injured or killed in the line of duty are an archetypal cause of CIS and should routinely induce a critical incident stress management (CISM) response.

IMPACT OF PSYCHOLOGICAL STRESS ON EHCWs

Critical incidents cause a variety of reactions, depending on the substrate on which the stress occurs. Typically, individuals first try at once to react and deny the event. A well-seasoned emergency worker may effectively turn off any measured consideration of the trauma in order to function calmly and professionally. Many such responses are decidedly Pavlovian, learned distancing through drilling and repetitive simulation over time. Eventually, however, the automatic response must give way to a more human response. Ideally, this occurs after the job at hand is over. Serious stressors can cause PTSD-like intrusive thoughts and arousal and thereby overwhelm a worker's capacity for de-

nial and his or her valiant attempts to keep emotions at a distance. The breadth of possible responses is as unpredictable as the casualties themselves who present to EMS or hospitals during and after a major terrorist event. An individual's antecedent ego strength, mental hygiene, coping skills, social support, life experience, resilience, diet, and physical fitness can all influence the response to CIS.

STRESS REACTIONS

The signs and symptoms of a stress reaction in a health care worker can include physical, emotional, cognitive, and behavioral components as listed in Table 40-3. Physical manifestations may include palpitations, dyspepsia, diarrhea, breathlessness, headaches, chills, sweats, fatigue, dizziness, cramps, and chest pain, to name but a few. Emotional responses to stress include heightened anxiety, fear, panic, grief, denial, depression, and guilt. Cognitive impairment may manifest as decreased memory, disorientation, hypervigilance, nightmares, intrusive images, and diminished problem-solving skills. Critical stress may also be manifest by withdrawal, avoidance, blaming, restlessness, outbursts, and changes in appetite, hygiene, sleep, and sexual behavior. CIS can also usher in feelings of spiritual emptiness, hopelessness, anger toward God, despondency, and overwhelming negativity (Table 40-4).

MEMORY AND PERCEPTION

All senses can help encode traumatic memory, but none is stronger than smell. No emergency worker can deny the memory of alcohol on the breath of a trauma victim or the smell of blood on the floor of an ED. Most rescue multitasking proceeds uninterrupted, but memory can be stored and reactivated at a later time if the stimulus is unusual, unexpected, or grossly overwhelming. Memories can be triggered or linked to perceived stimuli in ways that are both primitive and complex, resulting in behavior and emotion that can be unpredictable, even for an experienced worker. Human thought often focuses more on the story and meaning of what has happened than on more impersonal, objective, or existential versions of what happened. Workers should be empowered to interpret the facts without a lot of excess story or added meaning in order to minimize the negative fallout of a critical stress.

It is important to distinguish that CIS involves unusual *stress* not unusual people. Within 24 hours of a CIS event, over 85% of emergency personnel experience stress reactions. Thus it is normative. Although it may be assumed that maladjusted workers who are dysfunctional before a critical event can exacerbate this dysfunction in the aftermath of disaster, it must also be understood that the preponderance of normal, functional workers may display a wide range of responses to an abnormally stressful event and such responses are in fact entirely normal, under the circumstances.

Coping skills can predetermine how a CIS is perceived and handled. Acute coping involves both threat appraisal and execution of a response to the threat. An individual's own sense of self-efficacy in being able to cope will inform the coping response. When faced with a stressor, personality

| TABLE 40-4 | Possible Manifestations of Critical Incident Stress |

PHYSICAL EFFECTS

- Nausea (upset stomach)
- Tremor (hands, lips)
- Feeling uncoordinated
- Profuse sweating
- Chills
- Dizziness
- Diarrhea
- Chest pains, rapid heartbeat
- Increased blood pressure

COGNITIVE EFFECTS

- Slowed thinking
- Confusion
- Disorientation
- Memory problems
- Seeing event over and over
- Distressing dreams

BEHAVIORAL EFFECTS

- Substance abuse
- Excessive checking and securing
- Angry outbursts
- Social withdrawal
- Marked changes in behavior
- Increased or decreased appetite

EMOTIONAL EFFECTS

- Fear
- Guilt
- Grief
- Depression
- Feeling abandoned
- Worry about others
- Despondency
- Shock/numbing

characteristics such as anxiety, anger, and depersonalization contribute to affective flight, fight, or freeze responses, respectively. Fatigue, frustration, helplessness, and personal risk can all threaten the ability to cope with a critical event. Sublimation, denial, and diversion may all have a role. Impulsive overreacting, avoidance, and acting out are counterproductive. Having support groups in place ahead of time is often the best prevention for posttraumatic stress. Planning a response to CIS in the aftermath of terrorism is also important and is discussed later.

CRITICAL INCIDENT STRESS MANAGEMENT (CISM)

Treatment for CIS

CISM seeks to modulate CIS before its effects are firmly established. The process requires the collaboration of emer-

gency service personnel with peers and mental health professionals who are cross-trained in each other's discipline. The goals of CISM are to minimize the impact and long-term effects of traumatic stress and enhance recovery from CIS. It achieves these goals through debriefing within 24 to 72 hours of the event. During the debriefing, individuals involved in the critical incident meet with a team of peer counselors and mental health professionals to disabuse themselves of myths around the incident and to recognize that the threat and the attendant need to react have both passed. The purpose of CISM is summarized in Table 40-5.

There are currently more than 350 CISM teams in the United States, and over 400 worldwide, but all function as emotional first aid for exposed workers. For very large disaster events, the CISM team may recommend demobilization for psychological purposes into a central unit for decompression. This is usually coupled with an education and nutrition break, avoiding the use of junk food, caffeine, and alcohol.

TABLE 40-5	Purpose of CISM = Prophylaxis and Treatment

- Provide professionally guided review of impact of the incident on the person's life
- Enable ventilation of emotions
- Provide reassurance and support
- Educate about trauma reactions
- Advise on symptom management
- Minimize the potential for the development of psychological problems
- Assist the person to return to normal levels of functioning
- Identify individuals who may need additional counseling

TABLE 40-6	Skills to Lead a Mini-Debriefing

- Good interpersonal skills
- Knowledge of crisis intervention
    Knowledge that CIS is a real and a normal reaction to acute trauma
- Comfortable with self emotional expression
- Be seen as an ally
    Debriefers should be at peer level
    Role as a supportive friend, not as a boss; validate what is shared
- Never criticize before emotionally debriefed
- Do not assume participants' feelings
- Everyone participates at least once in debriefing
- Stop criticism
    Do not permit tough or insensitive comments
- Watch for nonparticipants
    Especially one who appears visibly shaken
- Do not stop until all grief and pain are out
- Be sincere and be your best

When acute stressors or risk are great, CISM may involve early *defusing*, a special form of debriefing for those most at risk of CIS who cannot wait for group debriefing. This individualized, abbreviated form of CISM is more resource intensive; thus it operates in a more limited scope for those few individuals who are decompensating or at particularly high risk of doing so. During defusing, workers are educated about stress reactions and empowered with relaxation techniques and encouraged to vent their feelings rapidly, which aids in the more rapid processing and assimilation of experiences and emotions. This critical incident stress *defusion* may require pharmacological therapy or even hospitalization in some circumstances. It may be followed up with later debriefing under closely supervised conditions with a licensed therapist, psychologist, or psychiatrist.

Within days after an event, more formal *critical incident stress debriefing* (CISD) may take place in order to allow those involved with an incident to process the event and reflect on its impact (26). The purpose of CISD is to accelerate normal recovery, for normal people, having normal and necessary reactions to abnormal events (27). Earlier is usually better, but CISD may be useful even weeks after an event (28). It is generally held over 2 to 4 hours in one location without breaks within the first 1 to 2 days after an incident. The intensity of the process takes workers through the cognitive realm to the emotional realm and then back to the cognitive in order to speed recovery from a critical incident. It allows participants to normalize their experience and to become educated in stress management and healthy coping techniques.

Operationally, the debriefing room should have a circle of chairs and two peer counselors that should include one mental health professional and/or possibly a member of the clergy or similar support staff. Not just anyone can lead a debriefing, and certain skills, clinical characteristics, and general rules of engagement come into play when conducting a mini-debriefing (Table 40-6). CISD is conducted in seven phases, as described in Table 40-7.

CISD CAVEATS

Despite many anecdotal successes and its widespread use for the last 50 years, CISD has few rigorously controlled studies to recommend it. As length of time between exposure to the event and CISD are increased, CISD becomes less effective (29). Debriefing should only be used to address a limited aspect of victims' disaster experience and to educate participants about other critical factors affecting their stress response as well as to make referrals to other resources if necessary. Because the purpose of CISD is to accelerate normal recovery for normal people having normal reactions to abnormal events, the pathway for unstable persons or those already impaired would be decidedly different. Studies suggest that those in need of additional assistance may benefit from ongoing groups rather than a one time meeting (30).

An optimal debriefing should include everyone involved in the incident: nurses, EMS workers, fire, police, and other rescue professionals. In some cases it may be appropriate to include spouses because they are the ones left to pick up the pieces after their partner is exposed to CIS. Some people are scared by their own physical and emotional reactions, and those who are unusually quiet or leave early may not be handling it as well as they want to believe. It is very important to let them know that whatever they are experiencing is a natural reaction. CISD may provide some immediate opportunities for victims to talk with one another, but it is unlikely to be an effective treatment for complex, ongoing, or persistent problems that are the result of the disaster itself, predisaster vulnerabilities, or the variety of social conditions that surround a disaster's aftermath (28).

Knowledge of crisis intervention and grief management is essential for those doing the debriefing. The process must not be confused with critique, and the atmosphere must be completely unthreatening to personnel. No one should be criticized before they are emotionally debriefed, and sessions should not end until all the grief and pain is out. Critical, insensitive, or gallows humor should not be tolerated because this will squelch expression of any feelings. It is also important not to

TABLE 40-7	CISD Phases for Debriefing Groups

INTRODUCTION	TEACHING PHASE
• Establish agreements, confidentiality, rules, and roles	• Abnormal reactions are normal reactions to abnormal situations
FACT PHASE	• Assess work situation; do you need time off?
• Who was aware first?	• Watch for fixation on the incident and avert finding excuses for the tragedy
• What was person's role in situation?	• Take distance and allow time to pass
• Location when incident occurred	• Expect the incident to bother you and others
• Focus on event's facts and description; allow pieces to fall into place chronologically	• Learn about what you are going through
• Watch for cognitive and emotional reactions	• Set realistic long-term expectations for recovery
THOUGHTS PHASE	• Teach how to get additional help if necessary
• "When did you realize this was a bad event?"	• Importance of reassurance
FEELING PHASE	• Keep usual routines and structure
• Encourage emotional reactions: "How did you react?" or "What was the worst thing about this event for you?"	• Eat well, exercise, and avoid use of alcohol, drugs, and junk food to cope
• People discuss fears, anxieties, concerns, feelings of guilt, frustration, anger, and ambivalence	• Do not isolate yourself from friends, family, or coworkers
• Pay special attention to those who are withdrawn, overquiet, or leave early	• Prevent yourself from becoming obsessed with the incident
• Allow all feeling to be expressed	• Avoid making life-changing decisions
• Emotional expression: first step in learning to deal	**REENTRY PHASE**
• Revisit feelings initially expressed	• What is the next step? "Where do we go from here?"
SYMPTOM PHASE	• Is another debriefing needed?
• What did you notice about yourself immediately after the event?	**POSTDEBRIEFING**
• What are participants experiencing now (anger, guilt, insomnia)?	• Always debrief the debriefers
• How has your life changed? (activities, hobbies, intrusive thoughts)	• Discuss organizational issues discovered
	• Review entire process: start with positives, what worked, what didn't work
	• Allow participants to process reactions
	• Assign follow-up activities

assume how participants are feeling and to let everyone have an opportunity to express themselves. Reluctant participants who are visibly shaken often demand extra attention in a more private setting.

In summary, CISM works by enabling individuals to vent their reactions rapidly, which, in turn, promotes more rapid processing of experiences and resultant emotions from CIS. Stress, improperly managed, can shorten the career or life of a provider, and it is an occupational hazard of emergency response personnel. Although controversy still surrounds the impact of CISM, it remains the current standard of care for CIS and stands as an important immunization against the effects of severe stress, PTSD, and professional burnout. From the ashes of terrorism, such immunized providers may emerge wiser and emotionally stronger. They are better able to cope with the everyday stresses of their calling. It is frequently a turning point where, beyond the crucible of terror, they reevaluate the meaning and the value of life and appreciate the little things they had often overlooked.

PREPAREDNESS ESSENTIALS AT THE POPULATION (MACRO) LEVEL

In the aftermath of terrorist attacks, there may be substantial psychological morbidity in the population (5). These effects seem to be far reaching and worldwide because the planet has shrunk and events in one nation can more easily influence behavior in another. One example of these global effects are evidenced by the events of September 11, 2001, appearing to have had a brief, but significant inverse effect on the suicide rate in England and Wales. This transatlantic impact was thought to be related to the external threat of terrorism creating social cohesion among this group of people (31).

INDIRECT EXPOSURE AND MEDIA TOXICITY

For the population at large, most exposure to a terrorist event will be indirect. Geographical proximity to a catastrophic event is key, but the psychological or mental proximity is also an important factor in determining the stress-related impacts to psychosocial functioning and to symptoms of PTSD (19). Even those not directly involved or physically injured by a terrorist act or perceived threat can exhibit signs and symptoms of PTSD and emotional distress (32,33). Diagnostic classifications of acute stress and posttraumatic disorder affirm that people can be markedly affected by witnessing a trauma or through the indirect impact of a trauma happening to others.

Indirect exposure would also include all forms of media, such as radio, newspapers, the Internet, and particularly television. Recent work suggests that vicarious vicitimization can and does occur even through the medium of television (34) and appears more likely in the presence of repeated exposure to disturbing images and other trauma-related conditions (35). The terrorist attacks of September 11, 2001, were able to incite widespread despondency and fear through the use of the media. PTSD symptoms have been reported in children who have watched television coverage related to horror films, war, industrial disasters, and terrorist bombings. Television can be a source of unnecessary secondary exposure to traumatic details (36). A study of the Oklahoma City bombing concluded that bomb-related television exposure to middle and high school students was a primary predictor of elevated PTSD scores and also played a role in sustaining these symptoms (1). Because exposure to terrorism via media immersion can lead to significant symptoms of PTSD, such exposure must be limited, especially for children (37,38).

Research suggests that the media may be a common trigger of suppressed traumatic memories, reactivation of PTSD in veterans, and a cause of immediate physiological arousal. This is particularly true among vulnerable adults who have a history of past critical incident exposure (35). It has also been shown that particular images may be more disturbing to people and contribute more to postdisaster psychopathology than others. The viewing of images of people jumping and falling from the World Trade Center correlated strongly with PTSD symptoms and depression more so than other images (35). After the terrorist attacks on the WTC, several experts have reaffirmed the negative effects of television exposure leading to psychological dysfunction (39). In both children and adults there was a statistically significant correlation between hours of television watched and the number and magnitude of significant stress symptoms. The notion that repeated viewing of disturbing images might correlate with psychopathology is unsurprising given the voluminous research on the deleterious effects of television violence on children. Most authorities believe repeated viewing of disturbing images can have lasting negative effects on children (40).

HARNESSING THE POWER OF THE MEDIA FOR GOOD

Because it is through the use of modern media that terrorists depend to maximize their negative impact on the psyche, the media must be properly managed to optimize societal outcome. Ideally, the media must inform the public

with discretion and restraint. The media will usually oblige if treated with respect, recognizing that like other rescue workers, they serve an important and complementary role in disaster work and recovery. Mental health officials and community leaders should warn the public of the emotional and mental health hazards of intensive disaster exposure via the news media (35). Contacts with the news media, for example, need to be coordinated early, and rules, guidelines, and policies need to be firmly established in advance. Webmasters and other media personnel must be educated to understand that news coverage of terrorist attacks can contribute to PTSD symptoms (37). A policy of full disclosure about truth in reporting and what information is relevant to public safety and which is sensationalistic muckraking must be discussed a priori. Being prepared both decreases the worry that precedes crisis and the turmoil that follows. Speculation must be avoided. Detailed accounting of what is being done to counter any terrorist threat needs to be relayed to the public. Recommendations for specific steps that the public needs to take to protect themselves must also be expressed. Compliance with all standard privacy policies should be established because invasions of privacy can exacerbate the psychological stress of victims (41). Speculation, tabloid hearsay, and other rumors that commonly fill the information gaps in times of crisis can be destructive to global mental hygiene and must be avoided (42,43).

COMMUNITY APPROACHES TO MENTAL HEALTH

A recurring lesson in any effective trauma and disaster response is that all intervention needs to be based on an understanding of and respect for local culture. A systematic assessment of trauma and loss exposure as well as current levels of distress experienced by individuals throughout the affected community is also important. Understanding the vulnerabilities of subpopulations such as children and the elderly and gaining an appreciation of the range and severity of posttraumatic stresses, secondary adversities, and trauma reminders that exert a lasting impact on the community is also useful (36). It is important to conduct risk assessment early and reach as many affected people as possible, especially those who report high-intensity or repeated exposure, display a heightened fear response, report peritraumatic dissociation, or those reluctant to seek professional help (4). Broad-scale outreach programs should be implemented no later than 1 to 3 months after a disaster (2). General guidelines and recommendations for intervention by mental health professionals in disastrous events can be found in Table 40-8 (2).

Getting back to everyday routines is very helpful to posttraumatic recovery (44). Rest, respite, sleep, food, and water are the primary tools of early and successful intervention. To cope with terrorism, anxious individuals should continue normal everyday activities to maintain balance in their lives. Familiar environments decrease anxiety and help anchor emotion. In crisis, the therapeutic value of family and friends cannot be overestimated (45).

TABLE 40-8	AREST Principles of Systemic Intervention by Mental Health Professionals in Disastrous Events

ANTICIPATE

- Provide an integrated vision
- Foresee different scenarios and develop contingency plans
- Train professionals and paraprofessionals
- Allocate human and economic resources
- Create treatment protocols
- Develop local, national, and international networks
- Facilitate collaboration among agencies
- Gain sponsorship and legitimacy

REDIFFERENTIATE

- Identity extent of social loss in terms of institutional role dysfunction
- Plan role redifferentiation within and between systems
- Initiate interdisciplinary teams

EMPOWER

- Debrief, educate, empower social agents in related fields that are in direct contact with survivors
- Help these agents adapt and restore original roles
- Delegate therapeutic responsibilities to these agents

SUPERVISE AND ASSESS

- Define boundaries and provide knowledge, expertise, and support to therapeutic agents
- Assess program deployment and needs by feedback

TREAT AND FOLLOW UP

- Focus on individual and family rehabilitation
- Consider delayed responses and deal with tertiary disaster

From Laor N, et al. With permission. (2)

Other stress-reducing activities should be added, such as regular exercise, social outings, family support, spiritual services, yoga, breathing exercises, or other forms of relaxation therapy. Community members should be told to trust their instincts about suspicious people or things but not to become paranoid. They should also try to control what they can by taking steps to ensure they feel safe in their homes and community. Although mass panic is unlikely, individuals should avoid overreacting to or becoming obsessed with perceived threats of terrorism. Thoughts of hatred, revenge, racist stereotyping, and xenophobia that commonly arise can become crippling and should be resisted (44). It should be recommended that people stay informed but tune out the constant news coverage. With the passage of time, there should be fewer cases of PTSD and related stress reactions. Unfortunately, the intense media coverage surrounding the anniversary of terrorist attacks can reawaken traumatic memories and even result in new-onset PTSD and MDD in susceptible groups of citizens (39). Safe ways of information acquisition should be recommended to the community such as radio listening and periodical reading where the ingestion of information may be more readily titrated. Primary and secondary prevention through education and restraint by both the media and the general public can help safeguard mental health from future terrorist events.

There are important roles for media personnel, teachers, parents, religious leaders, and clinicians to assist emotionally as many survivors as possible. Teachers and religious, business, and civic leaders need to be vigilant for those who show signs of social withdrawal and dangerous coping after such traumatic events. Clinging behavior in older children suggests regression and has been reported in children with PTSD symptoms (37). Schools have been shown to constitute an effective and cost-efficient setting in which to provide postdisaster or postwar mental health assistance to children and their families and should be considered for this purpose (36).

In order to signal security, promote public health, and foster resiliency within an affected population, coordinated community initiatives should be used to provide specific public health updates, provide suggestions and direction for self-care, as well as educate the populace on when and how to seek institutional care (45). City and local government, hospital officials, public health officials, and key community contacts chosen in advance may coordinate such initiatives through schools, faith communities, businesses, web sites, e-mail broadcasting, telephone hotlines, television, radio, and print updates, electronic town meetings, telemedicine, hospitals, and designated mental health clinics (45). Not only will these outlets be useful in dispelling rumors, but they will also offer a sense of community cohesion that has been shown to be helpful, even when direct contact is contraindicated (31). When prepared to face crisis with strong leadership, solid information, preestablished support networks, and a familiar stable environment, the public is best able to handle the uncertainty and chaos surrounding the threat of terrorism.

RESOURCES

The many resources for dealing with the psychological effects of terrorism offer up-to-date information as well as directions on how to obtain further assistance. Listed here are some of the recommended places to obtain more information related to terrorism and its psychological effects.

1. Coping with Terrorism. Web site: http://www.helping.apa.org/daily/terrorism.html. American Psychological Association: Helpful resource with fact sheets describing psychological consequences of terrorist attack and ways of coping with stress induced by it.

2. Tips for Talking About Disaster. Web site: http://www.mentalhealth.org/cmhs/emergencyservices/after.asp. The Center for Mental Health Services: Guidelines for teachers, parents, and service providers on how to help children, adolescents, families, and adults cope with stress after terrorist events.

3. Family Physicians Respond. Web site: http://www.aafp.org/x7472.xml. American Academy of

Family Physicians: Information to help children and parents cope with terrorism and the effects of PTSD.

4. Resources for Coping with Terrorism. Web site: http://www.icn.ch/terrorism.htm. International Council of Nurses: Provides information and manuals for assisting in coping and proving care in the aftermath of a terrorist attack.

5. Disaster Mental Health Institute. Web site: http://www.usd.edu/dmhi/Pubs/availability.html. University of South Dakota: Contains short booklets on coping with disaster that can be printed from the web site.

6. Disaster Handouts and Links. Web site: http://www.trauma-pages.com/pg5.htm. David Baldwin's Trauma Information: A cache of 14 disaster handouts at this site are categorized into material for adult victims, families and child victims, and disaster workers and their families.

7. Publications dealing with Psychology and Terrorism. Web site: http://www.ncdpt.org/publications.htm. The National Center on Disaster Psychology and Terrorism: Listing of multiple publications that deal with the psychological effects of terrorism and disasters.

8. International Critical Incident Stress Foundation, Inc. Web site: http://www.icisf.org/. International Critical Incident Stress Foundation: Resource for information and education associated with critical incident stress debriefing.

REFERENCES

1. Pfefferbaum D, Nixon S, Krug R. Clinical needs assessment of the middle and high school students following the 1995 Oklahoma City bombing. Am J Psychiatry 1999;156:1069-74.
2. Laor N ed. Facing war, terrorism, and disaster. Toward a child oriented comprehensive emergency care system. 2003.
3. Klitzman S, Freudenberg N. Implications of the World Trade Center attack for the public health and health care infrastructures. Am J Public Health 2003;93(3):400-6.
4. Martino C. Psychological consequences of terrorism. Int J Emerg Ment Health 2002;4(2):105-11.
5. Galea S, Ahern J, Resnick H, et al. Psychological sequelae of the September 11 terrorist attacks in New York City. N Engl J Med 2002;346(13):982-7.
6. Kleber R, Brom D, Defares PB. Coping with trauma: Theory, prevention and treatment. Amsterdam: Swets and Zeitlinger International, 1992.
7. Kulka RA, Schlenger WE, Fairbank JA. Trauma and the Vietnam War generation; report of findings from the National Vietnam Veterans Readjustment Study. New York: Brunner/Mazel, 1990.
8. O'Toole BI, Marshall RP, Grayson DA. The Australian Vietnam Veterans Health Study. III. Psychological health of Australian Vietnam veterans and its relationship to combat. Intl J Epidemiol 1996;25:331-40).
9. American Psychiatric Association. DSM-IV: diagnostic and statistical manual of mental disorders. 4th ed. Washington, DC: Author, 1994.
10. Gidron Y. Posttraumatic stress disorder after terrorist attacks: a review. J Nerv Ment Dis 2002;190(2):118-21.
11. Chen H, Chung H, Chen T, et al. The emotional distress in a community after the terrorist attack on the World Trade Center. Community Ment Health J 2003;39(2):157-65.
12. North CS, Pfefferbaum B. Research on the mental health effects of terrorism. JAMA 2002;288(5):633-6.
13. Schlenger WE, Caddell JM, Ebert L, et al. Psychological reactions to terrorist attacks: findings from the National Study of Americans' Reactions to September 11. JAMA 2002;288 (5):581-8.
14. Boscarina JA, Galea S, Ahern J. Psychiatric medication use among Manhattan residents following the World Trade Center disaster. J Trauma Stress 2003;16:301-6.
15. Kramer T, Booth B. Service utilization and outcomes in medically ill veterans with posttraumatic stress and depressive disorders. J Trauma Stress 2003;16:211-9.
16. Horowitz M. Stress response syndrome: a review of posttraumatic and adjustment disorders. Hosp Community Psychiatry 1986;37:241-9.
17. Bromet E, Sonnega A, Kessler RC. Risk factors for DSM-III-R posttraumatic stress disorder. Findings from a national comorbidity survey. Am J Epidemiol 1998;147:353-61.
18. Kessler RC, Little RJ, Groves RM. Advances in strategies for minimizing and adjusting for survey nonresponse. Epidemiol Rev 1995;17(1):192-204.
19. Cardenas J, Williams K, Wilson JP, et al. PTSD, major depressive symptoms, and substance abuse following September 11, 2001, in a midwestern university population. Int J Emerg Ment Health 2003;5(1):15-28.
20. Bleich A, Belkopf M, Solomon Z. Exposure to terrorism, stress-related mental health symptoms and coping behaviors among a nationally representative sample in Israel. JAMA 2003;290:612-20.
21. Jaycoxhoro LH, Masrxhall GN, Orland M. Predictors of acute distress among young adults injured by community violence. J Trauma Stress 2003;16:237-45.
22. Van Loey H, Maas C, Faber AW. Predictors of chronic posttraumatic stress symptoms following burn injury. Results of a longitudinal study. J Trauma Stress 2003;16:361-9.
23. Bronze MS, Huycke MM, Machado LJ, et al. Viral agents as biological weapons and agents of bioterrorism. Am J Med Sci 2002;323(6):316-25.
24. Maunder R, Hunter J, Vincent L, et al. The immediate psychological and occupational impact of the 2003 SARS outbreak in a teaching hospital. CMAJ 2003;168(10):1245-51.
25. Benight CC, Harper M. Coping self-efficacy perceptions as a mediator between acute stress response and long-term distress following natural disasters. J Trauma Stress 2002;15: 177-86.
26. Mitchell J, Everly GS. Critical incident stress debriefing: An operations manual for the prevention of traumatic stress among emergency services and disaster workers. Ellicott City, MD: Chevron, 1995.
27. Hokanson M, Wirth B. The critical incident stress debriefing process for the Los Angeles County Fire Department: automatic and effective. Intl J Emerg Ment Health 2000;4:249-57.
28. Hiley-Young B. CISD: value and limitations in disaster response. NCP Clin Q 1994;4:2.
29. Mitchell J. Stress: the history and future of critical incident stress debriefing. J Emerg Med Services 1998:7-52.
30. Raphael B, Wilson J. Psychological debriefing. theory, practice and evidence. Cambridge, UK: Cambridge University Press, 2000.
31. Salib E. Effect of 11 September 2001 on suicide and homicide in England and Wales. Br J Psychiatry 2003;183(3):207-12.
32. Pfefferbaum B, North CS, Flynn BW, et al. The emotional impact of injury following an international terrorist incident. Public Health Rev 2001;29(2-4):271-80.
33. American Psychiatric Association. DSM-IV: diagnostic and statistical manual of mental disorders. Washington, DC: Author, 2000.
34. Schuster MA, Stein BD, Jaycox LH. A national survey of stress reactions after the September 11, 2001 terrorist attacks. N Engl J Med 2001;345:1507-12.

35. Ahern J, Galea S, Resnick H. Television images and psychological symptoms after the September 11 terrorist attacks. Psychiatry 2002;65:289-300.

36. Saltzman WR, Layne CM, Steinberg AM, et al. Developing a culturally and ecologically sound intervention program for youth exposed to war and terrorism. Child Adolesc Psychiatr Clin N Am 2003;12(2):319-42.

37. Duggal HS, Berezkin G, John V. PTSD and TV viewing of World Trade Center. J Am Acad Child Adolesc Psychiatry 2002;41(5):494-5.

38. Veenema TG, Schroeder-Bruce K. The aftermath of violence: children, disaster, and posttraumatic stress disorder. J Pediatr Health Care 2002;16(5):235-44.

39. The deadly effect of non-lethal weapons [editorial]. New Sci 2002;174(2342):3.

40. Putnam F. Televised trauma and viewer PTSD: implications for prevention. Psychiatry 2002;65(4):310-2.

41. Mullin S. Public health and the media: the challenge now faced by bioterrorism. J Urban Health 2002;79(1):12.

42. Glass TA. Understanding public response to disasters. Public Health Rep 2001;116(Suppl 2):69-73.

43. Njenga FG, Nyamai C, Kigamwa P. Terrorist bombing at the USA embassy in Nairobi: the media response. East Afr Med J 2003;80(3):159-64.

44. Scurfield RM. Commentary about the terrorist acts of September 11, 2001. Trauma Violence Abuse 2002;3(1):3-14.

45. Saathoff G, Everly GS Jr. Psychological challenges of bioterror: containing contagion. Int J Emerg Ment Health 2002;4(4):245-52.

41

Being a Child in the Midst of Terrorism

Richard Aghababian and Mariann Manno

INTRODUCTION

Terrorism—a planned, often politically motivated event designed to kill many innocent victims and inflict physical pain, psychological suffering, and fear on an entire community—is new to our Western culture, but not to children worldwide. Terrorism, violence, and disaster have involved children in the form of naturally occurring events; transportation accidents; exposure to war; social, ethnic and religious conflict; and as collateral damage in adult mass casualty incidents. Throughout childhood and adolescence, children are physically less capable and emotionally more vulnerable to the effects of terrorism. This fact may make children likely primary targets for terrorism in the future.

Children are unique from the perspective of their anatomy, physiology, emotional development, and response to specific physical and psychological insults. These unique needs of children have rarely been considered in disaster planning. Civilian emergency physicians and Emergency Medical Services (EMS) systems have learned about mass casualty incidents through military models, focused on the needs of adult victims; consequently, they have limited personal clinical experience with pediatric disaster medicine. A terrorist attack with predominately pediatric casualties would have a tremendous and far-reaching impact on all child survivors, family members, and the community at large. All facets of the EMS system must be aware of this potential and be prepared to meet the special and divergent needs of children in the setting of a chemical, biological, radiation, or explosive event that involves large numbers of children. A paradigm shift that deals with unaddressed issues of treatment, equipment, triage, and training is a critical step in preparing to address the needs of children in the midst of terrorism.

PREPAREDNESS ESSENTIALS

DEVELOPMENTAL STAGES: WHAT CHILDREN UNDERSTAND

Development from infancy through adolescence is a continuous, dynamic process heavily influenced by close personal experiences and circumstances in the child's community. It is a web of evolving language, behavioral, cognitive, anatomic, and physiologic changes. New skills are achieved and build on previous milestones. The child is at the center of a series of concentric circles that represent his environment. Closest to him is the family, friends, and school. Farther out is his town, city, and so on. Disruption of the environment will affect the child depending on its severity and the child's developmental stage. Severe disruption of several facets, as seen in natural disasters, war, and terrorism have serious implications for the well-being and normal development of children of all ages.

Major themes of child development include attachment between the child and caregiver (especially the parent), emotional maturity and self control, the ability to master fearful and anxiety-provoking situations, and the formation of independent relationships with peers. Specific tasks or achievements toward these goals are accomplished at different ages or stages. It is helpful to consider an overview of child development broken down into somewhat artificial categories based on the goals and accomplishments of each stage (21).

Birth to 18 months of age is a time of physical growth and physiologic change. Infants develop through motor and sensory exploration of their environment. Rolling over, midline play, transferring objects from hand to hand, crawling, sitting, and finally walking allow the baby to interact with the world around them. Attachment to caregivers progresses from complete dependence to reciprocal relationship. After 6 weeks of age, infants increasingly respond to their environment. They smile, coo, and visually track their caretaker. Separation anxiety that peaks late in the first year and coping with temporary absences of the caretaker are hallmarks of the emotional development of this age. Lasting absences of primary caretakers are associated with nonorganic failure to thrive and with increased risk of pathology.

Toddlers (18 months to 3 years) are curious, interested, and active. This is a time of early independence, stubbornness, and negotiating limits. Perceptual constancy becomes better developed so that children in this age group are better able to cope with the absence of a parent. Transitional objects (stuffed animal, favorite blanket) can be used to ease a toddler through a difficult situation.

The preschool years (3 to 5 years) begin a time of language maturation, developing social skills, and a sense of independence. They see themselves separate from but still closely connected to their primary caretaker. Just as motor development is the hallmark of the toddler, language and prelogical reasoning occurs in the preschooler. Magical thinking, an overextension of causality (e.g., My brother got sick because I did not eat my dinner), and exaggerated fears and fantasies are features of the way children of this age figure out their world. Pain is interpreted as punishment. Death is a temporary, reversal event. Time, in general, is a difficult concept so that periods of time spent waiting or holding still may be intolerable. Expressive language lags receptive language. Children at this age may understand more than expected and interpret language literally (e.g., I will draw your blood). The choice of words in new situations is important. Explanations of painful procedures should occur immediately before it happens. Honesty, simple and brief, about discomfort and capitalizing on the child's curiosity by including them in the process (holding bandages, touching equipment) may elicit the preschooler's cooperation.

School age years (6 to 11 years of age) are a time of mastering complex cognitive tasks, following the rules, and meeting expectations at home and in school. School begins to replace home as a place of central importance with peers, academics, and sports competing with time spent with parents and siblings. Specific learning disabilities, ADHD, oppositional deficient disorder (ODD), anxieties, and phobias may present during this period and may make these children seem out of synch with peers. School age children understand true causality and the permanent nature of death. In the medical setting, these children are generally logical and cooperative. They should be included in conversations about their health and encouraged to make choices when appropriate.

Adolescence is a time of tremendous transition. Puberty is a time of rapid growth and change in the body's appearance as these children achieve adult proportions and reproductive capability. They are capable of abstract thinking and complex reasoning but many retain egocentric, hypersensitive, or dramatic tendencies. The quest for autonomy is a source of stress in families. In the medical setting, adolescents deserve full and honest explanations. They should be encouraged to ask questions and participate in discussions and decisions. Their maturity and privacy should be respected.

Because they are in the process of leaning about and mastering their world, children are more physically and emotionally vulnerable to the effects of disaster and depravation than older counterparts. When tragedy strikes a family, community, or nation, helping children cope and regain a sense of safety is of critical importance. In the immediate postdisaster period, children benefit from rapid reestablishment of order, routine, and safety. Children should be encouraged to express their feelings in constructive ways through discussion, play, or art. Regressive or clingy behaviors, moodiness, poor sleep, and somatic complaints are normal. Events should be handled honestly in developmentally appropriate language. Deception about the well-being and whereabouts of loved ones should be avoided. Children should be shown images of the disaster so that they have an authentic picture of what happened, but this should be done in a developmentally appropriate manner and in an environment that permits discussion and understanding. Unsupervised or repeated exposure to media, especially television with displays of graphic images, is harmful.

ANATOMY AND PHYSIOLOGY: HOW CHILDREN ARE DIFFERENT

The Pediatric Airway

The airway is the most important difference between adult and pediatric resuscitation and emergency care. Respiratory failure precedes cardiopulmonary failure or cardiac arrest in most children. Respiratory failure may result from a primary respiratory problem (reactive airway disease, pneumonia, upper airway obstruction, and/or infection) or may occur secondary to a number of causes (inhalation, drowning, overwhelming sepsis, a toxicologic overdose, or traumatic insult). Airway management is the most important skill acquired in pediatric resuscitation. In the injured child, oxygenation, ventilation, and airway protection are vital. The approach to the pediatric airway must take into account anatomic uniqueness and different sizes of neonates, infants, and children.

For all providers, basic knowledge of pediatric airway anatomy, head positioning, techniques to open the airway and remove foreign bodies, and the use of airway adjuncts and effective bag-valve-mask ventilation are essential skills. Advanced providers should be proficient in endotracheal intubation, rapid sequence induction, and surgical methods to establish an airway. In the setting of trauma, cervical spine immobilization must be maintained during airway management.

Pediatric Airway Anatomy. Infants have a prominent occiput that promotes head and neck flexion when the infant is supine. This often results in functional airway obstruction in a sick, hypotonic infant as the tongue flops backward onto the posterior pharynx. The first step in airway management is to place the patient in a sniffing position, which brings the tongue forward. In addition, the epiglottis is a large, broad, and floppy structure that partly obscures the vocal cords. The larynx is cephalad, anterior and cone or funnel shaped. The narrowest part of the young child's airway is at the cricoid ring, not vocal cords as in children over 8 years of age. The cricoidthyroid membrane is smaller and difficult to locate in young patients with a short neck. The overall caliber of lower airway structures is smaller and shorter. Small degrees of edema, bronchospasm, or excess mucus production may result in significant obstruction.

Pediatric Airway Equipment. These anatomic differences, taken in aggregate, explain why the pediatric airway is highly vulnerable to obstruction and respiratory failure. They also are the reason why different equipment will be required to resuscitate critically ill and injured pediatric victims. Straight (Miller) blades should be used to directly lift up the epiglottis and compress the tongue and submandibular tissue. Endotracheal tubes are selected by patient size. The common rule of thumb for children over 2 years of age is 4 + age years/4. For example, an average 4 year old would require a 4 + 4/4 or size 5 tube. Uncuffed endotracheal tubes should be used in most settings in children less than 8 years old since the cricoid ring provides an anatomic cuff. Cricoid pressure (Sellick maneuver) is essential to gently push and stabilize the anterior larynx within view. Narrower airway structures and higher resistances may require higher pressures when ventilation is initiated. Short tracheal lengths (4 to 5 cm in a newborn) predispose for tube dislodgement and right mainstem intubation.

Bag-valve-mask ventilation. Tthe first maneuver used to provide ventilation and an essential skill for all pediatric providers is bag-valve-mask (BVM) ventilation. Correct equipment and training is needed. Self-inflating bags (manual resuscitators) are manufactured in several sizes: neonatal (250 cc, for newborns only), small child (450 cc, up to 5 years), large child (750 cc), and adult (1,000 cc). Correct size bag is essential in order to deliver adequate tidal volume. The mask must make a tight seal on the patient's face. A properly sized mask should cover the mouth and nose. The top of the mask should fit in the bridge of the nose and the bottom, in the cleft of the chin. The mask should be clear and the rim, soft and compressible.

The E-C clamp technique describes BMV ventilation by one provider. The thumb and index finger (forming a C) firmly secure the mask on the patient's face with the upper part of the mask in the bridge of the nose and the lower edge in the cleft of the chin. The third, fourth, and fifth fingers (forming an E) grip the mandible. Pressure on the submental triangle can compress and obstruct the airway. If this is ineffective, two people may be required to provide BVM ventilation. In this case, one person makes a seal with the mask making an E-C clamp with both hands. The second person provides ventilation. Ventilation should proceed at age-appropriate respiratory rates with sufficient time for exhalation. The technique of saying, "squeeze-release-release" is helpful in avoiding overventilation. Observing chest rise with bagging is essential to ensure adequate ventilation. Gentle cricoid pressure may be helpful to reduce gastric insufflation and prevent regurgitation of gastric materials. Poor chest rise may result from improperly sized mask and/or bag, inadequate mask seal or gastric distention. Gastric dilatation that restricts diaphragmatic excursion can make assisted ventilation ineffective. This can be avoided by the Sellick maneuver and placement of a nasal or oral gastric tube. Airway adjuncts such as the oral airway in an unconscious patient or nasopharyngeal airway in the setting of oral trauma should be considered.

The American Heart Association (AHA) Pediatric Advanced Life Support (PALS) guidelines recommend training in BVM ventilation for all prehospital providers and the BVM technique as a primary method of ventilatory support, particularly if transport time is short. In the prehospital setting,

effective BVM ventilation can be mastered through training programs by greater than 90% of students. In a large controlled study of prehospital pediatric airway management in Los Angeles and Orange Counties in California, Gauche showed that BVM ventilation was as effective as endotracheal intubation in managing the young patient's airway.

Endotracheal intubation. Ongoing ventilation is required in a subset of critically ill or injured patients with respiratory failure, severely altered mental status, and increased intracranial pressure, to protect the lower airway in settings following trauma, burns, anaphylaxis, and inhalation. A relative indication for endotracheal intubation is the requirement of definitive airway control before transport. Postintubation patients must be monitored with end-tidal $CO2$ and pulse oxymetry.

Assessment of Shock/Blood Volume

The presence of shock or circulatory failure in young children can be subtle. The recognition of shock relies upon a systematic evaluation of the end organs of perfusion rather than the interpretation of vital signs. Almost all hypoperfused young children will be tachycardic and normotensive until end-stage shock and cardiopulmonary failure occur. Hypotension is rare, in children even with significant blood loss, and ominous.

Determination of the severity of shock requires an assessment of central nervous system perfusion (mental status, recognition of parents, developmentally appropriate response to new environment, response to painful procedures), the presence and quality of peripheral and central pulses, and skin perfusion (capillary refill, skin color, skin temperature, presence of mottling). Signs of adequate fluid resuscitation include improvement in tachycardia, increase in systolic blood pressure, improved skin perfusion, improvement in mental status in nonsedated patients, and reestablishment of urine output at 1 to 2 cc/kg/hr. Failure to improve following fluid resuscitation should prompt immediate surgical involvement.

Vascular Access

Obtaining vascular access is often the most technically difficult aspect in pediatric resuscitation. Compensatory mechanisms of tachycardia and peripheral vasoconstriction are seen in response to hypovolemia. Vasoconstriction is more pronounced in infants who are exposed to a cold resuscitation environment. Visualizing venous landmarks is often impossible. In general, peripheral IVs should be attempted in anatomically reliable sites like the greater saphenous vein. In settings where an experienced provider and equipment are available, a central line, usually the femoral, may be the appropriate choice.

However, intraosseous (IO) access will be the most expeditious choice in most prehospital and initial resuscitation settings, especially when multiple victims are present. The AHA PALS recommendation is that IO access is appropriate in any age patient (formerly recommended for children 6 years old and younger). Initial attempts should be at the tibial plateau distal to the tibial growth plate. Alternative sites include distal femurs, anterior iliac crests, and sternum. IO should not be attempted in bones where an IO has been previously placed and created a hole in the bone or with fractures. Confirmation of IO placement includes ability to withdraw bloody fluid from the marrow, stability of the IO in the bone, and, most importantly, the ability to flush IV fluid without infiltration into the soft tissues. Any fluid, drug, or blood product necessary to resuscitate a patient can be given through an IO.

Surface Area

The young child has an increased surface area/volume ratio making him more susceptible to insensible fluid and heat loss. In addition, infants and young children have less insulating fat and muscle mass for shivering and are less able to generate heat. Exposure to a cool environment (outside decontamination, undressed during resuscitation, wet clothes or blankets) or administration of large volumes of IV fluids may result in hypothermia. The young child's temperature should be monitored and maintained throughout evaluation and resuscitation with infant warmers, overhead lamps, warm blankets, and warmed IV fluid.

Additional Considerations in Pediatric Trauma

Head injury is the leading cause of morbidity and mortality in pediatric trauma. Other serious injuries are associated with disaster-related trauma including crush injuries from collapsed structures and blunt or penetrating trauma from flying glass and debris. Fractures may result from falls on unstable or slippery footing. Minor trauma generally consists of abrasions, lacerations, and puncture wounds from nails and other sharp objects. Important considerations come into play in the resuscitation of the seriously injured pediatric trauma patient. Many of these are derived from the young child's small size, developing fat and musculature, and pliable skeleton.

Kinetic energy from a blunt injury is transmitted over a smaller mass. Most seriously injured children have multiple injuries including injury to the central nervous system.

Head injuries are common because of the child's disproportionately large head and small torso. When ejected in the air from a blast or thrown from a motor vehicle, the small child travels headfirst. Intraabdominal organs are highly susceptible to injury because of their relatively large size within the abdomen and the lack of protection afforded by ribs, fat, muscle, and connective tissue. The bladder is within the abdomen and is unprotected by the bony pelvis. Thoracic injuries are uncommon but, when present, are a source of significant morbidity. Unlike adults, injury to the heart, great vessels, and lung occur without coexistent fractures. Spinal cord injures, also rare, can occur without bony abnormalities visible on plain radiographs.

PEDIATRIC ASPECTS OF NUCLEAR, BIOLOGICAL, AND CHEMICAL TERRORISM

Biological, Chemical Agents

Biological agents and the chemicals commonly considered in terrorism, such as the nerve agents, are unusual poisonings in children (22-24). The approaches that have been developed for the treatment of these weapons of mass destruction (WMD) have focused on an adult, military model. Yet children are more vulnerable to the effects of these agents. In the setting of a large-scale disaster, children are compromised simply because they are young and less able or unable to recognize the danger of an exposure. Because children are physically less mature, they are limited in their ability to climb, run, or flee. Children are more susceptible to respiratory failure and dehydration. Children with chronic illness, especially those with diminished cardiopulmonary reserve, are at greatest risk. Because they almost always congregate in groups at school and in day care and may be too young to practice prudent hygiene, they have a higher risk of person-to-person transmission. Finally, as large numbers of infected adults become unable to care for their children, the care of well and uninfected children becomes a greater burden to the community (Table 41-1).

TABLE 41-1	Agents Likely to Be Used in Chemical Terrorism		
TYPE OF EXPOSURE	**EXAMPLES**	**INTERVENTIONS**	**ANTIDOTES**
Nerve agents	Tabun Sarin Soman VX	Respiratory support, skin decontamination	Atropine, Pralidoxime, (Mark I)
Vesicants	Mustard gas Nitrogen mustard	Respiratory support, skin/mucous membrane decontamination	None
Irritants/Corrosives	Chlorine Bromine Ammonia	Respiratory support, skin/mucous membrane decontamination, nebulized albuterol	
Choking agents	Phosgene	Respiratory support	None
Cyanogens	Hydrogen cyanide	Cardiorespiratory support	Amyl nitrate, sodium thiosulfate, sodium nitrite

Source: AAP policy statement, chemical-biological terrorism and its impact on children. Pediatrics 2000 Mar;105(3):662-7.

TABLE 41-2	Mechanisms Through Which Children Could Be More Severely Affected by Chemical and Biologic Agents

1. Increased baseline respiratory rates place children at risk for absorbing larger amounts of aerosolized agents (sarin, anthrax, chlorine).
2. High vapor density agents are concentrated closer to the ground and within the breathing zone of children (sarin, chlorine) who are shorter and play for long periods on the floor.
3. Thinner, permeable skin and a large surface area allows for greater transdermal absorption of toxins.
4. Less keratinized skin may produce greater injury from vesicants.
5. High body surface promotes heat loss when exposed (prolonged periods with heat or outside) or wet (decontamination).
6. Increased risk of dehydration from gastrointestinal fluid losses.

Regarding biological or chemical agents used in terrorism, drug treatments and antidotes are not as well studied in children and commonly recommended adult medications are not approved for children. Weight based dosing regimens and dispensing mechanisms (e.g., autoinjectors for atropine and pralidoxime) are not available. First-line antibiotics (e.g., fluoroquinolones and tetracyclines) recommended for biologic agents are contraindicated in young children. In general, universal availability of equipment in the sizes needed to care for children of different ages is a pervasive problem encountered in emergency response. The technical aspects of airway management and vascular access may be obstacles in the setting of large numbers of younger patients.

A 2000 consensus statement of the American Academy of Pediatrics' Committee on Environmental Health and Committee on Infectious Disease entitled "Chemical-Biological Terrorism and its Impact on Children" highlighted mechanisms through which children could be more severely affected by chemical and biologic agents (Table 41-2) (24).

Chemical Agents. Readily available, chemical agents do not require sophisticated delivery devices for dispersion and are capable of rapidly causing illness. Nerve agents are well absorbed through intact skin. Impregnated clothing can release toxin for prolonged periods following initial contact. Health care and rescue workers must wear full protective gear including respiratory filers to avoid self-contamination. Sarin gas is concentrated closer to the ground and poses a special threat to children. Mustard gas, chlorine, and ammonia are corrosive and would injure skin, especially mucosa of the nose and eyes. Inhalation would cause chemical pneumonitis.

Atropine and 2-PAM (pralidoxime) are the antidotes used to treat these exposures. A Mark I injector kit administers an intramuscular injection of 2 mg of atropine and 600 g of 2-PAM. Preloaded injector sets for weight based dosing of pediatric patients are not available. Guidelines for the use of the standard autoinjector for pediatric ages and weights to approximate the desired dose ranges (0.02 mg/kg, atropine; 20 to 40 mg/kg, 2-PAM) have been developed (Table 41-3).

Biologic Agents. Biological agents may be used in their wild naturally occurring form or altered to increase antibiotic resistance and their spread (Table 41-4). Unlike chemical agents, biological agents may be associated with a delay in onset of illness. Since they may be unrecognized in early stages and are highly transmissible, biological agents can result in widespread secondary infection as heath care personnel, family members, and classrooms of contacts are exposed. Fever, malaise, headache, vomiting, and diarrhea are common early manifestations of many biologic WMD as well as the presentation of common pediatric emergent conditions from typical pathogens. Although many infections related to weaponized exposure may be treatable, the diagnosis may be delayed. A release of biological agents may be detected only after a pattern of illness is identified within a community.

The role of personal protective equipment (PPE) use in children is a concerning topic. To be effective, PPE outfits and masks would need to be properly sized and monitored while in use. Very limited research has been done in the area of benefit and risk of PPE equipment in children. Children were reported to have suffocated while wearing gas masks during Operation Desert Storm (25).

Anthrax is considered to be a significant biological agent threat to children. Experience with anthrax in children is extremely limited, making predictions about susceptibility or outcome difficult. Most strains of endemic anthrax are sensitive to penicillin G, the drug of choice. Alternative choices recommended for laboratory-produced antibiotic-resistant strains include ciprofloxacin and doxycycline (Table 41-5). Problems with recommendations for the treatment of anthrax with respect to pediatric patients are (a) anthrax vaccine is currently approved only for patients 18 to 65 years of age and (b) both quinolones and tetracycline are contraindicated in children (26).

Smallpox (variola) has a high rate of person-to-person transmission and case fatality rate. Smallpox was eradicated

TABLE 41-3	Autoinjector Administration and Dosing in Children

AGE	WEIGHT	# OF AUTOINJECTORS (OF EACH TYPE)	ATROPINE DOSE (MG/KG)	PRALIDOXIME DOSE (MG/KG)
3–7 years	13–25 kg	1	0.08–0.13	22–46
8-14 years	26–50 kg	2	0.08–0.13	22–46
>14 years	>51 kg	3	0.11 or less	35 or less

Source: Consensus Statement of 2003 Executive Committee.

TABLE 41-4	Biological Weapons of Mass Destruction

BACTERIA*	RICKETTSIA[a]	VIRUSES	FUNGI	TOXINS

Anthrax
Brucellosis
Botulism
Tularemia
Plague
	Q fever
	Epidemic typhus
	Rocky Mountain
	  spotted fever
		Smallpox
		Hemorrhagic
		  fevers
		Equine
		  encephalitis
		Yellow fever
		Hantavirus
		Ebola
			Coccidio	Aflatoxin
				• *C. botulinum*
				• *C. perfringens*
				• Ricin
				• Shigella
				• Staph
				• Tetrodotoxin

[a] Treatable with antibiotics

Source: Modified from AAP policy statement, chemical-biological terrorism and its impact on children. Pediatrics 2000 Mar;105(3):662-70.

in 1980, and children are no longer immunized for it. More than 80% of adults and close to 100% of children are susceptible to it. No antiviral therapy is available, and supportive therapy is the mainstay of treatment. Administration of the smallpox vaccine within the first several days postexposure may be useful for postexposure prophylaxis. Although the vaccine is currently contraindicated in children less than one year of age, many experts recommend vaccination of all children, even infants, following a true exposure to

weaponized smallpox. Research on new generations of smallpox vaccine should include children of all ages.

Toxins from biologic agents have the ability to produce symptoms quickly, without incubation period. Botulinum toxin is highly and quickly lethal. Patients initially develop difficulty seeing, speaking, and swallowing. As paralysis extends beyond the cranial nerves, generalized hypotonia and muscle weakness precede death from airway obstruction. Treatment includes ventilatory support and antitoxin,

TABLE 41-5	Therapy and Prophylaxis of Anthrax in Children

FORM	AGENT AND DOSE	COMMENT
Inhalational	*Therapy* Cipro 10–15 mg/kg IV q12h (max 400mg/dose) *or* Doxycycline 2.2 mg/kg IV q12h (max 100mg/dose) *and* Clindamycin 10–15 mg/kg q8h *and* Pen G 400–600 μ/kg/day divided q4h	• In MCI, oral route may be substituted for IV. Cipro is preferred because of better GI absorption. • Stable patients can be switched to single oral agent after 14 days to complete 60-day course.
	Postexposure prophylaxis Cipro 10–15 mg/kg PO q12h (max 500 mg/dose) *or* Doxycycline 2.2 mg/kg PO q12h (max 100 mg/dose)	• Children may be switched to PO amox to complete 60-day course. • Cipro and/or doxy recommended for first days of therapy or postexposure prophylaxis regardless of age.
Cutaneous, endemic	*Therapy* Penicillin V 40–80 /kg/d PO divided q6h *or* Amoxicillin 40–80 mg/kg/d PO divided q8h *or* Cipro 10–15 mg/kg PO q12h (max 500 mg/dose) *or* Doxycycline 2.2 mg/kg PO q12h (max 100 mg/dose)	• Ten days may be adequate for endemic cutaneous disease.
Cutaneous, terrorism	*Therapy* Cipro 10–15 mg/kg PO q12h (max 500mg/dose) *or* Doxycycline 2.2 mg/kg PO q12h (max 100 mg/dose)	• Cipro is preferred.
Gastrointestinal	*Therapy:* Same as inhalational	

Source: Consensus 2003 Executive Summary, based on recommendations from the American Academy of Pediatrics, Centers for Disease Control and Prevention, U.S. Food and Drug Administration, and Infectious Disease Society of America.

TABLE 41-6	Guidelines for KI Dosing		
AGE	**EXPOSURE, GY (RAD)**	**KI DOSE (MG)**	
> 40 years	>5 (500)	130	
1–49 years	0.1 (10)	130	
12–17 years	0.05(5)	65	
Adolescents > 70 kg	0.05(5)	130	
4–11 years	0.05 (5)	65	
1 month–3 years	0.05 (5)	32	
Birth–1 month	0.05 (5)	16	
Pregnant/lactating women	0.05 (5)	130	

Source: Consensus Conference and recommendations from the American Academy of Pediatrics, Centers for Disease Control and Prevention, and U.S. Food and Drug Administration.

Botulinum Immune Globulin. *Staphylococcus aureus* enterotoxic is capable of producing severe diarrhea in the very young that could least tolerate marked gastrointestinal fluid losses.

Radiation Exposure. Children are at greater risk than adults following radiation exposure. Appropriate doses and availability of potassium iodide (KI), marrow-simulating agents, and antiemetics are important considerations in preparing for a nuclear disaster. Communities must be prepared to make rapid assessments of the risk of their population's exposure and provide for immediate KI (within 2 hours) administration, preferably in a graded dosing regimen (Tables 41-6 and 41-7).

TREATMENT: EVENT AND POSTEVENT

The general principles of a pediatric mass casualty event are identical to one that involves few children. A unified command structure must be established; it should include local, state, and federal officials, hospital administrators, social workers, counselors, pediatric emergency medicine physicians, pediatric surgeons, and pediatric critical care and other subspeciality consultants.

Decontamination

If WMD is suspected, appropriate protective gear must be readily accessible and familiar to health care providers. Children present some unique challenges in decontamination. This process must be able to accommodate parentless children, nonambulatory children, children with complex medical needs, and technology dependent children. Young children lose heat quickly when wet and/or unclothed in large, open areas. Appropriate warmth must be provided during and following decontamination. Identification and surveillance of large numbers of children is difficult throughout this process. This is especially true if responsible adults (parents, teachers, chaperones) have been killed or injured or are missing.

Triage

An important role of the first responders to a multiple casualty incident (MCI) involving a large number of children will be to perform triage and initial patient assessments. The management of a large number of critically ill children will require access to well-trained and experienced pediatric practitioners capable of rapid pediatric cardiopulmonary assessment and interventions. In general, most EMS systems and emergency providers feel less comfortable with all aspects of pediatric emergency care than with adult emergencies. Several commercially available courses (Pediatric Advanced Life Support, Advanced Pediatric Life Support (APLS), and Pediatric Emergency for Prehospital Providers (PEPP)) teach fundamentals of pediatric assessment *of the individual patient*, including the pediatric trauma victim, and offer practice in pediatric procedures

TABLE 41-7	Guidelines for Home Preparation of KI Solution Using 65-mg Tablet

Grind 65-mg tablet into fine powder in a small bowl with the back of a spoon.
Add 4 tsp (20 ml) of water to the KI powder. Mix until dissolved.
Add 4 tsp (20 ml) of milk, juice, soda, or syrup to the KI/water mixture.
Mixture contains 8.125 mg KI/tsp (5 ml). Use age-based dosing guidelines:
   newborn to 1 month: 2 tsp
   1 month to 3 years: 4 tsp
   4 years to 17 years: 8 tsp or one 65-mg tablet
   children/adolescents >70 kg: two 65-mg tablets
Source: Consensus Conference recommendations.

but do not address mass casualty triage in depth. Pediatric triage in a disaster setting is further complicated by children with unfamiliar special needs and diagnoses, technology dependent children and parentless, psychologically distressed children of different ages.

In an MCI, decisions about destinations for pediatric patients would be dictated by pediatric capabilities in regional hospitals. In general, children in the immediate (or red) triage category should be transported to facilities with the most extensive pediatric capabilities. Children in the delayed (or yellow) category can be transported to closer hospitals with less sophisticated pediatric capabilities for stabilization, even if subsequent transfer to a children's hospital is expected. Minimal (or green) category patients should be distributed throughout the region, even transported to a more distant facility.

MCI triage has not been standardized in pediatrics. EMS regions may choose to use different triage systems. The START system (Simple Triage and Rapid Transport) is commonly accepted as a triage tool for adults and is applied to patients over 100 pounds or 8 to 10 years of age (Table 41-8; Figure 41-1). JumpSTART is a pediatric modification of START, which can be used in children between the ages of 1 and 8 years. The Jump START decision points reflect normal vital signs of young children and a child's likelihood of experiencing a respiratory arrest without cardiac standstill. Unlike adults who typically become apneic following a cardiac event, children suffer a respiratory arrest (apnea

TABLE 41-8	START Decision Points and Triage Categories

Ability to walk
Presence of spontaneous breathing
Respiratory rate (<30 *or* >30)
Capillary refill time (< 2 sec *or* > 2 sec)
Ability to obey commands

with a pulse) before a complete asystolic arrest occurs. Such children who are apneic but sill have a perfusing rhythm are likely to recover if their airway is opened and spontaneous respirations can be quickly reestablished. Infants (less than 1 year) are not included in JumpSTART.

Although untested in an actual MCI and more time consuming than START, JumpSTART provides an important tool for standardized pediatric triage. The many challenges involved in pediatric triage may cause the first responder's emotional response to the injured child to influence clinical judgment and waste valuable time and resources attempting to resuscitate children who are realistically not salvageable. Ongoing work in refining and validating a pediatric rapid assessment and triage tools is needed.

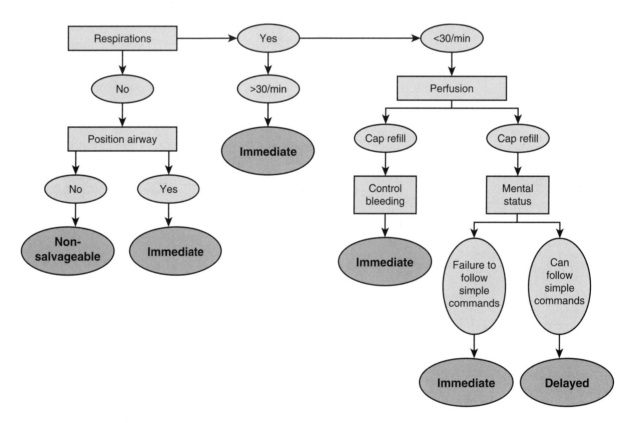

Figure 41–1. START Triage.

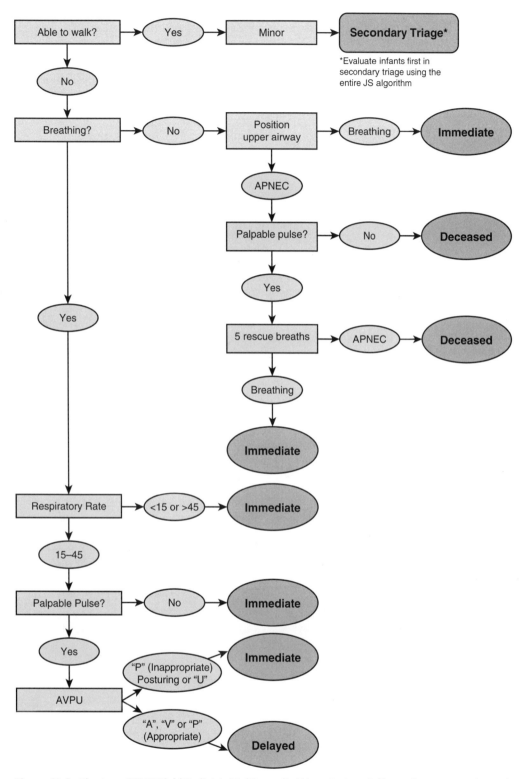

Figure 41–2. The JumpSTART Field Pediatric Multicasualty Triage System © (for patients ages 1–8 years). From Lou Romig MD, FAAP, FACEP, 2004; with permission.

TABLE 41-9	JumpSTART Decision Points

Ability to walk
Presence of spontaneous breathing
Presence of pulse in an apneic child
Respiratory rate <15 or >45
Palpable peripheral pulse
Appropriate response to painful stimulus

Transport

In small incidents, efforts to keep injured family members together are likely to be successful. In large MCI, this may not be possible or beneficial. Different types of injuries and the need for a variety of specialty care may require separating family members. Response vehicles must have pediatric-appropriate equipment and medication for resuscitation and decontamination.

Transition and Temporary Shelter

The postdisaster period may pose special hazards for children and requires detailed planning. A previously safe and structured environment has been destroyed, and adult supervision may be limited. An event during summer increases risks for dehydration, severe sunburn, and insect bites. Cold weather disasters may cause hypothermia and an increased risk of fire from candles and unsafe appliances. Children with chronic medical problems may suffer if their medications are not available. Technology dependent children may be compromised if power outages continue for long periods of time.

Housing families or children without parents in shelters is a complex task that takes careful planning (Table 41-10). Issues of safety (a childproof environment, drugs, alcohol, weapons, smoking), supervision (parentless children, lim-

ited numbers of adults to children), and illness (isolation, typical childhood illness exposure, infections caused by the disaster) must be considered. Documentation of health care provided while children are in shelters is important.

The development of an approach to the care of parentless children with regard to medical and mental health, shelter, guardianship, and placement is critical. "Displaced" children who exhibit signs of ongoing stress should undergo full medical and psychological evaluation.

PREVENTION AND MITIGATION

Disaster preparedness requires involvement of all members of a community. The entire community must educate itself about the types of disasters likely to affect them and should be encouraged to participate in disaster planning. Regional attention needs to be directed toward planning for children in a MCI event since an immediate response with local resources would occur before more sophisticated and distant (Federal Emergency Management Agency or disaster medical assistance teams (DMAT)) help would be available. Pediatric experts should be involved in disaster preparedness in all aspects: evacuation protocols, patient transport, and treatment policies for specific injuries. Pediatric equipment and medications should be included in National Disaster Medical System and DMAT supplies.

Hospitals

During a disaster, children will arrive in community hospitals, so all prehospital and emergency department personnel must be trained in basic disaster management as well as pediatric triage and decontamination. EMS systems and emergency departments must have adequate supplies of appropriate equipment for pediatric and newborn resuscitation and stabilization and transport of critically ill patients to destinations providing specialized pediatric trauma, burn and/or critical

TABLE 41-10	Pediatric Disaster Shelter Planning

- Supplies
  Diapers and other supplies for infant hygiene
  Infant formula and rehydration solutions
  Child-appropriate snacks and foods
  Games and other distractions for children
  Basic pediatric first aid equipment
- Staffing
  Train staff members in basic pediatric emergency care
  Provide staff to supervise children when parents are injured or unavailable
- Safety
  Childproof the shelter
  Appropriate supervision of children (especially parentless)
  Safety rules (set curfew; forbid alcohol, smoking, guns, candles, fire)
- Medical
  System for documentation of medical treatment
  Pediatric medical backup in place
  Contingency plans for children with special health care needs
  Plans for isolating sick children

care. Emergency departments with enhanced pediatric capabilities must have plans to alter usual functioning and enhanced ability to manage larger numbers of critically ill children. In their 2003 Executive Summary, the National Center for Disaster Preparedness recommends that hospitals keep a 48-hour supply of pediatric equipment and pharmaceuticals on hand for the hospital's average daily census plus an addition 100 patients. Each region should designate a children's hospital that would serve as a pediatric resource center.

Schools

Schools should figure prominently in community disaster planning. Sadly, schools may be the target of terrorism because children are highly concentrated there during predictable times. School personnel should be incorporated into disaster preparation efforts both from the standpoint of system preparedness and education of children. School may serve as a shelter for children, with or without their parents. Finally school, in some form, will be where children return following a disaster. Teachers and staff have important roles in postdisaster psychological evaluation and mental health support of children and serve as important constants in children's lives.

Families

All individuals and families should undergo some level of education and preparedness for a disaster (Table 41-11). Since distant resources may take 24 to 72 hours to mobilize, families should plan to be self-sufficient for several days. Anticipating the steps following a disaster will help children cope and retain some sense of control.

Primary Care Providers

Primary care physicians can function as community leaders encouraging involvement of all patients and parents in disaster planning. They should assist families in planning for the medical needs of chronically ill (including diabetes, asthma, immune deficiencies) and technology dependent children (ventilator support, supplemental oxygen, central line, gastrostomy tube). They should be used as a resource in planning for the medical and mental health of children in shelters and aid schools in disaster planning. They should serve as advocates for increased attention to the needs of children on regional and national levels and advocate for research in the pediatric aspects of nuclear, biological, and chemical terrorism.

Physicians who operate offices outside of hospitals need to develop and rehearse their own office disaster. This should include contingencies for (a) stockpiling medication and equipment, (b) dealing with emergent and continuing medical care for their own patients, and (c) relocating if the office must be evacuated.

Mental Health Resources

Mental health resources are a key component in the care of children during the acute phases and aftermath of a disaster. Mental health providers should serve as important resources in educating families and health care providers in the emotional needs of children of different developmental stages. Communities should have plans to augment current pediatric and family-centered mental health capabilities.

PREPAREDNESS HISTORIC EVENTS, SCENARIOS, AND RECOMMENDATIONS FOR THE FUTURE

CHILDREN IN WAR AND DISASTER: WHAT WE HAVE LEARNED FROM RECENT EVENTS

Children were not the primary target of the September 11 hijackers, but they were not spared from the traumatic aftermath. Eight children died on airplanes, many more lost a parent, some in New York City lost both parents or were displaced from their homes, thousands physically watched the event or were evacuated from their school, and millions watched television as horrifying images were broadcast by the media over and over again (9). Memories of this sentinel event emphasize the substantial and long-lasting effects of a large-scale disaster on a huge segment of the population and the importance of a widespread response from communities and schools in addressing children's mental health needs (10,11).

TABLE 41-11 Family Disaster Plan

- Understand disaster risks in your community.
- Undertake preventive measures to protect yourselves and property.
- Develop an evacuation plan.
- Develop a reunification plan with primary and secondary sites for the family to meet.
- Identify equipment and supplies needed to live independently for 3 days.
- Update disaster supplies on a yearly basis.
- Keep valuable documents (birth certificates, insurance information) in a safe place.
- Involve children in the family plan.
- Develop a plan for pets.
- Identify a family or friend in a different community with whom you can live if evacuated and homeless. Give them a copy of your plan.

School children from kindergarten, second, third, and fifth grades were among the thousands of people trapped in the World Trade Center in New York City following the 1993 bombing. For these children and their families, this was an incident of isolated psychological terrorism. The children believed themselves to be at risk of dying but did not suffer concomitant physical injury, loss of a parent and/or home, and disruption of daily life. Parents had no communication about their children's whereabouts for many hours. Koplewicz reported significant levels of Post Traumatic Stress Disorder (PTSD) symptoms and disaster-related fears in these children at one and nine months following the event (12,13). Interestingly, children in the control group, who attended the same or nearby schools but were not at the WTC on the day of the bombing, reported mild PTSD symptoms presumably because of media exposure (9).

The severe and widespread effect of war on children's mental health has been well established. Children exposed to long-standing political violence and civil wars suffer acute stress disorders and endure ongoing poverty and deprivation as refugees.

A prospective longitudinal study examined the posttraumatic stress of school aged Croatian children during and 30 months following the 1994 Yugoslavian attacks (14-16). Eighty percent of children reported moderate or severe symptoms of PTSD in 1994. This decreased to 60% three years later when the children were reassessed. Two factors that contributed to long-term symptomatology were actually witnessing violence in the form of killing and beating (exposure to "general wartime activities" was predictive only for short term symptoms) and younger age (17).

Beginning in September 2000, families and children in the Gaza strip have experienced traumatic events ranging from exposure to graphic media coverage of killings to actual helicopter bombardments of their homes. Among Palestinian children (9 to 18 years of age) who actually witnessed bombardments and the demolition of their homes, over 40% revealed severe to very severe symptoms of PTSD (images, flashbacks, nightmares) and fears. This was twice the rate reported by nonexposed children living in other parts of the Gaza strip. However, anxiety symptoms and disorders were high in children living in the Gaza strip not affected by shellings. The finding of high severity of symptoms related to close proximity and intensity of exposure is a pattern that has been described in natural disasters, like the Armenian earthquake (18). Emotional distress occurs not only in directly exposed children who actually view atrocities but also in nonexposed children who experience events through conversations with adults and the media (19).

Although treatment for psychological distress following disaster is recognized as a need for children, a standardized approach and research evaluating interventions have been lacking. Chemtob reported the results of screening and treatment of elementary school children in Hawaii following Hurricane Iniki (20). School-based, community-wide screening of all children in second through sixth grade identified a subset of children with highest degrees of psychological distress who were selected for individual or group treatment provided by school-based counselors. Children in the treated groups reported significant reductions in trauma-related symptoms at one-year follow-up. The authors concluded that school-based, community-wide screening and treatment effectively identified high-risk children and reduced psychological distress postdisaster in symptomatic children and suggested that this approach may be of benefit in other forms of large-scale disasters.

PREPAREDNESS HYPOTHETICAL SCENARIOS AND QUESTIONS TO CONSIDER

Scenario One. A bomb on a school bus explodes as it brings Boy Scouts to the Annual Jamboree on the Mall in Washington, D.C. The bus was destroyed with significant damage to surrounding buses. Five hundred Boy Scouts between the ages of 7 and 11 years were expected to attend the event and have traveled from all over the Eastern United States.

Scenario Two. Many school children and adult chaperones become nauseous and short of breath while on a school trip to the Museum of Science. More and more people, including museum staff, are developing symptoms.

Scenario Three. Police follow an "armed" man as he runs through a crowed suburban neighborhood toward a grade school. It is lunchtime on a warm sunny day. Most classes are at recess. Three buses are unloading the afternoon kindergarten classes. He runs between the buses and begins to shoot his weapon.

Questions to Consider

1. How would your local authorities and EMS systems handle each of these situations? Has there been community-wide disaster planning?

2. Could your emergency departments manage a significant influx of children? Does your emergency department have equipment to care for pediatric patients? Does your emergency department have access to pediatric subspecialty care?

3. What are the unique anatomic and physiologic characteristics of young children? Is your emergency department physician and nursing staff PALS trained? Have emergency medical technicians in your region received pediatric training (PALS, PEPP)?

4. What are pediatric considerations in treating chemical or biologic WMD exposure?

5. How would your community cope in the aftermath of these disasters?

6. What kind of support and counseling would be helpful for children at different ages?

RECOMMENDATIONS FOR THE FUTURE

1. Enhance capability of Emergency Medical Services.

   a. Teach (and drill) first responders a pediatric specific triage system (JumpSTART).

b. Equip EMS vehicles with pediatric-appropriate equipment and medications.

c. Increase numbers of paramedics with PALS training.

2. Enhance capability of hospitals.

a. Equip all hospital emergency departments with pediatric-appropriate equipment and medications.

b. Augment levels of supplies for equipment and medication beyond usual patient load.

c. Increase number of nurses and emergency physicians with PALS training.

d. Augment mental heath capabilities for patients, parents, and health care professionals.

3. Regionalize and integrate efforts.

a. Use tertiary care children's hospitals to assist in coordination of pediatric subspecialty care resources (pediatric emergency medicine, surgery, critical care, burn services).

b. Designate a regional pediatric resource center.

c. Incorporate pediatric expertise in DMAT planning and training.

d. Practice region-wide pediatric disaster drills, integrate pediatric components into all disaster drills, and include schools in community drills.

e. Involve pediatricians, families, and schools in planning with special attention to shelters and mental health needs of children.

f. Establish a community-wide approach to evaluation and treatment of mental health issues in children and families.

4. Commit to research and reevaluation leading to standardization.

a. Develop research and models to study the vulnerabilities of children in disasters.

b. Develop decontamination systems appropriate for all pediatric age groups.

c. Research pediatric disaster triage tools.

d. Research vaccines in spectrum of pediatric age groups.

e. Make weight-based doses of antidotes (atropine autoinjector) and pediatric-appropriate antibiotics and drugs (KI) available

PREPAREDNESS SUMMARY

PEDIATRIC CONSIDERATIONS IN TERRORISM AND DISASTER PLANNING

1. Special requirement for children. The unique needs of children throughout infancy, childhood, and adolescence have received little actual attention in disaster planning. It is important to consider the following important considerations that are critical to satisfactory pediatric disaster preparedness. Because children have unique needs related to size, anatomy, and physiology (1–4), they

a. Have thinner, less keratinized skin

b. Have increased susceptibility to shock and respiratory failure

c. Require appropriate equipment for resuscitation and decontamination for all ages/sizes

d. Require weight-based dosing for antibiotics and antidotes

2. Developmental and cognitive abilities precluding escape and/or self care

3. EMS system issues (5,6)

a. Lack of universal pediatric ALS training in EMS systems and emergency departments

b. Limited pediatric subspecialty care

c. Limited experience with coordination of pediatric emergency medicine, pediatric surgery, and pediatric critical care following pediatric MCI

d. Limited experience with rapid pediatric triage system in an MCI

4. Limited planning in families, schools, and communities for the medical and psychological care of children following a MCI with many pediatric victims (7).

5. Limited data, research, published literature regarding the special needs of children in disaster (8)

RESOURCES

1. American Academy of Pediatrics. Family Readiness Kit. Web site: www.aap.org.

2. American Red Cross. Web site: www.redcross.org.

3. Extension Disaster Education Network (EDEN). Web site: www.agctr.lsu.edu/eden.

4. Federal Emergency Management Association (for Kids). Web site: www.fema.gov/kids.

5. U.S. Geological Survey. Preparedness for natural disasters. Web site: www.usgs.gov.

6. National Weather Service. Web site: www.nws.noaa.gov.

7. Institute for Business and Home Safety. Web site: www.ibhs.org.

REFERENCES

1. Lee BS, Gausche-Hill M. Advances in pediatric resuscitation. Clin Ped Emerg Med 2001;2(2):91-106.
2. Stafford PW, Blinman TA, Nance ML. Practical points in evaluation and resuscitation of the injured child. Surg Clin N Am 2002;82(2):273-302.
3. Levy RJ, Helfaer MA. Managing the airway in the critically ill patient. Crit Care Cl 2000;16(3):489-504.

4. Stallion A. Initial assessment and management of pediatric trauma patient. Respir Care Clin N Am 2001;7(l):1-11.

5. Lovejoy J. Clinical approach to patient management after large-scale disasters. Clin Ped Emerg Med 2002;3(4):2117-223.

6. Maxson RT. Management of pediatric trauma: blast victims in a mass casualty incident. Clin Ped Emerg Med 2002;3: 256-61.

7. Gurian SK, Goodman A. Helping children and teens cope with traumatic events and death: the role of school health professionals. School Nurse News 2002;19(1):32-5.

8. Stoddard F, Saxe G. Ten-year research review of physical injuries. J Am Acad Child Adolesc Psych 2001;40(10):1128-45.

9. PTSD and TV viewing of World Trade Center. J Am Acad Child Adolesc Psych 2002;41(5):494-7.

10. Chen H, Chung H, Chen T, et al. The emotional distress in a community after the terrorist attach on the World Trade Center. Comm Mental Health J 2003;39(2):157-64.

11. Stuber J, Fairbrother G, Galea S, et al. Determinants of counseling for children in Manhattan after the September 11 attacks. Psych Serv 2002;53:815-22.

12. Kiplewicz HS, Vogel JM, Solanto MV, et al. Child and parent response to the 1993 World Trade Center bombing. J Traum Stress 2002;15(l):77-85.

13. Cardenas I, Williams K, Wilson JR., et al. PSTD, major depressive symptoms, and substance abuse following September 11, 2001, in a midwestern university population. Int J Emerg Ment Health 2003;5(l):15-28.

14. Smith P, Perrin S, Yule W, et al. War exposure among children from Bosnia-Hercegovina: psychological adjustment in a community sample. J Traum Stress 2002;15(2):147-56.

15. Fazel M, Stein A. The mental health of refugee children. Arch Dis Child 2002;87:366-70.

16. Kuterovac-Jagodic G. Post-traumatic stress symptoms in Croatian children exposed to war: a prospective study. J Clin Psych 2003;59(1):9-25.

17. Treating children exposed to disasters. Arch Ped Adolesc Med 2002;156(3):208.

18. Goenjian AK, Pynoos RS, Steinberg AM, et al. J Am Acad Child Adolesc Psych 1995;34(9):1174-84.

19. Thabet AA, Abed Y, Vostanis P. Emotional problems in Palestinian children living in a war zone: a cross-sectional study. Lancet 2002;359(9320):1801-4.

20. Chemtob CM, Nakashima JP, Hamada RS. Psychosocial intervention for postdisaster trauma symptoms in elementary school children. Arch Ped Adolesc Med 2002:156(3): 211-16.

21. Culbertson IL, Newman JE, Willis DJ. Childhood and adolescent psychologic development. Ped Clin N Am 2003; 50(4): 741-64.

22. Henretig FM, Cieslak TJ. Bioterrorism and pediatric emergency medicine. Clin Ped Emerg Med 2001;2(3):211-22.

23. Henretig FM, Cieslak TJ, Eitzen EM. Biological and chemical terrorism. J Ped 2002;141:311-26.

24. Chemical-biological terrorism and its impact on children: a subject review. Ped 2000;105(3):662-70.

25. Meier E. Effects of trauma and war on children. Ped Nurs 2002;28(6):626-9.

26. Blueprints guide to pediatric infectious diseases. Malden, MA: Blackwell Publishing.

42

Agricultural Terrorism and its Implications for the Health Care System

Timothy Rupp and Shane Zatkalik

INTRODUCTION

The first thing that would catch your notice would be the withered crop in the fields. Acres upon acres of stunted plants—in many areas reduced to a crunchy tan carpet of withered stalks and wrinkled leaves because the irrigation spigots had been turned off—would extend across huge vistas. Untended plots, overgrown fields, and rotting harvests would add to the impression of a ghostly landscape where nature itself had gone awry. Emaciated cattle, staggering aimlessly as if possessed, would bring home the reality that some catastrophe had occurred. What had been a bountiful, idyllic landscape had within the space of a single growing season been transformed into a demented nightmare. The pervasive sense of eeriness would be heightened by the pitiful sight of pigs unable to walk or eat due to sores on their feet, teats, and inside their mouths. Sows would refuse to nurse their young. In this scenario, the terrorists have used a "twin venom" cocktail of different plant pathogens and livestock diseases (foot-and-mouth disease, corn blight, karnal bunt, and rice blast) that has caught the country's agricultural experts, counterterrorism officials, and farmers off guard. (1)

The term "agricultural terrorism," or "agroterrorism," may be defined as the introduction of an agent, either biological or chemical, engineered to cause widespread devastation of natural resources, such as water supplies, soil, crops, or livestock, the result of which is damage to the economical, political, and social fabric of the affected society. In contrast to the so-called traditional forms of terrorism, namely the terrorist attacks of September 11, 2001, agricultural terrorism is considered less likely to mount direct human casualties. Acts of agricultural terrorism are seen as means by which the entire infrastructure of agrarian society, from the individual farmer to the large industrial manufacturers of agricultural products to the industries that rely on the products of agriculture for their success, may be crippled. The damage would not be limited to the eco-

nomic and industrial sectors; rather, the result of agricultural terrorism would impact the state and federal governments, resulting in a loss of confidence in both the administration and the government departments specifically created to oversee the safety of U.S. agriculture.

This chapter entertains the topic of agricultural terrorism and its impact on the health care system. Traditionally, agricultural terrorism is not expected to have a direct impact on human life, so the health care system's preparation for an agroterrorism attack must be equally nontraditional. That is to say, it is less important for the clinician to expect mass casualties from an act of agroterrorism; rather, the clinician needs to be vigilant and in close communication with local and regional health-monitoring agencies, in an effort to provide a network of surveillance and early warning against the possibility of an attack promulgated against the agricultural industry.

PREPAREDNESS ESSENTIALS

The best way to deal with threats to the national food supply and agricultural infrastructure is to prevent and deter intentional or unintentional introduction of plant and animal diseases into the United States. I have said many times that pests and animal disease prevention and eradication programs are central to the USDA's ability to protect the Nation's food supply and agricultural infrastructure. Simply put, the best defense is a good offense. (2)

To understand how greatly a terrorist attack against the agricultural industry might impact the United States, it is first essential to understand the effects a terrorist attack is expected to have. First, a terrorist attack, in general, is successful if it cripples the economy of the threatened country. In the case of agricultural terrorism, the target is the agrarian economy. Second, success depends on the ability to destroy the livelihood of as many people as possible. In the event of agricultural terrorism, the disruption of the agricultural industry would have far-reaching effects, not only to agriculture itself, but also throughout other industries that rely on agriculture for supplies. Third, an attack directed against the agricultural industry would likely put the food supply at risk for an indefinite period of time. And fourth, an attack directed against the agricultural industry would likely go undetected before it was recognized and contained (3).

When one considers the impact of zoonotic diseases in the recent past, it is easy to see how agriculture would be an attractive target for economic destabilization by a terrorist attack. Although not an attack of terrorism, the mad cow disease outbreak in the 1990s cost the English government between $9 and $14 billion U.S. dollars in compensation costs to farmers and laid-off employees of the beef and dairy industries (4). It is estimated, moreover, that an outbreak of foot-and-mouth disease within the United States would cost the nation more than $27 billion in trade losses alone each year (3).

The United States commercially produced 47,169 million pounds of red meat, 38,500 million pounds of poultry, 7,221 million dozen eggs, and 170 billion pounds of milk in 2002. The cash receipts for livestock and crops in 2003 are estimated to be $202 billion. The total gross domestic product, consisting of both the food and fiber sector and the farm sector, was $10,082 billion in 2001. In terms of employment, 129 million people are employed in the agricultural industry, 1.9 million of which are employed directly within the farm sector (5). It is clear that the United States is a world leader in food production, and many states' economies thrive because of the direct success of the agriculture industry.

The success of the agriculture industry fosters the success of other industries as well, namely the grocery, food service, restaurant, and lodging and tourism industries, and an attack on the agriculture industry would send ripples through those industries, causing economic catastrophe similar to the economic impact of the terrorist attacks of September 11, 2001, on the airline and lodging industries. It is estimated that 2003 sales for the restaurant industry will reach $426.1 billion (6), and that by 2008, the restaurant industry will employ 12.5 million workers and will likely reach 13 million by 2010 (7). This estimate takes into consideration commercial restaurant services as well as noncommercial restaurant services, such as school cafeterias, colleges and universities, hospitals and nursing facilities, and camps and community centers.

Food-based retail is estimated to capture 22.7% of the $3.489 trillion U.S. retail trade, with milk and cheese the second and third highest sellers ($10.6 and $8 billion, respectively) (8). The lodging industry grossed $14.2 billion in 2002, and tourism is currently the third largest retail industry, behind automotive and grocery, employing 2 million hotel property workers, as well as supporting more than 7.8 million travel and tourism jobs (9). Both in terms of economic destabilization and disruption of livelihood across many facets of American society, it is easy to see how attractive the agriculture industry would be to prospective terrorists.

Why, however, would one utilize agricultural terrorism, either in the form of a biological or a chemical agent, as a means of terrorism when so many other forms of weapons, with the capability of producing a direct effect in the form of loss of life and disruption of government activity, are so readily available? The answer, according to Singh, is simple. "While conventional weapons can be detected in metal detectors and other machines, biological warfare agents cannot be detected easily nor do they arouse suspicion. What's more

interesting is that they can be easily targeted. Creating bioweapons to kill livestock and crops is far easier than devising a missile to kill a few. A study suggests that livestock, particularly in developed countries, have become more susceptible as a result of intensive antibiotic and steroid programs" (10). Another reason why agricultural terrorism is so attractive is that the attack represents a danger to the perpetrator neither during nor after the attack. Chalk notes,

> Quite apart from their relative ease, bioattacks against agricultural targets are also comparatively risk free in the sense that they neither cross the threshold of mass killings (at least directly), nor, in most cases, do they represent a danger to the perpetrator him/herself. Destroying wheat or corn production or decimating a country's pig population would not attract unfettered state action in the way that a more "conventional" bioattack against humans would. Indeed in most countries, there is not even a deterrent against "agroterror" in the form of basic criminal punishment, and there has certainly been no great appreciation of the need to include agriculture in general counter-terrorism plans. Equally, because there is no large-scale loss of human life, perpetrators are unlikely to be affected by residual feelings of moral guilt or weakened by a loss of substantial political support. (4)

In his manuscript entitled "Agricultural Biowarfare and Bioterrorism," University of California at Davis microbiologist Mark Wheelis recognizes the special features that an attack on the agricultural sector would have (11). First, like Chalk and Singh, Wheelis notes that with the exception of a small number of zoonotic illnesses, most of the diseases a terrorist might introduce are not harmful to humans, making them much less lethal to produce and disseminate. Second, the equipment necessary to launch an agroterrorist attack is available on the open market, requires no specialized training to use, and costs very little. Third, the targets of agroterrorist attack, namely fields of crops or large areas of soil or animals, are largely unguarded and remarkably widespread. Fourth, the use of a biological or chemical agent against an animal or a plant population, although nevertheless an act of biowarfare, may be more easily justified both morally and punitively. The civil and criminal penalties for such crimes are much less severe than those meted against a perpetrator of an attack in which human lives are lost. Fifth, the number of cases necessary to create turmoil may be relatively few, and although few, the impact may be quite far reaching in terms of economic consequences. Sixth, it is possible to create the appearance of a naturally occurring event. Terrorist groups may evade detection if their activity resembles a naturally occurring event. A number of groups, moreover, had even claimed responsibility for natural disasters that befell the United States: namely, a 1989 fly infestation in Southern California and an outbreak of citrus canker in Florida, which had been attributed to a Cuban biological weapons program (12). Lastly, a terrorist act can be perpetrated without the criminal even entering the United States. The importation of large volumes of contaminated materials used in the agriculture industry, such as straw, animal feed, and fertilizer, may be spread over a large geographical area and may even mimic a naturally occurring event, thus evading detection.

HISTORIC EVENTS AND CASE HISTORIES

The Lord said to Moses, "Go to the king and tell him that the Lord, the God of the Hebrews, says, 'Let my people go, so that they may worship me. If you again refuse to let them go, I will punish you by sending a terrible disease on all your animals—your horses, donkeys, camels, cattle, sheep, and goats.'" (13)

Since antiquity there have been stories of poisoned well water, crops devastated by fire, and livestock either infected or killed during warfare. There exist many reports of biological terrorism during the world wars. The Germans and Japanese had attempted to introduce a variety of plant and animal pathogens, including anthrax, during conflicts surrounding the First World War. During the Second World War, the British accused the Germans of attempting to introduce Colorado beetles in to the potato fields of southern England (10). The United States had even been accused of agricultural terrorism by Cuba during the Cold War, when the Cuban government accused the United States of introducing a variety of biological agents into Cuba's crops and livestock (14).

Yet in spite of the apparent historical prevalence of the use of biological and chemical forms of agricultural terrorism, and the understanding of the ease and minimal expense with which an act of agricultural terrorism may be perpetrated, it is recognized that very few actual acts of agricultural terrorism have taken place. Carus's *Bioterrorism and Biocrimes: The Illicit Use of Biological Agents since 1900* recognizes only three cases in which biological agents targeted against plants and animals have occurred (15). The first took place in 1952 when African bush milk toxin was introduced into the livestock population of the Kenyan Kikuyu tribe by the terrorist organization Mau Mau (10,12). The second occurred in the 1980s when Tamil militants threatened to infect rubber and tea plants in Sri Lanka to destabilize the Sinhalese government of that country. The third occurred when the Dark Harvest group threatened to spread anthrax-infected soil throughout the United Kingdom to raise public awareness of the ecological dangers of germ warfare (4,15).

It is recognized, however, that a number of governments throughout the world have experimented with the use of agricultural terrorism during times of conflict. The British government experimented with anthrax-laced cow cakes for use against the Germans during World War I. During World War II, the German, British, Canadian, Japanese, and U.S. governments had biological weapons programs that conducted research on antianimal and anticrop agents including foot-and-mouth disease, rinderpest, and potato beetles (14). The United States had experimented with the use of a number of plant pathogens prior to termination of its biological warfare program in the early 1970s. The South African apartheid government had experimented with agricultural biowarfare in the form of antiplant and anticrop agents for use against neighboring countries (4).

Kadlec, contributing author to the textbook *Battlefield of the Future: 21st Century Warfare Issues*, writes in his chapter "Biological Weapons for Waging Economic Warfare" that the historical context for the use of biological agents had led to the creation of an international treaty. In 1972 the Biological Warfare Treaty prohibited the research, development, production, and use of biological agents for offensive use (16). The Office of Technology Assessment, although no longer a government agency today, in 1993 offered *Proliferation of Weapons of Mass Destruction: Assessing the Risks.* In its report, the office noted that although 162 countries had signed the treaty, there was no means to ensure compliance. The assessment further listed the nations suspected of pursuing bioweapons and bioterrorist activities, including Russia, China, Iran, Iraq, Syria, Israel, North Korea, and Taiwan (17).

Policy analyst Greco, in his report *Agricultural Terrorism in the Midwest: Risks, Threats, and State Responses,* makes note of the fact that the number of terrorist events targeting ecological and environmental sites in the United States over the past 5 years is greater than 500. He notes that the incidents, including the 2001 contamination of an Oregon tree farm by environmental activists and the 1999 destruction of a crop of genetically modified corn in California, may have eluded public attention but nevertheless represented an assault against the integrity of the U.S. agriculture industry (12).

PREPAREDNESS CHECKLIST TABLES AND SUMMARY

IDENTIFICATION OF POTENTIAL PLANT AND ANIMAL PATHOGENS

It is important to understand the characteristics of a pathogen used effectively against a plant or animal population as a form of agroterrorism. The antianimal agent must be highly contagious, highly virulent, and able to survive well in the environment. Its dissemination must result in economic hardship and an import ban by other countries (3). Some examples include foot-and-mouth disease, hog cholera, velogenic Newcastle disease, African swine fever, highly pathogenic avian influenza, and rinderpest. An antiplant agent is more difficult to characterize, although the majority of antiplant agents is from the fungus family. Weather, season, and growth stage, in addition to the choice of agent itself, play a role in the successful destruction of crops (3). Some examples of antiplant agents include wheat smut and rice blast.

The Office International des Epizooties (OIE) is an agency comprised of 155 member countries and has presented lists of zoonotic diseases with the potential for use in agroterrorist activity targeting animals (18). The diseases in List A are defined as "transmissible diseases that have the potential for very serious and rapid spread, irrespective of national borders, that are of serious socio-economic or public health consequence and that are of major importance in the international trade of animals and animal products" (Table 42-1). The diseases on List B are defined as "transmissible diseases that are considered to be of socio-economic and/or public health importance within countries and that are significant in the international trade of animals and animal products" (Tables 42-1 and 42-2). A number of the diseases on List B are considered agents that might be used against humans. The expectation would be that considerable human medical consequences might accompany an

TABLE 42-1 The World Organization for Animal Health Classification of Diseases

CATEGORY A: EPIZOOTIC DISEASES	
• Foot-and-mouth disease	• Vesicular stomatitis
• Swine vesicular disease	• Rinderpest
• Peste des petits ruminants	• Contagious bovine pleuropneumonia
• Lumpy skin disease	• Rift Valley fever
• Bluetongue	• Sheep pox and goat pox
• African horse sickness	• African swine fever
• Classical swine fever	• Highly pathogenic avian influenza
• Newcastle disease	

From The World Organization for Animal Health. Diseases Notifiable to the OIE: List A [online] April 23, 2004 [cited May 12, 2004]. Web site:http://www.oie.int/eng/maladies/en_classification.htm. With permission.

TABLE 42-2 The World Organization for Animal Health Classification of Diseases

CATEGORY B: EPIZOOTIC DISEASES (PART 1)	
MULTIPLE SPECIES DISEASES	**CATTLE DISEASES**
• Anthrax	• Bovine anaplasmosis
• Aujeszky's disease	• Bovine babesiosis
• Echinococcosis/hydatidosis	• Bovine brucellosis
• Heartwater	• Bovine cysticercosis
• Leptospirosis	• Bovine genital campylobacteriosis
• New world screwworm	• Bovine spongiform encephalopathy
(*Cochliomyia hominivorax*)	• Bovine tuberculosis
• Old world screwworm	• Dermatophilosis
(*Chrysomya bezziana*)	• Enzootic bovine leukosis
• Paratuberculosis	• Haemorrhagic septicaemia
• Q fever	• Infectious bovine rhinotracheitis/infectious pustular vulvovaginitis
• Rabies	• Malignant catarrhal fever
• Trichinellosis	• Theileriosis
	• Trichomonosis
	• Trypanosomosis (tsetse-transmitted)
SHEEP AND GOAT DISEASES	**EQUINE DISEASES**
• Caprine and ovine brucellosis (excluding *B. ovis*)	• Contagious equine metritis
• Caprine arthritis/encephalitis	• Dourine
• Contagious agalactia	• Epizootic, lymphangitis
• Contagious caprine pleuropneumonia	• Equine encephalomyelitis (Eastern and Western)
• Enzootic abortion of ewes (ovine chlamydiosis)	• Equine infectious anaemia
• Maedi-visna	• Equine influenza
• Nairobi sheep disease	• Equine piroplasmosis
• Ovine epididymitis (*Brucella ovis*)	• Equine rhinopneumonitis
• Ovine pulmonary adenomatosis	• Equine viral arteritis
• Salmonellosis (*S. abortusovis*)	• Glanders
	• Horse mange
	• Horse pox

TABLE 42-2 *(continued).*

• Scrapie	• Japanese encephalitis
	• Surra (*Trypanosoma evansi*)
	• Venezuelan equine encephalomyeliti
SWINE DISEASES	**AVIAN DISEASES**
• Atrophic rhinitis of swine	• Avian chlamydiosis
• Enterovirus encephalomyelitis	• Avian infectious bronchitis
• Porcine brucellosis	• Avian infectious laryngotracheitis
• Porcine cysticercosis	• Avian mycoplasmosis (*M. quallisepticum*)
• Porcine reproductive and	• Avian tuberculosis
respiratory syndrome	• Duck virus enteritis
• Transmissible gastroenteritis	• Duck virus hepatitis
	• Fowl cholera
	• Fowl pox
	• Fowl typhoid
	• Infectious bursal disease (Gumboro disease)
	• Marek's disease
	• Pullorum disease
LAGOMORPH DISEASES	**BEE DISEASES**
• Myxomatosis	• Acariosis of bees
• Rabbit haemorrhagic disease	• American foulbrood
• Tularemia	• European foulbrood
	• Nosemosis of bees
	• Varroosis
FISH DISEASES	**MOLLUSC DISEASES**
• Epizootic haematopoietic necrosis	• Bonamiosis (*Bonamia exitiosus, B. ostreae,*
• Infectious haematopoietic necrosis	*Mikrocytos roughleyi*)
• *Oncorhynchus masou* virus disease	• Marteiliosis (*Marteilia refringens, M. sydneyi*)
• Spring viraemia of carp	• Mikrocytosis (*Mikrocytos mackini*)
• Viral haemorrhagic septicaemia	• MSX disease (*Haplosporidium nelsoni*)
	• Perkinsosis (*Perkinsus marinus, P. olseni/atlanticus*)
CRUSTACEAN DISEASES	**OTHER LIST B DISEASES**
• Taura syndrome	• Leishmaniosis
• White spot disease	
• Yellowhead disease	

From The World Organization for Animal Health. Diseases Notifiable to the OIE: List B. [online] April 23, 2004 [cited May 12, 2004]. Web site: http://www.oie.int/eng/maladies/en_classification.htm. With permission.

animal-directed attack utilizing these agents (19). It is essential that clinicians who encounter a human case of any of these agents recognize the potential for the infection to be part of a much larger cluster, secondary to an agroterrorist event, and that clinical laboratory personnel, infection-control professionals, and local and regional health departments be notified as part of the chain of communication.

Kohnen notes that, with respect to the antiplant pathogens, outright death of the plant is not the purpose of attack. Rather, the diseased plants produce failed harvests by drastically reducing the quality and quantity of the plant's output (14). Once the plant has been infected, further transmission of the agents may be facilitated by airborne transmission, in the cases of fungal spores; by insect vectors, in the cases of plant viruses; or by water, in the case of bacterial pathogens. The crop diseases of particular agroterrorist concern can be found in Table 42-3.

ESSENTIALS FOR DETERRING AN AGROTERRORIST ATTACK

Wheelis observes that a number of steps may be taken to deter an agroterrorist attack (11). First, he recommends enacting appropriate legislation to penalize those who use biological or chemical agents against plants, animals, or humans and that this legislation provide for extradition of individuals charged with such offenses. An example of such legislation is the Agroterrorism Prevention Act of 2001. The bill, "to protect and promote the public safety and interstate commerce by establishing Federal criminal penalties and civil remedies for certain violent, threatening, obstructive and destructive conduct that is intended to injure, intimidate, or interfere with plant or animal enterprises, and for other purposes," was introduced in the U.S. House of Representatives in August 2001 by Representatives George Nethercutt

TABLE 42-3	Plant Pathogens

CROP AFFECTED	PATHOGEN TYPE	PATHOGEN	DISEASE	PRIMARY MODE OF TRANSMISSION
Cereals	Fungus	*Puccinia graminis**	Stem rust of wheat	Airborne spores
(wheat,	Fungus	*Puccinia glumarum**	Stripe rust of cereals	Airborne spores
barley, rye)	Fungus	*Erysiphe graminis*	Powdery mildew of cereals	Airborne spores
Corn	Bacteria	*Pseudomonas alboprecipitans*	Corn blight	Waterborne cells
Rice	Fungus	*Pyricularia oryzae**	Rice blast	Airborne spores
	Bacteria	*Xanthomonas oryzae*	Rice blight	Waterborne cells
	Fungus	*Helminthosporium oryzae*	Rice brown-spot disease	Airborne spores
Potato	Fungus	*Phytophthora infestans*	Late blight of potato	Airborne spores

From Piller C, Yamamoto K. Gene wars. New York: Beech Tree, 1998;246-7. With permission.

(R-WA), Saxby Chambliss (R-GA), and Randy Cunningham (R-CA) and referred to the House Subcommittee on Crime, Terrorism, and Homeland Security on September 10, 2001 (20).

Second, Wheelis recommends efforts to introduce new diagnostic agents for the early identification of outbreaks of exotic animal and plant diseases. Third, he recommends that the United States demonstrate it can, indeed, effectively control an outbreak of an exotic disease, thereby appearing less attractive to potential agroterrorists. Fourth, he recommends increased effective epidemiological investigations to determine the origin of outbreaks and ensure that terrorist activity is not misidentified as a naturally occurring event. Fifth, he recommends negotiation of an effective biological and toxin weapons convention protocol to ensure complete biological disarmament. The Biological and Toxin Weapons Convention renounced the use of all biological and toxin weapons, even those considered to be nonlethal. Finally, Wheelis recommends that the agricultural sector decrease its reliance on monoculture and expand the diversity of genotypes of plants cultured in an effort to reduce susceptibility to disease outbreaks (11).

PREPAREDNESS OF THE AGRICULTURAL SECTOR

Individual farmers within the agricultural sector might employ a number of steps to protect their farms from the risk of an agroterrorist attack. These measures, developed in 2001 by the Animal Agriculture Alliance (21), include the following:

1. Maintaining close relations with local police, fire, and emergency departments, informing them of the heightened security priority
2. Making sure public authorities have maps of the facilities in the area
3. Evaluating and scrutinizing requests for information about facilities, and replying only to those requests that have been submitted in writing and verified as authentic

4. Asking for references from those who request information about facilities and their management
5. Controlling and limiting public access to facilities and escorting all visitors to the facility
6. Maintaining basic security by locking file cabinets and doors to rooms where security equipment and information are housed
7. Maintaining appropriate lighting and alarm systems
8. Maintaining secure computer and information systems
9. Securing animal (and plant) health products
10. Thoroughly screening all job applicants, checking references carefully, and noting any hesitation by a prospective employee to a thorough investigation of his or her references
11. Observing employees for unusual patterns of behavior; not allowing employees to remove documents from the facility or to bring a video camera to the facility to record
12. Performing locker checks and installing surveillance in areas of unauthorized passage
13. Observing for signs that the facility may be a target for suspicious activity including requests for release of specific information or tours, calls, and letters criticizing or questioning the practices of the facility, harassing telephone calls and letters, increased media attention to issues related to the agriculture industry, and special interest by groups or campaigns, including those seeking employment
14. Developing a policy statement concerning care for livestock (and plants)
15. Routinely testing security systems and conducting mock drills
16. Developing a form of crisis communication and a plan of action in the event of a true emergency.

Essential to the early recognition and identification of a potential agroterrorist attack is communication with local, regional, state, and national agencies. Each farmer ought to be aware of the agencies in the area that might assist in responding to a potential agroterrorist attack. The Office of Emergency Preparedness provides telephone numbers and contact information for local and regional agencies that may be contacted in case of an emergency (22).

PREPAREDNESS OF THE MEDICAL COMMUNITY

The Centers for Disease Control and Prevention's *Morbidity and Mortality Weekly Report* has published a number of articles reflecting the preparedness and response of the medical community to biological and chemical terrorism and the recognition of illnesses associated with the intentional release of such agents (23,24). Reports such as these reinforce the fact that clinicians remain at the forefront of the recognition and response to a terrorist attack.

In June 2003 James James, the director of the American Medical Association's Center for Disaster Preparedness and Emergency Response, announced a coordinated program that will standardize training for physicians and other clinicians against bioterrorism and other mass casualty disasters, including naturally occurring disasters. The program, entitled Basic Disaster Life Support (BDLS) and Advanced Disaster Life Support (ADLS), will include didactic lectures, interactive presentations, and computer-generated simulations designed to educate and prepare those clinicians who are typically targeted for emergency medical situations, namely, emergency and critical care physicians and nurses and other primary care providers, paramedics, allied health professionals, medical students, emergency medical technicians, and pharmacists (25).

It is conceivable that BDLS and ADLS training provided might be germane to the veterinarian to a degree, in that the veterinarian may be one of the first links in the chain of recognition and response to a mass casualty event targeted specifically toward the agricultural sector. Radford Davis, DVM, comments that the reaction to an agroterrorist event depends on the rapidity with which the disease is discovered. This is supported by the fact that in the United Kingdom, the 2001 foot-and-mouth disease outbreak is thought to have been so severe because it was not noticed for a week after the initial introduction (11). Davis notes that at the farm level, the astute veterinarian will play a crucial role in the identification of a cluster of exotic diseases. He notes, moreover, that although over 350 are veterinarians trained as foreign animal disease diagnosticians, the thousands of veterinarians in private practice throughout the United States, as well as those in both state and federal positions, are not specifically trained in the diagnosis and management of exotic zoonotic illnesses (3). Because veterinarians as well as other clinicians are likely to be at the forefront of the response, it seems appropriate to allocate funds and to reinforce the education of those who may be key in thwarting an agroterrorist attack.

PREPAREDNESS OF THE STATE AND NATIONAL GOVERNMENTS

In her paper entitled "Responding to the Threat of Agroterrorism: Specific Recommendations for the United States Department of Agriculture (USDA)," Kohnen recommends a four-level approach to countering an agroterrorist attack: (a) at the level of the organism, through disease resistance; (b) at the farm level, through facility management techniques designed to prevent disease introduction or transmission; (c) at the level of the agricultural sector, through disease detection and response procedures, primarily under the auspice of the USDA; and (d) at the national level, through government policies designed to minimize the socioeconomic costs of a catastrophic disease outbreak (14). Kohnen recognizes, however, that the safety of the food supply is not dependent on the success of only one level of protection, but rather that the safety of the food supply rests on the success of all four levels acting in concert with one another. For example, although pest and disease control may be successful at the organism and the farm level, and thus reliance on the agricultural sector and the government for policy may not be necessary, the four levels must function together to ensure the safest food supply available.

Kohnen recommends the following steps to ensure the safety of the food supply: (a) the USDA should be ready to supply vaccines for all List A diseases (Table 42-1) in case of an outbreak; (b) the USDA should establish a biosecurity training program to educate farmers on biosecurity best practices. The program should extend to crop farmers in order to educate them on the risks of monoculture planting and suggest appropriate means of avoiding long-term harm; (c) the USDA should increase funding for disease detection and surveillance technology, such as linked human and animal disease databases and satellite surveillance. The agency should increase funding to the Agricultural Research Service or to private contractors for the development of rapid diagnostic technologies against foreign animal diseases, and these screening tests should be available at the state level. Kohnen comments that the Plum Island Animal Disease Center, located off the northeastern tip of Long Island, is currently certified as a level-3 biosafety laboratory. The U.S. level-4 biosafety facilities, located at the Centers for Disease Control and Prevention in Atlanta, Georgia, and at the National Institute of Health in Bethesda, Maryland, specialize in the research and management of diseases that are lethal to humans or have no known human vaccine available. There is no level-4 biosecurity facility in the United States for the study of farm animals, although animal diseases such as West Nile and Nipah viruses can be fatal to humans. Kohnen recommends, therefore, (d) that the funds be allocated to upgrade the Plum Island Animal Disease Center to a biosafety level-4 facility. She further recommends, (e) that the USDA establish a contingency network of accredited veterinarians in case of an outbreak of a catastrophic disease; (f) that the USDA prepare a contingency public relations campaign to restore/promote confidence in U.S. agricultural products; (g) that the USDA establish a contingency budget to fund disease eradication efforts and compensation costs; and finally, (h) that the USDA devise a strategy for obtaining very large amounts of money as preparation for a major disease outbreak and eradication effort.

The recognition of pathogens and the identification of clusters of disease outbreaks represent a significant step in thwarting an agroterrorist attack, but this does represent a retrospective approach to the problem. It has long been recognized that the food supply for the nation is remarkably poorly protected from corruption by terrorism; it is rather recently, however, that government agencies have made preventing an agroterrorist attack a fundamental part of their agenda, as reflected by changes in budget allocation and heightened legislative measures enacted at the state and national levels.

Note that only a percentage of the money requested to ensure the safety of the nation's food supply is allocated to the USDA. In the budget for fiscal year (FY) 2000, $8 billion had been allocated to a variety of government agencies to combat terrorism. The USDA received only 0.15% of that allocation, about $12 million. The budget for FY 2001, however, tripled the allocation to the USDA to about $41 million (14,26). The budget for FY 2004 is anticipated to provide the USDA with $368 million for the purpose of combating terrorism (27).

Secretary of Health and Human Services Tommy G. Thompson has led the effort to encourage Congress to increase Food and Drug Administration (FDA) funding to protect the nation's families from an attack on the food supply. Nearly 20% of all imports into the United States are food and food products. The FDA anticipates that the United States will receive over 8 million food shipments from over 200,000 foreign manufacturers in 2004—a huge volume that continues to grow rapidly. In FYs 2002 and 2003, Congress budgeted more than $195 million for food safety programs. In President Bush's FY 2004 budget, the Department of Health and Human Services (DHHS) is requesting $116.3 million, an increase of $20.5 million over FY 2003, to further protect the nation's food supply (28). Although augmenting the finances available to counter a terrorist attack and to heighten the safety of the food supply are steps of paramount importance in the preparedness against agricultural terrorism, it represents only a fraction of the necessary measures.

A number of states have enacted legislation in an effort to counter the possibility of agricultural terrorism. The Biological, Chemical, and Agricultural Terrorism Legislation Database contains a state-by-state synopsis of the legislation that has been proposed, the sponsoring legislator, and the status of the bill within the state's legislature. To date, 53 records of proposed legislation have been found, indicating a heightened awareness of the potential for an agroterrorist attack and an understanding of the means necessary to thwart it at the state level (29).

RESOURCES

The Office of Emergency Preparedness' National Disaster Medical System section is located within the Operations Branch of the Response Division of the Federal Emergency Management Agency, U.S. Department of Homeland Security. It is primarily responsible for responding to the medical needs of disaster-affected populations in major emergencies and federally declared disasters. By entering the geographical location into the search site on the web page, one is provided emergency contact numbers both locally and regionally (22).

The U.S. Department of Agriculture's web site contains both contact information for use in the event of an emergency and also updated information on current topics of interest; in particular, information on outbreaks of zoonotic illnesses and food safety (30).

The references in this chapter contain a number of entries on published articles and current information that may provide a great deal of detailed information to clinicians and veterinarians. The web pages cited are updated as information is obtained and reflect the ever-changing nature of the world in which we live.

SUMMARY

Experts in the field of agricultural terrorism have recognized the ease with which a terrorist attack against the agricultural sector may be promulgated. Most zoonoses and plant pathogens are not lethal to humans, making their dissemination less risky to the perpetrator. The materials necessary to carry out an agroterrorist attack are readily available, and their use is neither restricted nor challenging. The surveillance of livestock and crops is rather poor, making it likely that an attack will go unnoticed for a period of time. An agroterrorist attack may be made to mimic a naturally occurring event and even be promulgated without the perpetrator entering the United States. There exist few ramifications for the perpetrator of an agroterrorist attack, both legally and morally.

Traditionally, agricultural terrorism is not expected to have a direct impact on human life. The health care system's preparation and response to an agroterrorism attack must be equally nontraditional. The initial recognition of a successful agroterrorist attack will likely be achieved by those working at the individual level within the agricultural sector, namely farm laborers and owners, veterinarians, and local physicians caring for ill farm workers. Diseases commonly encountered among plants and animals may suggest a naturally occurring event; diseases commonly encountered among farm workers may suggest a naturally occurring event as well. The diagnosis and recognition of patterns of illness among individuals within a distinct geographical location or region will be the initial evidence that suggests an offensive. Patterns of disease that suggest agroterrorist attack may be manufactured to mimic naturally occurring plagues and disasters. Only with vigilance and close communication among local and regional health-monitoring agencies will the initial recognition of an agroterrorist attack be made. Once the offense has been recognized, local and regional health-monitoring agencies will intervene to quarantine and to treat the infected, to limit the interaction between exposed livestock and plants and their respective markets, and lastly to heighten the security surrounding the uninfected in an effort to maintain a safe and reliable market. On a larger level, agricultural and governmental agencies will work hand in hand in an effort to secure the safety of the agricultural goods available, as well as to encourage confidence in the safety and security of U.S. agriculture.

REFERENCES

1. Foxell JW. Agro-terrorism: the terrorist threat to U.S. food and agriculture. Web site: http://www.vddipharmaceuticals.com/agroterrorism.htm. Accessed September 7, 2003.
2. Current topics: selected issues in American agriculture today. In: The United States Department of Agriculture Fact Book 2001-2002. Web site: http://www.usda.gov/factbook/chapter1.htm. Accessed September 16, 2003.
3. Davis RG. Agricultural bioterrorism. Web site: http://www.actionbioscience.org/newfrontiers/davis.html. Accessed September 15, 2003.
4. Chalk P. RAND bioterrorism conference. Web site: http://www.rand.org.nsrd/bioterr/chalk.htm. Accessed September 15, 2003.
5. Key statistical indicators of the food & fiber sector. Web site: http://www.ers.usda.gov/publications/agoutlook/aotables/aug 2003 /aotab01.xls. Accessed September 15, 2003.
6. Industry at a glance. The National Restaurant Association. Web site: http://www.restaurant.org/research/ind_glance.cfm. Accessed September 15, 2003.
7. Restaurant employment on the rise. Restaurants USA. October 2000. Web site: http://www.restaurant.org/research/magarticle.cfm. Accessed September 15, 2003.
8. 2002-2003 progress report. Grocery Manufacturers of America. Web site: http://www.gmabrands.com/publications/docs/2002 PROGRESS.pdf. Accessed September 16, 2003.
9. 2003 lodging industry profile. American Hotel & Lodging Association. Web site: http://www.ahma.com/products_info_center_lip.asp. Accessed September 16, 2003.
10. Singh P. All about agricultural terrorism. Agriculture Online. Web site: http://www.agriculture.com/default.sph/agNotebook.class?FNC=ArticleList_Aarticle2_html. Accessed September 7, 2003.
11. Wheelis M. Agricultural biowarfare & bioterrorism. The Federation of American Scientists Chemical & Biological Arms Control Program. Web site: http://www.fas.org/bwc/agr/ main.htm. Accessed September 7, 2003.
12. Greco J. Agricultural terrorism in the Midwest: risks, threats, and state responses. The Agriculture Committee of the Midwestern Legislative Conference. Web site: http://stars.csg.org/csg-midwest/reports/2002/2002_mw_Ag_Terrorism.pdf. Accessed September 7, 2003.
13. Good News Bible. American Bible Society, 1976;71.
14. Kohnen A. Responding to the threat of agroterrorism: specific recommendations for the United States Department of Agriculture. BCSIA Discussion Paper 2000-29, ESDP Discussion Paper ESDP 2000-24, John F. Kennedy School of Government, Harvard University, October 2000. Web site: http://bcsia.ksg.harvard.edu/publication_list.cfm?program = CORE&ln=recent&gma=1. Accessed September 7, 2003.
15. Carus WS. Bioterrorism and biocrimes: the illicit use of biological agents since 1900. Amsterdam: Fredonia Books, 2002.
16. Kadlec RP. Biological weapons for waging economic warfare. In: Battlefield of the future: 21st century warfare issues. Web site: htttp://www.airpower.Maxwell.af.mil/airchronicles/battle/bftoc.html. Accessed September 16, 2003.
17. Office of Technology Assessment of the United States Congress. Proliferation of weapons of mass destruction: assessing the risks. Web site: http://www.wws.princeton.edu/~ota/disk1/1993/9341_n.html. Accessed October 8, 2003.
18. Classification of diseases. Office International des Epizooties. Web site: http://www.oie.int/eng/maladies/en_classification.htm. Accessed September 7, 2003.
19. Greenfield RA, Lutz BD, Huycke MM, et al. Unconventional biological threats and the molecular biological response to biological threats. Am J Med Sci 2002;323(6):350-7.
20. The United States House of Representatives. 107th Legislative Session. Web site: http://thomas.loc.gov/cgi-bin/bdquery/D?d107:1:./temp/~bdFG7g:21. Agroterrorism: Facing the threat. Farm Bureau News 2001;(80):19. Web site: http://www.fb.com/fbn/html/agriculturalterrorism.html. Accessed September 7, 2003.
22. The Office of Emergency Preparedness. Web site: http://ndms.dhhs.gov/Contacts/contacts.html. Accessed October 15, 2003.
23. Khan AS, Levitt AM, Sage MJ, et al. Biological and chemical terrorism: strategic plan for preparedness and response. Recommendations of the CDC Strategic Planning Workgroup. MMWR Morb Mortal Wkly Rep 2000;49(RR04):1-14. Web site: http://www.cdc.gov/mmwr/preview/mmwrhtml/rr4904a1.htm. Accessed September 7, 2003.
24. Recognition of illness associated with the intentional release of a biologic agent. MMWR Morb Mortal Wkly Rep 2001; 50(41):893-7. Web site: http://www.cdc.gov/mmwr/preview/mmwrhtml/mm5041a2.htm. Accessed September 7, 2003.
25. Basic Disaster Life Support (BDLS) and Advanced Disaster Life Support (ADLS): a brief program overview from the National Disaster Life Support Educational Consortium (NDLSEC). Web site: http://www.ama-assn.org/ama/pub/category/6206.html. Accessed October 15, 2003.
26. Annual report to Congress on combating terrorism: including defense against weapons of mass destruction/domestic preparedness and critical infrastructure protection. Washington, DC: Office of Management and Budget, 2000;47.
27. Annual report to Congress on combating terrorism: including defense against weapons of mass destruction/domestic preparedness and critical infrastructure protection. Washington, DC: Office of Management and Budget, 2003;15. Web site: http://www.whitehouse.gov/omb/inforeg/2003_combat_terr.pdf. Accessed October 16, 2003.
28. Progress report to Secretary Tommy G. Thompson: ensuring the safety and security of the nation's food supply. The United States Food and Drug Administration Center for Food Safety and Applied Nutrition, 2003. Web site: http://www.cfsan.fda.gov/~dms/fssrep.html. Accessed October 1, 2003.
29. The Biological, Chemical, and Agricultural Terrorism Legislation Database. The National Conference of State Legislatures. Web site: http://www.ncls.org/programs/esnr/terrorismdb.cfm. Accessed September 7, 2003.
30. The United States Department of Agriculture website. Web site: http://www.usda.gov. Accessed October 16, 2003.

43

Mass Fatality Incidents

Lynn Roppolo and Kathy J. Rinnert

INTRODUCTION

A *mass fatality incident* is a situation resulting in loss of life that exceeds death investigation resources in the local community (1). Both natural and humanmade disasters may potentially produce this level of devastation. In 2001, an earthquake in India killed over 20,000 people (2). The crash of TWA flight 800 in Long Island in 1996 resulted in 230 deaths (3). Terrorism is a growing threat to human life around the world, and the United States is not immune. In 1995, the bombing of the Alfred P. Murrah Federal Building in Oklahoma City, Oklahoma, claimed 168 lives (4). The terrorist attacks of September 11, 2001, took thousands of innocent lives at three locations in Washington, D.C., New York, and Pennsylvania. In this event, one of the worst terrorist events in recorded history, more than 3,000 individuals of varied racial and ethnic background lost their lives. (5). This horrific attack laid credence to the devastating and widespread impact mass fatality events can have on survivors, rescue workers, the community, the nation, and the world at large.

Management of the fatally wounded is an often overlooked but important part of disaster preparedness and response. As in all cases of unnatural death, there are a number of legal implications for mass fatalities including the identification of the deceased, the determination of the cause of death, and the assignment of responsibility for the disaster event (6). A mass fatality incident due to terrorism may have additional ramifications such as protection of rescue personnel and decontamination of human remains and typically involves a more complex investigative response. Every community must be aware of the implications of a mass fatality incident and the specialized support services required. Such an event may overwhelm local response efforts. Therefore, jurisdictions should establish prearranged plans for dealing with this situation that must include coordinated efforts with other agencies.

The purpose of this chapter is to

1. Describe how mass fatality management is integrated into the overall disaster response.

2. Describe the operational areas of a mass fatality response and key areas to be included in disaster preparedness plans.

3. Discuss special considerations in mass fatality management due to terrorism.

4. Identify local, state, and federal resources used in mass fatality incidents.

PREPAREDNESS ESSENTIALS

OVERVIEW OF A MASS FATALITY INCIDENT

The overall response to a mass fatality incident can be divided into three phases (1). The initial phase begins when the first responder arrives at the location of the disaster. This person, usually a public safety officer (police, fire, or emergency medical services), may become the incident commander of the event. The incident commander assesses the situation, activates the disaster plan, and coordinates the activities of the responding agencies. After the community disaster plan is activated, the second phase of response begins. At this point the incident command system (ICS) becomes operational, and senior public safety officers assume lead roles. Law enforcement and fire department personnel secure the scene, control environmental hazards, and assist with rescue efforts. Emergency medical services (EMS) personnel perform triage, provide stabilizing medical care, and transport survivors to nearby medical facilities. Additional resources are obtained as needed. During the first two phases of the response, rescue efforts are focused on the safe rescue of potentially living victims. The final phase is the resolution phase, which involves removal and transport of any human remains, coordination of morgue services, notification of relatives, and community support. Unlike previous phases of the response, this phase is no longer focused on life and property preservation (7). It is during this last phase that the local medical examiner or coroner (MEC) acts as incident commander to coordinate these activities.

A disaster becomes a mass fatality incident when local resources are overwhelmed and unable to manage the numbers or types of fatalities created by the event. The MEC is central to managing such events and is responsible for the following:

- Scene operations: search and recovery of human remains; initial evidence recovery
- Morgue operations: identification and processing of human remains, including the determination of the cause of death
- Family assistance center (FAC): antemortem information, identification notification, care of families (8)

After it is determined that an event involves fatalities, the information shown in Table 43-1 should be conveyed to the MEC during the initial notification process.

OPERATIONAL AREAS IN A MASS FATALITY INCIDENT RESPONSE

After the incident commander has determined that the disaster site is safe, the initial evaluation team (consisting of at least the MEC, the operations director, and the chief investigator from the local medical examiner's office) should proceed to the location (8).

There are three major operational areas of a mass fatality response: search and recovery, morgue operations, and family assistance (9).

Search and Recovery

During mass fatality events, search and recovery activities usually involve locating and removing bodies, body parts, and personal effects. Personal effects are those items carried by, or being transported with, an individual. Every mass fatality site should be regarded as a crime scene unless otherwise indicated by the MEC. Only authorized individuals should be allowed within the secure perimeter. Relatives of victims should be referred to the FAC.

The appropriate authorities must readily identify safety issues, such as the stability of a building in a structural collapse. The MEC should work with the incident command center and other agencies (i.e., hazmat) to determine the existence of any hazards and what actions should be taken to mitigate them, including the level of personal protective equipment required by rescue/recovery personnel. The MEC must have a sufficient number of people capable of functioning in a contaminated area. Universal precautions should be maintained at all times. Search and recovery of the remains should not take place until it is determined that the site is safe.

Every body, body part, or personal belonging is identified and tagged with a unique number. During all operations, bodies and body parts should be treated in a respectful and dignified manner. If possible, human remains should be covered or shielded from public view. If the bodies are scattered over an extensive area, a grid system is utilized in an effort to document the location, assist in recreation of the scene, and further the investigative process (7). Recovery and removal of the remains occurs after the search and tagging of a grid sector has been completed. Unless the remains are in danger of destruction, disintegration, or decomposition, bodies should not be moved from the scene until after the arrival of the MEC. If any of these dangers exist, bodies should be moved immediately to a safe fatality collection point (6). The fatality collection point is a location where the bodies can be temporarily placed until a temporary morgue can be established. The temporary morgue is used as a holding area until the morgue examination center (for morgue operations) is established (8). Some sources refer to the temporary morgue as the site for morgue operations (6). Sometimes the MEC's existing facilities may be the optimal site for morgue operations (7). For example, during the terrorist attack on the World Trade Center, additional morgue facilities were not needed as most human remains were crushed, fragmented, or commingled. Instead, innovative methods for DNA analysis were implemented using new computer software to assist with the identification process of every bit of human remains recovered (10).

Morgue Operations

Morgue operations are divided into several different stations to record and provide information about the deceased for eventual comparison to antemortem records. This information is used to confirm identification and establish the facts surrounding the death. Each body is escorted through each of the stations to ensure that (a) the remains are not mixed up with other remains, (b) documentation is complete, and (c) proper respect is paid to the deceased at all times (7). Any form of identification (i.e., driver's license) found in the vicinity of a body may provide information useful in

TABLE 43-1	Information Provided to the Medical Examiner or Coroner During Notification of a Mass Fatality Incident (7)

- Type of incident (i.e., structural collapse, biochemical hazard, explosive device, fire)
- Location
- Estimated number of fatalities
- Condition of bodies (i.e., fragmented, burned)
- Demographics of those killed including any hazardous conditions (i.e., entrapment, chemical contamination)
- Ongoing response actions
- Response agencies currently involved

uncovering the identity of the victim. Such findings, however, do not confirm the victim's identification (9). Traumatic injury resulting from the disaster event may cause significant distortion of body habitus and facial features, thereby complicating the timely and accurate identification of the victim. The MEC may request assistance from experts in pathology, anthropology, dentistry, mortuary affairs, search and recovery, and others as needed to assist with the identification process.

In the mass fatality morgue, identification procedures are initiated as follows (1):

- *In-processing station*—initiates all chain-of-custody documents, which allows the tracking of remains
- *Photography and full-body radiology station*—photograph remains as they are received; full-body radiology may be done to locate any objects or personal effects embedded within the remains
- *Personal effects station*—clothing and jewelry are collected, documented, and stored
- *Fingerprint station*—digit and foot impressions are taken
- *Medical radiology station*—additional radiography may be done as indicated to assist with determining the cause of death
- *Pathology station*—an autopsy is performed to establish the manner of death during which tissue samples may be taken for laboratory tests and DNA analysis (as indicated by protocol only)
- *Dental station*—postmortem dental films are taken and compared to antemortem dental records to assist in victim identification
- *Physical anthropology station*—skeletal measurements and anthropomorphic tables are utilized to determine approximate age, sex, and racial origin

- *Mortuary science station*—the remains are prepared for repatriation; embalming or other preservative process may also be indicated

After identification of the remains is completed, relatives should be contacted in an expedient fashion by the MEC or a designee. Psychosocial and religious support services should be readily available. If cremation is necessary to avoid secondary contamination or spread of disease, it should not be undertaken in the mass fatality morgue (6). In most circumstances, as soon as the identification is confirmed, the remains should be released and moved to a place designated by the family. Personal effects should be returned to the family as soon as possible. Unidentifiable bodies can be embalmed and stored pending further investigation (6).

Family Assistance Center

The site for the family assistance center should be established quickly utilizing locations such as in a hotel, conference center, school, or church. While the FAC should not be too close to the disaster scene, it should be easily accessible to families and provide adequate accommodations for those relatives coming from distant locations. Access to the FAC should be secure and limited to family members of victims only while providing adequate privacy and protection from media representatives. Individual meetings are conducted with families of the victims to collect antemortem data, which may be utilized in the identification process. Briefings by the MEC or staff should be performed at least twice daily to keep the families informed about the progress of the investigation and identification process. Grief counselors or religious support personnel should be present when the MEC notifies the family that victim's identification has been confirmed. The American Red Cross (ARC) or other appropriate

TABLE 43-2	Preparedness Essentials for Mass Fatality Incidents	
OPERATIONAL AREA	**TASKS**	**RESOURCES**[a]
Search and recovery	Safety	Law enforcement, fire, hazmat teams
	Search and recovery	Local: police, fire, rescue personnel, MEC Federal: USAR , DMORT
	Transportation	Contract services (refrigerated trucks), funeral homes, military, other government agencies
Morgue operations	Location	Local morgue. If temporary morgue facility needed—large building with adequate ventilation, basic utilities, and controlled access
	Additional resources	Local: pathology, anthropology, dentistry, mortuary affairs staff Federal: FBI, DMORT
Family assistance center	Location	Hotel, conference room, or church
	Support services	Mental health, religious, social support groups; volunteer agencies such as ARC, SA

[a]hazmat, hazardous materials; MEC, medical examiner or coroner; USAR, urban search and rescue; DMORT, Disaster Mortuary Operations Response Team; FBI, Federal Bureau of Investigation; ARC, American Red Cross; SA, Salvation Army.

agency may assist with family support, transportation, housing, supplies, and volunteer coordination. Medical and mental health professionals as well as religious clergy should be readily available. In addition, phone banks, computer/Internet access, and meal service may be provided to families at the FAC. Table 43-2 provides an overview of preparedness essentials for mass fatality incidents.

LOCAL, STATE, AND FEDERAL RESOURCES FOR MASS FATALITY MANAGEMENT

If it is determined that additional resources are needed, the county should declare a local emergency and call upon state resources for assistance that in turn may petition for federal resources as needed. Several local organizations may be a valuable resource in any mass fatality response. Twenty-four-hour contact information for the following agencies or resources should be included in the mass fatality response plan (7,11):

Local Resources

- MEC and staff
- Local urban search and rescue group
- Refrigerated truck service
- Utility services—phone, water, gas, electricity
- Food services
- Mental health support services
- Religious support services
- National Guard or Army Reserve unit
- Forensic anthropologist
- Site support services—for custodial and site maintenance
- Communications and information systems support
- Media services—to disseminate information
- Public health department

State Resources

- State emergency management
- Department of public safety—crime lab
- State health laboratory—coordinates with Centers for Disease Control and Prevention
- State board of funeral directors and embalmers
- State funeral directors association

Federal Resources

- National Disaster Medical System—Disaster Mortuary Operations Response Team (DMORT)
- Department of Justice—Federal Bureau of Investigation (FBI)
- Department of Defense—Office of the Armed Forces Medical Examiner (OAFME)
- National Transportation and Safety Board (NTSB)
- Bureau of Alcohol, Tobacco, and Firearms (ATF)
- Centers for Disease Control and Prevention (CDC)

Volunteer Resources

- American Red Cross
- Salvation Army

- Critical incident stress debriefing network
- Private: dental association-disaster team
- National Funeral Directors Association
- National Association of Medical Examiners

Federal resources may be called on to assist with state and local efforts in a mass fatality incident. Within the U.S. government's Federal Response Plan, under the direction of the Federal Emergency Management Agency (FEMA), the National Disaster Medical System (NDMS) provides medical assistance, victim identification, and mortuary services during mass fatality events. Disaster Mortuary Operations Response Teams (DMORT) are a critical component of the NDMS and consist of forensic scientists (anthropologists, dentists, and pathologists), funeral directors, embalmers, medical records technicians, medico-legal investigators, and specialists in mass fatality management. DMORT teams may only be activated for disaster events with presidential declarations providing functional support to the local MEC. However, via mandate, OAFME is required to investigate all federal and military crashes and deaths (12). Therefore, OAFME was the lead agency for the fatality investigation at the Pentagon on September 11, 2001, and the MEC in Arlington, Virginia, was not involved. OAFME maintains the right of first refusal for incidents involving nonmilitary federal buildings such as in the Oklahoma City bombing where the local MEC was in charge of the fatality investigation. OAFME's staff can respond to nonmilitary mass fatality incidents if a special request is made (12). The FBI may be involved to assist with the identification of victims and to investigate criminal acts such as terrorism (13). NTSB is tasked with assisting the recovery of fatalities from aviation accidents as mandated by the Family Assistance Act of 1996. The identification process for these fatalities however, remains under the jurisdiction of the local MEC (14).

SPECIAL CONSIDERATIONS IN MASS FATALITY MANAGEMENT DUE TO TERRORISM

Chemical Contamination

All personnel working with the MEC must be appropriately trained and equipped to operate in hazardous conditions. With proper handling and decontamination, the majority of chemically contaminated remains may be safely returned to their families for burial. All personnel should be trained in the proper use of Level C personal protective equipment (PPE), and a select number of individuals should be trained in the use of Levels A and B PPE. The MEC may train personnel to use PPE through mutual aid agreements with local fire departments, hazmat teams, or local/state environmental protection agencies. Additional assistance can be provided from the FBI, local law enforcement, the fire department, and/or specialized military teams. At the current time, DMORT has one weapons of mass destruction team for the nation capable of decontaminating chemically contaminated remains and monitoring them to ensure they are free of chemical agents. DMORT should be included in any mass fatality response, and chemical incidents due to terrorism are no exception. In their disaster plan, MEC should have an annex that outlines the specialized equipment and

TABLE 43-3	Mass Fatality Management in Terrorist Incidents	

TYPE OF THREAT	RESOURCES[a]	SUPPLIES[a]
Chemical	Mutual agreements for training with local fire departments, hazmat teams, local private industrial hazmat teams, or local/state environmental protection agencies or subcontractors; FBI, local law enforcement, fire department, and/or supporting specialized military teams; DMORT	PPE, ventilation fans, decontamination supplies, water run-off containers, waterproof tracking tags, refrigerated storage units, chemical detection monitors
Nuclear	Radiation safety officials	PPE, decontamination supplies, radiation detection monitors
Biological	Public health department; CDC	PPE, infection control supplies

[a]PPE, personal protective equipment; hazmat, hazardous materials; FBI, Federal Bureau of Investigation; DMORT, Disaster Mortuary Operations Response Team; CDC, Centers for Disease Control and Prevention.

procedures to be used for these events. The annex should include a list of PPE, ventilation fans, decontamination supplies, water run-off containers, waterproof tracking tags, and refrigerated storage units (15).

In the event of an incident involving chemical agents, the MEC should consult with the incident commander at the scene to determine the appropriate level of PPE required. The MEC must be prepared to establish a preliminary morgue at the incident site in order to gather evidence from the remains before they undergo decontamination during which evidence may be lost or obliterated. An initial evaluation team should enter the potentially contaminated zone or hot zone and make an assessment to develop a plan for the best approach for processing the remains. It is recommended that this team include the MEC or designee, an FBI hazmat technician, a law enforcement evidence collection technician, and a forensic odontologist (15). Common additives to the decontamination solution utilized for the gross decontamination process include soap and bleach (sodium hypochlorite) (16).

The off-site mass fatality morgue for a chemical incident requires specific modifications in the traditional morgue set-up. In addition to an autopsy area and identification station, the off-site morgue must have adequate room for (a) a detailed decontamination station, (b) an embalming station, and (c) a final rinse station. All remains must undergo a detailed decontamination, using bleach or a soap solution, prior to the performance of an autopsy or embalming. If the decontamination is performed in a closed area, it must be well ventilated. Decontamination activities should take place in an area separate from the embalming activities as some decontamination solvents (such as bleach) create toxic reactants when mixed with embalming fluid. Embalming not only allows easier storage of remains but also provides for a more accurate contamination reading from chemical agent monitors (15). After remains are decontaminated, there should be little threat to mortuary workers for chemical off-gassing or secondary contamination as most chemicals (with the exception of cyanide) are metabolized, hydrolyzed, or tightly bound in the body's tissues (15).

TABLE 43-4	Examples of Significant Fatal Terrorist Incidents (5, 21, 22)		

DATE	LOCATION	TYPE OF ATTACK	NUMBER OF FATALITIES
2001	World Trade Center, Pentagon, and site in Pennsylvania—United States	Crashing of hijacked aircraft	3,031
2001	Eastern seaboard—United States	Biological (anthrax)	5
2000	*U.S.S. Cole*	Explosive device	17
2000	Church bombing—Tajikstan	Explosive device	7
1998	Pipeline bombing—Columbia	Explosive device	71
1998	U.S. Embassy—East Africa	Explosive device	291
1997	Tourist killings—Egypt	Shooting	58
1996	Bus attack—Jerusalem	Explosive device	26
1995	Oklahoma federal building—United States	Explosive device	166
1995	Tokyo subway—Japan	Chemical (sarin)	12

During the autopsy of chemically contaminated remains, the performance of specialized testing may be necessary to detect chemical contaminants or residual metabolites. If the integrity of evidence is suspect, it should be packaged in a manner that prevents cross-contamination but does not destroy the evidence (15).

Nuclear Contamination

Deaths from nuclear contamination may occur as a result of the initial blast effect that occurs with the detonation of a nuclear device. On arrival to the incident scene, at the direction of the incident commander, the MEC should approach the scene with a radiation authority escort, an individual who is knowledgeable and experienced in radiation safety. This person has the capability to monitor and provide advice on contamination and exposure control for radiation incidents. If PPE is recommended, the clothing will likely be similar to the clothing worn for protection of air- and blood-borne pathogens. Remains should not be touched during the initial evaluation until a radiation survey has been completed and the areas of contamination are identified. Gross decontamination of the remains is then performed by removal of all outer clothing that essentially removes the majority of radioactive contaminants. Removed clothing should remain at the incident site for proper disposal by a clean-up team. The radiation authority will use standard contamination control practices such as dosimetry monitoring, double bagging, and tagging. Following gross decontamination, the radiation authority performs a second radiation contamination survey. If contamination is still present, the remains are placed in a body bag and labeled with a radiation tag that identifies the level of contamination. Remains that are free of radiation after gross decontamination are turned over

TABLE 43-5   Mass Fatality Management Preparedness Checklist

	TASK TO PERFORM[a]	COMPLETED
Communication	• Establish a notification system and mechanism for contracting the MEC • Establish a system to communicate between scene operations, morgue operations, and FAC • Establish a computer system to assist with documentation and tracking	
Hazard detection and decontamination	• Establish training in use of PPE for MEC and staff • Develop decontamination plan related to scene and morgue operations • Maintain additional resources for a hazardous event (i.e., additional biohazard bags, PPE)	
Safety and security	• Work with police, fire department, and local hazmat teams to identify potential safety and security issues and mechanisms to handle them	
Scene operations (search and recovery)	• Establish mutual agreements with local agencies for supplies and human resources • Develop a mechanism for additional resources specific to the recovery and care of the deceased (i.e., substantial body bags) • Establish documentation system for search and recovery • Establish a mechanism for search and recovery of the deceased • Establish a mechanism for transportation of bodies to the site of morgue operations • Identify mechanism to solicit support from state and federal resources such as DMORT to assist with all aspects of the mass fatality response	
Morgue operations	• Establish mutual agreements with local agencies or supplies and personnel assistance • Identify potential locations for temporary morgue • Identify resources for additional supplies and personnel for morgue operations	
Recovery operations (FAC)	• Identify lead agency such as the ARC to take charge of FAC • Identify and establish mutual agreements with other support resources for FAC	

[a]FAC, family assistance center; MEC, medical examiner or coroner; PPE, personal protective equipment; hazmat, hazardous materials; DMORT, Disaster Mortuary Operations Response Team; ARC, American Red Cross.

to the MEC for processing. Contaminated remains are transferred to an additional facility for further decontamination. Dry decontamination is first attempted. This process first involves removing clothing and then particulate matter either by brushing it off or applying sticky tape to the affected areas. If this process is not successful, wash and rinse is conducted. If it is determined that internal contamination exists, the MEC should work closely with the radiation authority to determine the optimal method of decontaminating, processing, and disposing of the remains. A higher medical authority such as the Radiation Emergency Assistance Center/Training Site (REAC/TS) may be consulted as needed (17).

Biological Weapons

Biological weapons have the potential to cause a mass number of fatalities. The mortality rate from untreated anthrax is 20% (18). Smallpox is one of the highest-threat bioterrorism agents, with a fatality rate of 30% (18).

In a bioterrorist attack, signs and symptoms of illness may be delayed for hours to weeks and may mimic naturally occurring disease processes. Mass fatalities that occur as a result of a biological incident may present at different times and in different locations. Most initial diagnostic studies are often nonspecific, and few laboratories are equipped with the sophisticated tests required to definitively identify specific pathogens. Special safeguards need to be employed to prevent contamination in laboratory workers during the process of identifying the biological agent. For example, smallpox and various viral hemorrhagic fevers should only be isolated in laboratories with Biosafety Level (BSL) 4 capabilities. There are only two BSL 4 facilities in the United States: the Centers for Disease Control and Prevention (CDC) and the U.S. Army Medical Research Institute (USAMRIID) (19). All MEC and staff must adhere to strict

guidelines for wearing PPE when a biological hazard is suspected. Although active biological agents may persist within the remains, the survivability of pathogens in corpses has not been studied (19). Remains contaminated with certain agents such as cholera, tuberculosis, plague, smallpox, yellow fever, or viral hemorrhagic fever may require embalming (16). All remains suspected of biological contamination should be placed in body bags and tagged appropriately to indicate the type of contamination prior to disposition. In the case of smallpox, the body should be wrapped in a large, impervious plastic bag, or disaster pouch, and sealed airtight with tape. The body should be then sealed in a second large, impervious plastic bag prior to transportation (20). Final disposition of the bodies will be at the discretion of the CDC and other authorities. A summary of preparedness efforts in a mass fatality response is provided in Table 43-3.

PREPAREDNESS HISTORIC EVENTS AND CASE HISTORIES

Table 43-4 lists recent significant terrorist attacks resulting in fatalities.

These horrific acts of violence clearly demonstrate the willingness of terrorists to target large numbers of innocent people. Explosive devices are the most commonly used weapons resulting in fatal injuries. Although the potential to cause massive fatalities exists for nuclear terrorism, no significant events have occurred. This is most likely due to the difficulties encountered with obtaining isotopes, development, and successful detonation of such a device. The recent bioterrorism attacks utilizing letters to disseminate anthrax spores was unprecedented and was the first time a classical biological warfare agent was successfully used against a

TABLE 43-6	Internet Resources for Mass Fatality Management	
Mass fatality management (general)	National Mass Fatalities Institute	www.nmfi.org/index.htm
	Joint Tactics, Techniques, and Procedures for Mortuary Affairs in Joint Operations	www.dtic.mil/doctrine/jel/new_pubs/jp4_06.pdf
	National Association of Medical Examiners' Mass Fatality Plan and DMORT	www.dmort.org
Chemical	U.S. Army Soldier and Biological Chemical Command (SBCOM)	http://hld.sbccom.army.mil/downloads/cwirp/guidelines_mass_fatality_mgmt.pdf
Biological	Centers for Disease Control	www.cdc.gov
	Honolulu Biological Incident Response	www.bt.cdc.gov/documents/regmeetingslides/lraine.pdf
	Biological Warfare Mass Casualty Management	http://www.emedicine.com/emerg/topic896.htm
Radiation	Radiation Emergency Assistance Center/Training Site (REAC/TS)	http://www.orau.gov/reacts

civilian population (23). Although there were few fatalities, this was a rude awakening of the potential threat of bioterrorism and the use of unconventional methods in terrorist events.

PREPAREDNESS CHECKLIST AND SUMMARY FOR MASS FATALITY MANAGEMENT

The National Association of Medical Examiners' Mass Fatality Plan is an excellent resource for detailed information on logistical needs in a mass fatality response (8). A general mass fatality preparedness checklist is provided in Table 43-5.

RESOURCES FOR MASS FATALITY PREPAREDNESS AND RESPONSE TO TERRORISM

Refer to Table 43-6 for Internet resources for mass fatality management.

REFERENCES

1. Fixott RH, Arendt D, Chrz B, et al. Role of the dental team in mass fatality incidents. Dent Clin North Am 2001;45(2):271-92.
2. Roy N, Shah H, Patel V, Coughlin RR. The Gujarat earthquake (2001) experience in a seismically unprepared area: community hospital medical response. Prehosp Disaster Med 2002;17(4):186-95.
3. Vosswinkel JA, McCormack JE, Brathwaite CE, Geller ER. Critical analysis of injuries sustained in the TWA flight 800 midair disaster. J Trauma 1999;47(4):617-21.
4. Jordan FB. The role of the medical examiner in mass casualty situations with special reference to the Alfred P. Murrah Building bombing. J Okla State Med Assoc 1999;92(4):159-63.
5. Hirschkorn P. New York adjusts terrorist death toll downward. 2002. Available at: http://www.cnn.com/2002/US/08/22/911.toll/. Accessed August 1, 2003
6. Hooft PJ, Noji EK, Van de Voorde HP. Fatality management in mass casualty incidents. Forensic Sci Int 1989;40(1):3-14.
7. Jensen RA. Mass fatality and casualty incidents. Boca Raton: CRC Press LLC; 2000.
8. National Association of Medical Examiners. Mass fatality plan. 2003. Available at: http://www.thename.org/Library/NAME%20Mass%20Fatality%20Plan%20with%20appendices.pdf. Accessed October 1, 2003.
9. Ralph TH. Mass fatality management: what industry response teams should know. 1999. http://www.disaster-resource.com/cgi-bin/article_search.cgi?id='103'. Accessed June 1, 2003.
10. Corp GC. 9-11 victim identification project results in one-of-a-kind software for mass fatality situations. 2003. Available at: www.forensicfocusmag.com/hotnews/39h1610414.html. Accessed September 1, 2003.
11. Maricopa County A. Emergency Support Function #14 Mortuary Services Annex. 1998. Available at: http://www.dem.state.az.us/serrp/esf14.pdf. Accessed June 1, 2003.
12. Sledzik PS. Federal resources in mass disaster response. CRM; 1996.
13. Federal Bureau of Investigation. Congressional Statement. 2002. Available at: www.fbi.gov/congress/congress02/mefford040202.htm. Accessed August 1, 2003.
14. National Transportation Safety Board. Transportation disaster assistance. 2001. Available at: www.ntsb.gov/Family/family.htm. Accessed August 1, 2003.
15. U.S. Army Soldier and Biological Chemical Command. Guidelines for mass fatality management during terrorist incidents involving chemical agents. 2001. Available at: http:// www2.sbccom.army.mil/hld/downloads/cwirp/guidelines_mass_fatality_mgmt.pdf. Accessed June 1, 2003.
16. Fulford CW. Joint tactics, techniques, and procedures for mortuary affairs in joint operations. 1996. Available at: www.dtic.mil/doctrine/jel/new_pubs/jp4_06.pdf. Accessed August 1, 2003.
17. U.S. Department of Energy. Model procedure for medical examiner/coroner on the handling of a body/human remains that are potentially radiologically contaminated. 2002. Available at: http://www.em.doe.gov/otem/coronerv2.pdf. Accessed September 1, 2003.
18. Henderson DA, Inglesby TV, Bartlett JG, et al. Smallpox as a biological weapon: medical and public health management: Working group on civilian biodefense. JAMA 1999;281(22):2127-37.
19. Jagminas L, Marcozzi DE, Mothershead JL. CBRNE-biological warfare mass casualty management. 2001. Available at: http://www.emedicine.com/emerg/topic896.htm. Accessed September 1, 2003.
20. Centers for Disease Control and Prevention. Guide D: Specimen collection and transport guidelines. Available at: www.cdc.org. Accessed September 1, 2003.
21. U.S. Department of State. Significant terrorist incidents, 1961–2001: a brief chronology. 2001. Available at: http://www.state.gov/r/pa/ho/pubs/fs/5902.htm. Accessed August 1, 2003.
22. Johnston WR. Worst terrorist attacks-U.S. and Worldwide. 2003. Available at: http://www.johnstonsarchive.net/terrorism/wrjp255i.html. Accessed October 1, 2003.
23. Dolnik A, Jason P. 2001 WMD terrorism chronology. 2002. Available at: http://cns.miis.edu/pubs/reports/cbrn2k1.htm. Accessed August 1, 2003.

44

Cyberterrorism

Brian Krakover

INTRODUCTION

In the past, most terrorist attacks have aimed to directly kill, injure, or intimidate a target group for political purposes. This has usually meant a bomb or shooting, which health care professionals can readily identify and treat according to preexisting standards. There is a new threat that can be potentially devastating to a health care system already bursting at the seams with high patient volume and acuity that is evermore dependent on computer systems for patient management and safety: cyberterrorism (1).

PREPAREDNESS ESSENTIALS

Cyberspace is constantly under assault. Spies, thieves, saboteurs, and thrill seekers break into computer systems, steal personal data and trade secrets, vandalize web sites, disrupt service, sabotage data and systems, launch computer viruses and worms, conduct fraudulent transactions, and harass individuals and companies (2). These attacks are facilitated with increasingly powerful and easy-to-use software tools, which are readily available for free from thousands of web sites on the Internet (3).

Cyberterrorism involves attacks on computers and networks and the information they contain. Computer networks have been attacked during recent conflicts in Kosovo, Kashmir, and the Middle East. However, with American society increasingly interconnected and ever more dependent on information technology, terrorism experts worry that cyberterrorist attacks could cause as much devastation as more familiar forms of terrorism (4). "Terrorists could cause a hell of a lot more damage taking out a power grid than blowing up a building," says Matt Yarbrough, former head of the Cybercrimes Task Force in the Justice Department (5).

Experts believe there are two major cyberterror scenarios we should be concerned with:

1. *The physical threat*: compromising critical systems to severely affect critical physical infrastructure, such as power grids, water and sewer systems, dams, hospital equipment, pipelines, communications, global positioning satellites, air traffic systems, or any other networked system, which would result in death and/or destruction.

2. *The critical data threat*: compromising critical computer systems to steal or irreversibly damage vital data, such as the Social Security database, a large financial institution's records, or secret military documents, which would result in death, destruction, and/or catastrophic economic turmoil (3).

Terrorists might also try to use cyberattacks to amplify the effect of other attacks. For example, they might try to block emergency communications or cut off public utilities in the wake of a bombing or a biological, chemical, or radiation attack. Many experts say this kind of coordinated attack might be the most effective use of cyberterrorism (2-4).

Attacks launched in cyberspace could involve diverse methods of exploiting vulnerabilities in computer security: computer viruses, stolen passwords, insider collusion, software with secret "back doors" that intruders can penetrate undetected, and orchestrated torrents of electronic traffic that overwhelm computers—which are known as "denial of service" attacks (Table 44-1). A good example is the Code Red worm. On July 19, 2001, more than 359,000 computers connected to the Internet were denied service after being infected with the Code Red (CRv2) worm in less than 14 hours. The cost of this epidemic, including subsequent strains of Code Red, is estimated to be in excess of $2.6 billion (6) (Table 44-2). Attacks could also involve stealing classified files, altering the content of Web pages, disseminating false information, sabotaging operations, erasing data, or threatening to divulge confidential information or system weaknesses unless a payment or political concession is made (6).

TERRORIST THREATS

The Al Qaeda network uses the Internet, encryption software, and other current information technologies to link its

TABLE 44-1	Types of Computer Attacks (13)
Computer viruses	Programs that could be fed into an enemy's computers either remotely or by "mercenary" technicians.
Logic bombs	A type of virus that can lie dormant for years, until, upon receiving a particular signal, it wakes up and begin attacking the host system.
"Chipping"	Placing booby-trapped computer chips into critical systems sold by foreign contractors to potentially hostile third parties (or recalcitrant allies?).
Worms	Programs whose purpose is to self-replicate ad infinitum, thus eating up a system's resources.
Trojan horses	Malevolent code inserted into legitimate programming in order to perform a disguised function.
Back doors and trap doors	A mechanism built into a system by the designer, in order to give the manufacturer or others the ability to "sneak back into the system" at a later date by circumventing the need for access privileges.
Denial of service	Blocking network access to a group of computers or even entire domains on the Internet.

members, plan attacks, raise funds, and spread propaganda (6,7). Other designated terrorist groups such as Hamas and the Lebanese Hezbollah have publicly accessible web sites for espousing propaganda and perhaps for command and control purposes as well (6). Using the Internet for communication, command and control is much easier than inflicting damage through the Internet. U.S. officials reportedly believe al-Qaeda has been training members in cyberattack techniques, and U.S. computer logs and intelligence gathered in Afghanistan both indicate that the group has scouted systems that control American energy facilities, water distribution, communication systems, and other critical infrastructure (6).

Admittedly, cyberattacks often lack the drama of traditional terrorist attacks, so they might not be attractive to some terrorist groups. Hackers who dislike America might also decide to perpetrate an attack independently. Following the April 2001 collision of a U.S. Navy spy plane and a Chinese fighter jet, Chinese hackers launched denial of service attacks against American web sites (8).

FEDERAL SECURITY EFFORTS

One of the first moves in America's new war on terrorism took place September 5, 2001, six days before the attacks on the World Trade Center and the Pentagon. The target was a Richardson, Texas, company called InfoCom that hosts Arabic web sites. An 80-person terrorism task force launched a three-day raid that closed 500 Internet sites, froze bank accounts, and seized information from the company's hard drives (9).

In February 2003 the White House released its National Strategy to Defend Cyberspace (1). It is intended to be a comprehensive plan to protect the nation's critical resources from cyberattack. The Department of Homeland Security is the lead agent for state, local, private sector, and academic outreach efforts. In June 2003 the Department of Homeland Security created the National Cyber Security Division (NCSD) to deal specifically with cyberterrorist threats (11). The FBI has created a National Infrastructure Protection Center, or NIPC, specifically to deal with cyberterror (10). The CIA created its own group, the Information Warfare Center, staffed with 1,000 people and a 24-hour response team. The Air Force created Electronic Security Engineering Teams, ESETs, in which teams of two to three members go to random Air Force sites and try to gain control of their computers. The teams have had a success rate of 30% in gaining complete control of the systems (10). NASA created the Automated Systems Incident Response Capability (NASIRC) to assist in complying with a range of federal policies, laws, and regulations pertaining to unclassified and classified information technology security. NASIRC provides security

TABLE 44-2	Estimated Economic Damages from Recent Computer Attacks	
YEAR	**VIRUS/ WORM**	**ESTIMATED DAMAGE IN U.S. DOLLARS**
1999	Melissa virus	$80 million
2000	Love bug virus	$10 billion
2001	Code Red I and II worms	$2.6 billion
2001	Nimda virus	$590 million–$2 billion
2002	Klez worm	$9 billion
2003	Slammer worm	$1 billion
Source: Swartz R. Cops take a bite, or maybe a nibble, out of cybercrime. USA Today, September 2, 2003.		

management, analysis, and technical support for the establishment of an agencywide computer network systems incident response and coordination capability (4,10).

WHAT DOES IT MEAN TO THE HEALTH CARE SECTOR?

The U.S. health care sector relies heavily on computer networks for bed tracking, laboratory and radiology studies, telecommunications, and medical records, all of which require the utmost security. Health care infrastructure, however, has not been a major focus of any of the previously mentioned national cybersecurity strategies.

IMPACT ON PREHOSPITAL CARE

Emergency medical personnel rely on a variety of emergency management systems. Historically, these systems were manual, for the most part. Today, emergency management has become both an art and advanced science, relying heavily on a variety of technologies for command, control, and intelligence. As we have discussed here, virtually any technology can be exploited or disabled. Let us look at some examples of systems used by emergency responders that can be disrupted or destroyed by a cyberattack (4).

Radio forms the basis of communications for emergency management teams. Older radio systems that do not rely on any sort of digital controls or repeaters may be attacked by methodologies that are a part of electronic warfare. Jamming requires little technical sophistication but is usually traceable to its place of origin. More sophisticated techniques, such as HERF (High Energy Radio Frequency) and EMP (Electro-Magnetic Pulse) devices, can quickly render radio communications useless (11).

Global positioning systems are becoming vital to emergency response efforts. GPS-based locators linked to online mapping equipment are increasingly being used by first responders in guiding them accurately and quickly to disasters. These systems are also utilized by air support. Such systems may fall prey to cyberattacks, preventing first responders from reaching the target site (12).

HEALTH CARE FACILITY CYBERATTACK RESPONSE

A coordinated response to a computer-based attack need not be different from the response to a nuclear, biological, radiological, or explosive attack. The DISASTER paradigm in the American Medical Association's Basic Disaster Life Support course utilizes an all-hazards approach that is useful to a cyberattack scenario. Furthermore, disaster response

exercises for conventional attacks or weapons of mass destruction (WMD) attacks should all be designed to include changes in procedure to accommodate the failure of the hospital's information system.

RESPONSE ESSENTIALS (FIG. 44–1)

D: DETECT

Detection of a cyberattack is fraught with many difficulties. Like a biological or chemical attack, the signs of attack may not be readily available. For example, a denial of service attack may be indistinguishable from everyday downtime or network errors. The results of an attack may be subtle and not readily noticeable to those inside the facility. All employees who either utilize the hospital or clinic information system must be vigilant for unusual error messages or suspicious personnel. Any suspicion of security violation or abnormal network or computer activity should be reported to the information technology (IT) Help Desk as soon as possible. Upon notification, each report should be investigated and taken seriously. A log system needs to be in place to track complaints because multiple small issues may be clues to a more widespread incident.

I: INCIDENT COMMAND

When a cyberthreat is deemed credible, the hospital's incident command system (ICS) needs to be activated. The chief IT officer should be involved in the incident command structure to coordinate internal protection measures, activate backup clinical systems, and coordinate with unit managers and care providers to ensure patient safety.

S: SCENE SECURITY AND SAFETY

Once the ICS has been activated, the health care facility must be secured from physical attack as well as physically securing essential information technology infrastructure

Detect
Incident Command
Scene Security and Safety
Assessment of Hazards
Support
Triage/ Treatment
Evacuate
Recovery

Figure 44–1. DISASTER Acronym for Disaster Planning (14). (From Basic Disaster Life Support (BDLS) Provider Manual. Dallas CE, Coule PL, James JJ, Lillibridge S, Pepe PE, Schwartz RB, Swienton RE, Editors. American Medical Association, Chicago IL 2003.1-9. With permission.)

like mainframes, exposed data lines, environmental controls, and super user/administrator access to network servers. Additionally, clinical areas need to be notified in order to activate redundant or protective systems that do not depend on the compromised network. These could include manual registration of patients, utilizing plain films instead of digital images, confirmation of lab test results, and ensuring availability of portable or manual equipment for critically ill patients.

A: ASSESS HAZARDS

The information technology personnel should assess the nature of the threat, the persistence of the threat (the difference between a single unauthorized access of medical records or the launching of a worm program that disrupts clinical lab information), who is affected, and what measures need to be taken to either ensure the rest of the health care organization remains functional or to prevent harm to patients.

S: SUPPORT

The ICS needs to move resources to the site of the disaster as well as provide accurate and timely information to the public, patients, employees, and law enforcement in the most secure manner available. The EMS command must rapidly identify the nearest secure locations and available transportation in the event that patients with critical needs must be evacuated.

T: TRIAGE/TREATMENT

The most vulnerable elements in a computer-based attack are patients with the greatest dependence on information technology, that is, critical care patients. Monitoring equipment must be calibrated and verified to be accurate, or, if this is not possible, the patients must be transferred to a higher level of care. Hospital personnel should switch to using bedside diagnostic equipment where possible and careful attention must be paid to documentation of times and quantities because many of these functions are performed automatically by computer software.

E: EVACUATION

Evacuation may only be indicated for the most critical of patients because information security may only be temporarily compromised. The chief information officer needs to provide timely assessment to the ICS in order to allow for transfer of patients or to prevent panic or undue or excessive response. That is to say, the response should be proportional to the threat. The disruption of a power grid is of greater significance than the hacking of a print server, for example.

R: RECOVERY

Once information security has been restored, standard operating procedures should be followed for debriefing of involved personnel and follow-up with law enforcement as well as with patients to identify any possible injuries. The IT office must continue its vigilance to ensure the same "back door" does not get used again and to make sure appropriate changes to security policy, practices, and software are remedied in response to the identified breach.

REVIEW

- Cyberterror can by itself or in combination with other attacks cause significant damage and should be integrated in all areas of disaster planning.
- People, not machines, are the best defense against computer or network compromise.
- There are two factors in computer security planning: physical threat and critical data threat.
- Good daily security habits are the best prevention against malicious users.
- A variety of federal resources are available to help with disaster planning with regard to computer and network security. Integrating the cyberattack scenario in an all-hazards approach to disaster planning will provide optimal results when a terrorist attack hits the community.

SUMMARY

To a health care organization, defense against cyberattack means more than just protecting computers and networks. It means protecting patients. Most hospitals rely on computer networks for lab data, bed tracking data, online medical records, radiology, pharmacy data, and even personnel scheduling. Nowhere is this more crucial than the emergency department (ED). In today's environment of overcrowded, understaffed EDs, how long would it take to notice that all of the serum potassium levels are coming back low or serum glucose levels are too high or always normal? Imagine the potential medical errors when the names on radiology imaging reports have been changed. One of the best ways to defend or prevent a cyberattack are the standard health care information security practices already mandated by HIPAA and other regulations. Good practices during normal operating conditions play an important role in protecting health care systems from cyberterrorism. A health care system that keeps patient information secure on a day-to-day basis stands a good chance of repelling a cyberattack successfully. Vigilant employees, realistic drills and preparation, and a management culture willing to ask hard questions and make tough changes in the future are key ingredients to a formidable cyberdefense (Table 44-3).

TABLE 44-3	Safe and Effective Methods for Gathering Intelligence on the Internet (13)

- Do not surf from an Internet address that ends with .gov or .mil.
- If possible, use a nondescript user name. Avoid names that indicate any belief, position, interest, etc.
- Surf from an innocuous domain from an Internet service provider (ISP) in your area.
- If possible, request that your ISP change your user name periodically.
- Never use that account for personal business, particularly home banking, stock trading, and other electronic commerce.
- Do not enter your real name or any real information in the mail preferences section of your browser. Use a consistent, innocuous name that changes only when your user name changes. Do not list an organization or affiliation.
- Never send a document, complete a form, request information, or send e-mail that includes any real personal information.
- Turn off Active-X, Java, and JavaScript on your browser. You will lose some of the functionality but will be preventing rogue programming code, or "applets," from damaging your system or extracting critical information.
- Do not download unknown programs from the Internet.
- Do not download documents into Microsoft Word unless you have properly installed the Word Virus prevention utility, available from www.microsoft.com.
- Do purchase, install, use, and regularly update a quality virus protection program.
- Do explore web guides like Yahoo, Lycos, and others, for sites that are relevant. Also look for "metasites," or those sites that include links to other sites.
- Do searches using Infoseek, Alta Vista, Hotbot, and others, on terms of which you are interested, including terrorism, particular names of groups or individuals you are interested in tracking, as well as your own organization to see what information is out there. Also check Usenet search engines, like dejanews.com, to see what is being posted in Usenet groups.
- Do fully explore sites that you find are relevant, including links to other sites.
- Do try anonymous ftp in place of http to possibly find additional files and directories to peruse.
- Do not assume the activities and information on sites is correct. Disinformation is a common practice on the Internet. Beware of propaganda.
- Do keep your eyes open for anything hacker challenges—where someone, or a company, puts out a challenge to crack a site. These may lead you to possible crossovers.
- Do examine cracker and extremist sites. Determine if there are ties between any of them.
- Do subscribe to Usenet groups within your area of interest, including selected cracker, political, and religious extremist sites.
- Do attend chat rooms in your areas of interest. Do not engage in the conversation if at all possible.
- Do consider active intelligence gathering. Send e-mail to sites you wish to track, and see if they will put you on their mailing list.
- Do think clearly before responding to any e-mail from anyone with whom you are not familiar. Consider all strangers foes until proven otherwise. Remember that e-mail addresses (the FROM: category in particular) can be forged.
- Remain in character as your alias in your intelligence-gathering process. This means, quite literally, developing an alter ego, with a profile you develop. Thus if you should elect to perform active intelligence gathering, you can remain consistent and less susceptible to being tripped up and losing your cover.

RESOURCES

1. InfraGard: www.infragard.net.

2. The Defense Information Systems Agency (DISA): http://www.disa.mil.

3. Executive Office of the President. Defending America's Cyberspace: National Plan for information systems protection. Version 1.0. November 1999.

4. Network Associates, Inc. An introduction to computer viruses (and other destructive programs). McAfee White Paper. Available online at http://www.nai.com/common/media/vil/pdf/av_white.pdf.

REFERENCES

1. The national strategy to secure cyberspace. White House, February 2003. Web site http://www.whitehouse.gov/pcipb/cyberspace_strategy.pdf.

2. Kirkpatrick D. Securing cyberspace. Fortune, September 10, 2002. Web site: http://www.fortune.com/fortune/fastforward/0,15704,370954,00.html. Accessed October 23, 2003.

3. U.S. Navy Center for the Study of Terrorism and Irregular Warfare. Cyberterror: prospects and implications [white paper]. U.S. Navy Postgraduate School, Monterey, CA, October 1999. Web site: http://www.nps.navy.mil/ctiw. Accessed October 23, 2003.

4. Council on Foreign Relations. Terrorism Q&A. Web site: http://www.cfrterrorism.org/terrorism/cyberterrorism.html.

5. Swartz J. Cops take a bite, or maybe a nibble, out of cybercrime. USA Today, September 22, 2003. Web site: http://www.usatoday.

com/money/industries/technology/2003-09-01-blaster-cover_x.htm. Accessed October 23, 2003.

6. Moore D, Shannon C, Brown J. Code Red: a case study on the spread and victims of an Internet worm. Presented at the Internet Measurement Workshop, Marseille, France, November 6-8, 2002.

7. Gellman B. FBI fears Al-Qaeda cyber attacks. San Francisco Chronicle, June 28, 2002, pp. 1, 10.

8. Thomas TL. Al-Qaeda and the Internet: the danger of cyber-planning. Parameters 2003; 112-24. Web site: http://carlisle-www.army.mil/usawc/parameters/03spring/thomas.pdf. Accessed September 1, 2003.

9. Behar R. Fear along the firewall. Fortune, October 1, 2001. Web site: http://www.fortune.com/fortune/articles/0,15114,368010,00. html. Accessed October 23, 2003.

10. Smith C. Get American troops ready to march on cyber battlefield. Insight Magazine, December 1, 1997. Web site: http://www.insightmag.com/main.cfm?include=detail&storyid=211938. Accessed October 23, 2003.

11. Cyberattacks during the war on terrorism: a predictive analysis. Institute for Security Studies, Dartmouth College, September 22, 2001. Web site: www.globaldisaster.org.

12. Collin BC. Cyberterrorism: from virtual darkness: new weapons in a timeless battle. National Interagency Civil-Military Institute (NICI). Web site: http://www.nici.org/Research/Pubs/98-5.htm. Accessed September 1, 2003.

13. Shabar Y. Information warfare. Institute for Counter Terrorism Studies, February 26, 1997. Web site: www.ict.org.il. Accessed October 23, 2003.

14. Copyright National Disaster Life Support Education Consortium.

INDEX